PRINCIPLES OF
Food Science

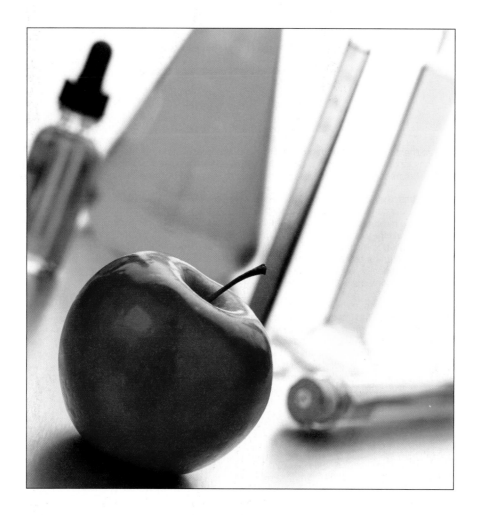

Janet D. Ward
Family and Consumer Sciences Teacher and Consultant
Hickory, North Carolina

Contributing Author
Larry T. Ward
Chairman,
Division of Mathematics, Science, and Computer Science
Catawba Valley Community College
Hickory, North Carolina

Publisher
The Goodheart-Willcox Company, Inc.
Tinley Park, Illinois
www.g-w.com

Library of Congress Cataloging-in-Publication Data
Ward, Janet D.
   Principles of food science / Janet D. Ward; contributing author Larry T. Ward.
     p.cm.
  Includes index.
  ISBN-13 978-1-59070-653-4
  ISBN-10 1-59070-653-6
   1. Food industry and trade. 2. Food--Composition I. Ward, Larry T. II. Title.

TP370.w37 2007
664--dc22
                                                                2005046790

Periodic Table of the Elements

Key:
- Element — Hydrogen
- Atomic Number — 1
- Symbol — H
- Atomic mass — 1.008

Legend: Metal | Nonmetal

Groups (1–18), Periods (1–7)

Group	Element
1	Hydrogen, 1, H, 1.008; Lithium, 3, Li, 6.941; Sodium, 11, Na, 22.990; Potassium, 19, K, 39.098; Rubidium, 37, Rb, 85.468; Cesium, 55, Cs, 132.905; Francium, 87, Fr, 223.020
2	Beryllium, 4, Be, 9.012; Magnesium, 12, Mg, 24.305; Calcium, 20, Ca, 40.078; Strontium, 38, Sr, 87.62; Barium, 56, Ba, 137.327; Radium, 88, Ra, 226.025
3	Scandium, 21, Sc, 44.956; Yttrium, 39, Y, 88.906; Lanthanum, 57, La, 138.906; Actinium, 89, Ac, 227.028
4	Titanium, 22, Ti, 47.88; Zirconium, 40, Zr, 91.224; Hafnium, 72, Hf, 180.948; Rutherfordium, 104, Rf, (261)
5	Vanadium, 23, V, 50.942; Niobium, 41, Nb, 92.906; Tantalum, 73, Ta, 180.948; Dubnium, 105, Db, (262)
6	Chromium, 24, Cr, 51.996; Molybdenum, 42, Mo, 95.94; Tungsten, 74, W, 183.85; Seaborgium, 106, Sg, (263)
7	Manganese, 25, Mn, 54.938; Technetium, 43, Tc, 97.907; Rhenium, 75, Re, 186.207; Bohrium, 107, Bh, (262)
8	Iron, 26, Fe, 55.847; Ruthenium, 44, Ru, 101.07; Osmium, 76, Os, 190.2; Hassium, 108, Hs, (265)
9	Cobalt, 27, Co, 58.933; Rhodium, 45, Rh, 102.906; Iridium, 77, Ir, 192.22; Meitnerium, 109, Mt, (266)
10	Nickel, 28, Ni, 58.693; Palladium, 46, Pd, 106.42; Platinum, 78, Pt, 195.08; (unnamed), 110, Uun
11	Copper, 29, Cu, 63.546; Silver, 47, Ag, 107.868; Gold, 79, Au, 196.967; (unnamed), 111, Uuu
12	Zinc, 30, Zn, 65.39; Cadmium, 48, Cd, 112.411; Mercury, 80, Hg, 200.59; (unnamed), 112, Uub
13	Boron, 5, B, 10.811; Aluminum, 13, Al, 26.982; Gallium, 31, Ga, 69.723; Indium, 49, In, 114.82; Thallium, 81, Tl, 204.383
14	Carbon, 6, C, 12.011; Silicon, 14, Si, 28.086; Germanium, 32, Ge, 72.61; Tin, 50, Sn, 118.710; Lead, 82, Pb, 207.2
15	Nitrogen, 7, N, 14.007; Phosphorous, 15, P, 30.974; Arsenic, 33, As, 74.922; Antimony, 51, Sb, 121.757; Bismuth, 83, Bi, 208.980
16	Oxygen, 8, O, 15.999; Sulfur, 16, S, 32.066; Selenium, 34, Se, 78.96; Tellurium, 52, Te, 127.60; Polonium, 84, Po, 208.982
17	Fluorine, 9, F, 18.998; Chlorine, 17, Cl, 35.453; Bromine, 35, Br, 79.904; Iodine, 53, I, 126.904; Astatine, 85, At, 209.987
18	Helium, 2, He, 4.003; Neon, 10, Ne, 20.180; Argon, 18, Ar, 39.948; Krypton, 36, Kr, 83.80; Xenon, 54, Xe, 131.290; Radon, 86, Rn, 222.018

Lanthanides:

Cerium, 58, Ce, 140.115; Praseodymium, 59, Pr, 140.908; Neodymium, 60, Nd, 144.24; Promethium, 61, Pm, 144.913; Samarium, 62, Sm, 150.36; Europium, 63, Eu, 151.965; Gadolinium, 64, Gd, 157.25; Terbium, 65, Tb, 158.925; Dysprosium, 66, Dy, 162.50; Holmium, 67, Ho, 164.930; Erbium, 68, Er, 167.26; Thulium, 69, Tm, 168.934; Ytterbium, 70, Yb, 173.04; Lutetium, 71, Lu, 174.967

Actinides:

Thorium, 90, Th, 232.038; Protactinium, 91, Pa, 231.036; Uranium, 92, U, 238.029; Neptunium, 93, Np, 237.048; Plutonium, 94, Pu, 244.064; Americium, 95, Am, 243.061; Curium, 96, Cm, 247.070; Berkelium, 97, Bk, 247.070; Californium, 98, Cf, 251.080; Einsteinium, 99, Es, 252.083; Fermium, 100, Fm, 257.095; Mendelevium, 101, Md, 258.099; Nobelium, 102, No, 259.101; Lawrencium, 103, Lr, 260.105

Introduction

Principles of Food Science is designed to help you learn about the relationships among science, food, and nutrition. Basic laws of chemistry, microbiology, and physics are applied to the production, processing, preservation, and packaging of food. You will explore the characteristics of each component found in food. You will examine the helpful and harmful effects of microorganisms on the food supply. You will also find out how the complex mixtures in foods are combined and separated.

Throughout the text, you will find features, such as Recent Research, Nutrition News, and Items of Interest. These features will help you evaluate the impact of science and technology on the food supply. You will also come across cooking, health, and storage tips that connect the science basics to your daily encounters with foods. Experiments at the end of each chapter will allow you to see how scientific principles are involved in food preparation. These experiments will help you build skills in teamwork, critical thinking, and problem solving. Questions and activities in each chapter are designed to help you expand your science vocabulary. These features will also help you apply basic math and technical writing skills to real-world food problems.

Understanding the relationship between science and food can help you reach goals in life. This text explores the world of opportunities in food science related careers. You can apply knowledge from this class in such career roles as nutritionist, chef, food chemist, or process engineer. Even if you decide a food science career is not for you, you can use what you learn to become a creative home cook. You will learn how to make wiser food choices and be aware of the health impact of those choices. You will gain the knowledge needed to evaluate future technological advances as they are applied to foods. You will also understand how the scientific process is used to develop new products in any field.

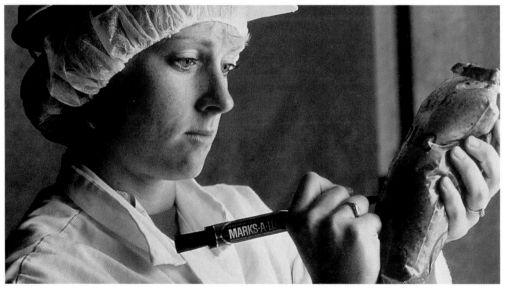

USDA

4

About the Authors

Janet Ward has 23 years of experience in the consumer and family sciences classroom. Her interest and expertise in the area of food science led to her involvement in developing the food science curriculum for the state of North Carolina. She has also written a multimedia and safety supplement to the food science curriculum and conducted a number of workshops on food science instruction. Janet is a member of several honorary societies and professional organizations, including the American Association of Family and Consumer Sciences. She has twice been a Carl Perkins grant recipient. She is a Christa McAuliffe Fellow and a former teacher of the year in her local school district.

Larry Ward has taught math and science at the secondary level for over 10 years. He has 22 years of experience teaching physics at the community college level and currently serves as Chairman of the Division of Mathematics, Science, and Computer Science at Catawba Valley Community College. He has published works on technology and physics and served as a member of a computer science curriculum writing team. Larry is a member of the American Association of Physics Teachers.

Technical Reviewers

Walter L. Hempenius, PhD
Food Industry Consultant
Cary, Illinois

Diane R. McComber
Emeritus Associated Professor (retired)
Food Science and Human Nutrition
Iowa State University
Ames, Iowa

Virginia Richards, EdD, CFCS
Assistant Professor
Georgia Southern University
Statesboro, Georgia

Lynn Turner, PhD
Professor of Food Science
North Carolina State University
Raleigh, North Carolina

Teacher Reviewers

Ronald E. Anderson
Science Instructor
Lyons Township High School
LaGrange, Illinois

Patricia Brinegar
Family and Consumer Sciences Teacher
Carmel High School
Carmel, Indiana

Martha Elliott
Family and Consumer Sciences Teacher
Lyons Township High School
LaGrange, Illinois

JoAnn Fredrikson
Family and Consumer Sciences Teacher
North High School
Sioux City, Iowa

Kathy Fullenwider
Family and Consumer Sciences Teacher
Earl Wooster High School
Reno, Nevada

Contents in Brief

Unit I
The Science of Food

Chapter 1
Food Science: An Old but New Subject   18

Chapter 2
Scientific Evaluation: Being Objective   35

Chapter 3
Sensory Evaluation: The Human Factor   58

Unit II
Basic Chemistry

Chapter 4
Basic Food Chemistry: The Nature of
Matter   78

Chapter 5
Energy: Matter in Motion   99

Chapter 6
Ions: Charged Particles in Solution   120

Chapter 7
Water: The Universal Solvent   144

Unit III
Organic Chemistry: The Macronutrients

Chapter 8
Sugar: The Simplest of Carbohydrates   170

Chapter 9
The Complex Carbohydrates: Starches,
Cellulose, Gums, and Pectins   196

Chapter 10
Lipids: Nature's Flavor Enhancers   216

Chapter 11
Proteins: Amino Acids and Peptides   241

Chapter 12
Enzymes: The Protein Catalyst   265

Unit IV
Food Chemistry: The Microcomponents

Chapter 13
The Micronutrients: Vitamins and Minerals   288

Chapter 14
Phytochemicals: The Other Food
Components   312

Chapter 15
Food Analogs: Substitute Ingredients   336

Chapter 16
Additives: Producing Desired Characteristics
in Foods   355

Unit V
**Food Microbiology: Living Organisms in
Food**

Chapter 17
Fermentation: Desirable Effects of Microbes   380

Chapter 18
Food Safety: Sources of Contamination   406

Unit VI
Food Preservation and Packaging

Chapter 19
Thermal Preservation: Hot and Cold
Processing   434

Chapter 20
Dehydration and Concentration: Controlling
Water Activity   459

Chapter 21
Current Trends in Food Preservation:
Irradiation, Packaging, and Biotechnology   479

Unit VII
Working with Complex Food Systems

Chapter 22
Mixtures: Solutions, Colloidal Dispersions, and
Suspensions   504

Chapter 23
Separation Techniques: Mechanical and
Chemical Methods   528

Chapter 24
Research: Developing New Food Products   547

Chapter 25
Food Science Related Careers: A World of
Opportunities   567

Contents

Unit I
The Science of Food

Chapter 1
Food Science: An Old but New Subject   18
   What Is Food Science?   19
Historical Highlight: George Washington Carver   22
   Recent Contributions of Food Scientists   26
Technology Tidbit: Twentieth Century Food Innovations That Changed the
      World   28
   Why Study Food Science?   29
Activity 1A: Developing Data Tables   32
Activity 1B: Using Data for Calculations   33
Activity 1C: Using Data to Create Graphs   34

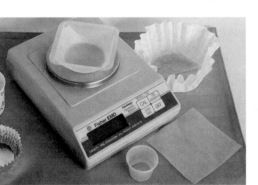

Chapter 2
Scientific Evaluation: Being Objective   35
   Science in the Food Industry   36
   Measurements   37
International Issue: The Metric System and Foreign Trade   38
   The Scientific Method   43
   Evaluating Scientific Studies   49
Experiment 2A: Balancing Chewing Gum   53
Experiment 2B: Measuring Accurately   54
Experiment 2C: Measuring Volumes of Irregularly Shaped
      Objects   56

Chapter 3
Sensory Evaluation: The Human Factor   58
   Influences on Food Likes and Dislikes   59
   Sensory Characteristics of Food Products   61
Recent Research: The Fifth Taste   63
Recent Research: Senses and Aging   65
   Taste Test Panels   66
Technology Tidbit: Computers and
      Sensory Evaluation   70
Experiment 3A: Odor Recognition   72
Experiment 3B: Taste Test Panel   73
Experiment 3C: Imitation Apple Pie   74

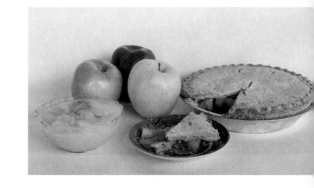

Unit II
Basic Chemistry

Chapter 4
Basic Food Chemistry: The Nature of Matter 78
The Basic Nature of Matter 79
Nutrition News: Elemental Nutrition 80
Chemical Bonding 83
The Classification of Matter 86
Physical and Chemical Changes 88
Item of Interest: Non-Newtonian Fluids 90
Experiment 4A: Physical Qualities of Food 94
Experiment 4B: Chemical Changes 96
Experiment 4C: The Chemical Detective 97

Chapter 5
Energy: Matter in Motion 99
Potential and Kinetic Energy 100
Forms of Energy 101
Technology Tidbit: Canning with Electrical Energy 104
Item of Interest: Electric Life Savers 105
Measuring Energy 106
How Heat Is Transferred 108
Historical Highlight: Temperature Scales 110
Factors That Affect Rates of Reaction in Food Preparation 112
Experiment 5A: The Boiling Point of Various Mixtures 115
Experiment 5B: Heat Transfer in Potatoes 116
Experiment 5C: Freezing Cream 118

Chapter 6
Ions: Charged Particles in Solution 120
Defining Acids and Bases 121
Nutrition News: Salt in the Diet 123
International Issue: Acid Rain 124
Measuring Acids and Bases 125
Item of Interest: pH and the Farmer 128
Applications of pH 130
Experiment 6A: Molarity of Sweetened Tea 139
Experiment 6B: Red Cabbage as an Acid-Base Indicator 140
Experiment 6C: pH and Chemical Leavening in Muffins 142

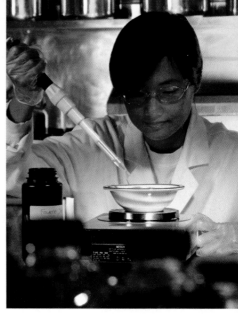

Agricultural Research Service, U

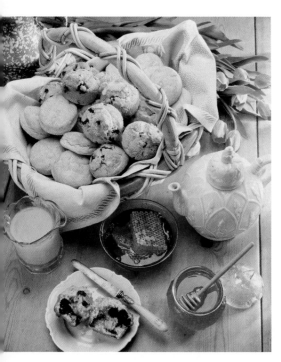

Chapter 7
Water: The Universal Solvent 144

The Structure of Water 145
Functions of Water in Food Preparation 150
Item of Interest: Cooking with Steam 151
Historical Highlight: How Soft Drinks Got Started 153
Water Content in Foods 154
Item of Interest: The Solution to Brewing the Perfect Cup 155
Functions of Water in the Body 157
A Safe Water Supply 159
Experiment 7A: Thermometer Calibration 163
Experiment 7B: Water in Hot Dogs 165
Experiment 7C: Water Purity 166

Unit III
Organic Chemistry: The Macronutrients

Chapter 8
Sugar: The Simplest of Carbohydrates 170

Carbohydrate Production 171
Sugars 172
Nutrition News: Lactose Intolerance 175
Sources of Sugar 176
Functions of Sugars in Food Preparation 179
The Nutritional Value of Sugar 184
Item of Interest: Controlling Tooth Decay 185
Nutrition News: Diabetic Diet Recommendations 186
Experiment 8A: Testing for Simple Sugars 190
Experiment 8B: Forming Sugar Crystals 192
Experiment 8C: Interfering with Crystal Formation 194

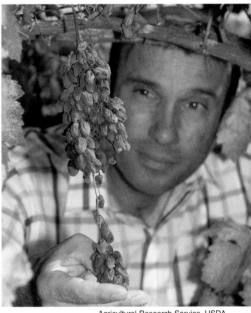

Agricultural Research Service, USDA

Chapter 9
The Complex Carbohydrates: Starches, Cellulose, Gums, and Pectins 196

The Types of Complex Carbohydrates 197
Functions of Complex Carbohydrates in Food Preparation 198
Physical Properties of Starch and Liquid Mixtures 200
Thickening Sauces with Starch 204
Technology Tidbit: Modified Corn Starches 205
Nutritional Impact of Complex Carbohydrates 206
Food Feature: The Trouble with Beans 207
Nutrition News: Carbohydrates and the Athlete 208
Experiment 9A: Characteristics of Starch 211
Experiment 9B: Which Fruits Contain Pectin? 213
Experiment 9C: Comparing Thickeners in Fruit Sauce 214

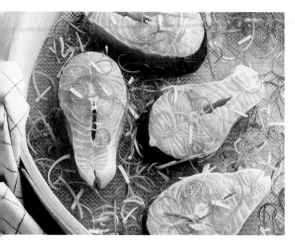

Chapter 10
Lipids: Nature's Flavor Enhancers   216
Chemical Structure of Lipids   217
Categories of Lipids   218
Nutrition News: What Are Trans-Fatty Acids?   221
Physical Characteristics of Lipids   224
Item of Interest: Melt in Your Mouth…   225
Functions of Lipids in Food Preparation   226
Lipids in Your Diet   230
Nutrition News: Carbohydrates vs Fats   231
Technology Tidbit: Measuring Fat Content   233
Experiment 10A: Testing Vegetable Oils for Frying   236
Experiment 10B: Fat in Ground Meat Products   237
Experiment 10C: Fats in Dropped Cookies   239

Chapter 11
Proteins: Amino Acids and Peptides   241
The Structure of Protein   242
Denaturation of Proteins   247
Functions of Protein in Food   249
Item of Interest: The "Bare Bone" Facts About Gelatin   251
Cooking High-Protein Foods   253
Technology Tidbit: "Eggs"actly Stable   254
Food Feature: Is My Chicken Done?   255
The Nutritional Contributions of Proteins   256
Item of Interest: What Causes Light and Dark Meat?   257
Recent Research: Browned Foods and Carcinogens   258
Experiment 11A: Working with Egg White Foams   261
Experiment 11B: Making Gluten Balls   263
Experiment 11C: Proteins, pH, and Coagulation   264

Chapter 12
Enzymes: The Protein Catalyst   265
Historical Highlight: Enzymes and Insulin Production   266
Enzymes Are Specialized Catalysts   266
Item of Interest: Enzymes Keep Going and Going…   267
Factors That Affect Enzyme Activity   270
Enzymes and the Food Supply   273
Food Feature: How Do They Make the Cherry Centers?   276
Recent Research: Enzyme-Producing Gene   278
Item of Interest: Produce Stabilizer   279
Experiment 12A: Catalase in Potatoes   282
Experiment 12B: Enzymatic Browning   283
Experiment 12C: Proteolytic Enzymes in Fruit   284

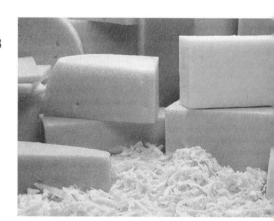

Unit IV
Food Chemistry: The Microcomponents

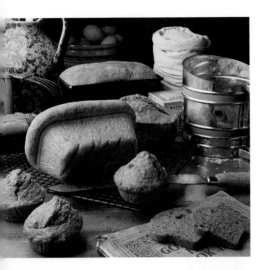

Chapter 13
The Micronutrients: Vitamins and Minerals   288

Vitamins   289
Minerals   293
Nutrition News: Conserving Calcium   295
Effects of Processing and Preservation   298
Nutrition News: MyPyramid   301
Recent Research: Tea with Lemon Please!   302
Vitamins and Minerals as Food Additives   302
Technology Tidbit: Packaging May Decrease Vitamin Loss   303
Preserving Vitamins and Minerals at Home   303
Experiment 13A: Minerals in Milk   307
Experiment 13B: Effects of Calcium on Coagulation   309
Experiment 13C: Determining Vitamin C Content   310

Chapter 14
Phytochemicals: The Other Food Components   312

Phytochemicals   313
Technology Tidbit: A Designer Tomato   317
Nutrition News: Organics—Are They Worth the Cost   319
Phytochemicals and Food Processing   321
Potential Health Benefits of Phytochemicals   324
International Issue: Prescribing Food in Japan   327
Experiment 14A: Effect of pH Changes on Chlorophyll   330
Experiment 14B: Effect of pH Changes on Flavonoids   332
Experiment 14C: Effect of Blanching on Chlorophyll   334

Chapter 15
Food Analogs: Substitute Ingredients   336

Functions of Food Analogs   337
Sugar Substitutes   339
Nutrition News: Do Artificial Sweeteners Help People Lose Weight?   341
Fat Substitutes   342
Historical Highlight: Margarine—A Modified Fat   343
Salt Substitutes   346
Recent Research: Can You Tell the Difference?   347
Experiment 15A: Artificial Sweeteners   349
Experiment 15B: Lowfat Ice Cream   351
Experiment 15C: Fat Replacers in Muffins   353

Chapter 16
Additives: Producing Desired Characteristics in Foods   355
What Is a Food Additive?   356
Regulating Additive Use   356
Recent Research: Caffeine: The Good, the Bad, and the Ugly   359
Functions of Additives   360
Nutrition News: Cholesterol-Lowering Spreads   369
Balancing Benefits and Risks   370
Experiment 16A: Pectin as a Texturizer   374
Experiment 16B: Emulsifiers in Process Cheese   375
Experiment 16C: Preservatives in Cured Meat   376

Unit V
Food Microbiology: Living Organisms in Food

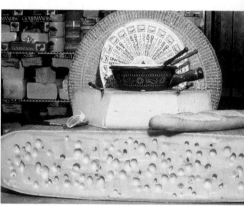

Chapter 17
Fermentation: Desirable Effects of Microbes   380
The Types of Single-Celled
    Organisms   381
Historical Highlight: Food Poisoning in
    Salem, MA?   383
Factors Affecting Microbe Growth   386
Recent Research: Bacteria Turns Pollution into
    Protein   387
Fermentation   389
Item of Interest: The Color Is in the Skin   392
Historical Highlight: Louis Pasteur: One of the
    World's Greatest Scientists   397
Experiment 17A: Factors Affecting Yeast Growth   401
Experiment 17B: Making Sourdough Starter   402
Experiment 17B Extension: Comparing Traditional Pancakes to Sourdough
    Pancakes   403
Experiment 17C: Lactic Acid Bacteria and Yogurt   405

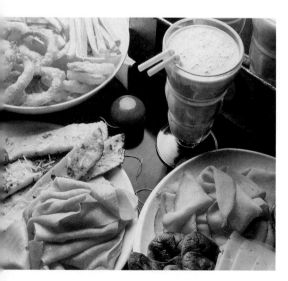

Chapter 18
Food Safety: Sources of Contamination   406
Types of Food Contamination   407
Types of Foodborne Illness   410
Item of Interest: Outbreaks of E. Coli   414
Item of Interest: Salmonellae—Who's the Culprit?   417
How Pathogens Enter the Food Supply   419
Food Industry Sanitation Procedures   421
Experiment 18A: Mold Growth in Foods   426
Experiment 18B: Growing Bacterial Cultures   428
Experiment 18C: The Gram's Stain Test for Bacteria   430

Unit VI
Food Preservation and Packaging

Chapter 19
Thermal Preservation: Hot and Cold Processing   434

Heat Processing   435
Historical Highlight: History of Canning   439
Cold Processing   442
Historical Highlight: A Brief History of Frozen Food   447
Technology Tidbit: Magnetic Resonance Imaging   451
Recent Research: Aseptic Packaging   451
Experiment 19A: Comparing Canned and Frozen Foods   454
Experiment 19B: Canning Food and pH Levels   456
Experiment 19C: Blanching Vegetables   457

Chapter 20
Dehydration and Concentration: Controlling Water Activity   459

Dehydration   460
Historical Highlight: Smoking as a Means of Preserving Foods   466
Item of Interest: Making Fruit Leather   468
Concentration   468
Intermediate-Moisture Foods   470
Experiment 20A: Dehydrating Meat   474
Experiment 20B: Concentrating Soup Stock   476
Experiment 20C: Backpacker's Dehydrated Soup   477

Chapter 21
Current Trends in Food Preservation: Irradiation, Packaging, and Biotechnology   479

Food Irradiation   480
Packaging   485
Recent Research: High-Dose Irradiation   485
Recent Research: Sensory Evaluation of Package Flavors   490
Biotechnology   492
Experiment 21A: Simulating Irradiation   498
Experiment 21B: Packaging to Prevent Oxidative Rancidity   499
Experiment 21C: The Permeability of Plastic   501

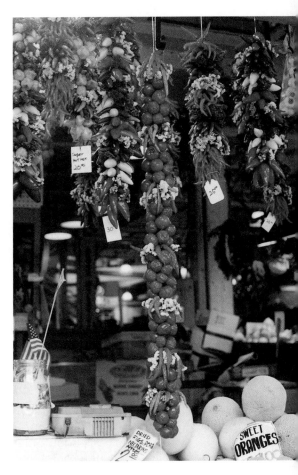

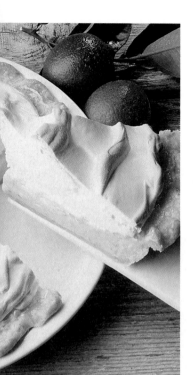

Unit VII
Working with Complex Food Systems

Chapter 22
Mixtures: Solutions, Colloidal Dispersions, and Suspensions 504
Solutions   505
Colloidal Dispersions   510
Item of Interest: Emulsifiers   513
Historical Highlight: Chocolate: A Complex Mixture   516
Suspensions   518
Experiment 22A: Creating a Water-in-Oil Emulsion   522
Experiment 22B: Measuring Calories in a Complex Mixture   524
Experiment 22C: Foam Variations   526

Chapter 23
Separation Techniques: Mechanical and Chemical Methods   528
Mechanical Separation   529
Chemical Separation   532
Selective Separation Through Barriers   533
Technology Tidbit: The Chemical Separation of Lactic Acid   534
Nutrition News: Athletes Under Pressure   536
Item of Interest: Cell Walls Versus Cell Membranes   538
Digestion and Metabolism   538
Experiment 23A: Filtration   543
Experiment 23B: Extracting Gelatin and Fat   544
Experiment 23C: Osmosis and Egg Membranes   546

Chapter 24
Research: Developing New Food Products   547
Research in the Food Industry   548
Developing Food Science Experiments   551
Recent Research: The Connection Between Fruit and Flowers   552
Developing a New Food Product   556
Item of Interest: Flavor Trends Guide Food Research   559
Activity 24A: Developing a Food Science Experiment   562
Activity 24B: Analyzing a Complex Food System   563
Activity 24C: Developing a New Food Product   565

Chapter 25
Food Science Related Careers: A World of Opportunities   567
Careers, Food, and You   568
Food Science Careers in the Food Industry   570
Item of Interest: Defining the Food Industry   571
Item of Interest: The Importance of Quality Control   575
Technology Tidbit: The Cook/Chill Foodservice System   577
Types of Employers   578
Activity 25A: Developing a Resume   583
Activity 25B: Preparing for a Job Interview   585
Activity 25C: Developing Career Goals   586

Appendix: Measurement Conversion Charts   587

Glossary   589

Index   603

Special Features

Historical Highlights

George Washington Carver   22
Temperature Scales   110
How Soft Drinks Got Started   153
Enzymes and Insulin Production   266
Margarine—A Modified Fat   343
Food Poisoning in Salem, MA?   383
Louis Pasteur: One of the World's Greatest
    Scientists   397
History of Canning   439
A Brief History of Frozen Food   447
Smoking as a Means of Preserving Foods   466
Chocolate: A Complex Mixture   516

Technology Tidbits

Twentieth Century Food Innovations That Have
    Changed the World   28
Computers and Sensory Evaluation   70
Canning with Electrical Energy   104
Modified Corn Starches   205
Measuring Fat Content   233
"Eggs"actly Stable   254
Packaging May Decrease Vitamin Loss   303
A Designer Tomato   317
Magnetic Resonance Imaging   451
The Chemical Separation of Lactic Acid   534
The Cook/Chill Foodservice System   577

International Issues

The Metric System and Foreign Trade   38
Acid Rain   124
Prescribing Food in Japan   327

Recent Research

The Fifth Taste   63
Senses and Aging   65
Browned Foods and Carcinogens   258
Enzyme-Producing Gene   278
Tea with Lemon Please!   302
Can You Tell the Difference?   347
Caffeine: The Good, the Bad, and the Ugly   359
Bacteria Turns Pollution into Protein   387
Aseptic Packaging   451
High-Dose Irradiation   485
Sensory Evaluation of Package Flavors   490
The Connection Between Fruit and Flowers   552

Nutrition News

Elemental Nutrition   80
Salt in the Diet   123
Lactose Intolerance   175
Diabetic Diet Recommendations   186
Carbohydrates and the Athlete   208
What Are Trans-Fatty Acids?   221
Carbohydrates vs Fats   231
Conserving Calcium   295
MyPyramid   301
Organics—Are They Worth the Cost?   319
Do Artificial Sweeteners Help People Lose Weight?
    341
Cholesterol-Lowering Spreads   369
Athletes Under Pressure   536

Items of Interest

Non-Newtonian Fluids   90
Electric Life Savers   105
pH and the Farmer   128
Cooking with Steam   151
The Solution to Brewing the Perfect Cup   155
Controlling Tooth Decay   185
Melt in Your Mouth…   225
The "Bare Bone" Facts About Gelatin   251
What Causes Light and Dark Meat?   257
Enzymes Keep Going and Going…   267
Produce Stabilizer   279
The Color Is in the Skin   392
Outbreaks of E. Coli   414
Salmonellae—Who's the Culprit?   417
Making Fruit Leather   468
Emulsifiers   513
Cell Walls Versus Cell Membranes   538
Flavor Trends Guide Food Research   559
Defining the Food Industry   571
The Importance of Quality Control   575

Food Features

The Trouble with Beans   207
Is My Chicken Done?   255
How Do They Make the Cherry Centers?   276

15

Food science is a rapidly changing field. It has grown along with the world's demands for safe, tasty, nutritious, convenient, mass-produced food. Food science applies basic principles of chemistry, physics, and biology to the processing and storage of food.

As you begin your study of food science, Chapter 1 traces some of the history of this field. You will explore recent contributions of food scientists and consider the benefits of this course of study.

Science involves experimentation, and experiments require measurements. Chapter 2 explores the types of measurements used in food science and the basic equipment you will work with in the lab. You will examine how the scientific method is used in food science labs. You will also learn safe and proper laboratory procedures.

Chapter 3 explores how food scientists measure the human response to food. Considering what people like and dislike is an important factor in developing new food products. Measuring human preferences is a type of scientific evaluation that is unique to food science.

Unit I
The Science of Food

1 Food Science: An Old but New Subject

2 Scientific Evaluation: Being Objective

3 Sensory Evaluation: The Human Factor

This is a photomicrograph—a photograph taken through an optical microscope—of artificial strawberry flavoring. Evaluating sensory characteristics, such as flavors, colors, and textures, is an important part of studying food products from a food science perspective.

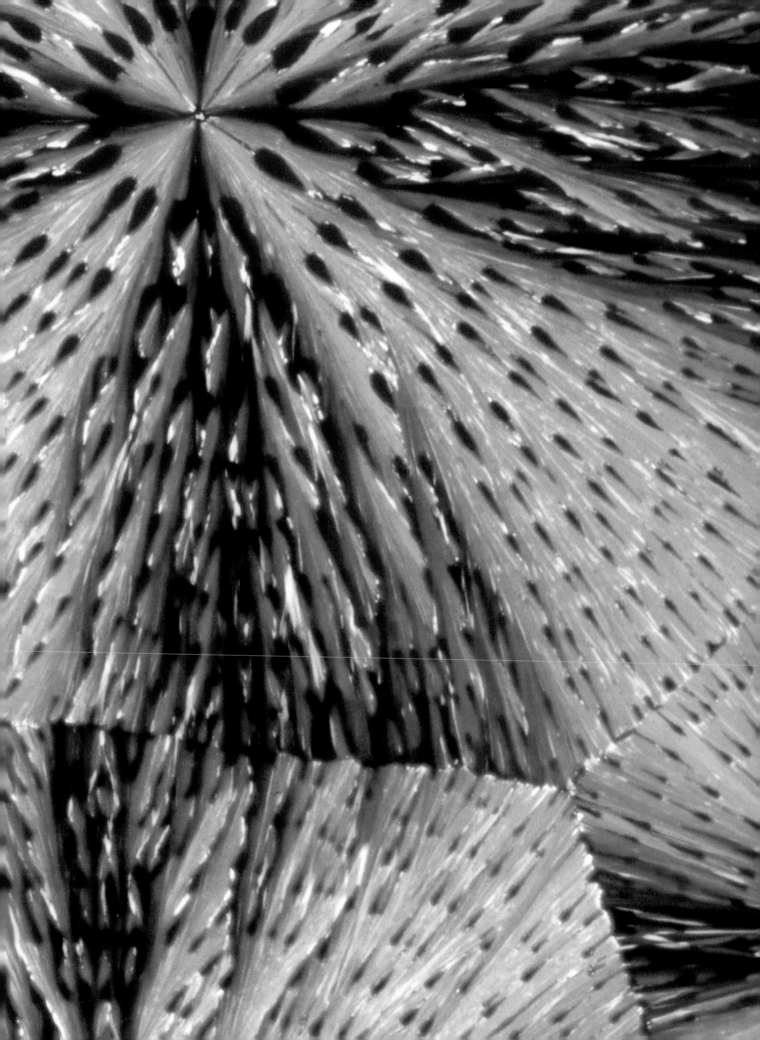

Food Science: An Old but New Subject

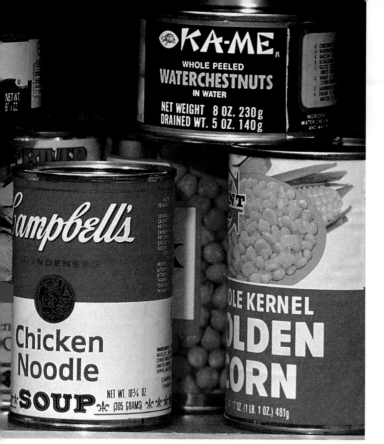

USDA

The development of safe canning procedures is considered one of the top food innovations of the twentieth century.

Objectives

After studying this chapter,
you will be able to

describe the three periods in the development of foods.

summarize how food products and processing methods have changed in modern history due to contributions of food scientists.

analyze how studying food science now can benefit you in the future.

Key Terms

food science

nutrition

hydroponic crops

food analogs

cryogenic liquids

adulteration

Whoever you are, wherever you live, you eat. Few things impact the quality of your life like the food choices you make each day. For your ancestors, there were few choices. Finding, growing, storing, and preserving food occupied most of the day. Since early history, what and how people eat has changed dramatically. Today, people have almost unlimited access to tens of thousands of fresh and processed food products. Many items are labeled *fast*, *quick*, *instant*, or *microwavable*. These products are all the result of research and technology.

As you make daily decisions about food products, you may find yourself asking a number of questions. What will I eat? How will I fix it? Should I eat out? Where could I go? Is this food safe? Is it nutritious? After studying this text, these questions will be easier for you to answer. See 1-1.

The first question you will address in this chapter is, What is food science? A little background will help you understand how this field has grown and why it is worth studying.

What Is Food Science?

Food science is the study of the nature of food and the principles of its production, processing, preservation, and packaging. People throughout history have been intrigued by the study of food. When technology moved food preparation from the home to the factory, however, food science began to evolve as a field of its own.

Food science is an example of an integrated course of study. It involves related topics from a variety of subjects. To understand food science, you need to be familiar with concepts from the "traditional" science courses—biology, chemistry, and physics. You need to be acquainted with nutrition and food preparation skills taught in family and consumer sciences classes. You need to be informed about health topics, such as physical fitness and the functions of body systems. An understanding of basic algebra concepts will help you complete many food science experiments. You will also use technical writing skills to list procedures and record observations. Developing these skills through your study of food science will prepare you for many careers.

Having some general nutrition knowledge will help you in your study of food science. *Nutrition* is the study of components of food and how they are used by the body to sustain life and health. Nutrition focuses on what happens to foods after you eat them. On the other hand, food science also focuses on what happens to foods before you eat them. Food scientists need to understand how the body converts food products into usable nutrients. This enables the scientists to develop foods that will meet people's nutritional needs.

Food science is a hands-on course. Most people learn best by doing. You can observe many of the principles of food science firsthand through experimentation. As you work with food products in experiments, you will better understand food preparation principles. You will learn why and how the ingredients in a recipe work together to make the foods you enjoy each day. See 1-2.

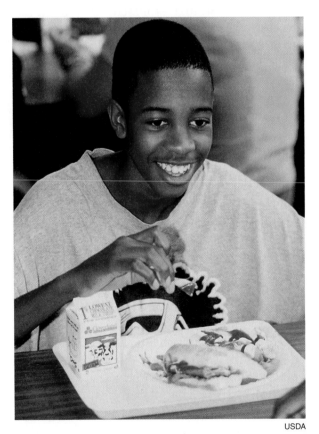

USDA

1-1 Most teens make the majority of their own food choices. Knowing about food products and how they affect the body can make these choices easier.

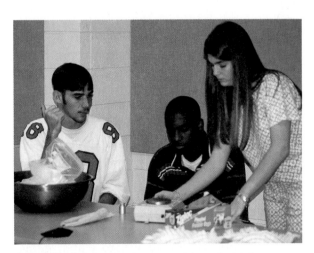

1-2 A food science class provides students many opportunities to learn by doing.

A Brief History

Imagine a world where an orange is so rare and expensive it is viewed as a highly valued gift. Do you find it hard to picture being excited about eating an orange? Only two generations ago, it was that way in most of the United States. In those days, people could preserve foods only by drying, salting, or pickling. Fresh produce was available only during the few short months of the growing season. A life without machinery made the planting, harvesting, and preparing of food long, hard work. Laura Ingalls Wilder's book *Farmer Boy* gives the following perspective of a young boy in the late 1800s:

> Then the rush of harvest came. There was no rest and no play for anyone now. They all worked from candlelight to candlelight. Everything must be saved, nothing wasted of the summer's bounty.

This type of struggle to meet daily food needs is still seen today in Third World countries. However, life in the United States has changed dramatically since the 1800s. Then, 9 out of 10 people were farmers. Today, technology makes it possible for only 2 people to produce enough food for 100.

Three Periods in the Development of Food

The history of food can be broken into three broad periods. The first period focuses on food discoveries of early peoples. The second period began with the invention of modern machines and the development of mass production processes. The third period is marked by government regulation to keep the food supply safe.

Early Food Discoveries

Throughout most of history, people ate whatever was naturally available in the areas where they lived. Through experimentation, people discovered which plants were tasty and safe to eat. Variety was limited by location and seasons.

Civilizations formed where water, game, and land would provide abundant food supplies. Men often hunted and fished for the meat portion of the diet. Women and children foraged for fruits and nuts.

Changing seasons required people to identify foods they could store for cold months when plants would not grow. Gradually, foods that were favored because of their keeping qualities were cultivated and farming began. Among these foods were high-energy grains, such as wheat, oats, rye, barley, and corn. People also looked for ways to extend the storage life of foods. They discovered that drying grains and other foods enabled them to be stored and used throughout the winter.

Many foods were discovered by accident. For example, it is believed that cheese was discovered in the hot desert areas of the Middle East. In this region, stomachs taken from animals were scraped, cleaned, and tied off to use as containers for liquids. When goat's milk was placed in these containers, something surprising happened. The milk would curdle because the animal stomachs contained an enzyme called *rennin*. Curdling was further promoted by warm temperatures and jostling motions as the milk was carried across the desert on camelback. Middle Eastern peoples discovered the curds, or "cheese," were quite tasty and would keep for a long time.

The Industrial Revolution

Much of the food you eat is prepared and preserved in ways that have been used for hundreds of years. Through trial and error, people learned techniques that would preserve foods, but they did not know why these techniques worked. It was not until the 1700s that tools and procedures for understanding the "whys" came into being. It was during this century that researchers began to discover chemicals and their relationships to life. The microscope was improved in the early 1800s. As a result, scientists began to understand bacteria and their effects on food spoilage and human health. The canning process was invented, and the first canning plant was opened in Boston in 1820. See 1-3.

Along with advances in scientific knowledge, the late eighteenth century brought major changes in the economy. These changes

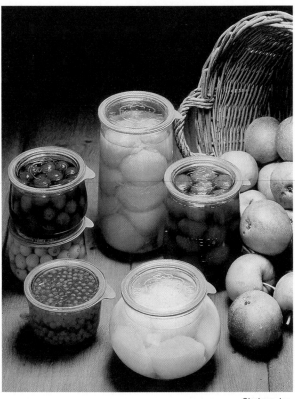

Glashaus, Inc.

1-3 The invention of the canning process made it possible to safely preserve large quantities of food.

were the result of the harnessing of steam and coal power and the development of power-driven machines. This period is referred to as the *industrial revolution.*

The use of steam and coal power sources enabled machines to do the work of many people. In the 1830s, the invention of such farm machinery as the thresher, reaper, and steel plow increased food production. The invention of specialized factory equipment sped food processing procedures. These developments led to the start of many food processing companies. Armour foods opened in 1867, and Pillsbury and Campbell were founded in 1869.

Ingredients began to be developed to make food manufacturing more profitable. Baking powder was mass-produced in 1856. Commercial yeast became available in 1868. Self-rising flour was first marketed in the 1890s.

World Wars I and II encouraged the development and acceptance of a number of food products. Some convenience foods were developed first for the military. An example is pancake mixes, which were developed during World War I. Pancake mixes were followed to the consumer market by biscuit and cake mixes in the 1930s. However, the majority of consumers initially snubbed these early convenience foods, considering them vastly inferior to homemade products.

As a result of World War II, many women entered the workforce to replace men who had enlisted in the armed services. These women had less time for food preparation. Thus, the demand for foods that could be prepared easily increased. Wartime rationing of sugar and butter made it difficult to have ample supplies for home baking. These two factors fostered the popularity of mixes that had been poorly received by consumers in the 1930s.

Government Regulation of the Food Industry

As with most new developments, the commercial mass production of food led to some problems. Government regulation was needed to address these problems. This has resulted in the consistent, economic, and convenient food supply you enjoy today.

Early Regulation

Before the 1820s, the main concern regarding food safety was spoilage. With the arrival of mass food production and canning in the 1820s, adulteration became a widespread problem. **Adulteration** is a lowering of the quality and safety of a product by adding inferior or toxic ingredients. The following are a few nineteenth and early twentieth century examples of adulterated food products:

❖ *Ground pepper* contained gravel, leaves, and twigs.

❖ *Vinegar* was diluted with sulfuric acid.

❖ *Coffee* contained roasted grain, scorched beans and peas, and baked horse liver.

❖ *Milk* was watered down or had chalk, starch, gelatin, or borax added.

❖ *Sugar* contained sand, dust, and lime.

A number of factors probably contributed to tampering with food ingredients. These include centralized food processing, greed, and declining personal accountability.

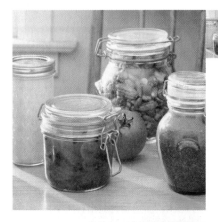

Historical Highlight
George Washington Carver

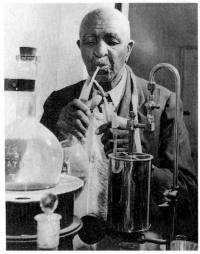

Through research in his chemistry lab, George Washington Carver developed hundreds of food products.

George Washington Carver (1860–1943) was a freed slave, artist, botanist, chemist, professor, pianist, and food scientist. George Washington Carver completed his high school education in his late 20s in Minneapolis, Kansas, while working as a farmhand. He continued his studies at Iowa State College. He received a degree in agricultural studies in 1894 and a master of science degree in 1896. Iowa State offered him an appointment as assistant botanist where he was responsible for the school's greenhouse. This was where he started a fungus collection that grew to 20,000 species and brought him his initial professional fame.

In 1896, Booker T. Washington offered Carver a position on the staff at Tuskegee Institute. As the director of agricultural research, Carver worked to improve the lot of the Southern farmer. He developed products derived from soil-enriching crops like peanuts and sweet potatoes. These products helped revolutionize the economy of the South. They freed the South from exclusive dependence on cotton, which depleted the soil.

Carver's work resulted in the development of hundreds of food and industrial products. Products derived from peanuts include flour, cheese, milk, coffee, ink, dyes, plastics, soap, and linoleum. Products derived from sweet potatoes include flour, vinegar, molasses, rubber, and a postage stamp glue.

Carver encouraged improved farming methods and conservation. He sought to change the lot of African American people through education. He paved the way for a better life for the entire South.

The United States Department of Agriculture (USDA) was established in 1862 to oversee food production and agricultural research. However, the chemistry division was given little authority to monitor or enforce the safety of the food supply. Harvey Wiley was appointed head chemist of the USDA in 1883. He began a campaign to eliminate misnamed and adulterated foods.

Wiley's work led to the Pure Food and Drug Act of 1906. This act established the Food and Drug Administration (FDA) to regulate and monitor the food supply in the United States. In 1938, Congress expanded the authority of the FDA in the Food, Drug, and Cosmetic Act. These two laws are the basis for all the rules and regulations written by the FDA. See 1-4.

Government Regulation Today

The Food, Drug, and Cosmetic Act contains detailed regulations regarding the production and interstate trade of foods. Over the years, the act has been updated to better

Milestones in Government Food Regulation

Date	Law	Actions
1862		❖ USDA is established.
		❖ President Lincoln appoints Charles M. Wetherill as first head of the Bureau of Chemistry in the USDA, which later becomes the FDA.
1879		❖ Investigation of food adulteration begins.
		❖ Peter Collier, chief chemist for USDA, begins research.
1880		Collier submits the first of over 100 food and drug laws attempted over the next 25 years to Congress.
1883		Dr. Harvey Wiley is appointed as chief chemist of USDA and expands the food adulteration studies.
1898		The Association of Official Agriculture Chemists is established as a committee on food standards with Dr. Wiley as head.
1906	❖ Pure Food and Drug Act	Congress passes the act because of Wiley's research. The bill prohibits interstate commerce of misbranded and adulterated food, drinks, and drugs.
	❖ Meat Inspection Act	Requires inspection of all meat sold across state lines.
1907	1st Certified Color Regulations	Seven colors are certified as acceptable for use in processed foods and drugs.
1913	Gould Amendment	Requires accurate labeling of food packages with weight, measure, or numerical count.
1930		❖ The name of the Food, Drug, and Insecticide Administration is shortened to Food and Drug Administration (FDA).
	McNary-Mapes Amendment	❖ Authorizes FDA standards of quality and fill-of-container for canned food, excluding meat and milk products.
1938	Food, Drug, and Cosmetic Act	The 1906 Food and Drug Act is expanded to cover cosmetics and give FDA authority to establish regulations and guidelines for the food industry.
1948		FDA publishes *Guide to Industry,* the first guidelines for the food industry referred to as the "black book."
1958		❖ The first GRAS list was published, establishing a list of food additives that were generally recognized as safe.
	❖ Food Additives Amendment	❖ Requires the safety of new additives to be established.
	❖ Delaney Clause	❖ Prohibits the use of any additive in food that is found to cause cancer.

(Continued)

1-4 Government regulation has ensured the safety and wholesomeness of the food supply for consumers in the United States.

Milestones in Government Food Regulation *(Continued)*

Date	Law	Actions
1960	Color Additives Amendment	Requires the safety of any new color additives for food, drugs, or cosmetics to be established before use is approved.
1966	Fair Packaging and Labeling Act	Requires all consumer products in interstate commerce to be honestly and informatively labeled.
1969		In the White House Conference on Food, Nutrition, and Health, President Nixon orders FDA to review its GRAS list.
1977	Saccharin Study and Labeling Act	Stops FDA from banning the chemical sweetener but requires a label warning that saccharin has been found to cause cancer in laboratory animals.
1988	Food and Drug Administration Act	Broadly spells out the responsibilities of the Secretary and the Commissioner of the FDA for research, enforcement, education, and information.
1990	Nutrition Labeling and Education Act	❖ Requires all packaged foods to bear nutrition labeling. ❖ Requires all health claims for foods to be consistent. ❖ Authorizes some health claims for foods. ❖ Standardizes the food ingredient panel, serving sizes, and terms such as "low fat" and "light."
1994	Dietary Supplement Health and Education Act	❖ Defines dietary supplements. ❖ Places burden of proof for safety on FDA. ❖ Authorizes some health claims for dietary supplement. ❖ Establishes Office of Dietary Supplements.
1995	FDA Mandated HACCP Regulations for Seafood	❖ Mandates HACCP program be established by each seafood processing facility. ❖ Authorizes FDA regulation and monitoring of seafood industry's use of HACCP.
Ongoing	Pilot HACCP Programs	❖ Provide training on HACCP by FDA. ❖ Develop HACCP programs for fruit juice and dairy industries.

1-4 *(Continued)*

protect U.S. citizens. Such updates have been in response to new research findings.

The act has done more than provide a set of enforceable regulations. It has been used as a basis for developing recommendations for safe food handling. These recommendations are published in the FDA *Food Code.* This reference is available to anyone seeking information on how to prevent foodborne illness. Restaurants, grocery stores, and institutions such as schools and hospitals use the *Food Code* as a guide to handling food safely. State and local agencies also use it as a model for writing their own food safety rules.

The FDA and USDA are still key regulatory agencies for the food industry. The FDA controls the use of pesticides on food crops and additives in processed foods. They have set food labeling guidelines and created standards for the safety and wholesomeness of food products. The USDA is responsible for the inspection of meat and poultry products shipped across state lines. They also mandated a system to ensure the safety of the meat and poultry industry. See 1-5.

Food safety has greatly improved since the early days of mass production. This is due to new chemical analysis methods as well as government regulation. Substances in foods can now be identified and controlled in parts per million or parts per billion.

Watchdog Groups

There are organizations called watchdog groups that observe and report scientific developments, policy, and legislation related to the food industry. Some are *nonpartisan* (they do not have an agenda or goal other than unbiased communication). Others have agendas that are political in nature and may result in biased reporting. Two organizations that are considered nonpartisan are the International Food Information Council (IFIC) and the American Dietetic Association (ADA).

The IFIC was founded in 1985. They define themselves as a nonprofit organization whose mission is to provide information to professionals who communicate with consumers

regarding science-based information on agricultural industries. It does not represent any product or company and does not lobby for legislation or regulatory action. They publish the bimonthly newsletter *Food Insight* and have online resources.

The ADA is a professional association of nutritionists and nutrition research scientists that report summaries of current research on food related topics. These reports are called position papers and can be found on their Web site.

These types of organizations can help the public make sense of conflicting reports in the media. Although the information is available to the general public, these groups focus on providing information to professionals and educators.

Food Labeling

Another area of government regulation is food labeling. The U.S. Congress has established guidelines that all food manufacturers must follow to market their products. These guidelines are intended to help protect consumers from food fraud and mislabeling. The guidelines are also designed to help keep consumers informed about the nutritional content of food products.

The Nutrition Labeling and Education Act of 1990 restricted the use of nutrition claims on food labels. It defined terms like *low fat* and *fat free*. This act also led to the standardized Nutrition Facts panel that appears on food labels, 1-6.

Food scientists are required to analyze and properly label food products. To develop a label that meets federal regulations, a food scientist must

❖ understand the FDA and USDA regulations regarding manufactured foods and their labels

❖ carefully analyze all ingredients in a food item by nutrient category

❖ accurately calculate ingredients and nutrients

❖ keep thorough records that support labeling information

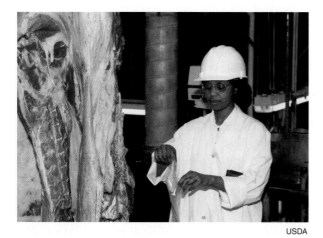

USDA

1-5 USDA inspectors evaluate meat for wholesomeness. They may also grade meat for quality.

Nutrition Facts

| Serving Size | 1 cup (56 g) |
| Servings Per Container | 9 |

Amount Per Serving

| Calories | 90 |
| Calories from Fat | 10 |

	% Daily Value
Total Fat 1g	2%
Saturated Fat 0g	0%
Trans Fat 0g	
Cholesterol 0mg	0%
Sodium 180mg	8%
Total Carb. 15g	5%
Fiber 2g	
Sugars 1g	
Protein 2g	

Vitamin A 15%	Vitamin C 15%
Calcium 2%	Iron 25%

Percent Daily Values are based on a 2,000 calorie diet. Your daily values may be higher or lower depending on your calorie needs:

		Calories:	2,000	2,500
Total Fat	Less than		65g	80g
Sat Fat	Less than		20g	25g
Cholesterol	Less than		300mg	300mg
Sodium	Less than		2,400mg	2,400mg
Total Carbohydrate			300mg	375mg
Dietary Fiber			25g	30g

Calories per gram:
Fat 9   Carbohydrate 4   Protein 4

1-6 Effective January 2006, food manufacturers are required to list *trans* fat on the Nutrition Facts panel.

Food manufacturers that fail to follow government regulations may have to pay large fines. They may also face expensive recalls of food products or forced closings of production plants.

Recent Contributions of Food Scientists

Many of the advances that have affected the world's food supply have been the result of the work of *food scientists.* These are professionals trained in the field of food science. In the last century, they have been involved in the identification of nutrients. They have helped establish links between the food supply and health. They have also developed thousands of new food products and ingredients.

Expanded Food Supply

One of the most urgent jobs of food scientists is to develop foods for hungry people throughout the world. Nearly two billion people do not have enough to eat. Research is being conducted to develop safe, tasty, nutritious, low-cost foods to meet the needs of these people. An example of such a food is incaparina. *Incaparina* is a cereal formulated from maize, sorghum, and cottonseed flour. It is economical and contains 28% protein. All the grains used to make it can grow in Central and South America, where there are large numbers of hungry people.

A second example of a product food scientists have studied to help feed the world's hungry people is amaranth. *Amaranth* is an ancient grain used by the Aztecs. Its high protein level and resistance to drought make it an economical option for people in many areas.

Another way food scientists are working to meet the needs of hungry people is to improve crop yields. Agricultural researchers are trying to develop new varieties of many food crops. They want to raise crops in regions where no crops would previously grow. Researchers are looking at raising hydroponic crops in some of these regions. **Hydroponic crops** are grown with their roots suspended in liquid nutrient solutions. Tomatoes, cucumbers, and lettuce grow well in this environment. Some hydroponic produce is presently available in U.S. grocery stores. See 1-7.

Biotechnology is an area of research that relates food science and agriculture. Biologists use technology to change a plant's genetic makeup. One example is a new variety of corn developed by Monsanto Chemical Company. This corn is not affected by a commonly used herbicide. An entire field of corn can be sprayed to kill weeds without damaging the corn. The advantages include lower production costs and a larger crop yield.

New Food Products

Food scientists are concerned about more than supplying food in regions where it is scarce. In areas where food is abundant, food scientists focus more on factors that affect the safety, cost, and quality of food products. Variety, ease of preparation, and nutrition are other factors food scientists study. They are trying to meet consumers' demands for inexpensive, tasty dishes that can be prepared and

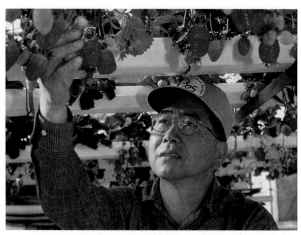

Agricultural Research Service, USDA

1-7 Hydroponically grown strawberries are cultivated with their roots suspended in a nutrient-rich liquid instead of soil.

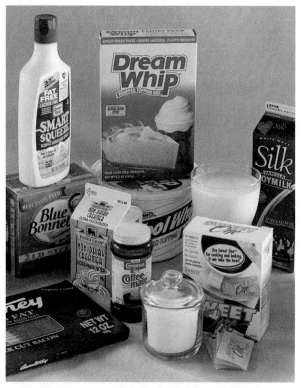

1-8 Food analogs often provide less costly or more healthful alternatives to traditional food products.

served quickly. This has led to the introduction of thousands of new food products in the last few decades. Food scientists can work two to three years on the development and test marketing of each new product.

Some of the food products food scientists have helped develop have been for use by the armed services. These foods needed to be compact and high in calories. The containers for these foods had to be lightweight, easy to open, soft, and durable. Much of what food scientists learned through work with the armed services has been applied to food products for backpackers.

Many food scientists are at work developing substitutes for natural ingredients. These substitutes are used because they are often healthier or less expensive. Examples include sugar and salt substitutes, nondairy creamers and toppings, and fat replacers. Such substitutes help reduce the need for dietary changes by people with conditions like diabetes and heart disease.

Food scientists have been involved in developing *food analogs.* These are natural or manufactured substances that are used in place of foods or food components. For instance, scientists have been using vegetable proteins to make products that look and taste like meat. One of these food analogs is bacon chips made from soybeans. This product looks and tastes like real bacon. Unlike real bacon bits, however, the food analog has a long shelf life and does not require refrigeration. See 1-8.

New Processing Techniques

Some of the food products designed to meet the needs of today's busy consumers are highly processed. Often, complex alterations make a food product quite different from its original source. For example, corn may be ground, powdered, liquefied, fermented, puffed, dried, fried, or popped. These processes can result in products that look and taste totally unlike corn. Food scientists are involved in developing production processes to achieve food products with the desired flavors, textures, and nutrient values.

Some production processes have been developed by food scientists who have worked for the NASA space program. For example, dehydrated foods and some special packaging techniques have resulted from work with NASA. These food processes have expanded food choices and helped reduce packaging costs. The space program has led to the development of vacuum packaging techniques, Teflon coatings, and freezer-to-oven cookware. The space program has also resulted

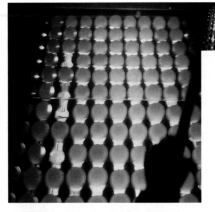

Technology Tidbit
Twentieth Century Food Innovations That Changed the World

What changes in food products, processing, preservation, and packaging have had the biggest impact on the way people eat today? Leading experts in

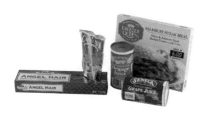

These products represent groundbreaking advances made by food scientists during the last century.

food science were asked their opinions to this question. Try to imagine life without their top 10 selections.

1. Juice in boxes and foil pouches
2. Safe canning procedures
3. The microwave oven
4. Frozen fruit juice concentrates
5. Prepackaged fruits, vegetables, and salads
6. Freeze-dried products like instant coffee and tea
7. TV dinners
8. Moisture control to prevent spoilage

9. Food fortification (adding nutrients to foods)
10. Milk in boxes (no refrigeration needed)

Other food innovations during this period that have had a large impact include

❖ margarine
❖ vegetable shortening
❖ corn syrup
❖ artificial sweeteners
❖ shaped cereals and snack foods
❖ artificial fats

Adapted from: Hayton, Bea, "50 Years of Food Innovations: The Hot, the Dry, and the Frozen," *Current Health*, Nov. 1990, pp. 17-19.

---

in improved water purification methods and microwave vacuum drying systems for agricultural crops.

Some of the new production processes developed by food scientists have a number of advantages. For example, using microwave vacuum drying to preserve rice limits energy use. The system is environmentally clean, and there is little or no sound pollution. Fire hazard is also reduced. In addition, the rice is dried without hardening or damage, and nutrients are preserved.

Researchers are studying quick-freezing as a food preservation technique. This research has led to higher-quality frozen food products.

Quick-freezing uses *cryogenic liquids*, which are substances that are in liquid form at extremely low temperatures. For example, nitrogen gas becomes liquid at –194°C (–317°F). Ordinary freezing techniques allow relatively large ice crystals to form. These ice crystals can rupture the cell walls of foods like fruits and vegetables. Cryogenic liquids are so cold that foods freeze almost on contact. This results in the formation of very small ice crystals, which cause minimal damage to cell structure. Products thus maintain much of the color, texture, and nutritive value of fresh foods.

Development of International Regulations

In the late 1980s, there was a big news story about the pesticide Alar. This pesticide was found on apples imported from Brazil. The problem was not as big as first believed. However, it awakened many people in the United States to the importance of monitoring imported foods for safety.

As technology has advanced, the globe has seemed to shrink. The increase in food exports and imports has led to a need for international food standards. Many food scientists are at work creating guidelines food producers all around the world can follow. Food scientists are working with members of the United Nations and legislative leaders from many countries to establish standards. Their goal is to ensure the safety and quality of the food supply worldwide.

Food scientists are involved in a broad range of activities. This section has addressed only a few of the ways food scientists are expanding and improving the food supply. Their efforts have enabled people today to eat better than was once thought possible.

Why Study Food Science?

Many food scientists focus on organic chemistry, microbiology, engineering, or nutrition. Others have received special training in one area of food production, such as poultry, animal, or dairy science. However, interest in one of these fields is not the only reason you might study food science.

Over half of all jobs in the world are linked to food in some way. Farmers, shippers, processors, food retailers, cooks, and waiters are among the people who must know how to handle food properly. There are jobs in every area and at every level of training and income that need some understanding of food.

Even if you never earn a living working with food, the problem-solving skills you develop in this class will be helpful. You can use these skills as you make consumer choices about food. Every time you buy a product, you are casting a vote. Every time you eat, you are affecting your health and potentially the

health of future generations. This course can give you the background and understanding you need to decide wisely.

Some food processing techniques reduce the nutrient content of some food products. Substitute ingredients, such as certain artificial sweeteners and fat substitutes, have been linked with health problems. Some food preservation methods have sparked concerns about the safety of the environment. By knowing about the science behind these issues, you will be able to make informed decisions.

Information from this class will help you understand food labels and analyze new products. This, in turn, will help you enjoy the benefits of today's food supply while avoiding potential hazards. You will feel equipped to make the best decisions when buying food for you and your family.

Understanding how scientific principles relate to food can also help you become a better cook. You might use knowledge from this class to create and adjust recipes. Even if you are not interested in preparing food, you will know the basic guidelines for maintaining food quality and safety. Knowing about food and its impact on the body will prepare you to make healthful choices. See 1-9.

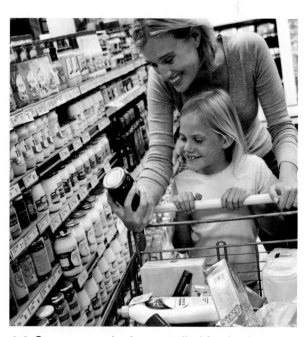

1-9 Consumers who have studied food science are better equipped to make informed choices about the foods they buy for their families.

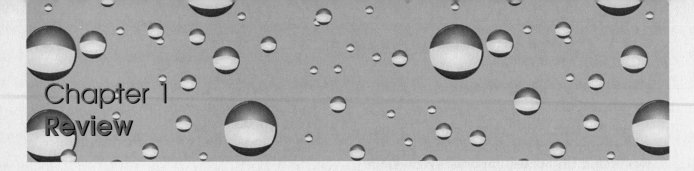

Chapter 1
Review

Summary

The field of food science applies knowledge to the production, processing, preservation, and packaging of food. All through early history, food products were discovered by trial and error. During the industrial revolution, advances in knowledge helped researchers start to grasp the science behind many food products. At this same time, mass production methods were developed and began to be used in the food industry. Problems resulting from mass production led the government to become involved in regulating the food industry.

In recent years, food scientists have made great strides in expanding the food supply. They have developed thousands of new food products and many food processing methods. They have also become involved in developing international food safety regulations.

Everyone who eats and makes food purchases can benefit from an understanding of food and how it affects the body. Studying food science can help you learn how ingredients function in food mixtures. This information can assist you in making wise decisions when buying, storing, and preparing foods.

Check Your Understanding

1. The study of the nature of food and the principle of its production, processing, preservation, and packaging is called _____.

2. Why is food science called an integrated course?

3. How did the food supply affect the development of early civilizations?

4. What tool was invented near the beginning of the industrial revolution that helped food scientists begin to understand food spoilage?

5. List the three major periods in the development of food.

6. What two laws are the basis for all the rules and regulations written by the FDA?

7. What is the reference used by restaurants, grocery stores, and institutions as a guide to safe food handling?

8. What are three results of the Nutrition Labeling and Education Act of 1990?

9. Give some examples of hydroponic crops and explain how they are grown.

10. Why might consumers choose to use food analogs instead of traditional food products?

11. What is the advantage of using cryogenic liquids in food production?

12. Name three benefits of studying food science.

Critical Thinking

1. Describe the major accomplishments regarding food during each of the three periods of history discussed in this chapter.

2. What benefits do adulterated food products have for food producers and what potential hazards do such products create for consumers?

3. What food analogs are regular parts of your diet?

4. Why is it necessary to have international food safety standards?

5. How can this course help you evaluate new developments in food products in the future?

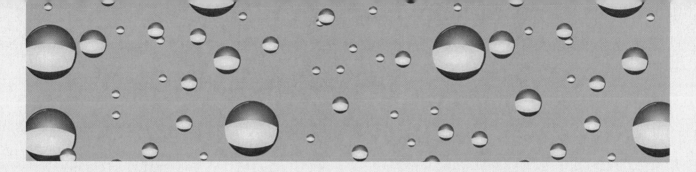

Explore Further

1. **Technology.** Use computer resources to research the contributions made by a historic food scientist. Subjects of your research might include Louis Pasteur, Clarence Birdseye, Charles Beck, Milton Hershey, Henri Nestle, or Nicholas Appert. Prepare an oral report describing the scientist's educational background and research. Also, describe the impact the scientist's invention or innovation has had on the food supply today. As an alternative, research contributions made by an organization such as NASA, FDA, or USDA that have affected today's food supply.

2. **Communication.** Debate problems humanity will face if the world hunger problem is not solved within the next 20 years. Address political, scientific, and economic problems.

3. **Writing.** Write a research report about what guidelines exist for foods shipped across national boundaries. What assurances do consumers have that imported foods have been produced safely?

4. **Math.** Collect nutrition labels from the packaging on foods from a meal you have eaten recently. Record how much of each food you consumed.

   A. Use the label information and your food record to calculate how many servings of each food you consumed.

   B. Calculate total calories consumed. (Multiply the number of servings by the calories per serving for each food eaten.)

   C. Calculate the percent of calories consumed from each of the energy nutrients—carbohydrates, fats, and proteins. (Percent equals total calories from an energy nutrient divided by the total calories consumed multiplied by 100.)

   D. Compare the percentage of calories from each energy nutrient to the recommended daily levels of 55% carbohydrates, 30% fat, and 15% protein. What changes could you make to improve your balance of energy nutrients in your diet?

Activity 1A
Developing Data Tables

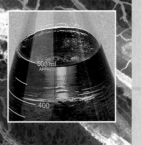

Purpose

Scientists conduct experiments to collect information. Scientists use data tables to organize information in a way that is easy to read. A well-designed data table will also help scientists see patterns and relationships in data they might miss otherwise. In this activity, you will set up a data table. This will prepare you to set up and use data tables in experiments throughout this course.

Equipment

ruler

Supplies

paper
pencil

Procedure

1. Data tables are made up of small boxes called *cells*, which are used for recording information. Cells are organized vertically into *columns*. Cells are organized horizontally into *rows*. Set up a data table that provides rows and columns to list the year and the total number of new products developed for each of five years.

2. *Headings* define the types of information that are listed in rows and columns. Headings for columns are written in the spaces of the first row or above the first row. Headings for rows are listed in a data table from top to bottom in the first column. Enter headings to define the types of information that will be recorded in your table.

3. Enter the years 1970, 1981, 1990, 1995, and 1996 into the appropriate cells of your data table.

4. The number of new food products developed each year in order are 1,041; 1,796; 10,301; 16,862; and 13,266. Enter these figures into the appropriate cells of your data table.

Questions

1. Does your data table have two rows with six columns or six rows with two columns?

2. What factors would help you determine if information should be entered into the rows or the columns?

3. Which year had the most new food products? Which year had the fewest?

4. What information would you lose if the data table listed information only for the beginning of each decade?

Activity 1B
Using Data for Calculations

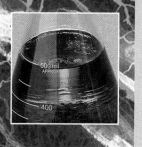

Purpose

In this activity, you will practice using information in data tables. You will be evaluating data on the types of health claims made on new food products between 1990 and 1996. During the last decade of the twentieth century, many new food products were a result of consumer demands for healthier foods. Health claims centered around the following topics: calories, fat, salt, cholesterol, fiber, calcium, additives, sugar, naturalness, and organics.

Equipment

ruler

calculator

Supplies

paper

pencil

Procedure

1. Set up a data table with 11 rows divided into 4 columns.

2. The headings for your columns are *Focus of Claims, 1990, 1995,* and *1996.*

3. Record the following types of health claims in your data table with the accompanying statistics, which are listed in order from 1990 to 1996. New products with claims focusing on additives (371, 167, 143), calcium (20, 21, 35), calories (1,165; 1,161; 776), cholesterol (694, 163, 223), fat (1,024; 1,914; 2,076), fiber (84, 40, 12), naturalness (754, 407, 645), and organics (324, 538, 645), salt (517, 205, 171), and sugar (331, 422, 373).

3. Add two rows to the bottom of your data table. The first row will list the total products with health claims each year. The second row will list the total other new products developed that year. (Hint: Use data from the table created in Activity 1A to complete the second row.)

Lab Extension

Create a second data table that will list the percentage of new products in each category for each year.

Calculations

Calculate the percentage of new products in each category for each year. Percentage equals part divided by the whole times 100. For example, in 1990 there were a total of 10,301 new products. Of those, 1,165 had claims regarding calories. Therefore, 11.3% of the new products introduced in 1990 had health claims focusing on calories.

$$1,165 \div 10,301 \times 100 = 11.3\%$$

Questions

1. Which health claims increased in number during each year listed?

2. Which health claims decreased in number during each year listed?

3. Which health claim has a greater number of new products in 1995 than in 1990 or 1996?

4. Did the total number of new products with health claims increase or decrease between 1990 and 1996?

Activity 1C
Using Data to Create Graphs

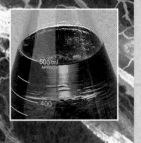

Purpose

When reporting experimental results, scientists often create graphs to help others picture the meaning of data. The three most common types of graphs used are bar graphs, line graphs, and pie charts. In this activity, you will use the data tables you created in Activities 1A and 1B to make several types of graphs. Computer spreadsheet programs can create graphs for you. Set up a spreadsheet to match your data table and enter the data. Then go to the *create graphs* item and follow the instructions.

Equipment

computer with spreadsheet program
    (optional)
ruler

Supplies

paper

Procedure

1. Line graphs are used to compare two variables. This type of graph is often used to show changes over the course of time or temperature. You will plot one variable along a horizontal axis. You will plot the second variable, which depends on the first, along a vertical axis. For instance, a line graph might be used to show changes in the number of grams of sugar that will dissolve in 1 L of water at different temperatures. Adding sugar to the water will not change the temperature of the water. However, increasing the temperature of the water will increase the amount of sugar that can be dissolved. Therefore, you would plot temperatures along the horizontal axis and grams of sugar along the vertical axis. Use the data table you created in Activity 1A to create a line graph showing the change in total new products developed from 1970 to 1996.

2. Bar graphs are used to compare totals between two or more categories. A bar with a different color or pattern is used to represent each category. Create a bar graph that compares the total number of new products with each type of health claim for each of the three years listed in the data table from Activity 1B.

3. Circle graphs, which are also called pie charts, are used to compare parts to a whole. A wedge of the circle is used to represent the relative percentage of each part. Use data from the table you prepared in Activity 1B to create a pie chart. This chart should compare the number of new products with each type of health claim to the total new number of products developed during the same year. You may chart data from 1990, 1995, or 1996.

Questions

1. Which type of graph was the easiest to generate?

2. Which type of graph would work best for three types of measurements taken on each five batches of pudding?

3. Describe information that would fit well into a pie chart.

4. What are the advantages of using computer programs to store and chart data?

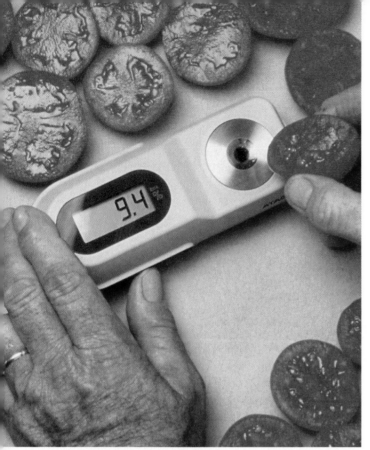

USDA

Food scientists have many measuring tools designed for specific tests. This digital refractometer is used to measure dissolved solids in commercial tomatoes.

Scientific Evaluation: Being Objective

Objectives

After studying this chapter,
you will be able to

describe the role of science in the development of new food products.

identify the function of measuring equipment used in the science laboratory.

demonstrate proper measurement techniques.

list the steps of the scientific method.

use proper safety procedures in the food science lab.

Key Terms

science	liter (L)
phenomenon	beaker
applied science	Erlenmeyer flask
experiment	graduated cylinder
formulation	buret
replicable	meniscus
International System	Celsius degree
of Units (SI)	scientific method
mass	hypothesis
gram (g)	variable
kilogram (kg)	control
weight	variation
calibrate	data
length	conclusion
meter (m)	meta-analysis
volume	

According to the dictionary, *science* is the systematic knowledge of natural and physical phenomena. A *phenomenon* is a fact, occurrence, circumstance, or process that can be observed. Scientists watch what occurs under controlled conditions to determine why things happen as they do. From study and observation, scientists discover the natural world has predictable patterns of behavior.

To be successful in the food science laboratory, you will need to follow some basic guidelines. You must make an effort to avoid biases, which can skew your results. You cannot base your conclusions on what you expect to happen. Instead, you must base them on what truly happens according to your careful observations. You will need to take accurate measurements. You will need to review literature on previous studies for ideas, hints, and procedures. You must keep detailed records of the steps you follow. You will also have to design procedures so you observe only one change at a time. Doing this allows you to know what causes the change in your results and how big the change is.

Science in the Food Industry

Because astronomers have recorded and plotted the movement of stars and planets, they can predict solar and lunar eclipses. Because chemists know how chemicals react to heat and light, they can recommend safe transportation methods for various chemicals. Because microbiologists know how molds grow, they have helped develop additives that can keep bread fresh longer. Because physicists understand thermodynamics (the study of heat), they have helped invent safer, more efficient ovens to cook food. See 2-1.

In each of these examples, knowledge gained by science has been put to a practical use. When basic scientific laws and theories are understood, they can be used to help people in their everyday lives. This process of putting scientific knowledge to practical use is called *applied science.*

Food science is an applied science. Basic laws of chemistry, physics, biology, and nutrition are applied to the production, processing, and packaging of the food supply. Through trial and error, your ancestors discovered effective ways to store and prepare food. Scientists can now explain why the methods your ancestors used worked. Scientists have also developed new and better methods of preserving and preparing foods.

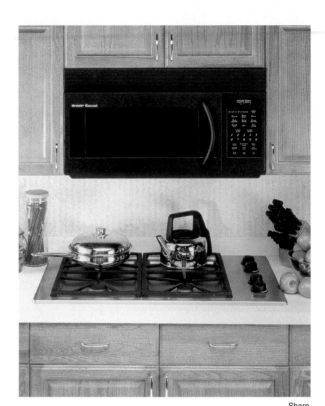
Sharp

2-1 Physicists have used their understanding of thermodynamics to help develop safe, powerful microwave ovens.

The development of new food products involves the application of scientific principles. Therefore, developments in the food industry have led to growth in the study of food science. Food scientists, like other types of scientists, experiment to learn what will work. An *experiment* is a controlled situation that allows a scientist or researcher to determine what causes a change to occur. For example, past experiments have produced the "best" way to prepare baked beans. The results of these types of food experiments are called recipes. In the food industry, recipes are called *formulations.*

Imagine the navy bean crop used by the Best Bean Company was destroyed by a plant disease this year. To keep the company from going broke, a substitute bean would be needed to produce their top-selling baked bean products. First, the food science team would study the characteristics of the navy bean. Next they would look for several beans that had similar physical characteristics. They would then experiment with each bean substitute. Their goal would be to find a bean and a recipe combination that looked and tasted like their original product.

Of course, you could experiment without being scientific. Suppose the Best Bean's food science team found a suitable substitute. However, they could not tell the production manager how to make their substitute product. Their experiments would not meet an important requirement. For an experiment to be scientific, it must be *replicable*, or repeatable.

Measurements

One guideline all researchers must follow is to take accurate measurement readings. To measure anything successfully, you must meet three requirements.

❖ You must identify what system of measurement or standard you are using.

❖ You must determine what you are trying to measure.

❖ You must decide what method of measurement will give you the most consistent results.

Scientists working all over the world share information. Therefore, they need a system of measurement that everyone can use. An international system has been developed that is based on the metric system. The metric system is a decimal system of measurement. Like the U.S. money system, which has cents, dimes, and dollars, all units in the metric system are divisible by ten. The internationally accepted version of the metric system is called the *International System of Units*, which is abbreviated *SI*. In this class, you will use basic metric units to measure mass, length, volume, time, and temperature. See 2-2.

To achieve success when preparing a recipe, you need to use the specified amount of each ingredient. Likewise, to obtain valid results when conducting an experiment, you need to use the specified amount of each substance. Precise numbers and units will help you use the correct amounts. You cannot accurately measure vague amounts, such as a "pinch" or a "sprinkle." Your pinch may be twice as large as another person's if your hands are the size of a professional basketball player's.

Prefixes make it easier to work with larger and smaller amounts of substances in the metric system. You must know these prefixes to follow the experiments in this class. See 2-3.

Besides being familiar with the metric system, you must know what types of measurements you need. You must also know how to take accurate measurements. (A table showing how to convert English units to metric and vice versa appears in the Appendix. The Appendix also includes a table listing standard metric equivalents for common measurements used in cooking and baking.)

Mass

Mass is a measure of the quantity of matter. When conducting food science experiments, you will often be measuring the mass of solid and liquid substances.

In this class, you will occasionally refer to kilograms. Most of the time, however, you will

Metric Base Units		
Type	**Name**	**Symbol**
Mass	gram	g
Length	meter	m
Volume	liter	L
Time	second	s
Temperature	Celsius degree	°C

2-2 All other units in the metric system are derived from these base units.

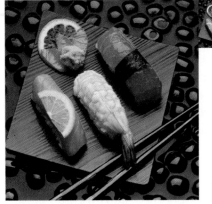

International Issue
The Metric System and Foreign Trade

The U.S. federal government is promoting *metrication*. This means changing from the English to the metric system of measurement. The metric system includes product standards and preferred sizes that are now being used by industries and governments worldwide.

Economics is a key reason the government is urging the switch. Products not measured in metric units are becoming increasingly unacceptable in world markets. The government realizes that switching to the metric system will improve U.S. standings in the global marketplace. Companies that have switched to metric units have increased their ability to sell products all over the world. U.S.

industries that have made this switch include the beverage and auto industries. Most people in the United States are now used to buying soft drinks in 1- and 2-liter bottles.

Congress first encouraged the change through the Metric Conversion Act of 1975. This act made switching to the metric system voluntary. In 1988, Congress passed amendments to the act. These amendments required any government function related to trade, industry, or commerce to use the metric system. Federal agencies are also required to seek ways to educate the public about the metric system.

A number of factors make the complete change to the metric

system difficult. One factor is reluctance of consumers to adopt the new system. Teaching the metric system in schools will gradually help the public feel more comfortable with metric terms and units. A second factor is the need to rewrite many legal definitions. Some state and federal regulations would also need to be rewritten. A third factor is the cost. Most businesses that use the English system are not willing to make expensive changes in production lines and equipment. However, many of these businesses plan to make the switch when they replace old equipment or build new plants.

Metric Prefixes

Prefix	Symbol	Meaning	Multiplier
Greater than 1			
kilo	k	thousand	1,000
hecto*	h	hundred	100
deka*	da	ten	10
Less than 1			
deci	d	tenth	0.1
centi	c	hundredth	0.01
milli	m	thousandth	0.001
micro	μ	millionth	0.000001

*These units are not used in this text.

2-3 These prefixes can be used to identify units greater than and less than one gram, meter, or liter (1,000 grams = 1 kilogram; 0.01 meters = 1 centimeter; 0.001 liters = 1 milliliter).

be massing substances between 0 and 300 g. A *gram (g)* is the mass of 1 cubic centimeter (cm³) of water at 4°C (39°F). A *kilogram (kg)* is the mass of 1 liter of water at 4°C (39°F). One kg equals 1,000 g.

Mass is often confused with weight. *Weight* is the measure of the force of gravity between two objects. Weight changes with location. Suppose a bag of flour weighs 5 pounds in Atlantic City, New Jersey, which is at sea level. The flour will weigh slightly less on Pike's Peak in Colorado, which is 4,301 m (14,110 feet) above sea level. The flour will weigh less than 1 pound on the moon. However, the mass will be 2.25 kg in all three locations.

To be accurate, scientists need a measurement that does not change from place to place. Massing a substance compares the substance to a standard mass.

Equipment for Measuring Mass

The two most common tools for measuring mass are the triple beam balance and the electronic balance. As the name implies, a triple beam balance has three beams. It works on the same principle as a seesaw. If a seesaw has the same amount of matter on each side, it will balance. On a triple beam balance, standard masses slide along the beams. These standard masses are used to equal the mass of an object put in the pan. Gravity will have the same effect on the standard masses as it has on the mass of the object. This will be true no matter what your location is.

Most laboratories today use an electronic balance. An electronic balance is faster and easier to use than a triple beam balance. When you turn on an electronic balance, you need to calibrate it. To *calibrate* is to adjust a measuring instrument to a standard. To calibrate an electronic balance, you measure a standard mass first. The balance will then compare all substances measured to that mass. See 2-4.

How to Measure Mass

It is easy to mass an apple. Massing milk or sugar is a bit more challenging. The apple stays where you put it. Milk and sugar would flow off the balance. You will often have to put substances in some kind of container before massing them. The container needs to be as

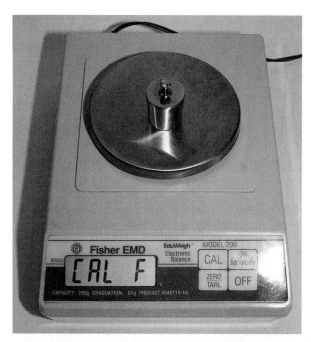

2-4 A 100-gram mass is placed on the weighing pan of an electronic balance. When the balance reads *CAL F*, the calibration is finished, and the balance can be used to mass other objects.

lightweight as possible and large enough to hold the substance you are massing. Weighing papers, plastic weighing dishes, and muffin cup liners work well for massing substances like salt, sugar, and flour. You can mass larger amounts of substances on coffee filters. You can mass liquids in beakers or plastic or paper cups. Using disposable containers and papers will save cleanup time in class.

You may have recognized a problem with massing objects in containers. How do you mass the substance without massing the container? There are two ways to handle this problem. With a triple beam balance, you must first mass the empty container and record the result. This mass is called the *tare*. Then you mass the container holding the substance and record the result. Subtract the first result from the second result. The difference is the mass of the substance. This process is called *taring*. When massing powders or liquids with a triple beam balance, you will record all three masses in your data table. See 2-5.

An electronic balance will do this math for you. Set the empty container on the calibrated electronic balance. Push the button labeled *Tare*. See 2-6. This will reset the balance to

Calculating Mass	
Mass of container and substance	*12.6 g*
Mass of empty container	*-1.2 g*
Mass of substance	*11.4 g*

2-5 To figure the mass of a substance, first mass an empty container. Then subtract this mass from the mass of the container with the substance in it.

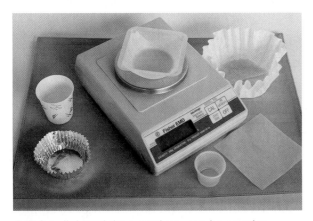

2-6 Any lightweight container can be used to mass powders and liquids on an electronic balance. The tare button can be used to erase the mass of the container before massing ingredients used in experiments.

zero. Add the substance you are massing to the container. The mass on the display screen will be the mass of the substance only.

When massing substances in this class, you need to be accurate to the nearest tenth of a gram. If your balance reads to the hundredth of a gram, round the number to the nearest tenth. For example, if the balance says 3.57 g, you will round to 3.6 g.

Length

Another type of measurement is length. *Length* is the distance between two points. This measurement allows you to evaluate the size of objects. For example, to evaluate different cake recipes, you will need to measure how high each one rises.

The standard unit of length in the metric system is the *meter (m)*. One meter is equal to 39.37 inches. Most objects you will measure in a food science lab are much shorter than a meter. You will usually record length measurements in centimeters (cm) and millimeters (mm). When you measure microorganisms in food, you will use micrometers (μm). One micrometer equals 0.000001 meter.

How to Measure Length

You will usually measure length with a ruler. You will need one with centimeter and millimeter divisions. The ends of rulers can be chipped, worn, or unevenly cut. Therefore, it is best to measure objects from another starting point. See 2-7.

What if the object you need to measure is a potato? You cannot accurately measure a round, uneven object by placing it next to a ruler and "eyeballing it." A more accurate method is to identify the endpoints of the object. To do this, you need a vertical surface that rises from a horizontal surface at a 90° angle. For instance, you might place the potato on a counter next to a wall. Position one end of the potato against the wall. Place a flat stick against the opposite end of the potato. The wall and the stick are the endpoints of the potato. Use your ruler to measure the distance between the endpoints. See 2-8.

Volume

Volume is a measurement derived from length. *Volume* is the amount of space occupied by an object. For example, the volume

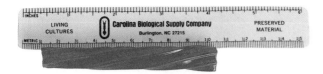

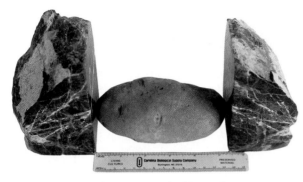

2-7 When measuring the length of an object, start at a mark other than the end of the ruler. This cherry licorice is 9.4 cm (3¹¹/₁₆ inches) long.

2-8 Place irregularly shaped objects between two parallel surfaces and measure the distance between the surfaces with a ruler. This potato is 13.5 cm (5⁵/₁₆ inches) long.

container are, the more accurately the container will measure volume.

Several types of containers are used for measuring volume in the food science lab. These include beakers, Erlenmeyer flasks, graduated cylinders, and burets. A *beaker* is a deep, wide-mouthed container with a pouring lip used to hold substances during experiments. An *Erlenmeyer flask* is a flat-bottomed, cone-shaped container used to mix and hold liquids. You can use beakers and Erlenmeyer flasks to measure volume when accuracy is not important. For example, measuring 500 mL of water for boiling a potato does not require great precision. A *graduated cylinder* is a tall container used to accurately measure the volume of liquids to the nearest milliliter. A *buret* is a graduated glass tube with a control valve at the bottom. It is used to pour an accurate amount of liquid. With practice, you can learn to control the flow so you can measure liquids a drop at a time. See 2-9.

of a box is calculated by multiplying the length times the width times the height. You can remember this calculation by the equation ($v = l \times w \times h$).

The metric unit for measuring fluid volume is the *liter (L).* A liter is just a little more than an English quart, or 4 cups. In this class, you will often use milliliters as well as liters to measure volume. You can use Table 2-3 to calculate that 1 L equals 1,000 mL.

A decimeter (dm) is one-tenth of a meter or 10 cm. This is a length of about 4 inches. A liter equals an amount of space 1 dm high by 1 dm wide by 1 dm deep (1 dm³). This means that 1 dm³ equals 1,000 cm³ (10 cm × 10 cm × 10 cm = 1,000 cm³). Therefore, a liter has 1,000 cm³ of volume. You can calculate that 1 mL = 1 cm³.

Equipment for Measuring Volume

You will usually measure liquids by their volume. You will use containers made of clear glass or plastic that have a graduated scale on the side. Containers are measured against a standard, and then marks are carefully placed on the side to show various volumes. Generally, the smaller the divisions on the

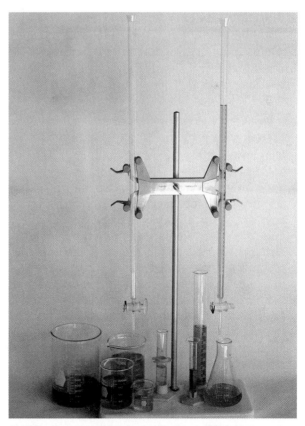

2-9 Beakers, graduated cylinders, Erlenmeyer flasks, and burets are used to measure the volume of liquids.

How to Measure Volume

The surface of a liquid in a measuring container does not appear to be flat. It appears to curve. This curve at the surface of the liquid is called the *meniscus.* The narrower a container is, the more obvious this curve will be. The meniscus is caused by liquid clinging to the sides of a container. To accurately measure liquid volume, place the container on a level surface. Read the volume at eye level from the bottom of the meniscus. See 2-10.

You must follow the correct procedures when measuring liquids for your measurements to be accurate. For instance, holding a measuring container at an angle alters the reading of liquid volume. It is easy to see if a container is tipped from side to side. However, it is difficult to tell if a container is tipped toward you or away from you. This is why containers for measuring volume should be set on a flat surface before you take a reading. You must also measure liquids at eye level. Looking down at a measuring container on a counter will cause you to view liquid in the container at an angle. This will make the volume of the liquid look larger than it really is. Small differences in the volumes of substances can affect the outcomes of some experiments and recipes.

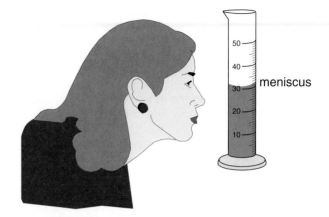

2-10 Take volume readings in a graduated cylinder or buret at eye level from the bottom of the meniscus. This liquid measures 31 mL.

Cooking Tip

Measuring the volume of solid and semi-solid fats presents a challenge. When you pack fat in a dry measuring cup, air pockets can form. The fat that clings to the cup afterwards is also difficult to clean out of the cup. The water displacement method solves both problems. Start by measuring a known volume of cool water. Use a large liquid measure so you will have room to add fat to the water. Calculate the total volume of the fat plus the water. Then gradually add fat to the water until the water level reaches the calculated total. For instance, suppose you start with 1½ cups of cool water and you need ½ cup of fat. The water will reach the 2-cup level when the correct volume of fat has been added. This method works for butter, hydrogenated shortening, and peanut butter.

Time

A fourth type of measurement is time. In most food science experiments, you will measure time in seconds. Whenever an experiment calls for time measurements, it will be critical to have someone act as a timer. Record start and stop times using a clock or watch. Failure to accurately monitor time can make your entire experiment invalid.

Temperature

Temperature is a measure of heat intensity. When you describe the temperature of a food, you probably think of words like *hot, warm, cool,* and *cold.* These terms give a general description of the heat intensity in an object. In food science experiments, however, you will need a more exact description of heat intensity.

The most commonly used unit of temperature in the laboratory is the Celsius degree (°C). The Celsius temperature scale is based on the boiling and freezing points of pure water. Water freezes at 0°C and boils at 100°C at 1 atmosphere of air pressure. The difference between these points is divided into 100 equal units. Therefore, a *Celsius degree* is 0.01 of the difference between the boiling and freezing points of water.

The United States still uses the Fahrenheit scale for most everyday temperature measurements. Therefore, most laboratory thermometers are marked with both the Celsius and Fahrenheit scales. It is important to locate the Celsius scale when taking temperature readings.

When recording any type of measurements, be sure to list the units in which you are measuring. Simply writing numbers does not provide enough information to anyone who is referring to your data table. It is important to clarify whether you measured items in metric or English units. You also need to specify which units of a measuring system you used. There is a big difference between grams and kilograms and between ounces and pounds. Anyone who is trying to follow your procedure will need to know what your measurements mean.

Remember that taking accurate measurements is only one aspect of scientific experiments. Scientists also use a process that helps guide the way they conduct experiments.

The Scientific Method

The *scientific method* is a system of steps used to solve problems. Scientists throughout the world use this method. However, you do not need to be a scientist to benefit from it. Solving problems using the scientific method is a useful skill no matter what your career choice might be.

Ask Questions

The scientific method begins when a question arises. Most four-year-olds have this step down pat. They ask questions such as Why is the sky blue? and How does a clock work? Scientists, like four-year-olds, are curious about what they observe. See 2-11.

Millions of lives have been saved because one scientist asked why bacteria on a petri dish had been killed. This scientist was Alexander Fleming. In answering the question, he discovered penicillin.

To approach a problem from a scientific angle, start by asking yourself such questions as what, why, and how. As you conduct experiments, you are likely to find as many unanswered questions as solutions. Each unanswered question could be developed into another scientific experiment.

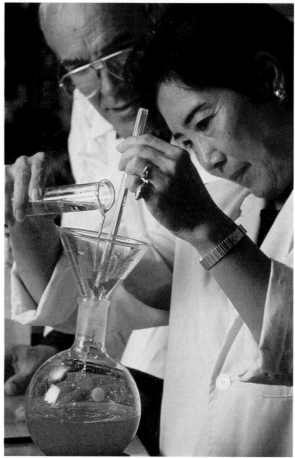

USDA

2-11 In the first step of the scientific method, food scientists ask questions about circumstances or events they have observed.

The food scientists at the Best Bean Company would use the scientific method to address their navy bean problem. Their question might be, Is there a substitute for navy beans that will be comparable in flavor, texture, color, and cost?

Define the Problem

The second step in the scientific method is to define what the problem is. In Fleming's discovery of penicillin, he began by asking why the bacteria had been killed. However, this question was too vague to be of much help. He defined the problem by asking, "What killed the bacteria in some spots and not others?" This question provided a clear statement of the observed event and the conditions under which it was observed. It set a goal and gave direction on how to solve the problem.

A student who finds he or she is failing math illustrates another example of defining a problem. This student has observed a problem. However, the student must specifically define what aspect of studying math is problematic. Perhaps the concepts are too complex. Maybe the examples in the book are confusing. Possibly the student is not studying enough. If the student does not define the problem, he or she will never pass the class. Although this step is very simple, it is critical to problem solving.

In this step of the scientific method, the Best Bean Company's problem is to find a substitute bean. This problem involves examining such factors as color, shape, texture, flavor, cooking characteristics, and cost. The company must also look at the impact a substitute bean will have on production techniques and customer approval.

In class experiments, the problem is the purpose for the experiment. This information is given in the introductory paragraph to each experiment.

Conduct Research

After defining the problem, you must list possible causes. This requires gathering as much information about the problem as possible. First you brainstorm, which means listing all ideas that come to mind.

Once you have listed ideas, it is time to do research. You can study books and articles on related subjects. Search the Internet for information. This is referred to as review of literature. Scientists check information such as patent applications published by other scientists. They look up scientific principles that are related. They examine questions other scientists have asked about a given topic. Food scientists often follow this path for clues about what types of procedures might help them answer their questions. See 2-12.

Think again about the example of the Best Bean Company mentioned early in this chapter. Best Bean's food science team might approach this step by finding names and descriptions of different kinds of beans. Another option would be to look for recipes that use other types of beans. Asking cooks what they have done about this problem would be an option, too.

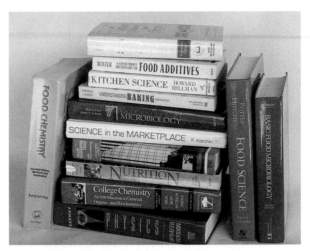

2-12 Books are just one resource to use when following the scientific method to conduct research about a problem.

In this class, your research will involve reading this textbook before conducting experiments. If you set up experiments outside class, you will need to find many information resources to assist you.

State the Hypothesis

From your research, you should be able to narrow your list of possible causes of the problem. As you proceed with the scientific method, you need to focus on a single cause. Select the cause that seems to be the most likely. Then state a hypothesis about this cause. A *hypothesis* is a possible solution to a problem. It is an educated guess based on available evidence.

After careful research, the food scientists at the Best Bean Company narrowed their options to three. Their hypothesis is that great northern beans, pink beans, and pinto beans are acceptable substitutes for navy beans.

Design the Experiment

The next step in the scientific method is to design an experiment to see if your hypothesis is correct. Designing an experiment involves answering questions like these

❖   How can I test this hypothesis?

❖   What steps will I need to take?

❖   Will this procedure prove or disprove my hypothesis?

❖   What equipment and supplies will I need?

- ❖ Will I need an assistant?
- ❖ What data will I need to collect?
- ❖ How long will it take?
- ❖ Do I need to take any safety precautions?
- ❖ How will I record the data?

In most science classes, this step is done for you. The laboratory experiment's procedure gives the experiment design. Read each experiment looking for the answers to the questions above. This will help you know how to conduct the experiment. It will also help you understand what you are looking for and why as you complete the experiment.

A well-designed experiment will have a control and a variable. A *variable* is a factor that is being changed. For the bean company, the variable is the kind of bean. Changing the bean may or may not change the quality of the product. The researchers must determine if the type of bean matters. They will do this by examining the quality of the finished baked beans against the control. See 2-13.

The *control* is the standard against which you measure all changes. In the baked bean example, the original recipe with the original bean would be the control. In this case, it is the result the bean company is seeking.

Each change made in an experiment is called a *variation.* For example, the bean company may have found three beans that are similar to the original bean. How many different batches of baked beans would the food science team need to make? They would need one batch with each type of new bean. They would also need a control to compare to the new baked bean recipes. This experiment would have a control and three variations.

When designing an experiment, you must control the number of variables. Analyze all the factors that could change your results. If your experiment includes more than one variable, you cannot tell which variable caused the changes. For example, changing the bean variety, the water content, and the spices in the same batch could skew the results. Even changing the source of water could affect the results.

In designing an experiment, you must decide what information you need to record. Look at your hypothesis and decide what kinds of measurements you need. The food scientists at the bean company would need to carefully measure the beans before and after soaking. This would allow the scientists to see which type of bean was closest to the original in size. Would they measure mass, volume, or both? They would record water volumes before and after soaking the beans. This would tell the researchers if the one bean variety absorbed the same, less, or more liquid than another variety. Cooking time records would allow the scientists to compare the heating time for the beans with the control. Best Bean does not want the beans to be tough from undercooking. On the other hand, the company does not want the beans to cook apart into a mush.

Conduct the Experiment

Carrying out your plan by conducting the experiment is the next step in the scientific method. In most experiments this year, each lab group will work with a different variation or control during the experiment. Each group will report its findings so the class can compare all the results. With different lab groups conducting different variations, it is critical that everyone follows the directions exactly, 2-14. Suppose your class was conducting an experiment to solve the problem at the Best Bean Company. What problems would develop if lab groups prepared the following variations of baked beans?

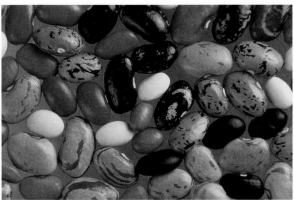

Agricultural Research Service, USDA

2-13 When researching a new formulation for a bean product, the type of bean is just one of many variables food scientists will investigate.

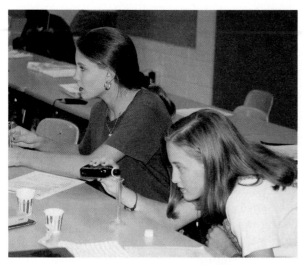

2-14 Following lab procedures carefully is essential to the successful outcome of experiments.

* Variation 1 is cooked twice as long as directed.
* Variation 2 includes 50 g brown sugar instead of 150 g.
* Variation 3 is cooked in an unmeasured volume of water.
* The control is prepared with twice the specified volume of molasses.

There would be no accurate way to tell if the beans made any difference. Failure to accurately follow the procedure would have allowed too many variables to be introduced. Changes could be caused by cooking time, sugar content, or water content. If the control is changed, there is no longer a standard against which to measure. How would you know what the quality is supposed to be? As you can see, following directions is important.

Besides carefully following directions, you must take precise measurements. However, it will not matter how precisely you measure if you do not keep accurate records. Records of your observations are of two basic types: numerical and descriptive.

Numerical observations are expressed in terms of numbers. When you take a measurement, you are making a numerical observation. As you record numerical observations, remember that numbers will be meaningless without units and a description of what you measured. A number scribbled on scrap paper could refer to the cooking temperature. However, the number might refer to the cooking time or mass of beans used in the recipe instead. Numerical records must include the units in which you took the measurements as well as the numbers.

Tables and charts can help you record and organize data. *Data* are measurable facts that are collected during an experiment. Make sure you record numbers neatly with any decimal points clearly marked. Reading and comparing data is easier if you neatly align numbers and decimal points. See 2-15.

The second type of observation is called a *descriptive observation*. Descriptions of what is happening that cannot be measured in numbers are often as important as numerical data. Descriptive observations may refer to such factors as color, texture, and odor. These factors can affect a person's willingness to try a food product. They can also indicate chemical and physical changes in a product.

When making descriptive observations, you may ask questions such as "How does the aroma of this variation compare to the control?" The following are examples of descriptive observations you may make in experiments this year:

* The liquid in Sample 2 has become cloudy.
* Sample 3 is sweeter than Sample 4.
* Solution 3 is releasing gas.
* Bubbles have formed along the surface of the vegetable.
* A film has formed on Sample 1.
* Variation 3 is a paler color than Variation 2.
* Sample 1 smells spicier and less earthy than Sample 2.

Practice increasing your observation skills. Look at little details and watch for changes that may occur. This part of conducting an experiment can be the hardest. It is easy to become distracted, daydream, or visit. This step requires self-discipline to make sure you stay alert.

Data Table

Trial	Mass of 250-mL cup	Mass of 125-mL cup	Mass of 50-mL cup
Scooped flour – A	146.4 g	78.6 g	34.9 g
B	104.9 g	48.8 g	19.8 g
C	124.7 g	57.0 g	24.0 g
Fluffed & spooned flour – A	107.6 g	56.4 g	21.7 g
B	102.0 g	55.3 g	20.9 g
C	104.8 g	50.1 g	19.0 g

Data Table

Trial	Mass of 250-mL cup	Mass of 125-mL cup	Mass of 50-mL cup
Scooped flour – A	146.4 g	78.6 g	34.9 g
B	104.9 g	48.9 g	19.8 g
C	129.7 g	57.0 g	24.0 g
Fluffed & spooned flour – A	107.6 g	56.4 g	21.7 g
B	102.0 g	55.3 g	20.9 g
C	104.8 g	50.1 g	19.0 g

2-15 It is important that data tables can be easily read. How easy is it to read the data table on the bottom as compared to the one on the top?

Evaluate the Results

Doing research and conducting experiments involves action. Evaluating the results mainly requires thinking. You must read through your data, observations, and notes. Look for patterns, common factors, changes, and questions. Look for answers to the questions and support for or against your hypothesis. Reach a conclusion about the accuracy of the hypothesis.

In this class, you will usually evaluate experiments the day after you conduct them. This allows your brain time to reflect on all the information you have gathered through research and experimentation.

As you go through the steps of the scientific method, keep in mind this is not a linear process. Sometimes a step can be skipped. Sometimes more information is needed. Testing a hypothesis often shows answering one question or solving one problem raises other questions or creates other problems. This means going back to a previous step.

Report the Results

The final step in the scientific method is to report your results. You must put your evaluation in writing so you can share it with others.

When writing conclusions, students will often simply rewrite their data and observations. This is not drawing a conclusion. A *conclusion* analyzes and applies data. For instance, you might describe ways you could apply the principle discovered in the experiment to other food situations. A conclusion will usually answer how, what, where, when, or why. It describes what the data and observations mean.

Another common problem in reporting results is stopping after reaching one conclusion. Many experiments could lead you to more than one conclusion. When this occurs, you might state ideas for further research that would be helpful. You might also state variables that should be better controlled. You often will not be aware of these variables

Lab Safety

Conducting experiments is an important and enjoyable part of any science class. For experiments to be successful, everyone needs to understand and follow some basic safety procedures. The following are general guidelines that will apply for most of the labs in this class. By learning these basic rules you can avoid the most common accidents that occur during food science experiments.

1. Follow lab rules and experiment procedures exactly.
   - ❖ Understanding and following rules and procedures is necessary for safe and successful experiments.
   - ❖ Do your homework. Read the experimental procedure before coming to class and review before proceeding.
   - ❖ Wash hands before and after experimental procedures.
   - ❖ To protect yourself and your lab partners, learn and follow all safety procedures.
   - ❖ Be sure all lab equipment is clean and is not chipped or broken.
2. Be serious.
   - ❖ Careless actions or horseplay can cause injuries to yourself or others.
3. Keep your hair under control. If it touches your shoulder, tie it back.
   - ❖ Loose hair can contaminate food samples that you will be taste testing.
   - ❖ Loose hair can block your vision, becoming a safety hazard.
   - ❖ Long, loose hair can easily catch fire when heat and open flames are used.
4. Be cautious around heated glass. It can explode.
   - ❖ When heating glassware, wear safety glasses to protect your eyes from flying glass.
   - ❖ When heating test tubes, point them away from people.
   - ❖ Cool hot glass slowly.
   - ❖ Call the instructor to assist in cleaning up any broken glass.
   - ❖ Use paper towels to pick up large pieces of broken glass. Sweep the area and then use wet paper towels to pick up small slivers of broken glass.
5. Remember that hot glassware looks the same as cold glassware.
   - ❖ Use tongs or oven mitts whenever you are using glassware to heat liquid mixtures.
   - ❖ When in doubt, assume glassware is hot.
   - ❖ If you should get burned, immediately put the burned area under cool running water. Send a lab partner to bring the instructor.
6. Protect eyes, skin, and clothing whenever you are working with strong acids and bases. Many of these substances look like water.
   - ❖ Wear splash goggles to prevent chemical burns to the eyes and protective gloves to prevent chemical burns to the skin.
   - ❖ If strong chemicals get on skin or eyes, flush the area immediately with cool running water. Have someone notify the instructor.
   - ❖ Plastic aprons or lab coats will help prevent damage to clothes. Wear older clothing on lab days.
   - ❖ Never taste a substance without permission from the instructor.
   - ❖ Use "food grade" ingredients. Maintain separate glassware for food use only.
7. Mix chemicals only as instructed.
   - ❖ Do not mix unknown chemicals. Poisonous fumes can be produced in some cases.
   - ❖ Always label containers containing chemicals to avoid errors in mixing.
8. Dispose of chemicals properly.
   - ❖ Follow directions given by your instructor.
   - ❖ A few chemicals used in this class may damage drain lines, septic systems, or contaminate water if handled incorrectly.
9. Plan time for lab cleanup.
   - ❖ Clean up spills immediately.
   - ❖ Return all supplies to their proper places.
   - ❖ Clean all glassware, equipment, and counter surfaces used during the lab.
   - ❖ Put away all equipment.

until after you have finished your initial experiment.

Your experiment may reveal more than one option for solving your problem. If this is the case, your conclusion needs to detail advantages and disadvantages of each option. Look again at the bean company's problem. What if all three bean variations were acceptable products? How would the production manager choose among the three? Suppose you were the production manager and the research team submitted the report in 2-16. Which variation would you choose?

Research is of little value if no one benefits from it. Scientists report their results in a variety of ways. They give oral presentations at professional meetings. They submit written reports for publication in scientific journals. Scientists often share with colleagues in discussion groups and through computer communications. They also write summaries to submit to employers. If their results include a major finding no one else has found, they may apply for a patent.

Your lab report is a simplified version of how scientists report their findings. Your report should be thorough and accurate. Future researchers may use it for their studies. Any research report needs to describe the purpose of the experiment, the procedure followed, and the data collected. Research reports need to specify observations made and questions answered. Major reports also include a review of related literature. Finally, these reports need to identify the researchers' conclusions.

Evaluating Scientific Studies

Vitamin A Prevents Cancer or *Vitamin A May Increase Cancer Risks*. Which headline is true? It is important to understand that scientific research is a process of discovery and debate. Because scientific research explores the unknown, there will be uncertainty and seemingly conflicting reports. New research published in journals should be viewed as discussions that give direction but not final answers. Knowing what is studied, how it was examined, what was controlled, and how it compares to real life situations can help consumers evaluate media hype. Researchers often examine hundreds of studies on the same issue before making recommendations to the public. When the results of several individual studies are pooled to yield overall conclusions it is called *meta-analysis*.

Research involving vitamin A found reduced risks of some cancers when diets contained recommended or higher levels of vitamin A (beta-carotene). In other studies when supplements were given and diets were low in vitamin A, there were no measurably significant benefits. One study had to be stopped because of increases in cancer rate when participants were given megadoses of vitamin A. This tells us that vitamin A may or may not impact your risk of cancer. These results could be due to vitamin A working in conjunction with other compounds found in foods that have not yet been identified. Perhaps errors in research may be causing these conflicting results.

When assessing new research, the following questions should be asked:

❖ Can the study be interpreted in another way?

❖ Are there any flaws or biases in the method or way the study was conducted?

❖ How does this study fit in with the current body of research on the subject?

❖ What are the limitations of this study?

It is important to remember that the scientific process requires ongoing discussion and debate.

Research Findings

Comparison Factor	Var. 1	Var. 2	Var. 3	Control
Type of Bean	great northern	pink	pinto	navy
Average Price	$25.75	$23.50	$19.75	$15.75
Bean Mass After Soaking	226 g	229 g	188 g	232 g
Cooking Time	1 hr, 15 min	1 hr, 30 min	1 hr, 10 min	1 hr, 5 min
Protein/Serving	8 g	7 g	7 g	7 g
Fiber/Serving	5 g	8 g	7 g	8 g
Appearance	Medium red	Rich red	Pale, muddy	Medium red
Texture	Tender	Tender	Tender	Tender
Flavor	Mild bean flavor	Mild bean flavor	Mild bean flavor	Mild bean flavor

Conclusion #1

Great northern beans have the highest supply cost. Pinto beans have the lowest supply cost, but they still cost 25% more than the navy beans in our standard formulation. Water absorption per 100 g of beans was as follows: great northern—126 g, pink—129 g, pinto—88 g, and navy—132 g. The pink beans took the longest time to become tender during the cooking process. Nutrition analysis revealed comparable protein levels, but great northern beans are significantly lower in fiber. The pink beans produced a product with a richer red color. The product made with pinto beans received the lowest appearance scores. Taste tests revealed no measurable differences in texture or flavor.

Conclusion #2

Gram for gram, navy beans had the largest increase in volume after soaking. This was followed by the pink, great northern, and pinto beans, in that order. The more water absorbed per gram of bean, the fewer beans needed per can. After navy beans, therefore, the pink beans should result in lowest supply costs. They are still 50% more than the navy beans in our standard formulation. This will result in an extra cost of 0.003 cents per can.

Supply cost, nutritional value, and product appearance make pink beans the best alternative to navy beans from a product standpoint. However, longer cooking time for the pink beans results in a 38% increase in energy and production costs. This would require a price increase of 10 cents per can.

Therefore, it is the recommendation of this team that great northern beans be used as a substitute for navy beans. The drawbacks of this substitution are high supply costs and low fiber content. Supply costs are well surpassed by production cost savings over pink beans. Though production costs are lower for the pinto bean product, it cannot compete in terms of appearance. Market research shows consumers will use price and appearance over nutritional value as pivotal factors in purchase decisions.

2-16 The first conclusion simply restates the data and observations. The second conclusion describes what the data and observations mean.

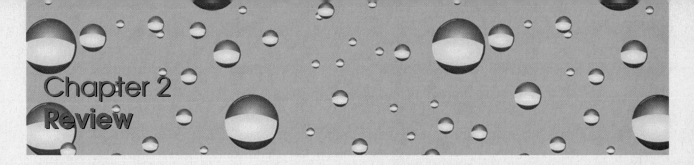

Chapter 2 Review

Summary

Food scientists apply their knowledge of basic scientific laws to solve problems in the food industry. They conduct experiments to develop new food products, processing methods, and packaging materials. The tools they use and the procedures they follow are basic to all scientists. You will use these same tools and procedures as you work in the food science lab.

In this class, you will often take measurements of mass, length, volume, time and temperature. You must become familiar with the measuring equipment you will be using. You must also learn how to measure accurately and record data and observations neatly.

The most important tool you will be using in this class is the scientific method. This process can help you solve most problems you face in life as well as in the food science lab. Through it you will ask questions, define problems, conduct research, and state hypotheses. These steps will help you design and conduct experiments and evaluate the results. Lastly, you must report your findings so others will benefit.

Check Your Understanding

1. Explain why food science is an applied science.
2. What are the metric base units for mass, length, volume, time, and temperature?
3. Describe how mass differs from weight.
4. Why is it best not to measure the length of an object from the end of a ruler?
5. How many cubic centimeters are in 55 milliliters?
6. On what is the Celsius temperature scale based?
7. List the steps of the scientific method.

8. What is the function of the control in an experiment?
9. Describe the two basic types of observations made during an experiment?
10. List 10 safety procedures you should follow when working in the food science lab.

Critical Thinking

1. The mass of a weighing paper is 1.2 g. The mass of the paper holding some salt is 13.8 g. What is the mass of the salt?
2. Explain how the measurements for length and volume are related.
3. Why is volume read from the bottom of a meniscus instead of the top?
4. What would happen if a researcher failed to realize a thermometer he or she was using has both Celsius and Fahrenheit scales?
5. What is the value of questions that arise during the experiment process?
6. Why would it be a problem to use only one resource when conducting research for a scientific experiment?
7. A food scientist bakes one cookie dough sample at 350°F for 13 minutes and a second sample at 375°F for 11 minutes. What is the problem with the scientist's procedure?
8. Explain how numeric and descriptive observations might both be used to evaluate the loss of water from tomato sauce during cooking.
9. Describe the difference between recording observations and writing a conclusion.
10. Describe how you could use the scientific method to develop the best time schedule for the nights your volleyball team has games.

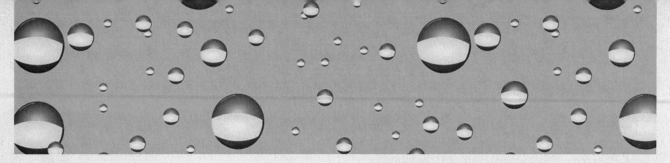

Explore Further

1. **Math.** Review the table in the Appendix that shows how to convert English measurements to metric. Convert the ingredient amounts and cooking temperatures specified in two of your favorite recipes to metric measurements.

2. **Technology.** Use the scientific method to design an experiment to compare the density of water, milk, and vegetable oil. Use a computer spreadsheet program to create a sample data table.

3. **History.** Investigate how and when the metric system was developed. Share your findings in a written report.

4. **Writing.** Using library or Internet resources select a recent research article to evaluate. After reading the article, write a paper that answers the questions listed in the *Evaluating Scientific Studies* section of this chapter.

Experiment 2A
Balancing Chewing Gum

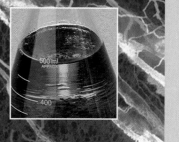

Purpose

You will be using an electronic balance to mass substances in most of the experiments in this class. This lab will help you become familiar with the electronic balance and how it is used. This lab is also designed to help you become familiar with proper procedure for experiments. Scientific procedure requires accuracy and consistency. Scientists usually conduct multiple trials and average their results to increase the validity of the results. You will be accomplishing this goal by averaging your results with the results of other lab groups. As you conduct this experiment, note anything that could cause error in your results.

Equipment

electronic balance
100-gram standard mass

Supplies

1 stick of regular chewing gum
1 stick of sugar-free chewing gum

Procedure

1. Use the 100-gram standard mass to calibrate your electronic balance.

2. Use the gum wrapper as weighing paper. Tare the gum wrapper.

3. Mass the regular gum. Record the mass in a data table.

4. Chew the gum for five minutes.

5. Place the chewed gum on the weighing paper and mass it. Record the mass in your data table.

6. Subtract the mass of the chewed gum from the original mass of the gum and record the difference.

7. Repeat the above procedure with the sugar-free gum.

Data

Record your data on a class data chart on an overhead projector.

Calculations

Calculate the class average for each type of gum. Do this by adding all the entries then dividing by the number of entries.

Questions

1. Which type of gum had a greater loss of mass after chewing? Why?

2. What substance caused the loss of mass during chewing?

3. Was there a difference in texture between the two types of gum? If so, why?

4. Given that sugar has 4 calories per gram, how many calories would you estimate are in a stick of gum? How does your estimate compare with the nutrition label on the gum package?

5. How would you determine the mass of 10 mL of milk?

Experiment 2B
Measuring Accurately

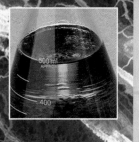

Purpose

For results of experiments to be consistent and valid, you must take all measurements carefully. In this experiment, you will compare methods and tools used for measuring liquid and dry volumes. You will measure liquid volumes in beakers, liquid measuring cups, and graduated cylinders. You will measure the dry volume of flour by scooping, spooning, fluffing, and massing. Hypothesize which method you believe will be the most accurate for measuring liquid and dry ingredients. See if this experiment proves or disproves your hypothesis.

Equipment

100-, 250-, and 400-mL beakers

2-cup liquid measuring cup with milliliter divisions

100-mL graduated cylinder

50-, 125-, and 250-mL dry measures

straight-edged spatula

electronic balance

Supplies

water

flour in canister

Procedure

Part I

1. Measure 50 mL of water in a 100-mL beaker.

2. Pour the water from the beaker in step 1 into the 2-cup liquid measuring cup. Place the measuring cup on a flat surface. View the amount of liquid in milliliters at eye level. Record the milliliter reading in a data table.

3. Pour the water from the measuring cup into a 100-mL graduated cylinder. Record the data in your data table. Empty the water from the graduated cylinder.

4. Repeat steps 1 through 3 twice. The first time, use a 250-mL beaker in place of the 100-mL beaker in step 1. The second time, use a 400-mL beaker in place of the 100-mL beaker in step 1.

Part II

1. Mass a 50-mL dry measuring cup. Tare the electronic balance.

2. Scoop flour from the canister with the 50-mL dry measuring cup. Level with a straight-edged spatula.

3. Mass the flour with an electronic balance. Record mass in the data table. Empty the dry measure.

4. Spoon flour into the 50-mL dry measuring cup until it is overfilled. Level with a straight-edged spatula.

5. Mass the flour with an electronic balance. Record mass in the data table. Empty the dry measure.

6. Stir the flour lightly with a fork to fluff it. Then spoon the flour into the 50-mL dry measuring cup until it is overfilled. Level with a straight-edged spatula.

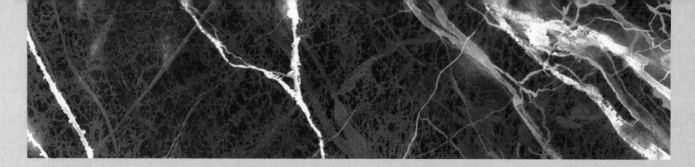

7. Mass the flour with an electronic balance. Record mass in the data table. Empty the dry measure.

8. Repeat steps 1 through 6 twice. The first time, use a 125-mL dry measuring cup in place of the 50-mL measuring cup in each step. The second time, use a 250-mL dry measuring cup in place of the 50-mL measuring cup in each step.

Data

Record your data on a class data chart on an overhead projector.

Calculations

Calculate the class average for each measuring method and each amount of flour in Part II. Look at the highest and lowest readings of the class data for each variation. Subtract the lowest reading from the highest to get the range. Calculate the percentage difference for each trial by dividing the range by the average and multiplying by 100.

range = highest reading – lowest reading

percentage = (range ÷ average) × 100

Questions

1. Which type of tool seems to be the most accurate for measuring liquids? Which size tool seems to be the most accurate? Explain your answers.

2. Predict how accurately a buret will measure liquids and explain why.

3. Which method of measuring the volume of dry ingredients produced the smallest spread in class data? Which size dry measuring cup produced the smallest spread in class data?

4. Would it be more accurate to measure 250 mL of flour in a 250-mL dry measure once or to measure 50 mL of flour in a 50-mL measure five times? Explain your answer.

5. How would changing the granule size of the dry ingredient affect the consistency of volume measurements?

6. What accounts for the differences in mass among the three methods used to measure flour?

Experiment 2C
Measuring Volumes of Irregularly Shaped Objects

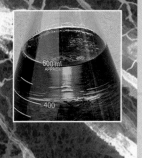

Purpose

In this lab, you will measure three types of substances commonly measured in the food industry. These are dry powders, liquids, and irregularly shaped objects. You will work with these three types of substances by making a small batch of self-rising biscuits. You will also practice working in a team, reading and following directions, and recording and manipulating data.

Equipment

electronic balance

small mixing bowl

fork

liquid measuring cup with milliliter markings

rubber scraper

2 1/2-inch thick cutting boards

rolling pin

2-inch biscuit cutter

pizza pan or cookie sheet

2 1000-mL graduated cylinders

wax pencil

Supplies

2 coffee filters

217 g self-rising flour

40 g shortening

175 mL milk

1000 mL rice

Procedure

Part I

1. Calibrate the electronic balance.

2. Tare a coffee filter to use as a weighing paper.

3. Mass 217 g of self-rising flour onto the coffee filter.

4. Tare a second coffee filter and mass 40 g of solid shortening.

5. Place the flour in a small mixing bowl. Cut the shortening into the flour with a fork until the mixture resembles coarse crumbs.

6. Measure 175 mL of milk. Add all at once to the flour mixture and stir with the fork until all flour is moistened.

7. Scrape the dough onto a floured surface. (The dough will be very sticky.) Flour the top of the dough and your hands. Fold, press, and turn the dough ball a quarter turn 10 times. Add flour as needed.

8. Shape the dough into a smooth ball. Place the dough between two cutting boards. Using a floured rolling pin, roll the dough out to a thickness of 1/2 inch.

9. Cut the biscuit dough with a 2-inch (5.2 mm) biscuit cutter.

10. Place biscuits so they are touching each other on an ungreased pizza pan or cookie sheet. Bake at 450°F for 12 minutes.

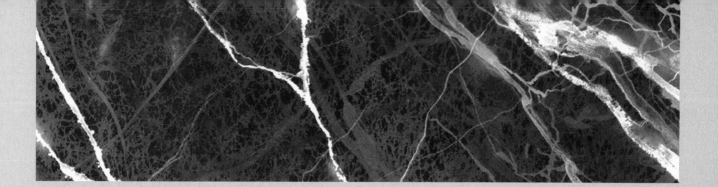

Part II

1. Use a wax pencil to label two 1000-mL graduated cylinders *A* and *B*.

2. After the biscuits have been baked, select three biscuits and mass them. Record this number in the data table.

3. Drop the same three biscuits, one at a time, into graduated cylinder A.

4. Pour 1000 mL of rice into graduated cylinder B. Record this volume in a data table.

5. Pour rice from graduated cylinder B on top of the biscuits in graduated cylinder A. Shake gently to ensure the rice completely surrounds the biscuits. Continue adding rice until the biscuits are completely covered.

6. In the data table, record the volume of rice remaining in graduated cylinder B.

7. In the data table, record the total volume of the rice and biscuits in graduated cylinder A.

8. Subtract the volume of rice in step 6 from the volume of rice in step 4. This is the volume of rice used.

9. Subtract the volume of rice calculated in step 8 from the volume reading in step 7. This is the volume of biscuits.

10. Discard all used rice and biscuits. If you wish to sample biscuits, taste only those that you did not use in the experiment.

Calculations

Calculate the density of the biscuits. (Density = mass ÷ volume.)

Data

Record the mass, volume, and density of your three biscuits in a class data table on an overhead projector.

Questions

1. What is the average density of your biscuits? The classes' biscuits?

2. Which is a more accurate measurement: mass or volume? Explain your answer.

3. How would you measure the volume of an irregularly shaped object in water?

4. What relationship is there between density and texture of the biscuits?

5. Which ingredient in the biscuits is related to density?

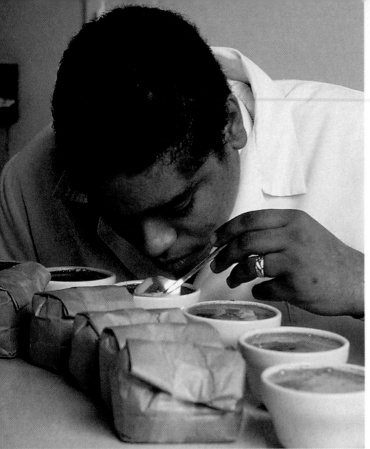

USDA

Checking the aroma is part of the inspection process for many foods. This researcher is smelling coffee as part of the inspection process.

Chapter 3

Sensory Evaluation: The Human Factor

Objectives

After studying this chapter,
you will be able to

compare reasons for evaluating food products subjectively and objectively.

list physical, psychological, cultural, and environmental influences on food likes and dislikes.

explain how taste and aroma combine to give foods their flavors.

conduct a taste test panel.

Key Terms

sensory evaluation	texture
taste bias	chewiness
appearance	graininess
colorimeter	brittleness
flavor	firmness
astringency	consistency
aroma	taste test panel
volatile	consumer taste panel
olfactory bulb	

You turn when you hear a thick steak sizzle as it hits a hot grill. Your mouth waters as you walk into Grandma's home and the smell of roast turkey surrounds you. You feel warmer just seeing the steam rise from a cup of hot cocoa on a cold winter day. You sigh as you bite into a just-baked chocolate chip cookie that seems to melt in your mouth. Your senses are all reacting to foods in your surroundings. See 3-1.

How would you feel about eating grubs, drinking rattlesnake's blood, or chewing raw

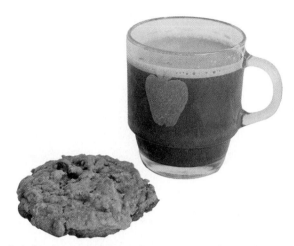

3-1 Seeing steam over hot cocoa and smelling a chocolate chip cookie are part of the sensory experience of sampling these foods.

fish eyes? People in some areas of the world consider these items to be delicacies. What makes you call one texture pleasant and another texture unappealing? Why does one person like chocolate and another person prefer vanilla?

Like all opinions, opinions about food are *subjective*. That is, they are affected by personal views and backgrounds. Your environment influences your food likes and dislikes. Personal experiences affect whether you like spaghetti sauce chunky or smooth, with mushrooms or meat, and spicy or mild.

A wide variety of foods is available, and people have differing opinions about what is good. Food scientists can use computerized equipment to measure such characteristics as volume and mass of food. However, evaluating taste, aroma, and texture is more difficult. There is no tool to accurately measure whether people will like or dislike a food. How then can food scientists forecast the success of new food products? As researchers develop food products, they try to look at the human factors that affect food choices. Then they make predictions about a product's potential for success or failure.

Food scientists have developed methods of evaluating the many factors affecting food choices. The subjective part of their evaluation is called sensory evaluation. *Sensory evaluation* is the human analysis of the taste, smell, sound, feel, and appearance of food. This chapter examines influences on a person's food likes and dislikes. It also discusses the way the human senses work and how researchers conduct sensory evaluations.

Influences on Food Likes and Dislikes

Bruce wants his apple soft and sweet. Jonathan wants one that is crisp and tart, and Larry wants his in a spicy apple pie. Larry finds blackberries enjoyable and Jonathan says they are bitter. Although these men are all related and have lived in the same home for years, they like different foods. See 3-2.

Physical Influences

Physiologists, who study the human body, have discovered that people inherit slightly different body chemistries. These differences in body chemistry affect people's perceptions of taste. You can demonstrate this by using taste test strips. One kind of taste test strip used in biology classes contains the chemical thiourea. Some people will say the strips have a distinctively unpleasant taste. Others will not taste anything.

Some people can see all the tints and shades of every color in the rainbow. Other people are born color-blind and are unable to tell whether an object is red or green. In the same way, a few people can identify every flavoring used in spicy fried chicken. However, some people are born "taste blind." They are unable to distinguish between tastes. Your body's genetic makeup will affect what you taste and how well you can identify flavors.

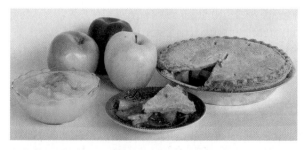

3-2 People have different food preferences. Which of these apple-based foods comes to your mind first when you are hungry for apples?

Number of taste buds, gender, health, and age play roles in your ability to detect flavors. Work at Yale University has demonstrated that people can be classified as "supertasters," "medium tasters," and "nontasters." A compound would be perceived as very bitter by the supertasters and nearly tasteless by the nontasters.

People's ability to taste is partially related to the number of taste buds inherited. A microscope reveals that supertasters can have as many as 1,100 taste buds per square centimeter on their tongues. The nontasters have been found to have as few as 40 taste buds per square centimeter.

Studies at Yale University show that women's ability to perceive bitter tastes varies with their hormone cycles. High levels of certain hormones cause bitter tastes to seem more intense. This may partially account for the change in food cravings and preferences for many women during pregnancy.

Psychological Influences

There is also a psychological aspect to food likes and dislikes. Research shows that many adults who detest a particular food became ill after eating that food as a young child. Although the food may not have caused the illness, the person will subconsciously link the two events. When food becomes linked with unpleasant memories, the food will become distasteful to one degree or another. This psychological factor is believed to be a protective mechanism of the brain. It keeps you from eating harmful substances again.

When negative experiences cause a person to dislike a food, the person has developed a *taste bias.* Taste bias can also be caused by positive experiences or taste preferences, 3-3. Imagine entering a lemon cake in a baking contest where your competition is all types of chocolate cakes. Suppose all the judges prefer chocolate to lemon. The judges would have trouble judging your cake fairly if they were not aware of their taste bias. Trained taste testers have to learn to put such food biases aside when evaluating food products.

Other factors that can cause bias in food products are label terms and brand names. Many students will state a brand preference

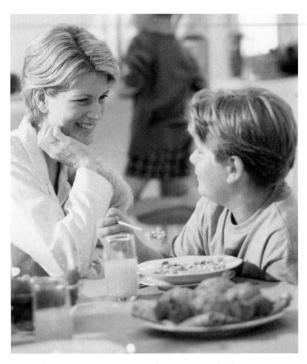

3-3 Many positive taste biases people have as adults are associated with happy memories of their childhood.

and then select a competitor's brand in a blind taste test. Advertising, peers, and setting influence this type of bias. Food manufacturers have found such biases very difficult to overcome in the marketplace.

Cultural Influences

The cultural patterns of people's lives strongly influence what and how people eat. *Culture* is the beliefs and behaviors followed by a group of people. These beliefs and behaviors are passed on from one generation to another. Region, lifestyle, religion, and holidays are all part of culture. For example, grits is a regional food that is more likely to be served in the South than the Midwest. The French lifestyle often includes daily shopping for fresh ingredients. In French culture, few people rely on convenience foods like frozen entrees for many meals. Traditionally, people of the Jewish religion do not eat pork, and Hindu followers do not eat beef. In the United States, the food most often eaten on Halloween is candy. In Mexico, a similar holiday is celebrated with the serving of pan de muerto, or bread of the dead.

Environmental Influences

People are more likely to eat what is available and economical. Environmental factors such as climate, geography, and fuel availability have much to do with food costs and obtainability. For instance, Jamaicans eat much fresh fruit, which grows abundantly in the warm local climate. Alaskans eat less fruit because it is not as readily available in their colder climate. People who live near rangelands are inclined to include a fair amount of meat in their diets. People who live in coastal regions tend to eat more seafood. In Asia, where fuel was scarce for centuries, raw fish and stir-fried dishes became common. In the United States, where fuel was plentiful, slowly cooked stews and roasted meats grew popular.

Food preferences are affected by your immediate surroundings as well as by the larger environment. This has been revealed in studies with young children. Most children learn to like the foods to which they are exposed. Adults who enjoy oysters are more likely to have eaten oysters as children than adults who do not enjoy oysters.

Sensory Characteristics of Food Products

To evaluate a food product, you first need to identify the desirable characteristics of that product. What is desirable will change from one product to the next. You want crackers to be crunchy, but cake should be moist, and gummy bears should be chewy. See 3-4.

There are three main sensory characteristics of food products: appearance, flavor, and texture. Understanding these characteristics will help you be more accurate in describing food products.

Appearance

Appearance refers to the shape, size, condition, and color of a product. In other words, it is what you see. Appearance is usually evaluated on both the exterior and interior of a product. For instance, you may cut a muffin in half and draw around it to show the outer shape. Note whether the shape is peaked or rounded. Then you may check to see if the

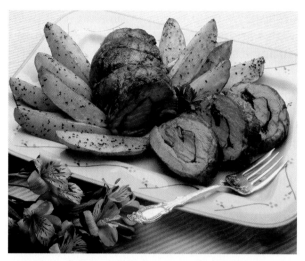

3-4 Desirable characteristics for roast potatoes are tender texture and golden brown color. However, roast beef should be slightly chewy and have pink coloring.

inside of the muffin is full of large tunnels or small, even holes. Both the shape of muffins and the size of air cells can indicate the quality of the product.

Color is one aspect of appearance that can be measured exactly. A *colorimeter* is a device that measures the color of foods in terms of hue, value, and chroma. *Hue* refers to whether the basic color is red, blue, or green. *Value* is the lightness or darkness of the color. Pink is a light value of red and burgundy is a dark value. *Chroma* is how intense the color is. Overcooked green beans become olive colored, which is a dull or low intensity of green. A lime has a bright or high intensity of green. With a colorimeter, the color of a product can be defined in numerical values. A new food product's color can then be described to distant manufacturing plants without sending samples. A year later, the color can also be compared with the next production run.

Color can influence a person's perception of other sensory characteristics. For instance, you might think a dark brown chocolate bar has a richer flavor than a light brown bar. When researchers do not want color to influence a taste panel, they use colored lights. Researchers may test chocolate bars first under red lights and then under green lights. This will help the researchers study the impact of flavor and texture differences more accurately. Taste testing rooms are equipped with various colored lights that can be used during a sensory evaluation. See 3-5.

Flavor

Flavor is the combined effect of taste and aroma. Taste starts in the mouth with the taste buds on the tongue. Each region of the tongue is designed to respond to one type of taste. The four basic tastes are salty, bitter, sour, and sweet. Each food will stimulate a combination of taste regions on the tongue. Sweet and sour sauce is a good example of how a food can be a combination of tastes.

Research indicates a food's taste is related to the shape of molecules in the food. These molecules bind to the taste bud. For example, a molecular shape that triggers sweetness has been identified. Suppose a molecule of a food matches up to a "sweetness" taste bud. This will cause nerve endings to begin sending messages to the brain. The brain knows that when nerve impulses come from that part of the tongue, the food is sweet. The more taste buds a food stimulates, the sweeter the food is perceived to be.

Sour foods are evaluated in terms of their astringency. *Astringency* is the ability of a substance to draw up the muscles in the mouth. You could look at astringency as the mouth-puckering power of a food. Tea, lemons, and sour balls are very astringent.

Your ability to taste foods is related to the temperatures of the foods. Flavors of some foods become more intense as the foods become warmer. However, some foods that are heated to high temperatures may lose some of their flavors.

Europeans serve cheese at room temperature rather than chilled to bring out the flavor of the cheese. Try this yourself. Taste fruit and cheese that are chilled. Then try a bite of each that has been allowed to stand at room temperature for 20 to 30 minutes. Which has the stronger flavor?

Cooking Tip
Mushrooms are a natural flavor enhancer. Add small amounts of finely minced mushrooms to soups, casseroles, sauces, and gravies for richer flavor.

Smell Impacts Flavor

The second component of flavor is aroma. The *aroma* is the odor of a food. The senses of taste and smell work together to give foods their characteristic flavors. Without seeing or tasting a cake, you can identify it as chocolate because of its aroma.

The nose is capable of identifying thousands of odors. Some people can identify odors better than others. Through training, however, most people can improve their ability to recognize odors. As your ability to identify odors improves, so will your ability to distinguish flavors.

Babies are born preferring sweet tastes. However, they do not seem to prefer one scent to another. Liking or disliking odors is related to experiences. Odors people like are often connected to home, holidays, and situations that make them feel secure. Odors people dislike may remind them of unpleasant events.

A substance's odor results from volatile particles coming in contact with the olfactory

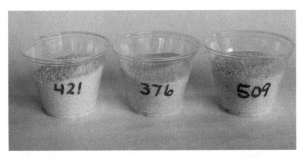
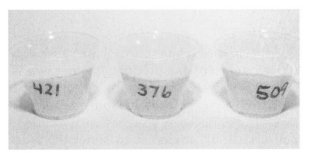

3-5 Numbering samples and using colored lights help eliminate taste tester bias based on the identity and appearance of food samples.

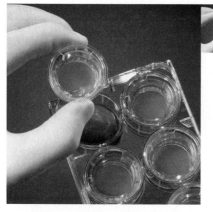

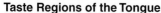

Recent Research
The Fifth Taste

Taste Regions of the Tongue

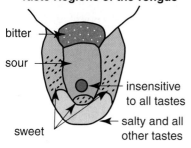

bitter

sour

insensitive
to all tastes

salty and all
other tastes

sweet

Maps like this have been used for
years to show regions of the tongue
that taste salty, sweet,
bitter, and sour. Researchers now
agree that the tongue responds to a
fifth taste—umami.

Experts working in taste
research have identified the fifth
taste quality called *umami*. It was
first identified in soy-based products. The term is Japanese
meaning delicious or savory.
Some people have described this
taste as brothy or meaty. Flavor
enhancers such as monosodium
glutamate (MSG) appear to
increase this savory flavor in
foods.

Researchers have found that
umami works with other flavors to
amplify taste sensations. One
researcher describes this quality
as 1 + 1 = 3. One theory is that
flavor enhancers help open
receptor sites on the tongue,
increasing stimulation. This not
only increases flavor sensations
but also seems to smooth out flavors. Another effect of MSG
seems to be a reduction in bitter
and sour qualities of foods like
citrus fruits.

Researchers have now identified the mechanism by which
taste occurs. Now that the compounds that cause taste messages to be sent to the brain
have been isolated, researchers
are working on ways to enhance
or block taste. It is projected that
within a few years researchers
will have found a way to increase
the sweet taste response so that
soft drinks, for example, will only
need 1/5 the sugar to taste as
sweet as they do today.

nerves deep in the nose. *Volatile* substances
contain particles that evaporate or become
gaseous quickly. These gaslike particles stimulate the olfactory bulb. The *olfactory bulb* is a
bundle of nerve fibers. It is located at the base
of the brain behind the bridge of the nose.
The brain learns to associate thousands of
types of nerve stimulation with specific foods
or experiences.

Odors can use two pathways to reach the
olfactory bulb. The first is through the nostrils.
This is why you can almost taste an apple pie
baking in the oven. Small gaseous particles of
the pie are released into the air during baking.
These gaseous particles trigger the sense of
smell, which contributes to your perception
of flavor.

The second pathway to the olfactory bulb
is through the back of the mouth. The nasal
and oral passages are connected at the top of
the throat. Volatile, gaslike substances are
pumped up into the nasal cavity during the
chewing process. When eating, take your time
to savor food by smelling it and chewing it
thoroughly. This allows more odors to reach
the olfactory bulb. Like the tongue, the more
the olfactory bulb is stimulated, the more
intense the flavor experience will be. See 3-6.

The brain registers the flavor of a food as a
combination of aromas and sour, sweet, bitter,
and salty tastes. The mind remembers the
combination of aromas and tastes and then
identifies the food based on experiences.

Texture

Texture is how a food product feels to the
fingers, tongue, teeth, and palate (roof of the
mouth). Texture of foods is evaluated in terms

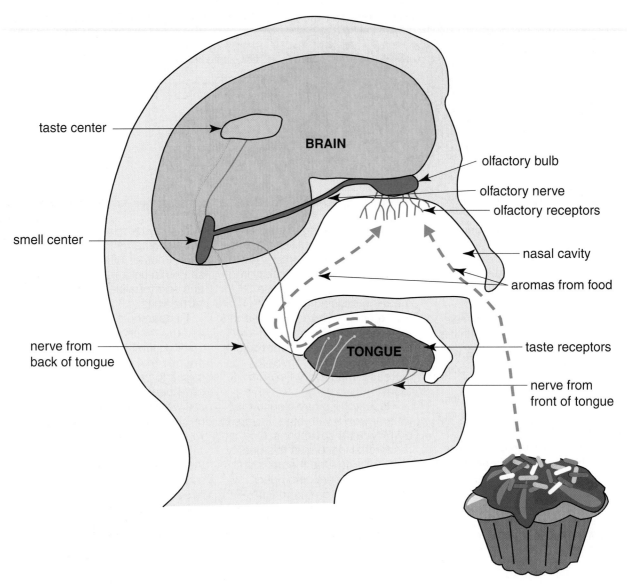

taste center

smell center

nerve from
back of tongue

BRAIN

TONGUE

olfactory bulb

olfactory nerve

olfactory receptors

nasal cavity

aromas from food

taste receptors

nerve from
front of tongue

3-6 The sense of smell has a great impact on the sense of taste.

of chewiness, graininess, brittleness, firmness, and consistency.

Chewiness refers to how well one part of a food slides past another without breaking. Taffy would rank high in chewiness and pudding would rank very low.

Graininess refers to the size of the particles in a food product. Cream is very smooth with microscopic particles. Grits, which are commonly served in the South, have a grainy or gritty feel, as their name implies.

Brittleness refers to how easily a food shatters or breaks apart. Pie crust and crackers are very brittle. Strawberries, cake, and caramels would not be considered brittle.

Firmness describes a food's resistance to pressure. Tough foods require considerable biting force to chew them. Beef jerky is a good example. Tender foods require so little force to chew, they almost seem to melt in your mouth. Tenderness is desired in most cakes and high-quality steaks. See 3-7.

Consistency describes the thinness or thickness of a product. It can be measured in terms of pourability. "Au jus," the flavored drippings from meat, is very thin. Milk gravy is usually thick enough to not soak into biscuits or toast.

As you evaluate foods in the lab, think about these characteristics that define texture.

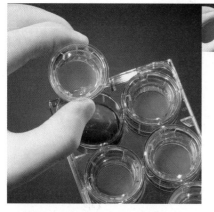

Recent Research
Senses and Aging

When you touch something, you sense texture. When you taste there is flavor. When you smell there is odor. All these senses have different names. However, the brain perceives them in the same way. Whether you touch, taste, or smell, you are stimulating nerve endings to send a message to the brain. When the right particle touches a nerve fiber, an electric impulse is sent to the brain. The location in the brain that receives the impulse and memories of similar experiences determines the sensation. These factors control whether you smell hot cocoa, feel its heat, or taste the bittersweet chocolate flavor.

Olfactory nerve cells at the ends of the neurons die and are replaced every 60 days. They are the only nerve cells the body remakes. However, there is a point at which smell nerve fibers become damaged and the body cannot repair them. The ability to taste salty, bitter, sour, and sweet remains. What people lose is the ability to identify the difference between the sour of vinegar and the sour of lemon.

The nerve endings in the nose are very sensitive and easily damaged. There appears to be a loss of olfactory function as a result of aging. Anyone who has worked with older adults knows that many have lost some to all of their ability to smell. Studies indicate that as many as 50% of people over age 65 are experiencing olfactory loss.

Experiencing food is a complex interaction of taste, sight, smell, and texture. People experiencing olfactory loss taste the sweet and sour of fruits without perceiving the orange, lemon, or strawberry flavor. This causes people with olfactory loss to consume fewer fruits and vegetables. In fact, older people may consume smaller amounts of many foods because their ability to enjoy food is reduced. When people start to lose their sense of smell, they are less likely to want to cook or eat. This may result in malnutrition if not corrected. This problem concerns family members and nursing home staffs as well as older adults.

Studies done at the University of Connecticut found another problem with olfactory loss. Older women with a reduced sense of taste and smell were more likely to be obese. They tended to eat more to get enough satisfying flavor. They also tended to choose more foods that had a creamy mouth-feel. These foods were often high in fat and sugar. Researchers believe such foods help people compensate for loss of flavor.

To help someone with olfactory loss increase his or her interest in a balanced diet, use the following tips:

❖ Serve fruits in sweet syrups. Most people prefer sweet tastes.

❖ Vary texture and color. Concentrate on the visual display.

❖ Increase the flavor of bland vegetables by adding olive oil, herbs, and/or spices.

❖ Increase cooking smells in the home by simmering foods the person can still smell.

❖ Make meals a social event. People eat poorer diets when they are alone.

❖ Make sure the person gets regular flu shots. Viral infections appear to damage the olfactory bulb.

"Making Sense of Taste and Smell," *Tufts University Diet & Nutrition Letter*, Vol.13:9, Nov. 1995, pp 3-6.

Remember that texture preferences are also subjective. Most French people, for instance, like their bread chewy. They want their bread to have a brittle, crunchy crust with a slightly chewy, moist center. Many people in the United States want a very tender bread with a soft crust.

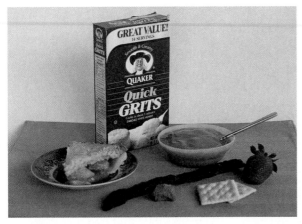

3-7 Each of these foods has a characteristic texture.

Measuring Texture Objectively

Food texture can be evaluated objectively by measuring its resistance to force. Physicists and engineers have developed an assortment of instruments that can measure how much force is needed to compress, tear, or juice a food. These types of measurements are used to evaluate uniformity, keeping quality, and packaging needs. However, they will not determine whether a consumer will like one variation of a food over another.

One example of an instrument that measures food texture is a compression machine. Compression machines show how much pressure it takes to compress one food compared to another. These machines may be used to determine how to modify ingredients or processing procedures to provide a standard texture for a food product. They can also tell a manufacturer how much packing is needed to allow a product to be shipped without being crushed.

A penetrating probe is another instrument that measures food texture. It is used to determine the quality of beef. Inspectors insert the probe into the meat carcass. The pressure needed to penetrate a given distance has been compared to how tender the meat will be after cooking. In this way, beef can be labeled as prime or choice before it is cut apart.

Like texture, other sensory characteristics of foods can be measured objectively. For instance, scientists can test flavor components by measuring a food's sugar, salt, and acid content. Appearance factors such as color, size, and shape can be measured, too. In the final analysis, however, what will matter is what the consumer wants. Manufacturers determine this by using taste test panels.

Taste Test Panels

Sensory evaluations involve more than stating whether you like a food. Your sense of smell, genetic makeup, and unique experiences create opinions about food that can interfere with controlled sensory evaluation. Once you recognize these factors, you are more likely to base an evaluation on measurable characteristics. For instance, you may or may not like chocolate. However, you can feel if the texture of chocolate is smooth, creamy, or gritty. Professional sensory evaluators have to be able to put aside personal taste biases to evaluate product quality.

Different types of sensory evaluation can be conducted depending on the information needed. A *taste test panel* is a group of people who evaluate the flavor, texture, appearance, and aroma of food products. Taste test panels can be composed of either trained professionals or untrained consumers. The type of panelists used depends on the purpose of the evaluation.

Trained sensory panelists are more likely to be used during a product's development, 3-8. This is the stage at which subtle differences must be identified if the product is to be successful. Trained individuals are also used for federal and state grading of such products as butter and cheese. The coffee and wine industries need tasters who are not only highly trained but also very sensitive to flavor differences. This requires "supertasters." Supertasters are people whose genetic makeup, health conditions, and experiences allow them to identify subtle differences in flavor and aroma.

Untrained consumers are used to evaluate products after the products have been developed. These consumers represent the buying public as members of consumer taste panels. *Consumer taste panels* are used to determine what the average consumer will prefer. These panels may test a new product and compare it to similar products on the market. Sometimes

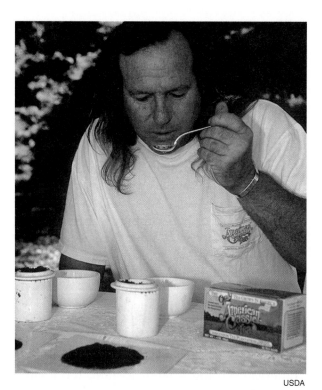

USDA

3-8 This trained taste tester is sampling tea at the South Carolina estate where it is grown.

consumer panelists evaluate whether they would buy a totally new type of product. They help manufacturers determine whether a food product will sell.

In this class, you will be using sensory evaluation to evaluate products in many laboratory experiments. You will base your evaluations on such factors as aroma, taste, feel, and appearance. Like any other skill, sensory evaluation improves with practice. Sensory evaluators have to learn to distinguish why they like or dislike specific food products. A food may have a pleasant taste but a disagreeable texture. A biscuit may look light and flaky but taste bitter. All these factors will need to be evaluated.

Setting up Taste Test Panels

Setting up a taste test panel requires thought and preparation. Researchers must try to remove any factors that could sway testers. Such factors include influences from other testers, the environment of the testing room, and psychological biases. Researchers must also create forms for testers to use in rating samples and recording responses.

Controlling Influences from Other Testers

The comments and body language of other panelists can easily affect the views of taste test panel members. Researchers can use a number of techniques to control such influences. Each tester may be isolated in a booth so he or she cannot see facial expressions of others. Products may be tested by one person at a time. Panelists may also receive strict instructions to make no comments or sounds that could sway other tasters.

Isolated taste testing can be hard to arrange in most classroom settings. For class experiments to be valid, students must do their evaluations alone. There should not be any talking or nonverbal signals until everyone has tasted and recorded his or her opinion. In most cases, controlling these variables will be based on an honor system. Whenever possible, arrange tasting stations in a circle with class members facing outward. This will reduce the accidental influences of others' facial expressions.

Controlling Environmental Factors

Environmental factors that should be controlled during taste tests include lighting and aromas in the testing room. Using colored lights during taste testing will not be possible in most classrooms. However, you can make sure light levels are similar in all testing areas. If masking color is important in a test, you can use blindfolds, 3-9.

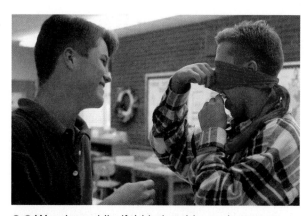

3-9 Wearing a blindfold helps this student more accurately measure his tasting ability. A partner hands him each sample and records the responses.

Aromas present in the classroom can strengthen or weaken your response to any given food. Suppose you eat a cooled chocolate chip cookie in a kitchen where more cookies are baking in the oven. You will be exposed to more volatiles in this setting than if you eat the same cookie in another place. You can control this variable to some extent by tasting samples the day after they are prepared.

Because tastes and aromas can linger, you should take a sip of warm water between each sample you taste. Professional taste testers do this to help rinse any food residue out of the mouth. The water needs to be warm to help remove any fats that may be present. Cold water can cause fats to cling to the tongue rather than wash away. Because fat is very flavorful, this step is critical in any food taste test. You might also eat plain soda crackers to help clear flavors from the mouth between food samples.

Another factor that should be controlled is the temperature of the food samples. Tests on perceiving sweetness show that maximum sweetness is perceived at different temperatures for different sweeteners. Maximum sweetness scores for table sugar are recorded at a temperature of 25°C (77°F). This is within normal room temperature ranges.

To help control this variable, have all samples at the same temperature. Take all chilled samples from the refrigerator at the same time. Also, allow baked goods time to reach room temperature before sampling.

Controlling Psychological Biases

Psychological biases can affect the way test panelists respond to various food samples. For instance, test samples are usually identified by codes. However, human response studies have shown that most people prefer samples with low numbers to samples with higher numbers. Likewise, people tend to prefer samples labeled with letters near the beginning of the alphabet. In other words, test panel members are likely to select sample 1 over sample 3. They are also likely to select sample A over sample B or C. When the order of samples is changed, panel members still prefer samples labeled *1* or *A*.

Researchers in taste testing have found this bias goes away when they use three-digit code numbers. For instance, people show no preference for sample 527 over sample 619. When you test samples in class, your teacher will randomly choose three-digit numbers to identify each product. He or she will keep a key to correctly identify each sample.

Another factor that can influence taste test panels is the number of samples provided. The number of samples a taster can reliably judge is limited. Four or five samples seems to be the most that tasters can evaluate at one time.

Tasters will tend to prefer the first samples presented to later ones. To help account for this factor, panelists will often taste the same samples in different orders.

Creating an Evaluation Form

Test panel members need some kind of numerical scoring system to rank food samples. Taste test panelists are often asked to rank products on a scale of 1 to 5, 1 to 7, or 1 to 9. A smaller scale does not allow enough choices to rank products. A numerical scale that goes above 9 gives too many choices. An odd number of choices provides a neutral point. This is the ranking respondents can use to indicate they neither like nor dislike a product.

Sometimes researchers will ask testers to use verbal labels to rank food samples. For instance, testers might rank samples using the labels *definitely like, mildly like, neither like nor dislike, mildly dislike,* and *definitely dislike.* Researchers can then assign the numbers 1 to 5 to these choices when assessing testers responses. See 3-10.

When a taste tester gives a food a high rating, he or she may not need to make any other comments. However, food manufacturers may want to know why panel members give a product a low rating. For this reason, numerical scores are often combined with descriptive observations. Panelists can use adjectives and descriptive phrases to indicate that a product was too brittle, creamy, or chewy. Panelists can describe the taste as too salty, sour, strong, or weak. These factors are critical in the early stages of a product's development. If researchers do not know what is wrong with a sample, they will have a hard time improving the product. See 3-11.

Universal Evaluation Form

When developing food products for children, manufacturers are likely to want some taste test panel members to be children. Similarly, when developing products for an ethnic market, manufacturers will want members of that market to be part of the test panel. However, problems can arise if panel members cannot read and write in the language used on an evaluation form. Below is an example of a testing form that could be used by any taste test panel member. Tasters simply mark the box below the face that is closest to the way they feel about the food.

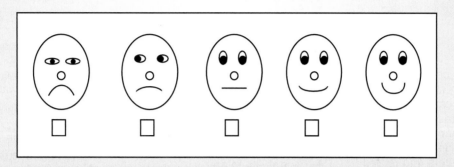

3-10 A universal evaluation form eliminates barriers that can be created by language on written forms.

Sample Evaluation Form

Characteristics	Sample # 382	Sample # 714	Sample # 569	Sample # 495
Appearance	4 Smooth and pale	4 Dark brown flecks	6 Flat top, golden top & bottom	5 Sloped top Yellowish
Texture	4 Tough	5 Greasy spots	7 Moist & flaky	6
Aroma	5 Faint	3 Almost burnt	6	5 Strong chemical smell
Flavor	4 Bland	4 Spotty, doughy	7	1 Bitter aftertaste
Overall eating quality	4	4	7	2
Comments	Overkneaded	Undermixed when shortening is added	Good quality	Cut out incorrectly and too much baking soda

3-11 These scores and comments might be typical of a taste tester who is sampling biscuits.

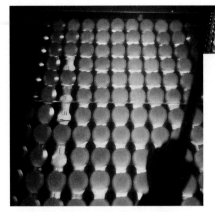

Technology Tidbit
Computers and Sensory Evaluation

Computers cannot replace human taste testers. However, new software can speed the evaluation of taste test results. Lightweight "pads" enable computers to recognize handwritten data. Taste testers can record their opinions directly into computers using screens that look like paper ballots.

Results that once took days and hours to tabulate can be computer generated in minutes. Other advantages food scientists find in using computers in sensory evaluation include

❖ portability to any environment

❖ ease of use and training

❖ flexibility for evaluating various food products

❖ reduction of incomplete ballots

❖ savings of time and money

❖ increased accuracy in tabulating results

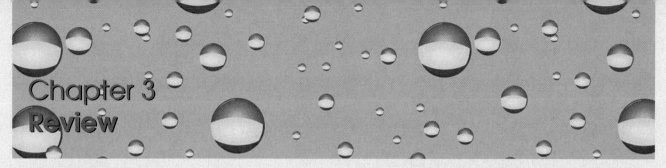

Chapter 3
Review

Summary

A number of factors influence your personal food likes and dislikes. These include your sense of taste and positive and negative experiences you have had with certain foods. Where and how you live, religion, and holidays are cultural factors that can affect how you feel about some foods. The impact of climate and geography on the availability and cost of products also shape your food preferences.

Understanding factors that affect your likes and dislikes will help you fairly evaluate samples in the food science lab. In the lab, you will be practicing sensory evaluation. This means you will be using your senses to judge the appearance, flavor, and texture of food products. You will develop sensory skills and learn to use descriptive words to make scientific observations. In time, you will find it easier to identify small differences among food samples.

Sensory evaluation is used by food scientists to assess how consumers will respond to new products. This type of evaluation is provided by taste test panels. Panels may be made up of trained testers or untrained consumers. In either case, food scientists need to carefully control factors that can trigger bias in panel members.

Check Your Understanding

1. List four main factors that influence taste preferences and give an example of each.
2. What factors affect a person's ability to detect flavors?
3. What is taste bias?
4. List the three main categories of sensory characteristics.
5. What three aspects of color are measured by a colorimeter?
6. What are the two components of flavor?
7. What four basic tastes can the human tongue sense?
8. What five qualities are used to evaluate the texture of a food?
9. When are trained and untrained test panelists most often used to evaluate the sensory characteristics of a food product?
10. List four factors that researchers must control when setting up a taste test panel.

Critical Thinking

1. Select a food that most members of your family like prepared differently. Describe each person's preference.
2. How do burning the tongue, catching a cold, and aging affect a person's ability to taste?
3. Describe the ideal sensory characteristics of a chocolate chip cookie.
4. Why do you think there seems to be a connection between eating rapidly and gaining excess weight?
5. With all the types of scientific testing that can be run on food, why are taste test panels necessary?

Explore Further

1. **Math.** Use three types of taste test strips to determine which class members can taste which chemicals. Tally the results and create a bar graph comparing the results of the three types of taste strips.
2. **Research.** Select several brands of one type of product and set up a taste test environment. Create a data table for evaluators to use for recording their responses. Then select a panel of taste testers and have them evaluate samples of each brand. Analyze the results and report your findings to the class.
3. **Communication.** Write an article for the school newspaper about the results of the taste test described above.

Experiment 3A
Odor Recognition

Safety

❖ **Do not taste samples.**

❖ **Do not smell samples directly when identifying aromas. Some foods are lightweight powders, which could easily be inhaled. Instead, wave your hand over the top of the container to direct the aroma toward your nose.**

❖ **Do not move around when blindfolded.**

Purpose

You usually use a combination of senses to identify foods. In this experiment, you will look at the role your sense of smell plays in evaluating food products. You will examine how accurately you can identify foods by only their aromas.

Equipment

blindfold

Supplies

a shoebox containing coded food samples in portion cups with lids

Procedure

Choose a lab partner or work with the partner your teacher assigns you. Determine which of you will identify aromas first and which will record the data. The partner who is recording the data will follow the steps of the procedure.

1. Blindfold the partner who will be identifying aromas.

2. Open the shoebox and remove one container. Open the lid and hold the container in front of your partner.

3. Have your partner wave his or her hand over the container to direct the aroma toward his or her nose. Ask your partner to identify the aroma he or she is smelling.

4. Record your partner's answer in a data table next to the appropriate code number. Do not name code numbers or give any indication as to whether your partner's answer is correct. Close the container and set it aside.

5. Repeat steps 2 through 4 until all samples have been tested.

6. Return all samples to the shoebox and exchange places with your partner.

7. Repeat steps 1 through 5.

Data

When all students have completed the lab, your teacher will read the key. Check to see how many aromas you correctly identified. Compile your responses with those of your classmates into a class data table. This table should show how many students in each test group correctly identified each sample. Compare your correct answers with those of your classmates.

Calculations

Use the information in the class data table to prepare a bar graph. This graph should compare the correct responses in each test group and the total correct responses for each sample.

Questions

1. Which aromas gave you the most difficulty? Which aromas gave your classmates the most difficulty?

2. Which food was most often identified correctly?

3. Why did some students have more difficulty than other students with this task?

4. Were the responses of the second member of each pair more or less accurate? Why?

5. Is taste or aroma more important in food identification? Explain your answer.

Experiment 3B
Taste Test Panel

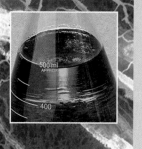

Purpose
Food preferences are based on experience, flavor, advertisements, peer pressure, culture, and habits. One goal of setting up a taste test is to prevent all these factors from affecting food choices of test panel members. After conducting taste tests, food scientists must determine how to overcome factors that may interfere with the sales of new products. In this lab, you will practice evaluating food samples.

Supplies
napkin

paper plate

3 numbered samples of soft drinks

3 numbered samples of crackers

3 numbered samples of chocolate chips

glass of lukewarm water

Procedure
1. Without any discussion with classmates, circulate through the tasting stations set up by your teacher or select one serving of each item as it is brought to you.
2. Take a small bite of a food sample and chew it for at least 20 seconds or take a small swallow of a drink sample and swirl it in your mouth for at least 20 seconds.
3. Evaluate the aroma, color, texture (or carbonation for soft drinks), and flavor of samples. Record your evaluations in a data table, using a ranking of 1 (worst) to 5 (best) for each characteristic. Also note any specific observations for each characteristic.
4. Take a small swallow of warm water to clear flavor compounds from your mouth.
5. Repeat steps 2 through 4 until you have tasted all samples. Make sure you taste all samples in each category before trying samples in another category. In other words, sample all the crackers before tasting any soft drinks.

Calculations
Calculate total evaluation scores for each sample. Then record your totals on a class data table. Use information from the class data table to calculate which soft drink, cracker, or chocolate chip was the class favorite. Your teacher will reveal the identities of the foods after all calculations are complete.

Questions
1. Did you prefer any food or drink brands other than those you usually purchase?
2. Were there clear class favorites in each sample category?
3. Why are there so many brands of the same types of foods available?
4. What variables may have influenced the results? How could you control these variables in future taste testing situations?

Experiment 3C
Imitation Apple Pie

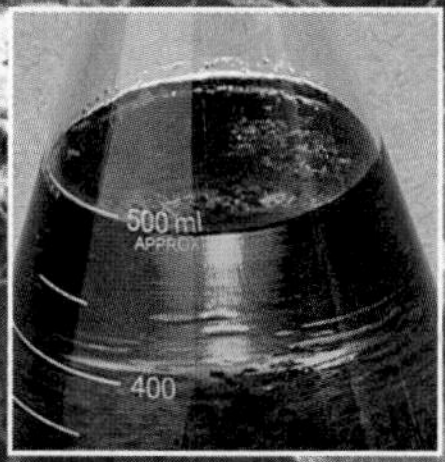

Safety

❖ Wash hands before handling food.

❖ Cut apples on a cutting board.

❖ Use hot pads to remove pies from the oven.

❖ Clean all work surfaces and utensils with hot soapy water.

Purpose

Human senses are limited and easily fooled. Chemists can create an imitation food product that looks and tastes like the real thing. The first frozen lemon pies contained neither lemon nor eggs. In this experiment, you will compare the taste of a real apple pie to the taste of an imitation apple pie.

For this lab, your teacher will divide the class into four groups. Group 1 will make a real apple pie. Group 2 will make an imitation apple pie. Group 3 will make a crumb topping for the real apple pie. Group 4 will make a crumb topping for the imitation apple pie. Choose the equipment and supplies and follow the procedure for the product your group is assigned to make.

Equipment
Real Apple Pie

paring knife

metric dry measuring cups

metric measuring spoons

2-quart saucepan

mixing spoon

pie pan

Imitation Apple Pie

metric liquid measuring cup

2-quart saucepan

metric dry measuring cups

metric measuring spoons

mixing spoon

pie pan

Crumb Topping

metric dry measuring cups

metric measuring spoons

mixing bowl

fork or pastry blender

Supplies
Real Apple Pie

7 to 8 medium golden delicious apples

125 mL (½ cup) flour

250 mL (1 cup) brown sugar

5 mL (1 teaspoon) cinnamon

1 mL (¼ teaspoon) nutmeg

125 mL (½ cup) water

pastry for one-crust pie

30 mL (2 tablespoons) margarine

Imitation Apple Pie

500 mL (2 cups) water

375 mL (1½ cups) sugar

7 mL (1½ teaspoons) cream of tartar

36 round snack crackers

pastry for one-crust pie

5 mL (1 teaspoon) cinnamon

1 mL (¼ teaspoon) nutmeg

30 mL (2 tablespoons) margarine

Crumb Topping

125 mL (½ cup) flour

125 mL (½ cup) brown sugar

2 mL (½ teaspoon) cinnamon

45 mL (3 tablespoons) margarine

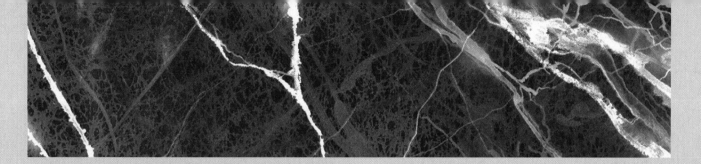

Procedure

Real Apple Pie

1. Peel, core, and slice 7 to 8 medium golden delicious apples.

2. Combine 125 mL flour, 250 mL brown sugar, 5 mL cinnamon, and 1 mL nutmeg in a saucepan.

3. Stir in 125 mL water.

4. Add the apples. Cook, stirring gently until the apple mixture comes to a boil.

5. Pour apple mixture into a pastry-lined pie pan.

6. Dot with slices of the 30 mL of margarine.

7. Cover with the crumb topping.

8. Bake at 400°F for 10 minutes. Then reduce heat to 350°F and bake for an additional 20 minutes or until the filling is bubbly.

Imitation Apple Pie

1. Heat 500 mL of water to the boiling point in a 2-quart saucepan.

2. Mix 375 mL of sugar with 7 mL of cream of tartar.

3. Add this mixture to the boiling water. Turn heat down to low.

4. Add 36 round snack crackers to the mixture, one at a time.

5. Simmer gently for 3 minutes but *do not stir.*

6. Pour this mixture into a pastry-lined pie pan.

7. Sprinkle with 5 mL of cinnamon and 1 mL of nutmeg.

8. Dot lightly with slices of the 30 mL of margarine.

9. Cover with the crumb topping.

10. Bake at 400°F for 30 minutes, or until the filling is bubbly.

Crumb Topping

1. Use a fork or pastry blender to combine 125 mL flour, 125 mL brown sugar, and 2 mL cinnamon in a mixing bowl.

2. Cut in 45 mL of margarine. Mixture should resemble coarse crumbs.

3. Sprinkle evenly over the top of the pie filling.

Data

Carefully examine a sample of each pie. Record your observations of the color, aroma, texture, and flavor in a data table.

Calculations

Convert the metric measurements in this experiment to English using the following equivalents:

$$250 \text{ mL} = 1 \text{ cup};$$

$$5 \text{ mL} = 1 \text{ teaspoon}.$$

Convert the English temperature measurements in this experiment to Celsius degrees using the following equation: $°C = \frac{5}{9}(°F-32)$.

Questions

1. How did the two pies compare in terms of color, aroma, and texture?

2. What flavors did you detect in the imitation apple pie?

3. List some examples of food products that contain artificial flavors and texturizers.

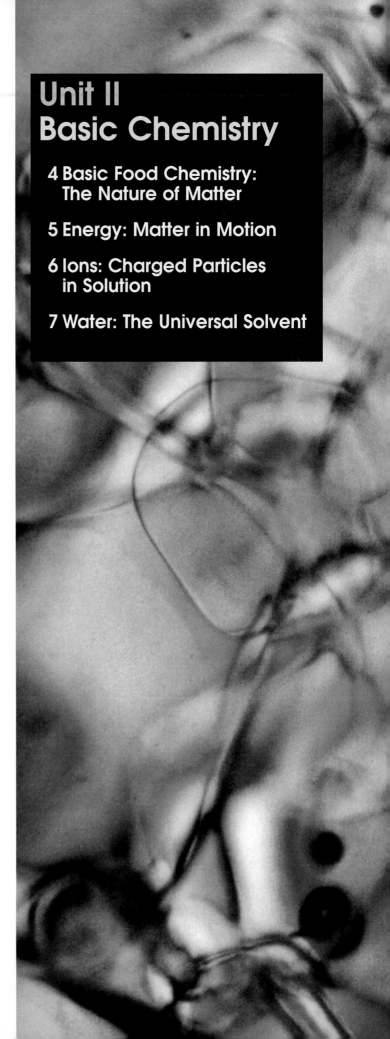

A food scientist must understand and predict how food will react in processing, packaging, and preservation. This requires an understanding of the nature of the particles in food. The branch of science that studies these particles and how they are categorized is chemistry.

Chapter 4 looks at the basics of chemistry needed for the study of food science. Particles are defined and classified according to their physical and chemical characteristics. You will study how these particles combine and break apart. You will also see how scientists describe chemical reactions in writing.

Change in the structure or position of these particles requires energy. Chapter 5 describes the types of energy. It describes how energy is transferred and measured. It also discusses energy's importance in food production.

Chapter 6 explores a category of particles called ions. The electrical nature of ions is basic to many reactions that occur in food mixtures. This chapter defines ions and describes how they are measured. It also examines some of the important applications of ions in the food industry.

Water is key to life and a main component of most foods. Chapter 7 identifies the unique chemical characteristics of the particles that make up water. It discusses water's role in chemical reactions. This chapter also examines how water functions in food preparation and in a nutritious diet.

This photomicrograph shows a substance that is essential in many chemical reactions in food products and in the human body—water.

Unit II
Basic Chemistry

4 Basic Food Chemistry: The Nature of Matter

5 Energy: Matter in Motion

6 Ions: Charged Particles in Solution

7 Water: The Universal Solvent

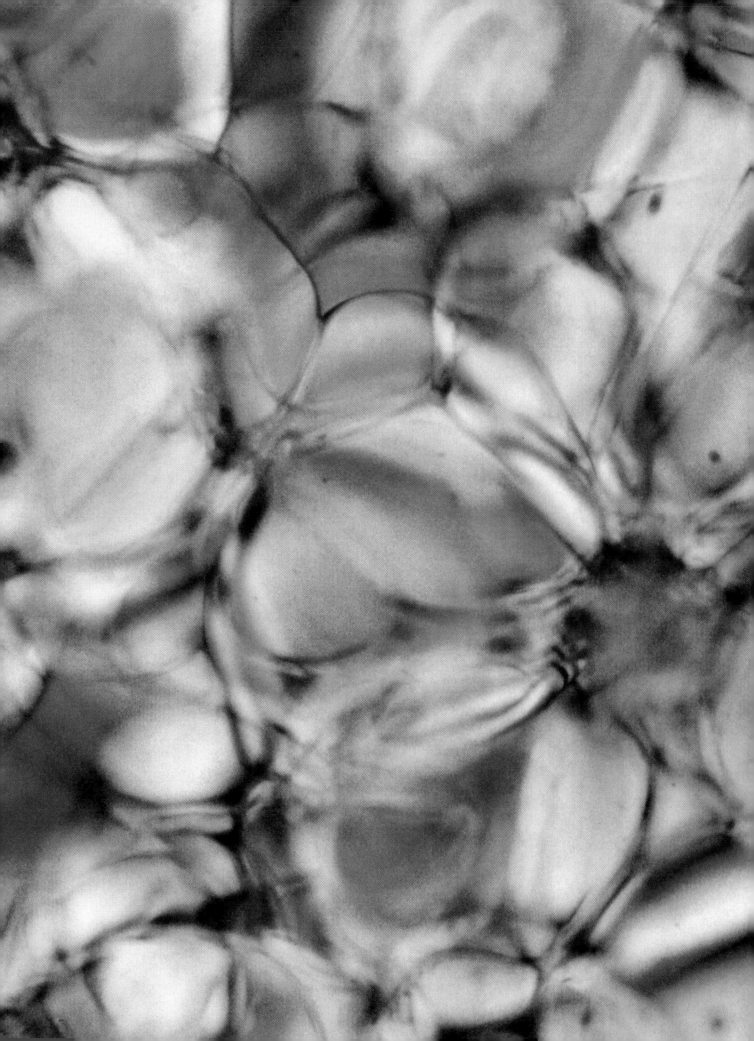

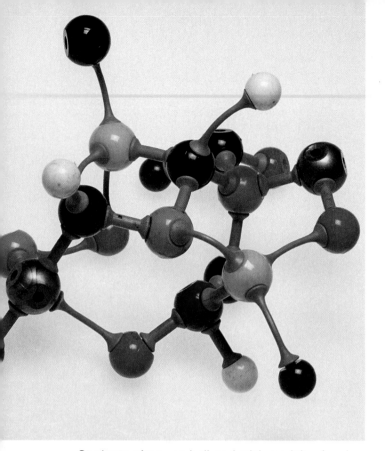

Chapter 4

Basic Food Chemistry: The Nature of Matter

Students often use ball-and-stick models of molecules to help them understand the basic nature of matter.

Objectives

After studying this chapter,
you will be able to

describe the basic structure of atoms.

identify symbols on the periodic table commonly used in food science.

define ionic and covalent bonding.

explain the difference between pure substances and mixtures.

compare physical and chemical reactions in laboratory experiments.

balance chemical equations to illustrate simple chemical reactions.

Key Terms

chemistry
matter
atom
subatomic particle
nucleus
proton
neutron
electron
orbital
element
atomic number
atomic mass
atomic mass unit
compound
molecule
chemical formula
chemical bond
shell
ionic bond
ion
covalent bond

Lewis structure
valence electron
double bond
pure substance
organic compound
inorganic compound
mixture
homogeneous
   mixture
heterogeneous
   mixture
solution
solute
solvent
physical change
phase change
chemical change
reactant
product
law of conservation
   of matter

To understand why ingredients react the way they do in recipes or formulations, you need to understand some basic chemistry. *Chemistry* is the study of the makeup, structure, and properties of substances and the changes that occur to them. It is the study of *matter,* which is anything that occupies space and has mass.

The Basic Nature of Matter

Everything you encounter, whether plant, animal, or mineral, is made up of atoms. An *atom* is the smallest unit of any elemental substance that maintains the characteristics of that substance. In other words, one atom of iron has the same physical characteristics as a chunk of iron. Atoms are extremely tiny. You cannot see them even through a powerful microscope.

Knowledge of atoms was once based on scientific theories and indirect experiments. Only recently have devices become available that allow scientists to map the individual locations and shapes of atoms. Fortunately, it is not necessary to see individual atoms to learn much about them.

Subatomic Particles

Although atoms are the smallest unit of any element, they are not the smallest particles known. Each atom is composed of smaller parts called *subatomic particles.* The *nucleus,* or central core of the atom, contains tightly clustered particles of protons and neutrons. A *proton* is a subatomic particle that has a positive electrical charge. A *neutron* is a subatomic particle that is electrically neutral. Protons and neutrons have about the same mass.

The third particle in an atom is called an electron. *Electrons* have a negative electrical charge that is equal to, but opposite of, the positive charge of protons. Electrons are much smaller than protons or neutrons. It takes approximately 1,836 electrons to equal the mass of one proton. The reaction between the positive and negative charges of protons and electrons causes the electrons to spin around the nucleus. Electrons prefer to move in pairs. The space occupied by a pair of electrons in an atom is called an *orbital.* See 4-1.

Parts of an Atom

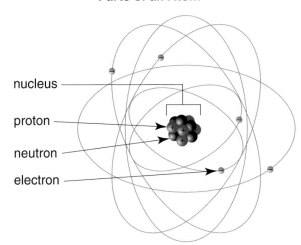

4-1 Protons and neutrons are tightly clustered in the nucleus of an atom. Electrons travel at tremendous speeds in the space outside the nucleus.

Elements

An *element* is a substance that contains only one kind of atom. There are 90 naturally occurring elements known on earth. All matter in the universe is composed of one or more of these elements. Scientists have even used some of these elements to create approximately 20 additional elements.

The number of protons in the nucleus determines which element an atom is. Pure oxygen is composed of atoms with 8 protons in the nucleus. Calcium, one of the main components of bone tissue, is composed of atoms with 24 protons in each nucleus.

A simple system of symbols is used to identify the elements. These symbols are a form of abbreviation. Learning these symbols will make it easier for you to record chemical reactions.

The symbol for many elements is the first letter of the element's name. This letter is capitalized. The symbol for carbon is C. The problem is that eleven elements begin with the letter C. A second letter from the name of the element is added in these cases. For example, calcium is represented as Ca. Note the second letter is lowercase.

You may wonder why the symbol for potassium is K and iron is Fe. Some of the elements' symbols come from their names in other languages. *Kalium* is Latin for potassium; *ferrum* is Latin for iron. See 4-2.

The Periodic Table

In the nineteenth century, researchers became aware of links between the physical and chemical characteristics of elements. These properties seemed to repeat in a regular fashion. In an effort to classify elements by these relationships, a Russian chemist, Dmitry Mendeleyev, developed the *periodic table.* This chart helps show how elements relate to and react with one another. He was able to use the chart to predict the existence and properties of elements that were unknown at the time.

Each cell of the periodic table gives information about one chemical element. The format of this information can vary somewhat from source to source. However, it will usually include the symbol for the element. It will also point out some physical features of the atoms of the element. These features help distinguish an atom of one element from an atom of another.

Two characteristics of atoms shown in many periodic tables are the atomic number and the atomic mass. The *atomic number* is the number of protons in the nucleus of each atom of the element. The *atomic mass* is

Elements Most Commonly Found in Foods	
Element	**Symbol**
Aluminum	Al
Calcium	Ca
Carbon	C
Chlorine	Cl
Fluorine	F
Hydrogen	H
Iron (Ferrum)	Fe
Magnesium	Mg
Nitrogen	N
Oxygen	O
Phosphorus	P
Potassium (Kalium)	K
Sodium (Natrium)	Na
Sulfur	S
Zinc	Zn

4-2 Learning symbols for elements commonly found in foods will help you read and write chemical equations in food science class.

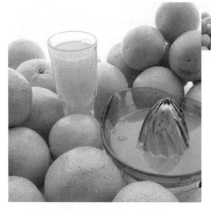

Nutrition News
Elemental Nutrition

A number of elements have been found to be essential for good health. Many of these are the nutrients dietitians and other health professionals call minerals. Each of these minerals has at least one important function in the body. Food processing can strip some foods of these vital elements. This is one reason everyone needs to include fresh fruits and vegetables and whole grain products in their daily diets.

Besides the dietary minerals, the elements carbon, hydrogen, and oxygen are vital to good nutrition. These elements make up carbohydrates, fats, and proteins. (Proteins also contain nitrogen, and they often contain sulfur, too.) These three nutrients have many functions in the body, including meeting all your energy needs.

approximately equal to the sum of the masses of protons and neutrons in an atom. The mass of a proton or neutron is defined as equal to one **atomic mass unit.** The mass of an electron is $\frac{1}{1,836}$ of an atomic mass unit. Electrons are so small their mass is insignificant.

Not all atoms of an element have the same number of neutrons. Scientists have calculated an average atomic mass for each element. This is the number used on periodic tables. The atomic number and atomic mass are not in the same places within the cells of all periodic tables. It is simplest to remember the atomic number is a smaller number than the atomic mass.

The organization of the cells in the periodic table is a key to how elements will interact chemically. The table is arranged in columns and rows. The columns, which are called *groups,* are often numbered left to right from 1 to 18. The rows, which are called *periods,* are numbered top to bottom from 1 to 7. See 4-3. Later in the chapter, you will read more about what an element's group and period tells you about the element.

Metals and Nonmetals

Many periodic tables use a color key to group elements into various classes. One main classification that is often used groups elements as metals and nonmetals. Elements in these groups have a number of properties in common. They also tend to react with other elements in similar ways.

Except for hydrogen, the elements on the left side of the periodic table are metals. (Even hydrogen is a metal at very low temperatures and very high pressures.) *Metals* are usually shiny solids at room temperature. (Mercury is an exception. It is a liquid at room temperature.) They are good conductors of heat and electricity. Metals can also be drawn into wires or pounded into sheets.

Nonmetals are found on the right side of the periodic table. Many of these elements are gases at room temperature. They tend to be poor conductors of heat and electricity, and they are generally brittle when solid.

Compounds and Chemical Formulas

When two elements combine, they form a new substance totally unlike the elements from which it was made. *Compounds* are substances in which two or more elements have chemically combined. The basic unit of any compound is a *molecule.* Sodium (Na) is a soft silver metal that is explosively reactive. Chlorine (Cl) is a yellowish-green gas that is poisonous. Both elements are dangerous in large amounts. When Na and Cl combine, they form sodium chloride. Do you recognize the name? It is the chemical name for table salt. This salt is a white granule that is safe to eat. The chemical formula that represents a single molecule of the compound sodium chloride is NaCl.

A *chemical formula* is a combination of symbols of the elements that make up a compound. The chemical formula represents one molecule of a compound. If you know how to read a chemical formula, you can quickly identify the elements in a substance. For instance, the chemical formula for water is H_2O. From this formula, you can see that water is composed of hydrogen and oxygen. See 4-4.

In some chemical formulas, you will see subscript numbers written to the right and slightly below some atomic symbols. These numbers tell how many atoms of each kind are in a molecule. The 2 in the formula for water indicates there are two atoms of hydrogen in a water molecule. If a number does not follow a symbol, the molecule contains only one atom of that element. Therefore, the formula H_2O tells you that a molecule of water has two atoms of hydrogen and one of oxygen.

Chemical formulas can also tell something about how the atoms are arranged in a molecule. A molecule of acetic acid (vinegar) contains two carbon atoms, four hydrogen atoms, and two oxygen atoms. The chemical formula could be written as $C_2H_4O_2$. However, each carbon atom can combine with up to four other atoms. Therefore, many arrangements of the atoms are possible. The structure of an acetic acid molecule is similar to the figure below.

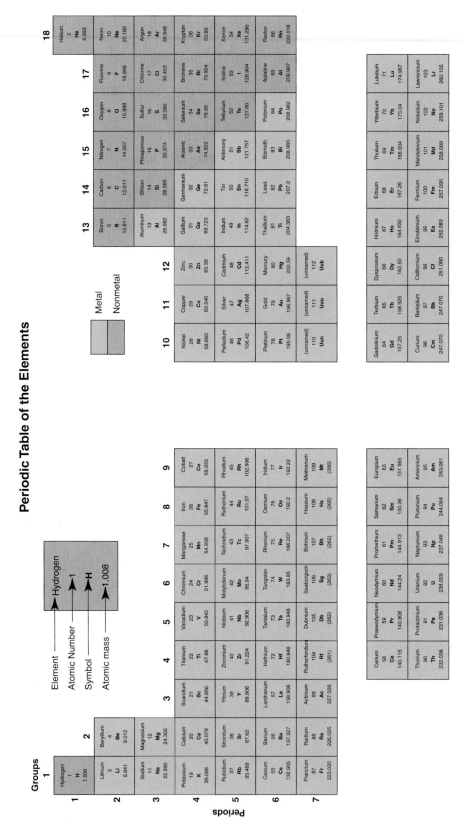

4-3 The periodic table helps researchers predict the chemical behavior of the elements. The elements outlined in red are those of greatest concern to dietitians.

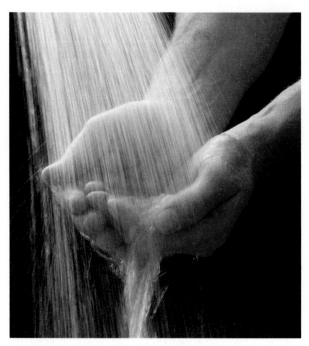

4-4 Water is a compound made up of the elements hydrogen and oxygen.

Electron Shells in a Calcium Atom

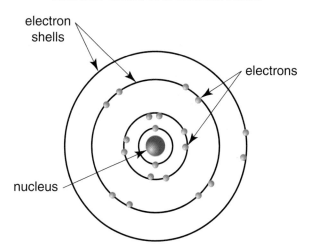

Note: The relative sizes of the particles and shells in this model are inaccurate.

4-5 This model represents a calcium atom, which has 20 electrons. These electrons are grouped in four shells surrounding the nucleus.

Formulas for carbon-based compounds are usually written in a way that shows how the atoms connect to the carbon. Thus, the formula for acetic acid is usually written as CH_3COOH. Note how this formula is similar to the arrangement of the atoms in the molecule.

Chemical Bonding

The lines in the diagram for an acetic acid molecule represent chemical bonds. A *chemical bond* is the force that holds two atoms together. The subatomic particle that forms the bond is the electron. Whether two elements will combine, and in what ratio, depends on their electrons.

Electrons move in orbitals about the nucleus of atoms in predictable patterns of space. An area of space surrounding the nucleus that has one or more orbitals is called a *shell.* (Shells are referred to by their energy levels or by their principle quantum number. This text will use the more visual term *shell.*) The first shell has one orbital and can hold two electrons. The next shell can hold up to eight electrons in four orbitals. See 4-5.

Atoms can have up to seven shells. The number of shells in the atoms of an element determines the element's period, or row, in the periodic table. In other words, all the elements in the third period have atoms with three shells.

Atoms are most stable when the outer shell of electrons is full. If the outer shell is one electron short of being full, the atom will try to gain an electron. If an atom has only one electron in its outer shell, the atom will try to give away the electron. This will cause the shell to be empty.

All the elements in a group, or column, of the periodic table will react with other elements in similar ways. This is because all the elements in a group have the same number of electrons in their outermost shells. For instance, each element in group 17 has one electron missing in its outer shell. The elements in group 16 are missing two electrons from their outer shells. Thus, an element's location in the periodic table helps to predict how it will combine with other elements.

The element at the top of group 1 in the periodic table is hydrogen. Hydrogen has one proton in its nucleus and one electron moving in a shell around the nucleus. All the other elements in group 1 also have only one electron in their outermost shells. These elements all bond readily with other elements.

The elements in group 18 of the periodic table have their outermost shells full of electrons. These elements are extremely stable. A *stable* element is one that is least likely to form chemical bonds.

Ionic Bonds

There are two basic types of chemical bonds. One type is an *ionic bond,* in which the electrons are transferred from one atom to another. This causes both atoms to have a charge. The atom receiving an electron will be negatively charged, while the one that loses the electron becomes positively charged. Therefore, the ionic bond is a result of the attraction between a positive charge and a negative charge, 4-6.

Ionic Bonding

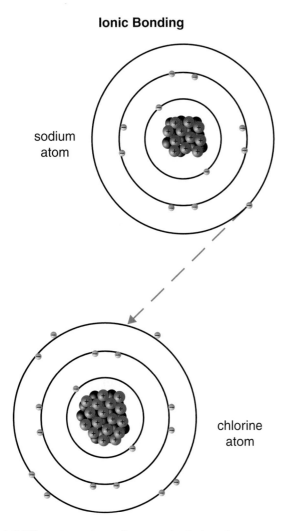

sodium atom

chlorine atom

4-6 When two atoms form an ionic bond, one atom gives an electron to the other.

Table salt is an example of a compound with an ionic bond. Remember that salt is made of Na and Cl. A sodium atom is electrically neutral. It has 11 positively charged protons and 11 negatively charged electrons. Its outer shell contains only one electron. A chlorine atom is also electrically neutral. It has 17 positively charged protons and 17 negatively charged electrons. Its outer shell is missing one electron.

The sodium atom transfers the electron in its outer shell to fill the outer shell of the chlorine atom. The sodium atom now has 11 positively charged protons and 10 negatively charged electrons. This gives the sodium atom a net positive charge. The chlorine atom that received the electron now has 18 electrons and 17 protons. It has a negative charge.

An atom or group of atoms that has a positive or negative electrical charge is called an *ion.* An ion with a positive electrical charge has a superscript plus sign (+) written beside the chemical symbol. An ion with a negative electrical charge has a superscript minus sign (–) written beside the chemical symbol. Thus, the sodium ion is written as Na^+, and the chlorine ion is written as Cl^-.

Like charges repel each other and opposite charges attract. Therefore, sodium ions will push away from other sodium ions and pull toward chlorine ions. This will cause sodium and chlorine atoms to form an alternating pattern or structure. This regular arrangement of atoms causes a crystalline structure or crystal. See 4-7.

Substances with ionic bonds will tend to dissolve in water. This is because one end of the water molecule is slightly positive, whereas the other end is slightly negative. The positive sodium ion is attracted to the negative end of the water molecule. The negative chlorine ion is attracted to the positive end of the water molecule. This results in the ionic bonds being pulled apart. The salt crystal is now a salt solution in water.

Sodium, like all elements except hydrogen in group 1 of the periodic table, is a metal. Chlorine, which is found in group 17 of the periodic table, is a nonmetal. Ionic bonds form between metals and nonmetals. Compounds like table salt that result from ionic bonds are

Salt Crystal

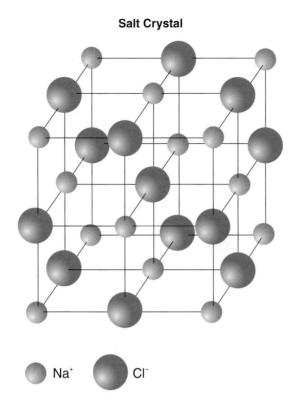

Na⁺   Cl⁻

4-7 Ionic bonding results in crystals. In a salt crystal, each chlorine ion is surrounded by six sodium ions.

crystalline in structure. The crystalline shape is a result of the interaction between the negative and positive ions.

The metals potassium and calcium will also combine with chlorine. Potassium chloride is the compound used to make no-salt seasonings. Calcium chloride is used as a drying agent. See 4-8.

Storage Tip

Some compounds will easily react with water. Because air contains water, dry powders, such as baking powder, need to be stored in airtight containers.

Covalent Bonds

The second type of chemical bond, a *covalent bond,* is formed when atoms share one or more pairs of electrons. Water molecules are formed by covalent bonds between two hydrogen atoms and one oxygen atom.

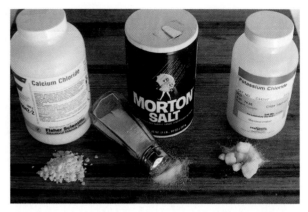

4-8 Calcium chloride, sodium chloride, and potassium chloride are all compounds formed by ionic bonds between metals and chlorine, a nonmetal.

Hydrogen atoms have only one electron. It is in a shell that can hold up to two electrons. Oxygen atoms have eight electrons. There are two electrons in the inner shell and six in the outer shell, which can hold up to eight. An oxygen atom will share one of the six electrons in its outer shell with each of two hydrogen atoms. At the same time, each of the hydrogen atoms will share its electron with the oxygen atom. Thus, both hydrogen atoms will have a full shell of two electrons. The oxygen atom will have a full shell of eight electrons. See 4-9.

This is shown better with the Lewis structure. The *Lewis structure* is a shorthand method of diagramming electrons that are likely to be shared. The Lewis structure helps scientists have a better picture of how atoms combine. This system was developed by Gilbert Newton Lewis, a chemist from the United States. It is another tool to help predict how elements will react.

The electrons that are likely to be shared or transferred are in partially full shells and are called *valence electrons.* In the Lewis structure, each valence electron is represented by a dot next to the symbol for the element. A shell can hold a maximum of eight electrons. Therefore, the dots are arranged in pairs on the four sides of the element symbol. The water molecule described earlier would be diagrammed in the following way:

H· plus H· plus :Ö· yields :Ö:H
                                            |
                                            H

Covalent Bonding

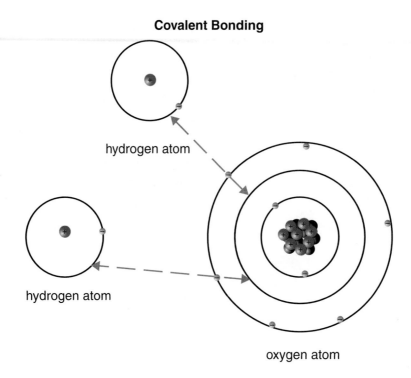

hydrogen atom

hydrogen atom

oxygen atom

4-9 Covalent bonds are formed when one atom shares an electron from its outer shell with another atom.

Another example of the Lewis structure is shown below for methane (CH_4). A molecule of CH_4 has four hydrogen atoms surrounding a carbon atom. Hydrogen is always on the outside or end of molecules. This is because it has only one electron and can only form one bond.

$$\begin{array}{c} H \\ H\!:\!\overset{..}{\underset{..}{C}}\!:\!H \\ H \end{array}$$

The definition for covalent bonds states that more than one pair of electrons can be shared. When two atoms share two pairs of electrons, a *double bond* is formed. An example of this is carbon dioxide, CO_2.

$\cdot\overset{\cdot}{C}\cdot$ plus $\cdot\overset{..}{\underset{..}{O}}\!:$ plus $\cdot\overset{..}{\underset{..}{O}}\!:$ yields $:\!\overset{..}{\underset{..}{O}}\!:\!:\!C\!:\!:\!\overset{..}{\underset{..}{O}}\!:$

The number of valence electrons around the atoms equals the number of valence electrons in the molecule. When shared pairs are counted, each of the atoms has eight electrons around it.

The Classification of Matter

Matter can be classified into the two general categories of pure substances and mixtures. Each of these general categories can be divided into two subcategories. Referring to Chart 4-10 can help you see how these categories break down.

Pure Substances

A *pure substance* is matter in which all the basic units are the same. You can group pure substances as elements and compounds. Elements important in food science are those needed for good health. These include iron, calcium, and potassium. Most of the pure substances food scientists work with are compounds. Common examples include salt (sodium chloride) and baking soda (sodium bicarbonate).

Organic and Inorganic Compounds

Chemists divide the study of pure substances even further by dividing compounds into two main groups. This method of classifying compounds is based on the source of the

The Classification of Matter

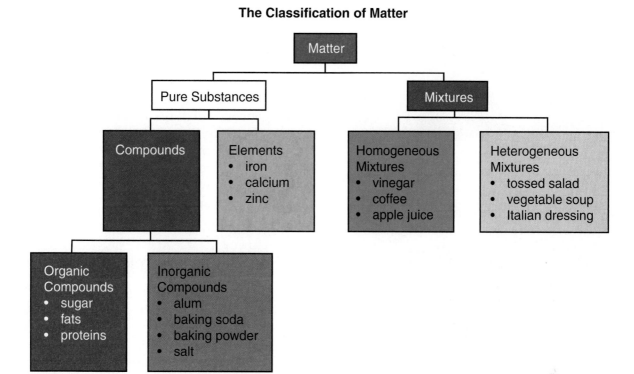

4-10 This chart illustrates how the various classifications of matter are related.

compound in nature: living or nonliving substances. Scientists have discovered that all living substances contain carbon. Most nonliving substances do not.

Chemists group compounds into two main categories: organic and inorganic. *Organic compounds* contain chains or rings of carbon. Most organic compounds also contain hydrogen and oxygen. All the sources of energy in your diet are organic compounds. These compounds (carbohydrates, fats, and proteins) are the main components of the food you eat. *Inorganic compounds* either contain no carbon or have only single carbon atoms. Examples of inorganic compounds in foods are table salt, water, and minerals.

Mixtures

Most of the substances you will work with in the foods lab are *not* pure substances. They are mixtures. *Mixtures* are substances that are put together but not chemically combined. Calcium is an element and table salt is a compound. Both are pure substances. However, few people sit and eat pure calcium or pure salt. A glass of milk contains both calcium and

salt. Milk is a mixture of these two substances plus many others.

You can categorize mixtures as homogeneous or heterogeneous. A *homogeneous mixture* has a uniform distribution of particles throughout the sample. Visually, you cannot tell one part of the mixture from another. Examples of homogeneous mixtures are tea, mayonnaise, and soft drinks. Homogenized milk is also an example of a homogeneous mixture.

A *heterogeneous mixture* has a non-uniform distribution of particles. A bowl of vegetable soup is a heterogeneous mixture. When you look at a spoonful of the soup, you can see corn, beans, carrots, and onions in a broth. If you pureed this soup in a blender, it would become a homogeneous mixture. See 4-11.

Sometimes, homogeneous and heterogeneous mixtures can be hard to tell apart. For instance, at first glance, hot cocoa appears to be a homogeneous mixture. However, when a cup of cocoa sits without stirring, the heavier cocoa molecules will gradually settle to the bottom. Although cocoa looks uniform, the

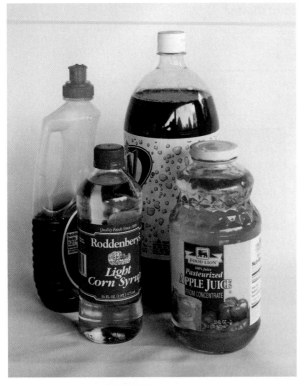

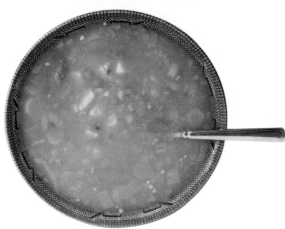

4-11 Maple syrup, corn syrup, soft drinks, and apple juice are examples of homogenous mixtures. Vegetable soup is an example of a heterogeneous mixture.

very small particles will not stay evenly distributed throughout the milk. Therefore, hot cocoa is a heterogeneous mixture.

Most homogeneous mixtures are solutions. A *solution* is a homogeneous mixture of one material dissolved in another. The material that is dissolved is called the *solute*. The material that does the dissolving is the *solvent*. In sweetened drinks, water is the solvent and

sugar is the solute. Water is also the solvent in plain coffee and fruit juice.

The substances in heterogeneous mixtures can be separated by mechanical means. For example, you could strain the vegetable soup and then hand sort the vegetables. Separating homogeneous mixtures is more difficult but not impossible. For instance, salt water is a homogeneous mixture. You cannot separate the salt from the water by hand. However, if you heat salt water, the water will turn to steam and evaporate, leaving salt crystals behind.

Physical and Chemical Changes

When scientists analyze what happens in the world around them, they describe changes they observe. Whether you are looking at chemicals or food, you will observe two basic kinds of changes. These are physical changes and chemical changes. It is important to understand how these changes differ to interpret what you see.

Physical Changes

When you chop onions, the pieces become smaller, but the substance is still onion. It has the same color, flavor, and aroma as onion. This is an example of a physical change. *Physical changes* involve changing shape, physical state, size, or temperature without changing the chemical identity. If you freeze water and then crush the ice, you still have H_2O. Melting ice is also a physical change. Water goes from a solid state to a liquid state, but it is still water. Dissolving salt in water is another physical change. You can still taste the salt and feel the wetness of the water.

Phase Changes

One example of a physical change is a change in the phase or physical state of a substance. The phases or states of matter are solids, liquids, and gases. A shift from one of these states to another is called a phase change. A *phase change* is a physical change in the visible structure of matter without changing the molecular structure.

In the *solid* state, atoms and molecules are close together in a rigid structure. Solids have a definite shape and volume. Examples include salt and ice.

As a solid is heated, the atoms and molecules begin to move farther apart as they gain energy. As a result, solids lose their structure and become *liquid*. The particles flow or slide past one another. The substance has no definite shape of its own. It will take the shape of the container. Liquids do have a definite volume. Examples are water, milk, and fruit juice.

As more heat is added to a liquid, the atoms and/or molecules gain enough energy to escape into the air. This represents a change to the *gas* phase of matter. Gases will expand to fit any closed container in which they are stored. They have no definite shape or volume. See 4-12.

Any phase change is an example of a reversible physical change. You can freeze water to make ice—the solid phase of water. When left at room temperature, the ice returns to the liquid phase. If more heat is added, the water boils and evaporates as steam—the gas phase. Steam, or water vapor, returns to the liquid state as it cools.

Chemical Changes

When bread is heated, it gets warmer. It may also lose some water content. These are physical changes. When bread is toasted, browning occurs. The color and flavor change because the starch molecules have undergone a chemical change.

A *chemical change* occurs whenever new substances with different chemical and physical properties are formed. Chemical changes can produce changes in color or odor. Other evidences of a chemical change include flavor changes and the release of gas. Mixing water and baking powder results in a chemical change. The mixture will foam and fizzle as a gas is released. Fermenting grapes is also an example of a chemical change. When grape juice is fermented to make wine, yeast changes the sugar in the juice into alcohol.

Identifying Physical Versus Chemical Changes

There are times when it will be difficult to tell physical and chemical changes apart. For example, when you open a carbonated beverage, it begins to fizz. This change is caused by the carbon dioxide physically separating from the water. If you combined baking soda and an acid ingredient to make muffins, the batter would begin to bubble. In this case, carbon dioxide is being formed through a chemical reaction. See 4-13. Chemical changes will often

States of Matter

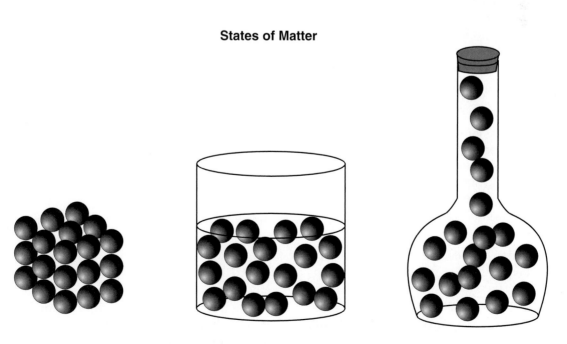

4-12 As a substance goes from the solid to the liquid to the gas state, the amount of space between molecules increases.

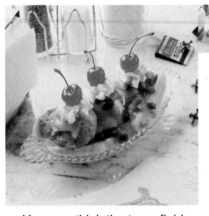

Item of Interest
Non-Newtonian Fluids

You may think the term *fluid* has the same meaning as the term *liquid.* However, *fluids* are substances that have characteristics of liquids and gases. A unique type of fluid is a non-Newtonian fluid. *Non-Newtonian fluids* have characteristics of liquids and solids. You can make a

substance that has these characteristics by combining two parts cornstarch with one part water. If you tried to pour this mixture from a beaker, it would act like a slow-moving liquid. However, suppose you placed this mixture on a lab table and struck it with your fist. It would instantly resist

the force and act like a solid. This is why stirring a mixture of cornstarch and liquid is difficult unless there are at least equal amounts of both substances. This is important to remember when dissolving cornstarch in a small amount of liquid before adding it to a gravy or sauce.

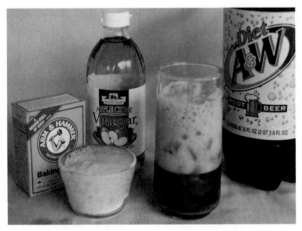

4-13 The fizz that forms on a soft drink is the result of dissolved carbon dioxide physically separating from the soft drink. The fizz that forms from combining baking soda and vinegar is the result of a chemical change.

involve other noticeable changes in odor, color, or taste.

Permanent and Reversible Changes

Physical and chemical changes are similar in that they may or may not be reversible. You can change fruit juice from liquid to solid back

to liquid and it is still fruit juice. That physical change is reversible. However, you cannot chop an onion and then put it back together again. Although the substance is still onion, its physical state has been permanently changed into tiny pieces.

The way your body uses food provides an example of a reversible chemical change. Your body breaks down carbohydrates from your diet into glucose, which can be used as a short-term energy source. If you do not have any short-term energy needs, your body can convert excess glucose into body fat for storage. Later, when you need more energy, your body can convert the body fat back into glucose.

Burning cookies illustrates a permanent chemical change. If you severely overbake cookies, they will turn black. You cannot reverse this chemical change to make the cookies edible again.

Chemical Equations

You can describe a chemical change using a *chemical equation.* In a chemical equation, chemical formulas are used to represent the compounds involved. Chemical formulas on the left side of the equation are called *reactants.* They are the substances that exist before a chemical change takes place. A plus symbol (+) is used to indicate that substances are combined. An arrow represents a chemical change, or *reaction.* One or more chemical formulas on the right side of the equation are the **products.** They are the substances that are formed.

When sodium hydroxide (NaOH) is mixed with hydrochloric acid (HCl), a reaction will occur. This reaction will produce salt (NaCl) and water (H_2O). The chemical equation representing this reaction would be written as follows:

$$NaOH + HCl \longrightarrow NaCl + H_2O$$

sodium hydroxide (lye) + hydrochloric acid   yields   salt + water

The *law of conservation of matter* states that matter can be changed but not created or destroyed. The conservation of matter is shown in chemical equations. There must always be the same number of atoms on the right side as there are on the left. Although elements can recombine to form new compounds, the atoms themselves will not change. Therefore, there must also be the same kind of atoms represented on the right as were on the left. Look at the following equation:

$$C_{12}H_{22}O_{11} + O_2 \longrightarrow CO_2 + H_2O$$

This formula represents a simplified version of the digestion of sugar. The left side of the equation has 12 carbon atoms and the right only 1. This equation is not balanced. There has not been a conservation of matter. Every time a sugar molecule is digested, there must be more than one molecule of CO_2 made. For the equation to balance, there must be 12 carbon atoms on each side.

$$C_{12}H_{22}O_{11} + O_2 \longrightarrow 12CO_2 + H_2O$$

Now the carbon atoms balance, but the oxygen atoms and hydrogen atoms still do not. If there will be 11 molecules of water for every molecule of sugar, the hydrogen atoms will balance.

$$C_{12}H_{22}O_{11} + O_2 \longrightarrow 12CO_2 + 11H_2O$$

12 Cs 22 Hs 13 Os   12 Cs 22 Hs 35 Os

As you can see, the carbon and hydrogen atoms are in balance, but the oxygen atoms are not.

Twenty-two more oxygen atoms on the left will balance the equation.

$$C_{12}H_{22}O_{11} + 12O_2 \longrightarrow 12CO_2 + 11H_2O$$

Now the equation balances. For every molecule of sugar, you need 12 molecules of oxygen. This will result in 12 molecules of carbon dioxide and 11 molecules of water.

Careful measurements and repeated trials of this reaction would show that this ratio is constant. There will always be 12 molecules of carbon dioxide for every molecule of sugar digested. When chemical formulas are known, scientists can use them like recipes or formulations to combine the exact amounts of ingredients needed. See 4-14.

Notice that in balancing the equation, the arrangement and number of atoms in the molecules was not changed. Only the number of each kind of molecule can be changed when balancing equations.

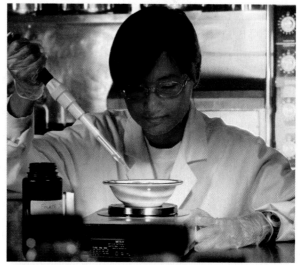

Agricultural Research Service, USDA

4-14 Food scientists use chemical formulas when preparing formulations of food products.

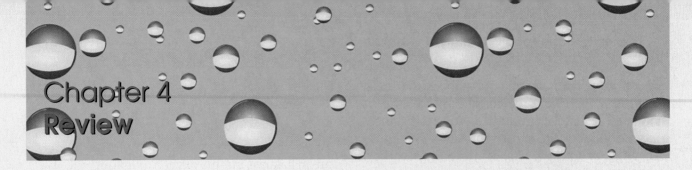

Chapter 4
Review

Summary

A study of food science requires knowledge of the basic nature of matter. You need a mental picture of how subatomic particles fit into the structure of atoms. You need to know that matter is made up of chemical elements, which are identified in the periodic table. This information will be your basis for understanding how atoms form ionic and covalent bonds to create molecules and compounds.

Food scientists must be able to predict how food products will perform during processing and preservation. Learning to classify products as pure substances or mixtures will help you make such predictions. As you observe the behavior of food compounds, you will need to identify physical and chemical changes. Then you will use chemical equations as you record what you observe. This course will help you see how food preparation techniques relate to the chemical structure of ingredients in foods.

Checking Your Understanding

1. Name the three subatomic particles. Give the atomic mass, charge, and location in the atom for each particle.

2. Describe the chemical symbols used to represent elements.

3. What is the difference between the atomic number and the atomic mass of an element?

4. What does the 2 in the formula CO_2 (carbon dioxide) indicate?

5. What is the most stable arrangement for electrons?

6. How can an element's location in the periodic table help predict how the element will combine with other elements?

7. How do ionic and covalent bonds differ?

8. Identify the two categories of pure substances and give an example of each.

9. Give two examples of homogeneous mixtures and two examples of heterogeneous mixtures.

10. Explain the main difference between physical and chemical changes.

11. Compare the shape and volume of the three states of matter.

12. How do you know that a chemical equation will always have the same number of atoms of each type on each side?

Critical Thinking

1. What is the Lewis dot structure for each of the following chemical formulas? Each of these compounds is formed with covalent bonds. The elements are all nonmetals.
   a. C_2H_6
   b. NH_3
   c. CH_3COOH

2. Chlorine is found in column 17 of the periodic table. The elements in column 17 are known as halogens. From your knowledge of chlorine, what characteristics would you expect to find in the other halogens?

3. Using the periodic table, identify how many bonds with other atoms can be formed by each of the following elements:
   a. calcium
   b. fluorine
   c. magnesium
   d. nitrogen
   e. phosphorus
   f. potassium
   g. sulfur

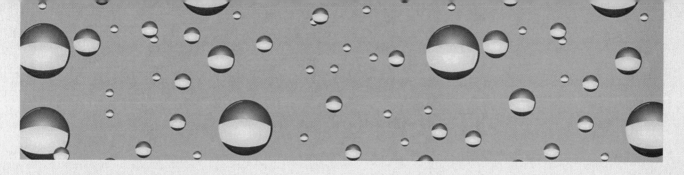

4. Identify whether each of the following is a physical or chemical change:
   a. brewing tea
   b. sweetening lemonade
   c. browning pork chops
   d. basting a turkey as it roasts
   e. slicing tomatoes
   f. caramelizing onions
   g. cooking pancake batter
   h. melting chocolate
   i. simmering spaghetti sauce

5. List 10 food items in your refrigerator. Identify whether they are compounds, heterogeneous mixtures, or homogeneous mixtures.

Explore Further

1. **Science.** Obtain a chemistry model kit or materials from home, such as marshmallows and toothpicks. Use these materials to construct models of each of the following molecules: water, acetic acid, and methane.

2. **Math.** Mass 100 mL of sugar. Combine the sugar with 100 mL of water. Water has a mass of 1 g/mL. What is the combined mass? What is the combined volume? Explain the results of conservation of mass and your understanding of molecules.

Experiment 4A
Physical Qualities of Food

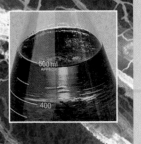

Purpose

All food products are made of chemical compounds. Each compound has measurable characteristics, including boiling point, freezing point, color, aroma, and density. Becoming familiar with these characteristics will help you predict how ingredients will react in food mixtures. In this experiment, you will examine the boiling points and densities of several common food products.

Equipment

2 or 3 100-mL graduated cylinders

5 cups or bowls

1 or 2 250-mL beakers

3 150-mL beakers

thermometer

beaker tongs

Supplies

100 mL water

100 mL corn syrup

100 mL vegetable oil

100 mL cooking sherry

6 chocolate chips

100 mL rice

3 miniature marshmallows

3 ice cubes

1 drop food coloring

Procedure

1. Tare a 100-mL graduated cylinder. Use this graduated cylinder to mass 100 mL of water, corn syrup, vegetable oil, and cooking sherry. Record measurements in a data table. After massing each liquid, pour it into a cup or bowl and set aside. Be sure to wash and dry the graduated cylinder after massing each liquid.

2. Mass the chocolate chips. Use rice to measure the displacement volume of the chocolate chips in a 100-mL graduated cylinder. (Review how to measure the volume of irregularly shaped objects from Experiment 2C.) Record measurements in the data table.

3. Mass the marshmallows. Use rice to measure the displacement volume of the marshmallows in a 100-mL graduated cylinder. Record measurements in the data table.

4. Working quickly to reduce melting, mass the ice cubes. Measure the volume of the ice cubes using the water displacement method in a 250-mL beaker. Record measurements in the data table. Then place the ice cubes in a cup or bowl and return them to the freezer until they are needed.

5. Heat 50 mL of the water measured in step 1 in one of the 150-mL beakers on a hot plate or burner until it boils. Measure and record the temperature. Discard the heated water.

6. Heat 50 mL of the corn syrup in another 150-mL beaker until it boils. Measure and record the temperature. Discard the heated corn syrup and wash the thermometer.

7. Heat 50 mL of the cooking sherry in a third 150-mL beaker until it boils. Measure and record the temperature. Discard the heated cooking sherry.

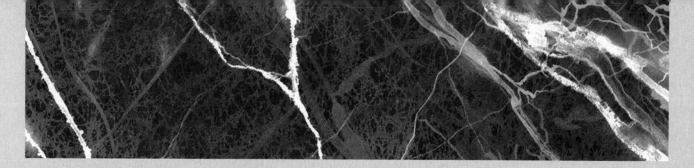

8. Using the formula *density = mass ÷ volume,* calculate the density of the four liquids and three solids.

9. Read steps 11 and 12 and predict what will happen.

10. Add a drop of food coloring to the remaining 50 mL of water and pour it into the 250-mL beaker.

11. Slowly pour the remaining 50 mL of corn syrup into the 250-mL beaker with the colored water. Then slowly pour 50 mL of the vegetable oil into the 250-mL beaker. Finally, slowly pour the remaining 50 mL of cooking sherry into the 250-mL beaker. Observe what happens.

12. Add the chocolate chips, marshmallows, and ice cubes to the liquids in the beaker.

Questions

1. Which of the liquids or solids is the densest?

2. Which of the liquids or solids is the least dense?

3. Was there a relationship between a liquid's density and its boiling point?

4. How accurate were the predictions you made in step 9?

5. How can you apply this information to food preparation?

Experiment 4B
Chemical Changes

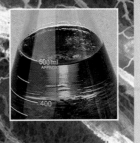

Purpose

When a chemical change occurs in a mixture, some signs of that change can be observed. Some of the signs that a chemical change has occurred include color changes, the forming of a gas (bubbling or foaming), temperature changes, and the forming of a precipitate (a solid settling out of a solution).

Equipment

magnifying glass or microscope

100-mL beaker

glass stirring rod

2 watch glasses

test-tube tongs

Supplies

1 g sodium chloride

1 vitamin C tablet, crushed

2 g sodium bicarbonate

40 mL distilled water

Procedure

1. Use the magnifying glass or microscope to examine a small amount of sodium chloride. Describe the appearance in your data table.

2. Taste a few crystals of sodium chloride. Describe the taste in your data table.

3. Repeat steps 1 and 2 twice, the first time with the crushed vitamin C tablet and the second time with the sodium bicarbonate.

4. Combine 1 g of sodium chloride, half of the vitamin C tablet, and 20 mL of distilled water in the 100-mL beaker. Stir with a glass rod until the sodium chloride has dissolved.

5. Pour a small amount of the solution on a watch glass. Discard the remaining solution and wash the beaker and glass rod with warm, soapy water.

6. Heat the watch glass on a range over medium heat until the liquid boils away.

7. Remove the watch glass from the heat with the test-tube tongs and allow it to cool.

8. Examine the residue on the watch glass with a magnifying glass or microscope. Taste the residue. Record your observations on appearance and flavor in your data table.

9. Combine 2 g of sodium bicarbonate, the remaining half of the crushed vitamin C tablet, and the remaining 20 mL of distilled water in the cleaned 100-mL beaker. Stir with the cleaned glass rod until the sodium bicarbonate has dissolved.

10. Repeat steps 5 through 8, being sure to use a clean watch glass in step 5.

Questions

1. What happened when water was added to the powders?

2. Describe any physical changes that occurred during this experiment.

3. Describe any chemical changes that occurred during this experiment.

4. How can you apply information from this experiment to food preparation?

Experiment 4C
The Chemical Detective

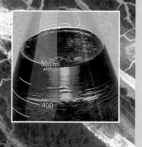

Purpose

During this experiment, you will observe the physical and chemical properties of four common household substances. You will be given four unknown powders and three liquid indicators. You are to record any changes you see after adding each indicator to each powder. You will then test an unknown mixture of two to four of the powders with the indicators and try to determine which powders your mixture contains. A good detective observes small details.

Equipment

glass plate
wax pencil
small scoop
magnifying glass

Supplies

indicators I, II, and III in eye dropper bottles
powders A, B, C, and D in small portion cups
mystery powder

Procedure

Part I

1. Use the wax pencil to draw a three-column, four-row table on the glass plate. Label the columns *I*, *II*, and *III*. Label the rows *A*, *B*, *C*, and *D*.

2. Use the small scoop to place a pea-sized sample of each powder in each cell of the appropriate row of the table.

3. Use a magnifying glass to examine each powder. Record your observations of its appearance in the physical properties column of your data table.

4. Place one drop of *Indicator I* on each powder in column I. Record any reaction observed in the column marked *Indicator I* on the data table.

5. Repeat the procedure with *Indicator II* in the second column and *Indicator III* in the third column. Record observations.

6. Clean the glass plate.

Part II

1. Obtain a mystery powder from your teacher.

2. Use the wax pencil to draw a three-column, two-row table on the glass plate. Label the columns *I*, *II*, and *III*. Label the rows *mystery* and *test mix*.

3. Place a pea-sized sample of the mystery powder in each of the cells in the first row of the table. Use a magnifying glass to examine the mystery powder. Record your observations of its appearance in the mystery powder data table.

4. Place a drop of each indicator on the mystery powder in the appropriate column. Record your observations in the mystery powder data table. Hypothesize which of powders A, B, C, and D are in the mystery powder.

5. Combine equal amounts of the powders you believe are in the mystery powder. Place a pea-sized sample of the mixture in each of the cells in the second row on the glass plate. Use a magnifying glass to examine the mixture. Compare the appearance with that of the mystery powder.

6. Place a drop of each indicator on the mixture in the appropriate column. Compare the results with the results for the mystery powder.

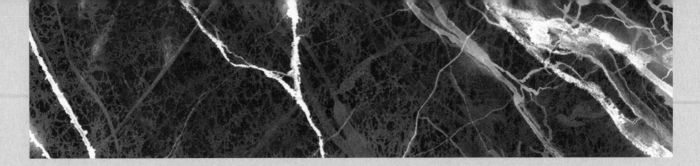

Questions

1. Which test, if any, was the most helpful in identifying the mystery powders? Explain your answer.

2. What other tests could be done to make identification of these powders easier or more accurate?

3. What differences, if any, were there in the mystery powder and the mix you prepared based on your hypothesis?

4. Name a career that would use these identification skills.

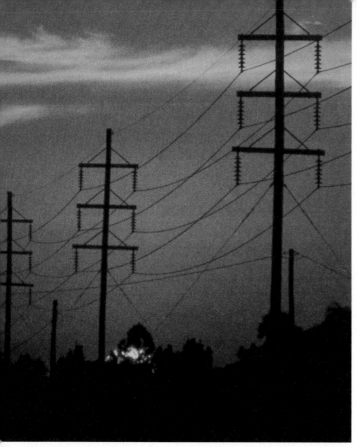

USDA

Power lines carry electrical energy to wherever it is needed.

Chapter 5

Energy: Matter in Motion

Objectives

After studying this chapter, you will be able to

identify sources of energy as potential or kinetic.

differentiate among the various forms of energy.

explain the relationship between heat and temperature.

summarize three basic ways heat is transferred.

list factors affecting the rate of reaction in food preparation.

Key Terms

energy
potential energy
kinetic energy
external energy
internal energy
mechanical energy
chemical energy
endothermic reaction
exothermic reaction
electrical energy
radiant energy
magnetron
microwave
nuclear energy
heat
calorie
heat capacity

specific heat
temperature
conduction
convection
radiation
fusion
crystallization
latent heat of fusion
evaporation
vaporization
condensation
liquefaction
latent heat of
    vaporization
latent heat
deposition
sublimation

You need energy to fuel your body, cook your food, and light your home. In fact, any change that takes place in the universe requires a transfer of energy. Because energy is important to all aspects of life, having a basic understanding of energy is useful. Simply defined, *energy* is the ability to do work. If you pick, peel, or eat an apple, you have used energy. You have used force to change the position, shape, or structure of the apple.

The food industry uses large amounts of energy in the processing and packaging of food products, 5-1. Food scientists need to understand how heat is transferred in cooking and preservation processes. Food scientists also need to consider how energy affects the structure of food during these operations. This type of knowledge about energy will help food scientists develop new food products to meet the needs of consumers.

The history of technological development parallels discoveries of new energy sources and ways to use them to improve living conditions. Since the discovery of fire, people have been learning new ways to harness energy. Prior to 1800, people thought energy was a fluid named *caloric.* It was during the nineteenth century that scientists began to understand the nature of energy.

Potential and Kinetic Energy

One way to categorize energy is by its state or position. Energy can be described as stored or in motion. Energy that is stored is called *potential energy.* It can also be called the energy of position or the measure of work done. If you hold a rock at the edge of a cliff, it has potential energy due to its position. Lifting the rock to the top of the cliff required an output of energy, or work. The potential energy of the rock can be thought of as the stored work done in the lifting. An apple sitting on a table has potential energy stored in it in the form of carbohydrates. This is a result of photosynthesis, which is work done by the tree that produced the apple. When you eat the apple, its potential energy is released in your body. All the energy you get from food is stored in the food in the form of chemical potential energy.

Kinetic energy is the energy of motion. Mass in motion possesses kinetic energy. The faster an object moves, the more kinetic energy it has. Energy is constantly changing from potential to kinetic energy and back again. An example of this is as simple as a child swinging faster and lower, higher and slower on a swing. The fastest speed at the bottom of the swinging motion is when maximum kinetic energy is reached. The slowest speed at the top of the swinging motion is when maximum potential energy is reached.

So far, you have read about potential and kinetic energy in terms of whether an object is in motion. The atoms and molecules that make up objects are always in motion. Therefore, you may wonder how the energy of any object can be all potential energy. Looking at whether motion is applied to objects or coming from within objects can help answer this question.

Kinetic and potential energy can be described as external or internal energy. *External energy* is energy applied to an object

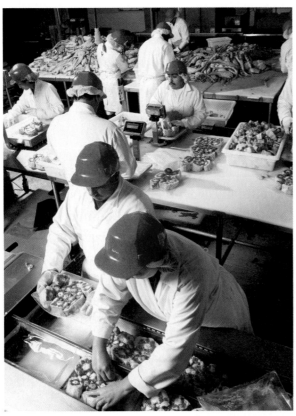

5-1 Food processing and packaging requires a lot of energy.

by another source. If you are sitting perfectly still, your body has *external potential energy*. No outside sources are causing you to move, but you are in position to do work. If a friend pulls you out of your chair, your body has *external kinetic energy*. Outside sources are causing you to move and do work.

Internal energy refers to energy within an object. It is a result of forces between the atoms and molecules of a system. Your body has *internal kinetic energy*. This is because the molecules within your body are moving and doing work. Your body also has *internal potential energy*. Fat within your body is a stored source of fuel that you can use to do work.

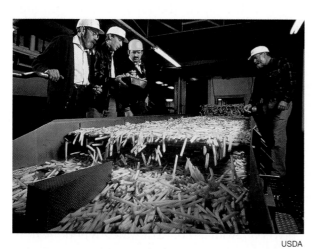

USDA

5-2 French fries have potential or internal energy, which is measured in calories. The conveyor belt and the French fries that are falling are examples of kinetic energy or energy of motion.

Food contains internal potential energy. A source of fuel your body could use to do work is stored within each piece of food. The food industry spends much time and effort analyzing, measuring, and studying the energy stored in food. See 5-2.

Forms of Energy

Another way to define or categorize energy is by the types or forms of energy used to do work. There are five main forms of energy in the universe: mechanical, chemical, electrical, nuclear, and radiant. See 5-3.

Energy has the ability to change from one form to another. This is one of energy's most important properties. Energy's versatility and people's ability to harness it is the basis of much human technological accomplishment.

Mechanical Energy

Mechanical energy is the total kinetic and potential energy of a system. A waterwheel provides a simple example of mechanical energy. The kinetic energy of falling water causes the wheel to turn as the water hits the paddles of the wheel. The wheel goes around, causing gears to turn. These gears turn the grinding stone, which performs the work of crushing grain into flour. The energy of the wheel as it rotates is a form of mechanical energy. See 5-4.

Much of the energy your body uses is mechanical energy. You can view the human

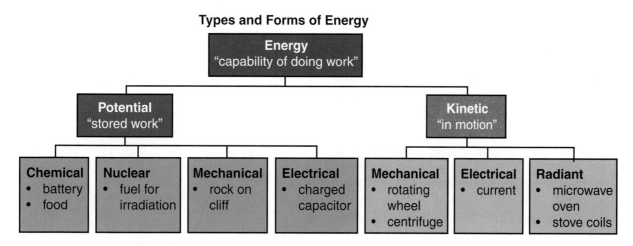

5-3 This flowchart shows one way to organize the types and forms of energy discussed in this chapter.

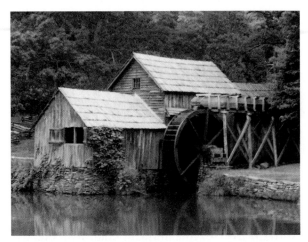

5-4 This mill once used the mechanical energy generated by the waterwheel to run a machine shop, corn mill, and sawmill.

body as a machine. When you move your arm, you are using a lever, which is a type of simple machine. For any motion to occur in the human body, stored energy has to be converted into kinetic energy. Each time you blink, walk to the refrigerator, or chew food, you are using mechanical energy.

Physicists and engineers who develop equipment for food processing are concerned with the efficient and safe use of mechanical energy. They must understand how to develop machinery that will successfully convert energy into a usable form. They must also understand how to perform processing functions without damaging the food product.

Chemical Energy

In chemical reactions, bonds between atoms are broken and/or formed. The forming and breaking of these bonds generates *chemical energy.*

Physical and chemical reactions may be either endothermic or exothermic. A reaction whose products have less total heat than the reactants is called an *endothermic reaction. Endo-* means within. *Thermic* refers to heat. Therefore, an endothermic reaction absorbs or stores energy. The result is a lower temperature after the reaction than before. This is why mixing salt and ice results in a lowering of temperature, as seen in making homemade ice cream. The ice and salt absorb heat energy from the ice cream mixture. This lowers the

temperature of the ice cream and allows it to freeze. The heat energy is used to melt the ice and break the bonds of the salt crystals. As the bonds break, the salt dissolves in the water from the melted ice.

In *exothermic reactions,* energy is released during the reaction. *Exo-* means outside. An exothermic reaction will have a higher temperature after the reaction than before. For example, when sodium hydroxide (NaOH) is dissolved in water, energy is released. This causes the temperature of the water to increase. Sodium hydroxide is commonly known as lye, and it is often used as a drain cleaner. It works by releasing heat when dissolved in water. The heat melts fat, which is the substance that most commonly causes blocked drains. As the fat melts, it combines with the NaOH to form soap. The combination of heat and slippery soap breaks up the clog. The substances that made up the clog can then be easily flushed through the drain pipes. See 5-5.

Digestion is another example of an exothermic reaction. When the food you eat is broken down during digestion, heat is released. Your body can use this heat for warmth.

Most chemical reactions involve a combination of breaking and forming bonds between atoms. For example, when heat is applied to charcoal briquettes (partially burned wood), bonds are broken between carbon and hydrogen atoms in the charcoal.

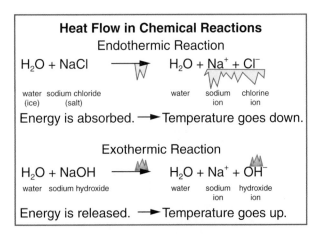

5-5 Many chemical reactions either store or give off heat energy, resulting in a temperature change in the products of the reactions.

Bonds are also broken between oxygen atoms in the air. Two products that are formed from the released atoms are carbon dioxide (CO_2) and water (steam, H_2O). Heat is released as the bonds break, resulting in fire. The energy released in the fire can then be used to cook food.

Chemical energy is the fuel for the human body. Energy for bodily functions comes from the breaking of chemical bonds in carbohydrates, proteins, and fats. The processes used by the body to convert this stored chemical energy in foods is called *metabolism.* Chemical energy is involved in all the processes from food preparation through digestion.

Electrical Energy

One way energy is transported is as **electrical energy,** which is produced by the movement of electrons. Electrical energy can be efficiently transported and changed from one form of energy to another. These characteristics make electrical energy very useful to the food scientist.

Electrical energy is transported through materials that are good conductors. These materials have atoms that remain relatively stationary while allowing electrons to move from negatively to positively charged atoms. Metals like copper and silver are good conductors of electricity.

The energy of falling water can be changed to mechanical energy through a waterwheel. This mechanical energy can then be changed to electrical energy. This is what happens at power electric dams. The electrical energy can then be transported through wires to electric appliances.

Appliances can convert electrical energy into other forms of energy. Lamps can convert electrical energy into light, a form of radiant energy. Toasters and ranges can convert it into heat, which is another form of radiant energy. Blenders, can openers, and electric mixers convert electrical energy back into mechanical energy that can perform work. Think of the many ways people use electricity in your home to help prepare and store food. See 5-6.

Radiant Energy

Radiant energy is energy transmitted in the form of waves through space or some

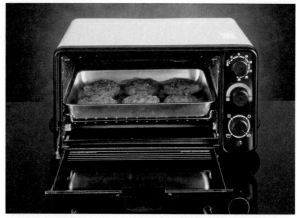

Hamilton Beach/Proctor-Silex, Inc.

5-6 A toaster-oven converts electrical energy to radiant energy.

medium. Radiant energy is also referred to as the electromagnetic spectrum. See 5-7. Visible radiant energy is called *light.* Other examples of radiant energy are radio waves, ultraviolet waves, and microwaves. Part of the energy used to cook food when using electric coils is in the form of radiant energy. Charcoal grills and gas flames use radiant energy to cook food, too.

Microwaves

Microwave ovens convert electrical energy into radiant energy to cook food. The microwave oven's energy source is an electron tube called a **magnetron.** This tube converts electrical energy into **microwaves,** which are low-frequency electromagnetic waves of radiant energy. Microwaves travel in straight lines. They are reflected by metals. However, microwaves pass through many types of glass, paper, and plastic materials. The microwave oven is designed so the interior surfaces reflect the waves toward the food.

Any polar compound will be agitated by microwaves to some extent. Water molecules are polar molecules that are prevalent in most food products. The more water there is present in a food, the faster the food will cook. Radiant energy agitates the water molecules throughout the food. The agitation provides friction, which heats the food. The water then conducts heat energy toward cooler portions of the food. If this food is in a broth, the liquid helps transfer heat, which speeds the heating

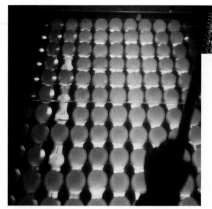

Technology Tidbit
Canning with Electrical Energy

What do you think Borden, McDonalds, General Mills, the U.S. Department of Defense, and NASA have in common? All have donated money and/or equipment to the Ohio State University for research into a new food preservation process. You might wonder why the armed services and NASA would be interested in food preservation. The armed services deliver more preprepared meals than most restaurant chains. These meals are called MREs for "meals ready to eat." NASA needs stable and nutritive lightweight foods for use in space programs.

Researchers at Ohio State are exposing food to rapid electrical pulses. The electrical pulses occur at a rate of 10,000 per second. These pulses are thought to inactivate or kill microorganisms and inactivate enzymes that are present in food. The electrical pulses do not add significant heat energy to the food. As a result, the food maintains near-fresh flavor and quality without the use of refrigeration or freezing.

This new preservation process could result in improved food quality with lower energy costs. This process will also conserve more nutrients than the present canning and freezing methods do.

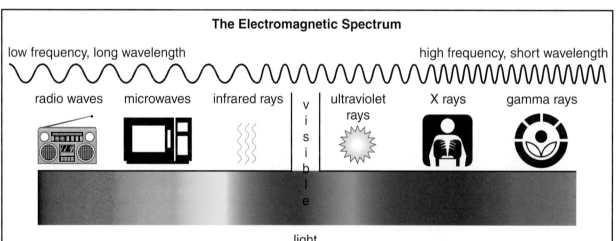

Among the shortest radio waves are microwaves used for cooking. The infrared region provides heat energy and is only absorbed at the surface. Ultraviolet light kills bacteria and can help in food preservation. Ultraviolet light also enables human skin to produce vitamin D. Gamma rays are used in the food preservation method known as irradiation. The gamma rays destroy living organisms present in the food that would cause food spoilage.

5-7 The electromagnetic spectrum shows the complete range of radiant energy.

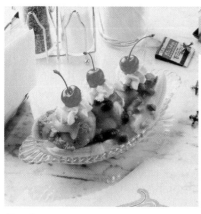

Item of Interest
Electric Life Savers

Equipment

pliers

Supplies

wintergreen Life Savers candies
resealable plastic bag

Procedure

Place the candy in the plastic bag and seal the bag. Take the sealed bag and the pliers into a closet or room without windows. Turn out the lights and wait five minutes for your eyes to adjust to the darkness. Crush the candy with the pliers.

What Happened and Why?

The sugar and menthol in the candy give off a blue-white light when crushed. Mechanical energy from the pliers breaks the candy structure. This breaks bonds between atoms, causing electrons to be separated unevenly. For example, the electron from a hydrogen atom that is shared with an oxygen atom remains with the oxygen atom. The hydrogen atom now has a positive charge and the oxygen atom has a negative charge.

Electrons jump across the gap between candy pieces to balance the positive and negative charges that result. As the electrons move through the air, powered by kinetic electrical energy, they strike or run into nitrogen molecules. The electrical energy from the moving electrons causes electrons in nitrogen to move to a higher orbital or shell. The "excited" nitrogen quickly releases this extra energy and the electrons in the nitrogen move back to their original orbital. The extra energy is released as radiant energy in the form of visible blue-white light. This is basically the same phenomenon that causes lightning.

Striking two sugar cubes together will have the same result to a lesser degree. However, you will not be able to observe this reaction with diabetic candy or clear suckers.

---

process. Foods that are high in fats and sugars also tend to heat rapidly in a microwave oven. These substances help conduct heat from other compounds in the food.

Cooking Tip
To avoid overcooking some areas of frozen foods when using a microwave oven, use low power to defrost. Water molecules locked in crystalline structure (ice) cannot absorb microwaves. Surface water that has melted will absorb energy and heat up; this transfers heat to the next layer of ice. High power will overcook foods on the outside before heat can be transferred to the frozen center of the food.

Induction Cooktops

Induction cooktops use electromagnetic waves to generate heat in food. Special pans are needed to conduct the energy. The bottoms of the pans must also be perfectly flat. Alternating currents create a magnetic field that excites molecules in the pan material. Induction cooktops can boil water in half the time of gas and electric stoves and the surface of the cooktop stays cool.

Nuclear Energy

The newest form of energy to be used in the food industry is nuclear energy. *Nuclear energy* is the result of splitting or combining atoms of certain elements, which then give off

Microwave Safety

Rapid buildup of steam can create pressure that can cause sealed foods to explode in a microwave oven. To help avoid this problem

❖ Vent plastic wrap used to cover food containers.

❖ Pierce whole fruits and vegetables that have tough, unbroken skins.

❖ Never hard-cook or soft-cook eggs in their shells.

Avoid using metal in a microwave oven because it reflects microwaves. Food placed in metal containers will be shielded and will not cook. Also, too many reflected microwaves can overload the oven's magnetron tube, resulting in expensive repairs. However, you can use small pieces of aluminum foil to shield food to prevent overcooking in a microwave oven. For instance, you might cover the ends of drumsticks and wings on chicken and turkey. However, do not allow aluminum foil to come within one inch of the inside walls of the microwave oven. This can cause sparks to jump from the foil to the walls, damaging the lining of the oven.

Researchers have observed that microwaves can superheat water up to 110°C with no sign of boiling. When water is heated on a range-top, boiling action is created by currents transferring heat in the fluid. In a microwave oven, this type of heat transfer cannot keep pace with the heat generated by microwaves. Therefore, the water can reach temperatures above the boiling point before any sign of boiling appears. To avoid injury from boilovers and explosions of superhot liquids,

use caution when heating liquids in a microwave oven. Rapid boiling will begin if any of the following is added to water immediately upon removing it from a microwave oven:

❖ tea bags

❖ powders, such as instant coffee, cocoa mixes, and other hot beverage mixes

❖ ice cubes

A related potential problem can occur when products such as pastries with a jellied filling are heated in a microwave oven. The filling becomes extremely hot, while the exterior of the pastry becomes only warm. This can result in severe burns when the product is eaten.

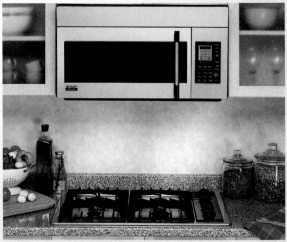
Sharp

Following safety precautions is important when using a microwave oven to prepare food.

radiation. This radiation may be used directly in medicine (X rays) or food preservation (irradiation). It is also used by nuclear power plants to generate electricity. See 5-8.

Measuring Energy

Most scientific understanding comes through studying measurements taken during experimentation. To understand how energy works in food preparation, you need to accurately measure energy and its flow. You need to know the definitions of two energy measurements you will be using in food science: heat and temperature.

Heat

Heat is an energy transfer from one body to another caused by a temperature difference

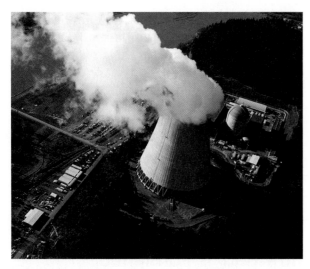

5-8 Nuclear power plants convert nuclear energy to electrical energy.

between the two bodies. The temperature difference is a result of the relative kinetic energies per atom of the two substances. Scientists can measure a substance's ability to produce or absorb heat.

Food scientists most often measure energy in terms of the capacity to produce heat. This unit of measurement is the calorie. One *calorie* is the heat required to raise the temperature of one gram of water one degree Celsius.

Do not confuse this calorie with the term *Calorie* used to measure the energy value of food. A Calorie with a capital *C* is also called a *kilocalorie.* This unit is 1,000 times greater than a calorie with a lowercase *c*. A Calorie is the amount of heat needed to raise the temperature of one kilogram of water one degree Celsius.

Dietitians found it difficult to work with traditional calories when calculating the large energy values of food. Dietitians also found people became depressed when hearing their food intakes associated with large calorie values. (How would you feel if someone told you there were 30,000 calories in one carrot instead of 30?) The Calories dietitians use measure the internal potential energy of foods.

The ability of a substance to absorb heat is called its *heat capacity.* Water has one of the greatest heat capacities of any known substance. This is one reason it makes an excellent cooking medium. Water will rapidly absorb heat and transfer it to any food suspended in the water. The water content of a food product

determines the food's heat capacity. Food with a large water content has a high heat capacity.

Specific heat is the ability of a substance to absorb or transfer heat as compared to water's ability to absorb or transfer heat. The specific heat of water is 1.0 cal/g °C. This means that each calorie of heat will raise the temperature of 1 g of water 1°C. Similarly, the specific heat of any substance is the amount of energy needed to raise the temperature of 1 g of that substance 1°C.

The physical property of specific heat is important in food storage. Cooling foods with low specific heats will require less heat energy to be removed than cooling foods with high specific heats. See 5-9.

Specific heat is one of the many factors researchers analyze when determining the best processing method for a given food. Knowing a food's specific heat will help researchers predict how a food product will react during processing.

Researchers also evaluate the heat produced or released by machinery used in food processing. They want to design processing methods that are *energy efficient.* This means getting the maximum work done for the lowest energy costs.

Temperature

Temperature is the measure of the average kinetic energy of a group of individual molecules. This means that temperature is an indirect measure of molecular motion.

People often confuse temperature with heat, which is the measure of all the kinetic energy in a substance. For example, a glass of water and a pitcher of water may have the same temperature. However, the pitcher holds more heat because it has a greater mass. You can test this by pouring a glass of iced tea from a full pitcher. Note how quickly the tea in the glass reaches room temperature. Compare this with the time required for the remaining tea in the pitcher to reach room temperature.

You can determine whether many foods have finished cooking by measuring their temperatures. Temperature is measured with various types of thermometers. In food preparation and storage, you may need to work with candy, deep-fat, freezer, meat, and oven thermometers.

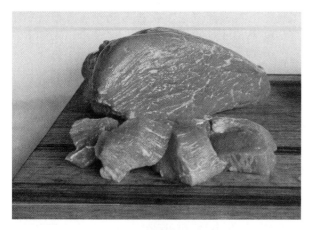

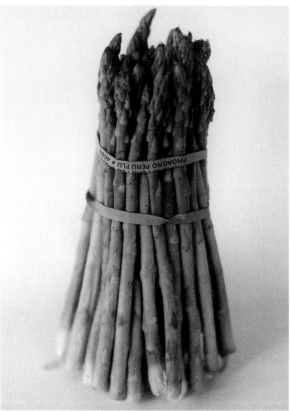

5-9 Lean beef has a lower specific heat than asparagus and thus requires less energy to reduce its temperature. This means less heat energy must be removed from beef than from an equal mass of asparagus during refrigeration.

Carefully monitoring temperature is important when preparing foods at home. A thermometer that is off by 2°C (3°F), can make the difference between creamy fudge candy and gooey fudge sauce. Therefore, it is important to check the accuracy of a candy thermometer before use. Thermometers are calibrated for accurate measurement. However,

mass production can result in calibration slippage. This could throw off the readings of the economical thermometers most people use in their kitchens. See 5-10.

Food companies use precision equipment to carefully monitor temperature during each step of production. Careful monitoring of temperature is especially important in pasteurization, fermentation, bread production, and candy and jelly making. Manufacturers know the difference just a few degrees can make in product quality.

How Heat Is Transferred

Heat flows naturally in only one direction: from hot objects to cooler ones. When the temperature is the same in both objects, heat flow stops. The amount of heat in an object will depend on its size and the material of which it is made. *Thermodynamics* is the branch of physics that studies heat flow and temperature in relation to material properties. Besides an understanding of heat flow and temperature, you need an understanding of the three basic ways heat is transferred. The three basic methods are conduction, convection, and radiation.

Conduction

Conduction is the transfer of heat through matter from particle-to-particle collisions. In conduction, there is no visible motion of the heated body. The movement that occurs is at the molecular level as molecules collide with each other. When a pan touches a heat source, rapidly moving molecules in the heat source collide with the pan's surface. Kinetic energy is transferred to the cooler, slower-moving molecules of the pan. As the molecules in the pan gain energy (heat), they move more rapidly. These molecules then collide with molecules deeper in the pan. Eventually, the inside of the pan transfers kinetic energy to the molecules on the surface of the food. This type of heat transfer also occurs within solid and semisolid food products. Conduction will continue until the heat source, the pan, and the food all have the same temperature. See 5-11.

Only metals make use of electron conduction and are, therefore, the best conductors of

Calibrating a Candy Thermometer

Candy making requires an accurate thermometer. The difference of one or two degrees can determine whether candy sets or remains a thick sugar syrup. For example, fudge that is only slightly overcooked will be dry and hard. If fudge is undercooked by just two degrees, you will have to eat it with a spoon.

You must check the accuracy of a thermometer against a known temperature under certain conditions. After you check the accuracy, you can calibrate, or adjust, the thermometer. To calibrate a thermometer

1. Bring a pot of water to a boil.
2. Insert the thermometer into the center of the boiling water. Do not allow the thermometer to touch the bottom of the pan.
3. Wait until the temperature reading stabilizes.
4. Read the temperature scale at eye level while the bulb is still in the water.
5. If the thermometer does not read 100°C or 212°F, make the proper calculations.
   a. If the thermometer reads too high a temperature, add degrees to the temperature in the recipe. For example, suppose the thermometer reads 103°C in boiling water. The difference between the thermometer and the temperature of boiling water is +3°C. Add 3°C to the temperature in the recipe. If the recipe says to cook to 113°C, you will cook the mixture to 116°C.
   b. If the thermometer reads too low a temperature, subtract degrees from the temperature in the recipe. For example, suppose the thermometer reads 95°C in boiling water. The difference between the thermometer and the temperature of boiling water is -5°C. Subtract 5°C from the temperature in the recipe. If the recipe says to cook to 113°C, you will cook the mixture to 108°C.

The above directions are for calibrating a thermometer at sea level, where water boils at 100°C (212°F). For every 150 meters (500 feet) you climb above sea level, however, the boiling point is lowered about 0.6°C (1°F). Therefore, if you live at an altitude of 2130 meters (7000 feet) above sea level, water would boil at 92°C (198°F). The method for calibrating a thermometer at this altitude would be the same. You would simply have to adjust your calculations to the appropriate boiling temperature.

5-10 Before making candy, calibrate your thermometer to be sure you are accurately measuring the temperature of candy ingredients.

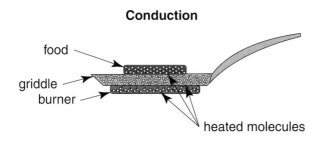

Conduction

food
griddle
burner
heated molecules

5-11 Energy is transferred in conduction through molecular collisions.

heat. In electron conduction, when the electrons collide, they speed up and may skip about the atomic framework of the metal. The next collision could be one, ten, or one hundred atoms from where the previous collision took place. It is because of this skipping of atoms during electron collisions that heat can

be conducted so rapidly through metal. Because metals are also easily shaped and durable, they are the substances most commonly used to make cookware.

Convection

Convection is the transfer of heat by the motion of fluids, such as water or air. It is much faster than conduction. As a fluid is heated, random motion of molecules increases and molecules are pushed farther apart. This decreases the density of the fluid and causes currents to form called *convection currents*. As the fluid heats and becomes less dense, it rises, pushing cooler particles aside. The cooler particles, being more densely packed, sink until they come in contact with the heat source. The cycle repeats until the fluid is the same temperature throughout. See 5-12.

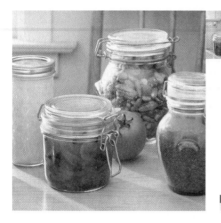

Historical Highlight
Temperature Scales

Reference Temperatures

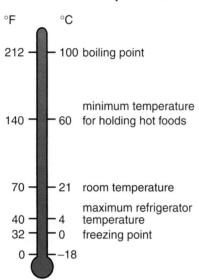

°F	°C	
212	100	boiling point
		minimum temperature
140	60	for holding hot foods
70	21	room temperature
		maximum refrigerator
40	4	temperature
32	0	freezing point
0	−18	

You are likely to use the Fahrenheit temperature scale when measuring food and cooking temperatures in your home kitchen. However, you will be using the Celsius temperature scale to measure temperatures in the food science lab.

Fahrenheit Scale

The Fahrenheit scale is used widely in Great Britain and the United States. It was introduced by Gabriel Daniel Fahrenheit. It is based on two fixed points. These points are the lowest temperature Fahrenheit could reach and his wife's body temperature, which at the time was 96°.

Celsius Scale

Formerly known as the centigrade scale, the Celsius scale was renamed by the Ninth World Conference on Weights and Measures. The name change was to honor the Swedish astronomer Anders Celsius, who first developed the scale in the eighteenth century. This scale is commonly used by scientists because it is based on the boiling and freezing points of water.

Use the following formulas to convert Fahrenheit temperatures to degrees Celsius and Celsius temperatures to degrees Fahrenheit:

$$\frac{5}{9}\,(°F − 32) = °C$$
$$\frac{9}{5}\,°C + 32 = °F$$

Convection

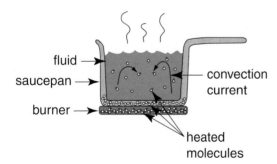

fluid →
saucepan →
burner →
← convection current
heated molecules

5-12 Energy is transferred in convection by molecular collisions and the movement of fluids. As gases and liquids are heated, the molecules move faster and farther apart, causing them to become less dense and rise.

This method of heat transfer is used every time food is cooked in boiling water. The water develops currents that move the energy more rapidly than can be accomplished through conduction alone. This principle is also at work in an oven during baking. The currents in the oven are in the air that is trapped when the door is closed. The coldest air comes in contact with the element at the bottom of the oven. This air rises as it is heated. Again, the convection currents enable heat to transfer at a more rapid rate than conduction alone would allow.

When you open an oven door or lift a pan lid on the range, you should stand to the side. Air currents will move the hottest air rapidly upwards. This could result in steam burns, fogged glasses, or damaged contact lenses.

Radiation

Radiation involves the transfer of heat by electromagnetic waves. Radiation does not require the presence of matter. This is why the energy of the sun can travel through the vacuum of space. Broiling and rotisserie cooking are common methods of using radiation in food production.

A solar oven also cooks food through radiation. Light, like other forms of radiant energy, travels in straight lines. Some materials, such as shiny metals, can reflect it. However, atoms and molecules on the surface of food can absorb light. By reflecting light from the sun into one location, solar ovens can raise temperatures to a point high enough to cook food.

All three forms of heat transfer are usually involved in the cooking of foods. Conduction and convection are responsible for cooking the inside of the food. Radiation is responsible for much of the browning.

Energy Flow in Phase Changes

Before phase change can occur in a substance, a flow of energy must take place. When a substance moves from a solid to a liquid phase, the phase change is called melting or *fusion.* This phase change requires energy to be added to a substance. When a substance moves from the liquid to the solid phase, the phase change is called freezing or *crystallization.* This phase change requires energy to be removed from a substance. The energy needed to melt or freeze a substance is called the *latent heat of fusion.*

When water boils, steam rises from the pan. Water is a liquid and steam is a gas. See 5-13. When a substance changes from the liquid to the gaseous phase, the phase change is called *evaporation* or *vaporization.* When energy is released from steam, the steam cools and condenses back into water. *Condensation* or *liquefaction* is the change of a gas to a liquid. The amount of heat needed to either evaporate or condense a substance is called the *latent heat of vaporization.*

You could make a graph of the temperature change in water as it moves from frozen to liquid to gas. This graph would show extended plateaus at the melting and boiling

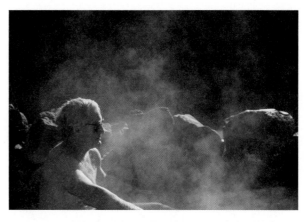

5-13 Steam is the gas phase of water.

points. This characteristic of the measure of temperature over time reveals another fact about energy flow. At the point of a phase change, the temperature will remain constant. The temperature will not change until all the molecules have organized themselves into a new pattern. For example, all water molecules must organize themselves into a crystal formation when water becomes ice. The energy needed to complete this rearranging of molecules is called *latent heat.* It is the energy required to complete a phase change without a change in temperature.

Under certain temperature and pressure conditions, the liquid phase can be skipped. For instance, you may have seen frost form on a window on a cold morning. This is an example of water vapor in the air (gas) changing directly to a solid state. Changing a substance directly from the gas phase to the solid phase is called *deposition.* Deposition requires energy to be released from a substance. The deposition of frost on an ice cream freezer indicates the freezer is cold enough to freeze ice cream.

Another process that skips the liquid phase is sublimation. *Sublimation* is changing a substance directly from a solid to a gas. It requires energy to be added to a substance. If you have ever seen gas rising from dry ice, you have seen sublimation. Dry ice is solid carbon dioxide. Instead of melting into a liquid, it sublimes directly into a gas. Sublimation is used in the food industry to freeze and dry foods at the same time. Freeze-dried coffee and instant tea are food products developed through sublimation.

If a substance is being cooled, latent heat is being released. This occurs during freezing, condensing, and deposition. If a substance is being heated, latent heat is being used or absorbed. This occurs during melting, vaporization, and sublimation. See 5-14.

Factors That Affect Rates of Reaction in Food Preparation

You have examined the forms, position, measurement, and flow of energy. In addition, there are several factors that will influence how energy works in food preparation. One of these factors is the presence of enzymes, which you will read about in Chapter 12. Other factors or variables that influence the rate of reaction are temperature, surface area, and thickness of the food.

Temperature of Reactants

As temperature increases, so does molecular motion. The faster molecules move, the more they collide. Collisions must occur before chemicals can react with each other. Therefore, the speed of a chemical reaction is directly related to the temperature of the reactants. The rate of a reaction approximately doubles for every 10°C increase in temperature. This is why a roast cooks faster in an oven than in a slow cooker, which uses lower temperatures.

Amount of Surface Area

The greater the surface area is, the faster the reaction will be. This is because so much heat transfer occurs through conduction. For conduction to work, molecules must come in contact with each other. The larger the surface area is, the greater the chance of contact. Increasing the surface area of a food exposed to a heat source is a way to speed up the rate of cooking. For example, a four-pound shoulder roast will take seven to eight hours in a slow cooker. The same roast cut into cubes and stewed in the same cooker would take three to five hours.

Thickness of the Food

A principle related to surface area is the thickness of the food. Obviously, the farther the center of a food is from the surface, the longer it will take the food to cook completely. When you cut food, you not only increase the surface area, you also decrease the distance to the center. See 5-15.

One reason microwaves can speed cooking is that microwaves can penetrate to a depth of 5 to 7.5 cm (2 to 3 inches). This penetration enables cooking to begin below the surface long before energy could be transferred from the surface inward. Foods that are thicker than 10 to 15 cm (4 to 6 inches) should be cooked at lower power levels. This will allow for the time needed to conduct energy into the center without overcooking the surface.

Phase Changes

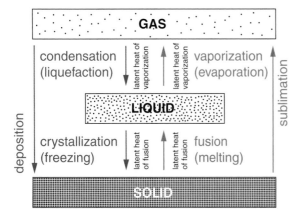

5-14 The phase changes shown in blue release energy and reflect a decrease in molecular disorder. The phase changes shown in red require added energy and reflect an increase in molecular disorder.

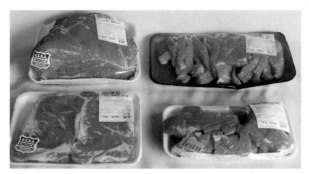

5-15 Smaller pieces of meat have more surface area and less distance to the center of each piece than larger pieces. Therefore, they will cook faster.

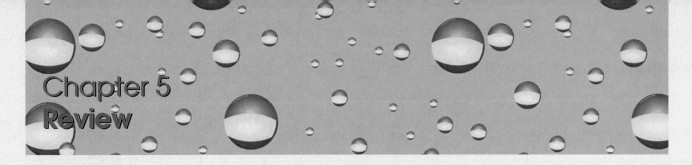

Chapter 5 Review

Summary

Energy is the ability to do work. Potential energy is stored energy, and kinetic energy is energy in motion. The five forms of energy—mechanical, chemical, electrical, radiant, or nuclear—can be converted from one form into another. Each form has important functions somewhere in the food chain.

Heat is the measure of the total kinetic energy of a substance. It is measured in calories. Temperature is the average kinetic energy of individual molecules. Temperature is measured in degrees Celsius or Fahrenheit.

Heat flows in one direction, from hot objects to cooler ones. However, it can flow in one of three ways. Conduction involves molecular collisions. Convection occurs through currents of fluids. Radiation uses electromagnetic waves. A good cook knows when and how to control all three types of heat flow. Other factors that must be controlled are the temperature of reactants, the surface area, and the thickness of the food.

An understanding of how energy relates to food can help you choose foods, preparation methods, and cookware. You can use your knowledge of energy to improve food quality and reduce waste.

Check Your Understanding

1. What is the difference between external potential energy and internal kinetic energy?
2. List the five forms of energy and give an example of each in relation to food.
3. Describe the difference between exothermic and endothermic reactions.
4. List three ways people cook food using radiant energy.
5. How does a calorie differ from a Calorie?
6. Explain the difference between heat transfer through conduction and convection.
7. How does heat transfer through radiation differ from conduction and convection?
8. Name the phase changes that require the addition of energy and give an example of each in food preparation.
9. Name the phase changes that require the removal of energy and give an example of each in food preparation.
10. List three factors that can affect the rate of reaction or energy flow in cooking. Give an example of each.

Critical Thinking

1. What kind of energy conversion is performed by a food processor and a waffle baker?
2. Would you use a thermometer to measure heat or temperature? Explain your answer.
3. Explain why it is important to calibrate a thermometer.
4. Explain how a microwave oven uses all three methods of heat transfer to cook food.
5. Assume you have all day to prepare a meal. Plan a menu using turkey, potatoes, broccoli, and apples. Plan a second menu with these foods that you could prepare in one hour. Apply what you know about factors that affect rates of reaction in food preparation.

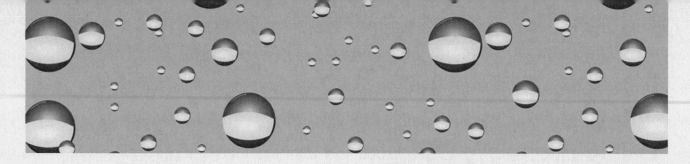

Explore Further

1. **Analytical skills.** Research the specific heats of various cookware materials. Recommend the best material for keeping cooked food warm and for rapid heating. Give reasons for your recommendations.

2. **Math.** Convert the Calories from three food labels to calories as defined by the scientific world.

3. **Communication.** Set up a class debate on the merits of microwave ovens versus conventional ovens. (A third group could prepare to debate the merits of convection ovens.)

4. **Reading.** Research the career field of thermodynamics, physics, thermochemistry, or mechanical engineering. List specific careers in the field related to food science. Describe the training needed for careers in the field.

5. **Science.** Set up a procedure that will determine which of three methods is the fastest for cooking a baked potato in a conventional oven. The methods are wrapped in foil, wrapped in foil with a heat pipe inserted vertically, and unwrapped with a heat pipe inserted horizontally. Report your findings to the class and explain the results in terms of the principles discussed in the chapter.

6. **Reading.** Research types of campfire or outdoor cookers. Using supplies from home, construct one of the cookers you investigated. Report to the class how and why your cooker works. Describe how effective it would be on a camping trip.

7. **Research.** Investigate new cooking appliances that use infrared, high-wattage bulbs and induction coil cooktops. Report to the class on the advantages and disadvantages compared to traditional gas and electric cooktops and microwaves.

Experiment 5A
The Boiling Point of Various Mixtures

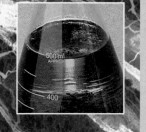

Purpose

During this lab, you will determine which substances lower or raise the boiling point of water. Pure water boils at 100°C. Adding other substances to water changes the boiling point.

Equipment

400-mL beaker

15-mL (1-tablespoon) metric measuring spoon

100-mL graduated cylinder

thermometer, calibrated

thermometer holder

Supplies

200 mL distilled water

assigned ingredient

Procedure

1. Measure 200 mL of distilled water in a 400-mL beaker.
2. Add the ingredient of your assigned variation.

Variation 1: 15 mL (1 tablespoon) flour

Variation 2: 15 mL (1 tablespoon) sugar

Variation 3: 15 mL (1 tablespoon) NaCl (table salt)

Variation 4: 15 mL (1 tablespoon) KCl (potassium chloride)

Variation 5: 25 mL isopropyl alcohol

Variation 6: 25 mL vinegar

3. Place a thermometer in the center of the mixture and place the beaker on the heat source.
4. Heat the mixture until it boils, using the glass rod to stir the mixture occassionally as it heats. Record the temperature of the boiling mixture.
5. Continue boiling the mixture for 2 minutes. Record the temperature.
6. Use a bar graph to chart the classes data.

Questions

1. What substances raised the boiling point of water?
2. What substances lowered the boiling point of water?
3. Did the boiling point change with continued heating for any substances?
4. Use the information you gathered in this experiment to write a hypothesis about the boiling points of mixtures.

Experiment 5B
Heat Transfer in Potatoes

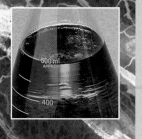

Purpose
In this experiment, you will observe how energy moves from water through food during cooking. You will be collecting data from thermometers placed at different depths in a potato. Then you will be presenting the data in a series of line graphs, with each line representing a different thermometer.

Equipment
1000-mL beaker
vegetable peeler
3 thermometers
wax pencil
vegetable brush
electronic balance
metric ruler
thermometer holder
beaker tongs
cooking tongs
saucer
terry cloth towel

Supplies
250- to 300-g potato
350 mL water
foil

Procedure
1. Clean a 1000-mL beaker, a potato peeler, and three thermometers with hot, soapy water.
2. Use a wax pencil to label the three thermometers A, B, and C.
3. Use a vegetable brush to wash the potato to remove soil from the surface.
4. Mass the potato and record the mass in a data table.
5. Measure and record the length and width of the potato. Use this data to calculate the center point on the top of the potato. Mark this point.
6. Measure and record the height of the potato. Use this measurement to determine half the depth of the potato. Use a wax pencil to mark this length on thermometer A, measuring from the center of the bulb up.
7. Use a vegetable peeler to make a slit down into the center of the potato at the point marked in step 5. Insert thermometer A to the mark measuring half the depth of the potato.
8. From the length measurement taken in step 5, determine one-fourth of the length of the potato. Mark this point on the top of the potato in a straight line from thermometer A to one end of the potato. Make a slit at this spot with the vegetable peeler.
9. Use the height measurement taken in step 6 to determine one-fourth of the depth of the potato. Use a wax pencil to mark this length on thermometer B, measuring from the center of the bulb up. Insert thermometer B into the slit made one-fourth of the way from the end of the potato in step 8. Insert thermometer B no further than the mark indicating one-fourth of the depth of the potato.

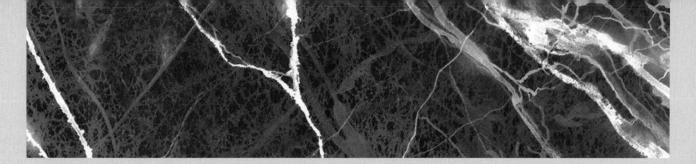

10. Pour 350 mL water into the 1000-mL beaker. Place the beaker on a medium-high heat source and bring the water to a boil.

11. Lower the potato with the inserted thermometers into the boiling water.

12. Insert thermometer C into a thermometer holder. Clip the holder with the thermometer to the side of the beaker. Position the thermometer in the water so it is suspended above the bottom of the beaker and the bulb is completely surrounded by water.

13. Continue to heat the beaker on medium-high heat. Record the temperature reading from each thermometer every minute until thermometer A has reached 90°C.

14. Remove the beaker from the heat with beaker tongs.

15. Carefully remove the potato from the beaker with cooking tongs. Handle the potato according to your assigned variation, making sure to keep thermometers A and B in place.

    Variation 1: Place the potato on a saucer.

    Variation 2: Wrap the potato in foil.

    Variation 3: Wrap the potato in a terry cloth towel.

    Variation 4: Wrap the potato in foil and then in a terry cloth towel.

16. Continue to record the temperature of the potato according to thermometers A and B for another ten minutes.

17. Remove the thermometers and mass the potato. Record the mass in the data table. Cut the potato in half. Observe the interior.

Calculations

Calculate the average cooking time for the potatoes among all the lab groups. Was there any relationship between length of cooking time and the intial mass of the potato?

Questions

1. Did the mass of the potato change during cooking? Why or why not?

2. Is there any relationship between the depth of the potato and the cooking time?

3. Plot the temperature readings from each of the thermometers on a line graph. Compare the graphed data and explain the differences.

4. Why did the temperature of the boiling water go down when the potato was first added? Why did the temperature of the water climb above 100°C after the potato was added?

5. What happened to the appearance of the water?

6. Where did the bubbles form as the potato cooked?

Experiment 5C
Freezing Cream

Safety

- ❖ Wash equipment and work surfaces before starting the lab.
- ❖ Check seals on bags to prevent leaks.
- ❖ Wrap the ice bag in a towel to insulate it and protect your hands from the cold.
- ❖ Avoid contaminating the ice cream with salt. Wash the thermometer used to measure the temperature of the ice-salt mixture before using it to measure the temperature of the ice cream. Also clean the outside of the ice cream bag before sampling the ice cream.

Purpose

During this lab, you will evaluate the role salt plays in the process of freezing ice cream. To prepare a smooth ice cream product, you must constantly mix the ingredients during the chilling process. You will be taking temperature readings to examine the flow of energy during the physical and chemical changes that occur as you mix the ingredients.

Equipment

100-mL graduated cylinder
metric measuring spoons
thermometer
electronic balance
terry cloth towel

Supplies

125 mL (½ cup) half-and-half
75 mL (⅓ cup) whipping cream
30 mL (2 tablespoons) sugar
3 mL (¾ teaspoon) vanilla
30 mL (2 tablespoons) pasteurized egg substitute

1-quart resealable plastic bag
dash of salt
230 g ice
1-gallon resealable plastic bag
rock salt or potassium chloride

Procedure

1. Measure half-and-half, whipping cream, sugar, vanilla, and egg substitute. Combine these ingredients in a 1-quart resealable plastic bag and add one dash of salt.
2. Measure and record the temperature of the mixture in the 1-quart bag.
3. Squeeze the excess air out of the bag and seal.
4. Mass 230 g of ice and
   Variation 1: 90 g of rock salt
   Variation 2: 45 g of rock salt
   Variation 3: 135 g of rock salt
   Variation 4: 45 g of potassium chloride
5. Place the ice in a 1-gallon resealable plastic bag.
6. Measure and record the temperature of the ice.
7. Add the rock salt or potassium chloride to the ice. Then place the 1-quart bag into the 1-gallon bag and seal.
8. Wrap the bags with a terry cloth towel and gently knead the bags for 10 minutes.
9. Check and record the temperature of the ice and salt mixture. Wash the thermometer.
10. Remove the 1-quart bag from the 1-gallon bag. Clean the outside of the 1-quart bag.
11. Check and record the temperature of the ice cream mixture.
12. Sample each of the ice cream variations. Describe the consistency of each variation.

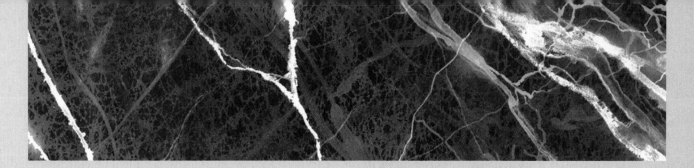

Questions

1. What difference did the amount of salt make to the ice cream?

2. What difference did the kind of salt make to the ice cream?

3. Which variation gave the best quality ice cream product?

4. How can you apply what you learned in this lab to other food situations?

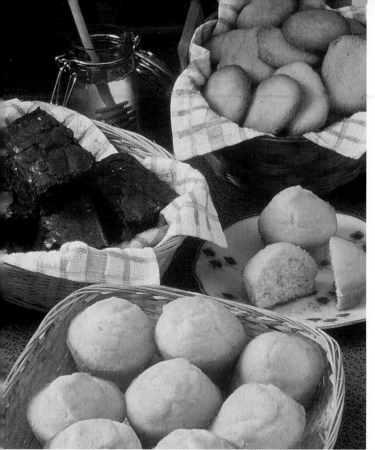

The acid and base levels of batters and doughs can affect the quality of baked goods.

Chapter 6

Ions: Charged Particles in Solution

Objectives

After studying this chapter, you will be able to

describe the ionization of water.

distinguish between the characteristics of acids and the characteristics of bases.

state how the pH scale is used to identify acids and bases.

explain the role of pH in food preservation and baking applications.

Key Terms

ionization

hydrogen ion

hydronium ion

hydroxide ion

acid

base

salt

neutral

proton donor

proton acceptor

Bronsted-Lowry theory

organic dye

pH scale

indicator

titration

endpoint

equivalence point

neutralization

concentration

Avogadro's number

mole

molarity (M)

buffer

botulism

chemical leavening agent

You have probably heard the terms *sour stomach, bitter herbs, buffered aspirin, heartburn,* and *acid rain.* What do these terms describe?

How are they related? To answer these questions, you need to take a close look at charged particles in solutions. You also need to define the terms *acids, bases,* and *salts.*

Acids, bases, and salts are a related group of compounds. The structure and function of these compounds could not be defined until the nineteenth and early twentieth centuries. However, these substances have been recognized as a fundamental category of chemical compounds since ancient times. These substances have been primary factors in food preservation and wine, cheese, and bread making throughout history, 6-1. Acids and bases also play a key role in digestion and many other bodily functions. Understanding how this classification of compounds function can improve your baking skills. Knowledge about acids, bases, and salts can also help you maintain a safer, healthier food supply.

Defining Acids and Bases

In Chapter 4, you read that ions are charged particles or particles that have an imbalance of electrons and protons. You also learned in Chapter 4 that ions of opposite charges can form ionic bonds. These concepts provide a basis for learning about acids and bases and how they react in foods. Looking at water molecules can also help you better understand acids, bases, and salts.

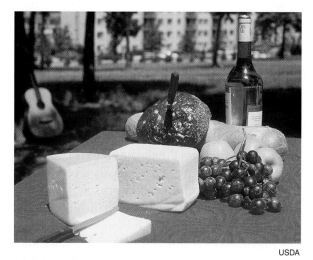

USDA

6-1 The production of these food products is based on principles of acid and base reactions.

The Ionization of Water

You will recall the chemical formula for water is H_2O. Two hydrogen atoms are bonded to one oxygen atom. However, a close analysis of water shows that pure water is not just a group of H_2O molecules. At any given time, a small number of molecules in a volume of water are separating into ions and then recombining. This process of forming ions is called *ionization.* It is represented by the chemical equation below. The ability of the reaction to move in either direction is represented by a double-ended arrow.

$$H_2O \longleftrightarrow H^+ + OH^-$$

During the ionization process, a hydrogen atom breaks away from the water molecule. It leaves its electron with the oxygen atom. Remember that atoms prefer to have their outermost electron shell either full or empty. When the hydrogen atom gives its only electron to the OH group, it has an empty electron shell. The hydrogen atom becomes a positively charged *hydrogen ion,* which is represented by the symbol H^+. However, scientists have found that hydrogen ions do not exist in water.

A hydrogen ion has no electrons. Therefore, it is immediately drawn to bond with a water molecule with which it can share a pair of electrons. This forms a group of three hydrogen atoms and one oxygen atom. The group has a total of 11 protons but only 10 electrons, giving the group a positive charge. A hydrogen atom bonded to a water molecule is called a *hydronium ion* and is represented by the symbol H_3O^+.

An oxygen atom has two empty spaces in its outer shell. The hydrogen atom remaining in the OH group shares its electron with the oxygen atom. The transfer of the electron from the hydrogen atom that broke away fills the oxygen atom's outer electron shell. This means the OH group has a total of 10 electrons. However, it has only nine protons, eight in the oxygen atom and one in the hydrogen atom. Therefore, the OH group becomes a negatively charged *hydroxide ion,* which is represented by the symbol OH⁻. See 6-2.

Hydrogen, hydronium, and hydroxide ions are used to define acids and bases. *Acids*

The Ionization of Water

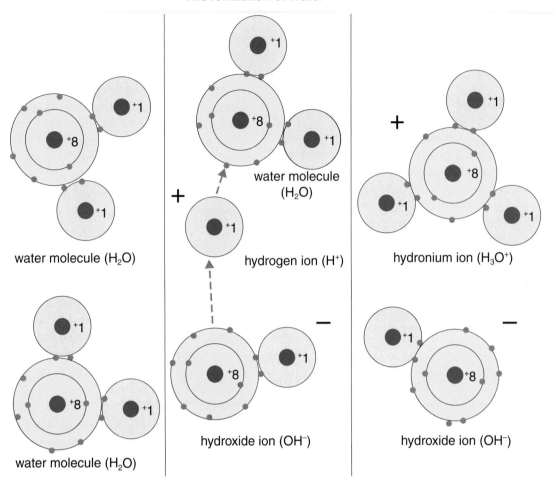

water molecule (H₂O)

hydrogen ion (H⁺)

water molecule (H₂O)

water molecule (H₂O)

hydronium ion (H₃O⁺)

hydroxide ion (OH⁻)

hydroxide ion (OH⁻)

6-2 When a hydrogen atom breaks away from a water molecule, the atom leaves its electron behind. This creates a positive hydrogen ion and a negative hydroxide ion. The hydrogen ion is immediately drawn to another water molecule, creating a hydronium ion.

are substances that create a surplus of hydrogen ions or hydronium ions. Acids have a positive charge. *Bases* are substances that produce a surplus of hydroxide ions. Bases have a negative charge. Bases are also called *alkalis*. If acids and bases combine to form a compound with ionic bonds, that compound is called a *salt.*

A substance is *neutral* when it has an equal number of positive and negative charges. Pure water is neutral because it always has an equal number of hydronium and hydroxide ions.

Theories of Acids and Bases

In 1923, two scientists independently developed a theory that explained how acids and bases work at the molecular level. The scientists who developed this theory were the

Danish chemist Johannes Bronsted and the English chemist Thomas Lowry. These chemists found that acids and bases separate in water to form ions.

In chemical reactions, acids donate hydrogen ions (H⁺) and bases accept hydrogen ions. Because a hydrogen atom only has one electron to give up, a hydrogen ion is a single proton. Therefore, acids are compounds that easily give up the proton from a hydrogen atom. They are *proton donors.* Acids have extra H⁺ ions they can contribute. Bases easily accept protons and are therefore called *proton acceptors.* Bases have a negative charge and will readily accept H⁺ ions.

These facts about the nature of acids and bases are summarized in the *Bronsted-Lowry theory.* This theory states that acids are proton donors and bases are proton acceptors. This

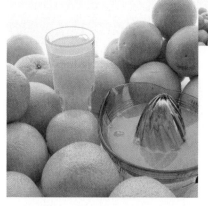

Nutrition News
Salt in the Diet

Nutrition Facts panels on food product labels recommend limiting your sodium intake to no more than 2,400 mg daily. However, many people in the United States consume well over 3,000 mg of sodium a day. The main dietary source of sodium is salt. Therefore, a diet high in salt is high in sodium.

There is some evidence that salt preference is established through exposure between the ages of one and three. Therefore, parents should limit the amount of sodium in the diets of young children. This may help those children control their salt intake when they grow older.

Research has linked excess sodium in the diet to a number of health problems. For some people, excess sodium can increase the risk of high blood pressure. Sodium also speeds calcium loss from bones. For each teaspoon of salt you consume in a day, you will lose 23 mg of calcium from your bones. This equals 10% of your total bone mass over each 10-year period. Bone loss is associated with fractures and related complications, especially in later life. A third health problem that may be tied to excess sodium intake is stomach cancer. Sodium appears to irritate the lining of the stomach, which increases the chances of cancer cells developing. Excess sodium has an additional risk for athletes. Too much salt causes dehydration of cells and increases potassium loss, which leads to chronic fatigue.

To reduce your risk of these health concerns, registered dietitians recommend that you avoid high-sodium foods. Besides salt, these foods include many processed foods, such as frozen dinners, canned soups and vegetables, and processed cheeses. Sauces and seasonings, such as soy sauce, ketchup, and chili powder, are high in salt, too.

Try flavoring foods without the use of salt and high-sodium seasonings. Ground pepper, fresh herbs, onion, cumin, and curry powder are all low in sodium. It will take you about four to six weeks to become used to foods with less salt.

---

scientific explanation also states that, whenever possible, acids and bases naturally react with their opposites to achieve a neutral charge. The Bronsted-Lowry theory defines acids and bases in terms of proton needs that will achieve this balance.

The Bronsted-Lowry theory is the most comprehensive theory about the nature of acids and bases. Even so, it does not explain the reaction in known acids like carbon dioxide (CO_2). Carbon dioxide is the source of carbonation for soft drinks. However, it does not have a hydrogen ion or proton to donate.

Another discovery about acids and bases was made in 1923 by an American chemist named Newton Lewis. Lewis discovered that acid/base reactions could be described in terms of the movement of electrons. In acids and bases where there is no hydrogen involved, ions are looking to donate or accept electrons. Substances that donate electrons are bases, and substances that accept electrons are acids. Carbon dioxide is an acid because it is an electron acceptor.

Identifying Acids and Bases

You can identify acids and bases in two common ways. One way is through sensory evaluation. You can also identify acids and bases with the use of organic dyes.

Sensory Evaluation of Acids and Bases

A simple way to identify many acids and bases is by sensory evaluation, such as taste testing. You must use caution, however, because not all acids and bases are safe to taste. Poisoning can result from tasting certain acids and bases. In those cases where testing can be done safely, you would find that acids taste sour. Lemons, grapefruit, cranberries, vinegar, and yogurt contain acids that are safe to taste, 6-3. Bases have a bitter flavor. Quinine water, milk of magnesia, and baking soda are examples of bases that are safe to taste.

Another type of sensory evaluation that can help you identify bases is to touch them with your fingers. Again, you must use caution. Some bases can cause severe chemical

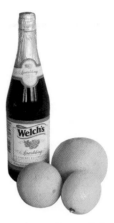

6-3 Citrus fruits and cranberry juice taste sour because they contain acids.

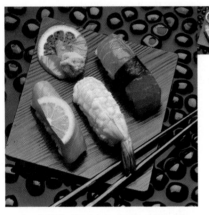

International Issue
Acid Rain

In 1852, Robert Angus Smith became Britain's first official Alkali Inspector. In this role, Smith was responsible for monitoring pollution. He reported on the chemistry of the air in Manchester, England, an industrial city. The closer Smith was to the city, the more acidic he found the air to be. However, he found that winds could carry acidic particles 100 to 2,000 kilometers from the city.

In 1872, Smith coined the term *acid rain*. He noted that acid rain damaged plants and materials. Smith also noted that people in affected areas had more cases of bronchitis and pneumonia.

In 1972, acid rain gained public attention at the United Nations Conference on the Human Environment.

What Is Acid Rain?

More study is needed for experts to agree on a clear definition for acid rain. They currently debate what level of pH constitutes acid rain. It may be easier to define acid rain by the kind of dissolved acids than by the pH level.

A number of factors have been found to affect the pH of rain. As rain falls to earth, it dissolves acids from pollutants and carbon dioxide from the air. These compounds lower the pH of rain to an acidic 5.6. Excess dust can raise the pH of rain to a pH of 7.0 or 8.0. Lightning, volcanoes, and decaying plants can lower the pH of rain to 4.5 to 5.0.

What Causes Acid Rain?

The main components in acid rain are linked to sulfur and nitrogen oxides. Sources of these

acidic compounds are fossil fuels and vehicle exhaust.

What Are the Effects of Acid Rain?

Acid rain damages materials, corrodes metals, and eats away buildings and statues. It has a possible negative impact on the health of people living in affected areas. It has effects on agricultural and aquatic ecosystems. Some forested areas have lost trees to excessive acid. Entire lakes and streams have become too acidic to support fish life.

Research during the 1970s and 1980s has been inconclusive. Balancing the possible dangers caused by acid rain against the economic costs of correcting the problem is difficult.

What concerns do you have about acid rain? What role can you play in helping to control it?

burns. When examining bases that are safe to touch, you will find they have a slippery feel. As you may have guessed, soaps and cleansers are bases.

Organic Dyes

Historically, the second method of identifying acids and bases is with organic dyes. *Organic dyes* are naturally occurring color pigments that change color when exposed to acids or bases. The most widely used organic dye in science classes is *litmus*. Litmus is extracted from a plant and added to paper strips. These strips are convenient and economical to use in science laboratories. When litmus paper is dipped in acids, it will turn red. When litmus paper is dipped in bases, it will turn blue. Another common indicator used in science labs is pHydrion paper. It turns shades of yellow to orange red in acids and yellow green to blue green in bases. See 6-4.

Acids and bases affect the colors of fruits and vegetables that contain organic dyes. These fruits and vegetables include plums, blueberries, cherries, red onions, and red cabbage. For instance, red cabbage retains its red color in cooking liquid that is acidic. If the cooking liquid is alkaline, however, the cabbage will turn bluish purple.

Red and purple fruits and vegetables are not the only foods affected by acids and bases. Green vegetables will be brighter green if you add baking soda while cooking. However, this is not a recommended practice. Remember that baking soda is a base. Therefore, you will neutralize the vitamin C (ascorbic acid) content of vegetables when you add baking soda.

It is easier to observe the color changes of organic dyes if they are dissolved in water. You can simmer fruit or vegetable skins or pieces in distilled water. When the dye leaves the food and colors the water, you will have an organic dye solution.

Measuring Acids and Bases

Stomach acid is described as a "strong" acid and tea as a "weak" acid. For a scientist, such descriptions are not very accurate. One person's definition of weak may be different from another's. Scientists need a way to accurately define and measure the acidity of a substance. This can be critical in the food industry. A small difference can determine whether harmful bacteria will be able to grow in a food product.

The *pH scale* was developed to express the degree of concentration of hydrogen or hydronium ions present in a solution. The larger the number of hydronium ions in a solution, the more concentrated the acid will be. A food scientist at a beverage bottling plant developed the pH scale. He was responsible for monitoring the acid level of the beverage during production. He found using the number representing the power of the hydronium ions in the mathematical formula would simplify his records. Thus the lowercase *p* stands for "power of" and the capital *H* stands for "hydronium ions." Chart 6-5 shows the relationship between pH scale, hydrogen or hydronium ions, and hydroxide ions. The pH scale is used to show how the acidity or alkalinity of solutions are related. Note that each number in the pH scale represents 10 times greater or fewer hydronium ions.

A solution with a pH of 1.0, such as the hydrochloric acid in the human stomach, is very concentrated. A cup of coffee with a pH of 5.0 is a dilute acid solution. Water has a pH of 7.0 and is neutral. It does not exhibit characteristics of either an acid or a base. That is because in *pure* water the hydronium and hydroxide ions are always in balance. A base

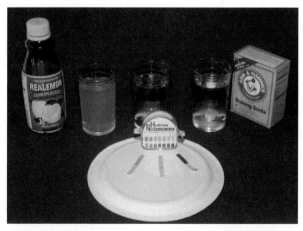

6-4 This pH paper turned orange in an acidic solution of lemon juice and green in a basic solution of baking soda.

has a pH of 7.1 to 14.0. Blood has a pH of 7.4 and is therefore slightly basic. Ammonia, a common household cleaner, has a pH of 11.0. Sodium hydroxide (NaOH) drain cleaner, which is commonly called lye, has a pH of 14.0. It is a very concentrated base. See 6-6.

It is important to understand the difference between strength and concentration of acids and bases. The stronger an acid or base is, the more completely it reacts with water to form ions. A pure acid or base is concentrated. The more water you add, the more dilute the

The pH Scale

pH	Concentration of Hydrogen or Hydronium Ions (molecules per liter)		Concentration of Hydroxide Ions (molecules per liter)
1	0.1	or 10^{-1}	10^{-13}
2	0.01	or 10^{-2}	10^{-12}
3	0.001	or 10^{-3}	10^{-11}
4	0.0001	or 10^{-4}	10^{-10}
5	0.00001	or 10^{-5}	10^{-9}
6	0.000001	or 10^{-6}	10^{-8}
7	0.0000001	or 10^{-7}	10^{-7}
8	0.00000001	or 10^{-8}	10^{-6}
9	0.000000001	or 10^{-9}	10^{-5}
10	0.0000000001	or 10^{-10}	10^{-4}
11	0.00000000001	or 10^{-11}	10^{-3}
12	0.000000000001	or 10^{-12}	10^{-2}
13	0.0000000000001	or 10^{-13}	10^{-1}
14	0.00000000000001	or 10^{-14}	10^{-0}

6-5 The pH scale is based on the number of hydronium ions present in a solution.

pH of Some Common Foods

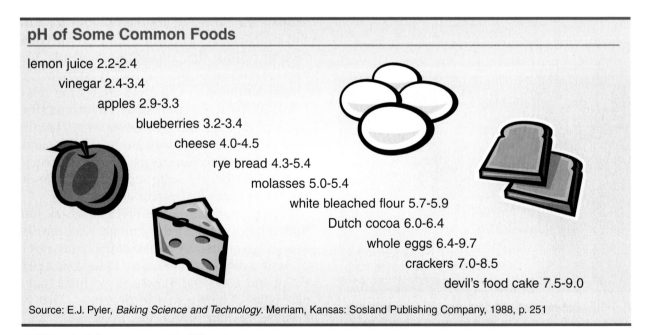

lemon juice 2.2-2.4
vinegar 2.4-3.4
apples 2.9-3.3
blueberries 3.2-3.4
cheese 4.0-4.5
rye bread 4.3-5.4
molasses 5.0-5.4
white bleached flour 5.7-5.9
Dutch cocoa 6.0-6.4
whole eggs 6.4-9.7
crackers 7.0-8.5
devil's food cake 7.5-9.0

Source: E.J. Pyler, *Baking Science and Technology*. Merriam, Kansas: Sosland Publishing Company, 1988, p. 251

6-6 Foods fall at a range of pH levels.

acid or base becomes. Hydrochloric acid is a strong acid whether it is concentrated or diluted with water.

In summary, the greater the hydrogen or hydronium ion concentration is, the more concentrated the acid and the lower the pH will be. The greater the hydroxide ion concentration is, the more concentrated the base and the higher the pH will be. See 6-7.

It is important to remember that very strong acids and very strong bases will cause severe burns. That is why you need to wear splash goggles whenever you are experimenting with acids and bases. If you splash any strong acid or base on skin, immediately flush the area with running water. This will dilute the acid or base and help prevent damage.

Measuring pH

Scientists have two methods of measuring pH. The most economical is using organic dyes. These organic dyes are called *indicators.* An indicator demonstrates through color change the degree of acidity of a solution. The problem with organic dyes is accuracy. Scientists know that litmus is blue at pH 8.0. However, it is also blue at pH 7.5 and pH 10.0. To get a more accurate reading, you need a pH meter. The meter has a probe that you insert into a solution. Most pH meters will give accurate readings to a tenth of a pH unit. See 6-8.

Food scientists often use another method to measure the pH of foods. This method is called *titration.* It is the process of adding a base with a known pH to an acid. Titration is also the process of adding an acid with a known pH to a base. An indicator is added to the unknown. Using a burette, the base or acid whose pH is known is dispensed into the unknown a drop at a time. Scientists look for a color change to occur. Then they can calculate how many acid molecules had to be present to neutralize all the base molecules.

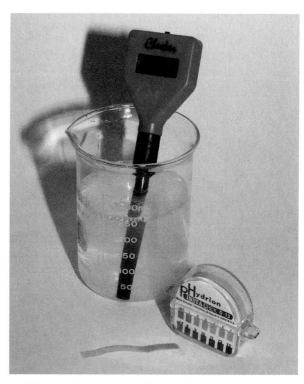

6-8 You can measure pH with pH paper. For more accurate pH readings, however, use a digital pH meter.

Characteristics of Acids and Bases

Acids are any substances that:	Bases are any substances that:
Produce excess hydronium or hydrogen ions	Produce excess hydroxide ions
Have a positive electrical charge	Have a negative electrical charge
Are proton donors	Are proton acceptors
Are electron acceptors	Are electron donors
Taste sour	Taste bitter
Turn litmus red	Turn litmus blue
Have a pH of 1.0 to 6.9	Have a pH of 7.1 to 14.0

6-7 Remembering these characteristics will help you distinguish acids from bases.

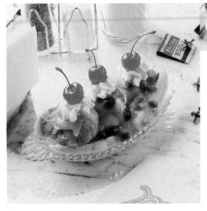

Item of Interest
pH and the Farmer

Your garden may consist of a tomato plant on the patio or acres of a food crop produced for market. In either case, pH is an important consideration. Food crops will grow in a soil pH of 5 to 8. However, most prefer a pH of 6 to 7. This is because microorganisms work best at a slightly acidic to neutral range. (*Microorganisms* are plants and animals too small to be seen by the human eye.) Microorganisms in the soil release nutrients from the soil so plants can absorb the nutrients needed through the root system.

The most important of these nutrients is nitrogen. Plants must have nitrogen to produce proteins. If the soil becomes too acidic, nitrogen is released more slowly and calcium becomes unavailable to the plants. Excess aluminum, iron, and manganese can reach toxic levels in acidic soil. Adding ground limestone *(lime)* in the fall will neutralize acidic soil for spring planting. If your soil is too alkaline, you can lower the pH. To do this, add gypsum *(calcium sulfate),* aluminum sulfate, or powdered sulfur.

Organic matter acts as a buffering agent. *Organic matter* can be well-rotted manure or *compost* (decomposed food scraps, plant clippings, leaves, etc.). A study found that soil around acid-loving plants would become acidic when 1 inch of compost was added annually. The soil on the same property around plants needing neutral pH would maintain a neutral pH when compost was added. Compost helps adjust the pH of the soil to the needs of the plant, whether acidic, neutral, or slightly alkaline. Although scientists know compost works, they have not identified all the chemical reactions that are taking place. Maintaining the proper pH for garden soil can usually be accomplished by adding 1 inch of compost each year.

Commercial farmers have the soil in fields analyzed for pH and mineral content. Commercial fertilizers and lime are added to maintain the ideal conditions for each type of crop.

It is easy and inexpensive to get an accurate pH reading of the soil in your garden. You can get pH strips from most local drugstores and nurseries. You can also have samples of soil tested by your local County Extension Service.

The point at which there is an equal number of acid and base molecules is called the **endpoint.** This is also called the **equivalence point.** The endpoint is where neutralization has occurred. **Neutralization** is the point at which all ions in a solution have combined chemically. For example, suppose you have a solution with 20 hydronium ions. You would have to add 20 hydroxide ions before neutralization would occur.

In neutralization processes, the reactants are an acid and a base. The products are water and a salt. The equation below shows what happens when two common chemical compounds, hydrochloric acid (HCl) and sodium hydroxide (NaOH), are combined.

$$\underset{\text{acid}}{HCl} + \underset{\text{base}}{NaOH} \longrightarrow \underset{\text{forms ions in solution}}{H^+ + Cl^- + Na^+ + OH^-} \longleftrightarrow \underset{\text{water}}{HOH} + \underset{\text{salt}}{Na^+Cl^-}$$

After neutralization occurs, it is impossible to tell how a solution was formed. It could have been made by mixing an acid and a base. The solution could also have been made by dissolving a salt in water.

Measuring Concentrations of Acids and Bases

Titration can work only if you have a known solution. You must know the volume and concentration of this solution. *Concentration* is the measure of parts of one substance to the known volume of another. You may wonder how a scientist knows how many molecules are in a known solution. Scientists cannot sit down and count out atoms of an element as a child counts out different colored candies. Atoms are too small.

In 1811, Amadeo Avogadro, an Italian physicist, made an observation about gases. He observed that equal volumes of different gases at the same temperature and pressure contained the same number of particles. This principle led scientists to discover that 22.4 liters of any gas at 0°C always contains 602,000,000,000,000,000,000,000 particles. This number is usually written in *scientific notation* as 6.02×10^{23}. This number is known as *Avogadro's number.* Avogadro's number of particles of any substance is known as a *mole.* A mole of one element always has the same number of atoms or particles as a mole of another element.

Avogadro's work led to another discovery. One mole of an element has a mass in grams equal to the atomic mass of the element. You can find the atomic mass of an element on the periodic table. When looking at the periodic table, you will note the atomic mass is the largest number describing each element. Remember the other number is the atomic number and represents the number of protons. The atomic mass is the average number of protons and neutrons for each element. Oxygen has an atomic mass of 15.9994. For the purposes of this class, round the atomic mass to the nearest tenth. Thus, one mole of oxygen has a mass of 16.0 grams. See 6-9.

The same principle applies to molecules. One mole of a compound has a mass in grams equal to the combined atomic masses of the elements in the compound. Think about water. Each water molecule contains two hydrogen atoms and one oxygen atom. Each hydrogen has an atomic mass of 1 for a total

Mole Mass of Elements

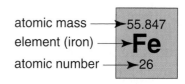

atomic mass ⟶ 55.847
element (iron) ⟶ **Fe**
atomic number ⟶ 26

6-9 By looking at the atomic mass of iron in a periodic table, you can calculate that one mole of iron equals 55.8.

of 2. Oxygen has an atomic mass of 16. These numbers are added together to get the atomic mass of a mole of water, which equals 18 grams. The following example illustrates how to determine the number of grams of $C_6H_8O_6$ (ascorbic acid) equal one mole.

1. Using the periodic table, find the atomic mass of each element in the compound.
$$C = 12$$
$$H = 1$$
$$O = 16$$
2. Multiply the atomic mass of each element by the number of atoms of that element in the compound.
$$C = 6 \times 12 = 72$$
$$H = 8 \times 1 = 8$$
$$O = 6 \times 16 = \underline{96}$$
$$176 \text{ grams}$$

Molarity

Suppose a scientist needs a known amount of sodium hydroxide (NaOH). He or she can simply calculate the number of grams in a mole. In titrations, however, the acid or base is in water solution. This is because diluted acids and bases are safer to work with in case of spills. Therefore, scientists measure solute concentrations in terms of *molarity (M).* The formula for molarity is

$$\text{molarity} = \frac{\text{moles}}{\text{liters}}$$

A one molar (1 *M*) solution is 1 mole of an element or compound dissolved in 1 liter of distilled water. You would write the chemical formula for a one molar solution of sodium hydroxide as 1 M NaOH. The steps to preparing this solution are as follows:

1. Determine the atomic mass of 1 mole of NaOH.

    Na = 23
    O = 16
    H = 1
    _____
    40 grams

2. Mass 1 mole or 40 grams of NaOH.
3. Dissolve 40 g NaOH in 1 liter of distilled water.

In Chapter 4, chemical equations were described as representing individual atoms or molecules. One mole of any substance always has the same number of particles. Therefore, chemical equations can also represent the number of moles of each of two combined substances. The number preceding the elements or molecules tells scientists how many moles to combine for the desired result. For example, look at the equation below. How many moles of oxygen are needed for the body to use 1 mole of glucose?

$$C_6H_{12}O_6 + 6O_2$$

The number 6 preceding the O_2 represents 6 moles.

Applications of pH

The relationship of acids and bases to pH is helpful in understanding how the body digests food. More important to the food scientist is the role of pH in food preservation and baking.

pH and Digestion

The balance of pH in the human body is critical for many life processes. It is especially critical for digestion. The digestive process begins in the mouth. There, food is mixed with saliva, which has a pH of about 6.5

After food is swallowed, it travels to the stomach. To digest proteins, the stomach produces one of nature's strongest acids—hydrochloric acid. The pH in the stomach is between 1.5 and 1.7. The stomach has a special lining that produces large amounts of mucus.

This mucus enables the acid to digest food without eating through the stomach wall.

The digestion process continues in the small intestines. Once food leaves the stomach, the pH is rapidly raised to around 7.0 by the addition of pancreatic juice. This juice is a base with a pH of about 8.0. Digestion in the small intestine is also aided by bile. This substance is stored in the gallbladder and has a pH of about 8.4. Once food is adequately digested, nutrients are absorbed into the bloodstream. The body maintains the pH of the bloodstream at about 7.4. See 6-10.

It is not possible for any food you eat to make the stomach more acidic. People who believe they have excess stomach acid may really have stomachs that are too full. A stomach that is too full can stretch the valve to the esophagus. This causes stomach acid to splash up into the esophagus, creating heartburn.

People have long believed that excess acid would cause ulcers. Recent research has revealed that people with ulcers may have bile salts in the stomach. Bile is normally found only in the *duodenum*, which is where the small intestine joins the stomach. Bile is fine in the duodenum, but it upsets the delicate chemical balance of the stomach. Bases can damage the mucous lining that protects the stomach from acid. When bile salts splash back into the stomach, the lining is weakened. This allows the hydrochloric acid to eat into the stomach lining and wall.

Stomach acids do cause damage for people with bulimia. *Bulimia* is an eating disorder that often involves induced vomiting. Unfortunately for bulimics, there is no way to prevent stomach acid from coming up with the food. The strong acid eats away at tooth enamel and the delicate skin lining the mouth. This can cause mouth sores and permanent tooth damage.

The Role of Buffers

A *buffer* is a compound that helps stabilize pH by absorbing excess acids or bases in a solution. A buffer solution is made by combining a weak acid or base and one of its salts. An example is acetic acid (CH_3COOH) and sodium acetate ($NaCH_3COO$). The salt (sodium acetate) ionizes in solution to form Na^+ and

pH of the Digestive Tract

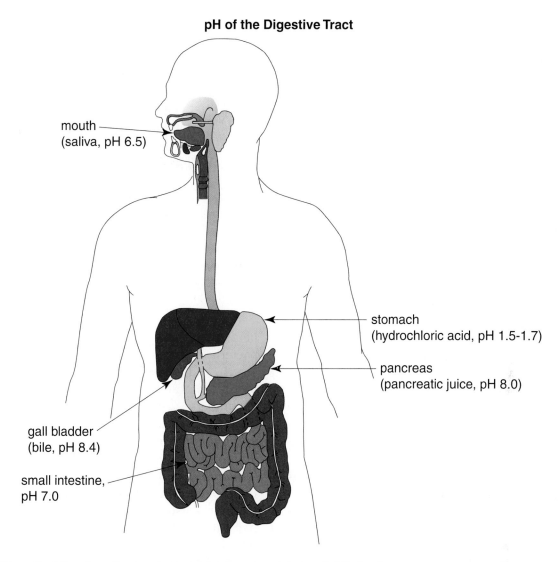

mouth
(saliva, pH 6.5)

stomach
(hydrochloric acid, pH 1.5-1.7)

pancreas
(pancreatic juice, pH 8.0)

gall bladder
(bile, pH 8.4)

small intestine,
pH 7.0

6-10 The pH of the digestive tract ranges from very acidic to slightly basic.

CH_3COO^- ions. If hydronium ions are added to the solution, the CH_3COO^- ions react with them to form acetic acid and water.

$$Na^+ + CH_3COO^- + H_3O \rightarrow Na^+ + CH_3COOH + H_2O$$
(ionized sodium acetate)   hydronium   sodium   acetic acid   water
ion   ion

If hydroxide ions were added to the acid-salt solution, the acetic acid would react. It would release a hydrogen atom and form CH_3COO^- ions and water.

$$CH_3COOH + OH^- \rightarrow CH_3COO^- + H_2O$$
acetic acid   hydroxide   acetate ion   water
ion

Buffers play a key role in blood chemistry. The stability of the blood pH is so important the body has three buffering systems to maintain the balance. In the body, lactic acid is a by-product of energy production. Ammonia is a result of protein digestion. These substances are balanced by phosphate ions (HPO_4^{-2}) and bicarbonate ions (HCO_3^-). The third buffering agent is proteins found in blood plasma. The structure of protein enables it to absorb either excess acids or bases. A fluctuation of as little as 0.2 in the blood pH can lead to death if not corrected. Buffers are also used to coat some aspirin tablets to make them easier to digest without damaging the digestive system.

Because most foods are complex biological systems, they contain substances that act as buffers. In plants, acids like citric and malic acid work with phosphate (PO_3^-) salts as buffering systems. Buffering salts are added to processed foods to stabilize pH. They include calcium phosphate, potassium phosphate, and sodium phosphate. Another group of compounds that can function as buffers is proteins. You will read more about these in Chapter 11.

Food Preservation

Food spoilage is caused by microorganisms growing in and feeding on food. Many foodborne illnesses are caused by bacteria growing in foods. Bacteria and other microorganisms grow best at a certain pH. For instance, most bacteria thrive in an environment that has a pH of 5.0 to 7.0. Preserving food and keeping it safe depend on an understanding of the pH environments of food products.

The deadliest type of foodborne illness is **botulism.** It is caused by a toxin produced by the bacteria *Clostridium botulinum.* This bacterium will not produce toxin at a pH of 4.6 or lower. Any food that naturally has a pH of less than 4.6 will not support growth of this bacterium. Such high-acid foods can be safely canned in a boiling water canner. These high-acid foods include most fruits and some varieties of tomatoes.

Clostridium botulinum is a spore-forming microorganism that lives naturally in the soil. This bacterium is commonly found in many foods with a pH above 4.6. Such foods, which are often called low-acid foods, include corn, green beans, and other vegetables. These foods must be canned at a very high temperature. Otherwise, the *Clostridium botulinum* multiplies rapidly in the oxygen-free environment of the sealed food container. The normal temperature of boiling water (100°C) is not hot enough to kill *Clostridium botulinum* if the pH is above 4.6. Therefore, low-acid foods have to be pressure canned. A pressure canner increases the temperature of boiling water to kill more microorganisms. See 6-11.

Many low-acid foods can be preserved by the pickling process. Through the pickling process, cucumbers become crisp with a sour bite. This process not only changes the texture and flavor of foods but the pH as well. Pickling involves soaking or heating foods in a vinegar (acetic acid) solution. The vinegar

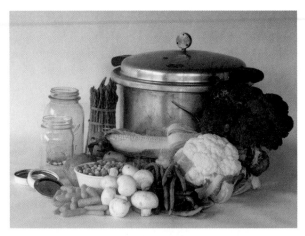

6-11 Low-acid vegetables, which have a pH of 4.6 or higher, must be pressure canned to ensure their safety.

helps lower the pH to below 4.6 so harmful bacteria cannot grow. Beets, cabbage (sauerkraut), and watermelon rinds are some of the foods commonly pickled in addition to cucumbers.

Buttermilk and yogurt have a naturally low pH. If stored properly, these and other low pH foods will generally stay fresh for long periods. However, even foods with low pH may be spoiled by the actions of some microorganisms. Yeasts can grow in a range of pH 4 to 7. They play a role in the making of wines and breads. Molds will grow in a wide range of pH from 2 to 8.5. Mold and pH monitoring are a part of the processing of tea, coffee, chocolate, cheese, and shelf-stable juices.

Salts are a by-product of neutralization. They help preserve foods. They work by killing bacteria through dehydration. Salt is abundant, inexpensive, and works without refrigeration or special canning. As a result, packing in salt was a common preservation method for pioneers in colonial America. Settlers in the United States often salt cured hams, bacon, and other pork products.

Baking

Batters and doughs used to prepare baked goods are complex food mixtures. Understanding the effects of pH on these mixtures can help a baker be more successful. The freshness and pH of ingredients will affect the flavor, color, and texture of finished products.

Chemical Leavening Agents

Chemical leavening agents are ingredients that are added to baked goods to lighten or aerate the finished product. Baking powder and baking soda are the chemical leavening agents used to make many baked goods light and fluffy, 6-12. These leaveners work because they contain a base. When they are combined with an acid and moistened in batter or dough, neutralization occurs. The by-products of the neutralization process are a salt, water, and carbon dioxide gas. The carbon dioxide becomes trapped in the batter or dough and creates air pockets. These air pockets swell and form a light, porous structure during baking.

Baking Soda

Baking soda, or sodium bicarbonate, is a salt. It is formed by combining sodium hydroxide (NaOH), a strong base, and carbonic acid (H_2CO_3), a weak acid.

Sodium bicarbonate is a base. When baking soda and an acid are combined in a baked product, carbon dioxide is released. Acids commonly used with baking soda include lemon juice, vinegar, sour cream, buttermilk, and cream of tartar (tartaric acid). The equation

below shows what happens when baking soda and vinegar (5% solution of acetic acid) are combined.

$$NaHCO_3 + CH_3COOH \longrightarrow Na(CH_3COO) + H_2O + CO_2$$
sodium bicarbonate + acetic acid → sodium acetate + water + carbon dioxide

Baking soda will leaven a product if acid is not present. However, the by-product, sodium carbonate, has a bitter flavor. The product will also have a yellowish color. Heat must be added for this reaction to occur.

$$2NaHCO_3 \xrightarrow{heat} CO_2 + Na_2CO_3 + H_2O$$
sodium bicarbonate   carbon + sodium + water
dioxide   carbonate

Baking Powder

Baking powder is a combination of baking soda, dry acids, and a filler. Most baking powders used in the United States have two dry acids. One acid reacts when exposed to moisture and the other acid reacts when heated. These baking powders are called *double-acting* baking powders. The filler in baking powder absorbs moisture to help prevent the baking soda and acids from reacting prematurely. The most common fillers are cornstarch and calcium carbonate.

Cream of tartar (potassium bitartrate) is one of the moisture-activated dry acids often used in baking powders. When liquid is added, the cream of tartar begins a two-step reaction with the baking soda. This reaction results in the release of some carbon dioxide before baking begins. If batter or dough is overmixed or baking is delayed, this carbon dioxide can be worked out of the mixture. Therefore, it is important to quickly finish mixing and begin the baking process after adding baking powder to a mixture.

The formula below shows the first step in the two-step reaction between the baking soda and cream of tartar.

$$NaHCO_3 + KHC_4H_4O_6 \xrightarrow{moisture} KNaC_4H_4O_6 + H_2CO_3$$
sodium   +   potassium   sodium potassium   +   carbonic
bicarbonate   bitartrate   tartrate   acid
(baking powder)

The following formula shows the second step in the two-step reaction between the baking soda and cream of tartar.

$$H_2CO_3 \longrightarrow H_2O + CO_2$$
carbonic acid   water + carbon dioxide

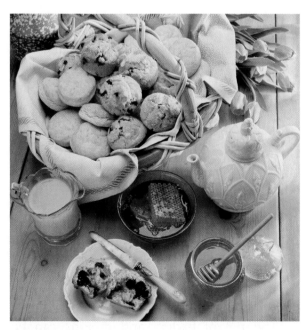

6-12 Biscuits are usually leavened with baking powder. Muffins may be leavened with baking soda.

In double-acting baking powder, most of the carbon dioxide is released after the product is exposed to heat. Several dry acids react slowly or only after heat is added. These include calcium dihydrogen phosphate, sodium aluminum sulfate, and sodium dihydrogen pyrophosphate. Most commercial baking powders are made with sodium dihydrogen pyrophosphate. These baking powders release about 30% to 40% of the carbon dioxide during mixing. They release another 10% if the product is allowed to stand more than 15 minutes. They release the remaining 50% to 60% during baking. These baking powders produce sodium pyrophosphate as a by-product. This substance does not give a bitter flavor to the finished product like the sodium carbonate produced by baking soda. See 6-13.

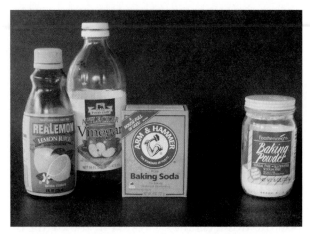

6-13 Baking soda must be used with an acid ingredient like vinegar or lemon juice. Baking powder contains a dry acid and needs only the addition of water and heat.

$$NaHCO_3 + Na_2H_2P_2O_7 \xrightarrow{heat} Na_3HP_2O_7 + CO_2 + H_2O$$

sodium bicarbonate   sodium dihydrogen pyrophosphate   sodium pyrophosphate   carbon dioxide   water

In each of the chemical leavening agents discussed so far, the gas that is produced is carbon dioxide. This is the only gas produced by chemical leavening agents available for retail sale in the United States. By law, baking powder must release 12 g of carbon dioxide per 100 g of baking powder.

Cooking Tip

If you run out of baking powder when preparing a favorite recipe, you can make an ingredient substitution. In place of 5 mL (1 teaspoon) baking powder, you can use 2 mL (½ teaspoon) cream of tartar plus 1 mL (¼ teaspoon) baking soda. You can also use 1 mL (¼ teaspoon) baking soda plus 125 mL (½ cup) buttermilk or other acidic liquid. This substitution will require you to reduce other liquid ingredients in the recipe by 125 mL (½ cup).

Ammonium Bicarbonate

Ammonium bicarbonate is a chemical leavening agent that does not form a solid product that remains in the dough. However, the ammonia gas that is produced can affect the taste of the product if it cannot escape. Therefore, ammonium bicarbonate is used only in thin baked goods with a large surface area, such as cookies and crackers. This shape allows the unwanted ammonia gas to escape during baking. Ammonium bicarbonate is only available to commercial bakers. It requires ventilation systems to remove ammonia gases.

$$NH_4HCO_3 \longrightarrow NH_3 + CO_2 + H_2O$$

ammonium bicarbonate   ammonia   carbon dioxide   water

Batters and Doughs

Analyzing batters and doughs before and after baking reveals that pH changes affect the color and texture of many products. For example, the more basic the batter for a particular type of cake is, the flatter and coarser the cake texture will become.

Acidity of batters and doughs is affected by the acid mix in the leavening agent. The various acids used in baking powders neutralize or react with the baking soda at different rates. For instance, sodium dihydrogen pyrophosphate is a slower acting acid. Baking powder containing this acid will give batters and doughs a high pH for a long period. On the other hand, monocalcium phosphate is a fast-acting acid. Baking powder containing monocalcium phosphate will give batters and doughs a high pH for a shorter period.

The pH of batters and doughs can be altered by adjusting the ingredients. Acidity can be increased by adding various acids such as acetic acid (vinegar) or cream of tartar. Batters can be made more basic by adding baking soda.

Different cakes have different pH needs. Angel food cakes are the most acidic. Egg whites form a more stable foam when beaten if they are acidic. The color pigment in flour, anthoxanthin, is whiter when the batter is acidic. This pigment is yellowish when the batter is basic. Many angel food cake recipes will call for lemon juice or cream of tartar. These ingredients provide sufficient acidity to maximize the volume of the beaten egg whites and promote a snowy white color.

Chocolate cakes will have a deeper, darker color and a smoother flavor if they are basic. Devil's food cake will be light brown at a pH of 7.5. It will be a deep red-brown at a pH of 8.8. This is why chocolate cake recipes will call for baking soda as the leavening agent. Milk or water will give the cake a deeper color than buttermilk, which is more acidic. This is why buttermilk is commonly used in German chocolate cakes, which have a lighter color. See 6-14.

Eggs and pH

Eggs have porous shells. Carbon dioxide, which is an acidic gas dissolved in eggs, will gradually escape through these shells. As the carbon dioxide escapes, the pH of the egg will climb. Therefore, eggs that have been stored for a while will have a higher pH than fresh eggs. Fresh whole eggs will have a pH of 6.4 to 7.0. Older eggs may have a pH as high as 9.7.

The pH, and thus the age, of eggs can affect the way eggs perform in baked goods. Fresh egg whites can have a pH as low as 5.6. These egg whites will be thicker than egg whites from older eggs. The thicker an egg white is, the more air it will trap and the greater volume it will attain when beaten. This means fresh egg whites will produce higher meringues and lighter angel food cakes. Adding cream of tartar to egg whites will also produce these qualities by lowering the pH. See 6-15.

The loss of carbon dioxide does not seem to affect the egg yolk. Yolks will maintain a fairly stable pH for several weeks.

Older eggs have their advantages. The loss of carbon dioxide releases the membrane around the egg white from the shell. Hard-cooked eggs will peel easily if they have been stored for several days before cooking. Fresh eggs are very difficult to peel without tearing the egg white.

pH and Fruit Maturity

As fruits mature, acids develop. These acids aid in the production of the fruits' characteristic flavor compounds. The acids improve juice quality, affect color development, and help increase sugar content. As ripening progresses, some acids are neutralized as others develop or increase. The ideal pH and the acid mix are different for each type of fruit.

Optimal pH Ranges for Various Cakes

Cake Type	pH Range
Fruitcake	4.4–5.0
Angel food cake	5.2–6.0
Pound cake	6.6–7.1
Yellow layer cake	6.7–7.5
White layer cake	7.0–7.5
Sponge cake	7.3–7.6
Chocolate cake	7.5–8.0

J. Amendola & D. Lundberg, *Understanding Baking*, 2nd ed. New York, Van Nostrand Reinhold, 1992, p.129.

6-14 The pH of cake differs from one type to another.

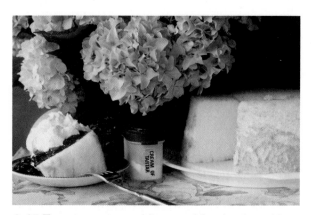

6-15 To get a snowy white angel food cake add lemon juice or cream of tartar to lower the pH.

Testing pH levels plays an important role in determining harvest time for many fruits. The pH of grapes is critical to successful wine making. Growers carefully test the pH of grape samples to see if the grapes have reached optimum pH.

The flavor of citrus fruits is a delicate balance between the sweetness of sugars and the sourness of acids. As citrus fruits ripen, sugars increase and acids decrease. The ripening process and the changes associated with it stop once citrus fruits are picked. Therefore, citrus growers test the pH of fruits to determine when to harvest for peak flavor.

The ideal mix of sweet and sour is different for every variety of citrus fruit. The ideal mix also varies, depending on the month and the location. To assist growers, food scientists have created charts showing the best ratios of sugars and acids for different citrus fruits.

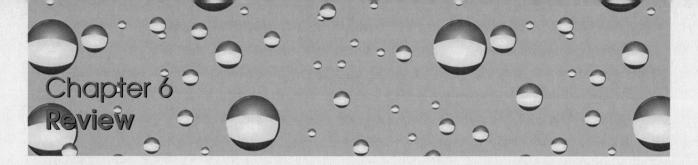

Chapter 6 Review

Summary

When water ionizes, negatively charged hydroxide ions and positively charged hydronium ions are formed. Because these ions are always in balance in pure water, water is neutral. Acids have a surplus of hydronium ions, which gives them a positive charge. Acids are proton donors or electron acceptors. They turn litmus paper red and have a sour taste. Bases have a surplus of hydroxide ions, which gives them a negative charge. Bases are proton acceptors or electron donors. They turn litmus paper blue and have a bitter taste. When acids and bases are combined, they neutralize each other by forming water and a salt.

The pH scale was developed to measure the concentration of hydronium ions in a solution. This scale is used to measure the relative strength and weakness of acids and bases. Through Avogadro's work, the mole was developed as a way to accurately measure equal numbers of molecules of any substance. Molarity is the number of moles of any substance per liter of water. These measurements assist scientists in combining the proper amounts of acids and bases.

Acids and bases play important roles in the body and in food products. The digestive process works because of carefully controlled pH levels in the body. The blood uses buffers to help maintain a constant pH. In the food industry, pH is related to the safe preservation of food. The development of chemical leavening agents and the production of baked goods also require an understanding of pH. Determining when to harvest many fruits is based on pH level, too.

Check Your Understanding

1. List three atoms or groups of atoms found in pure water.

2. What is the difference between the Bronsted-Lowry theory and the theory of acids and bases proposed by Newton Lewis?

3. Describe two common ways to identify acids and bases.

4. What does pH stand for?

5. Describe three ways to measure pH.

6. How many grams of acetic acid (CH_3COOH) equal 1 mole?

7. Calculate the amount of acetic acid and distilled water needed to make 0.6 M CH_3COOH.

8. Name one acid and one base involved in digestion and give the pH of each.

9. How do acids and salt help preserve food?

10. Explain how chemical leavening agents work.

11. Name three ingredients that can be added to a mixture when baking soda is the leavening agent used.

12. Describe how a double-acting baking powder works.

13. How does pH affect the quality of angel food cake?

14. How does the age of an egg affect its pH level?

15. How do acids affect the quality of fruit?

Critical Thinking

1. Your grandmother suggests you add a pinch of baking soda to broccoli during cooking to keep it bright green. What can you tell her about this tip?

2. You have discovered that one of your friends has started purging to help lose weight faster. How would you explain to your friend the dangers of pH as related to bulimia?

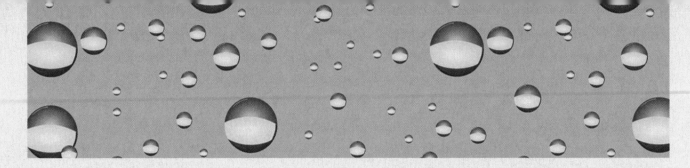

3. What is the advantage of taking a buffered aspirin?

4. Placing an open box of baking soda in a refrigerator helps neutralize odors from foods. What does this tell you about the pH of the volatile substances that cause food odors?

5. How would overmixing a batter or dough containing baking powder affect the quality of the baked product?

Explore Further

1. **Reading.** Research the use of vinegar and baking soda as cleaners. Is there a relationship to their use and the pH of the material being cleaned? Can you draw general conclusions about when to use vinegar and when baking soda would be better? Share your findings with the class.

2. **Math.** Measure the pH of at least seven of your favorite beverages. Create a bar graph that compares the pH of the seven beverages.

3. **Foods and nutrition.** Prepare two batches of chocolate chip cookies. Prepare one batch with baking soda, as listed in the recipe. Prepare the other batch with $1\frac{1}{2}$ teaspoons of baking powder. Conduct a taste test of the two types of cookies. Which do your classmates prefer? Why? What changes does the leavening agent make in the texture, flavor, and color of the cookie?

Experiment 6A
Molarity of Sweetened Tea

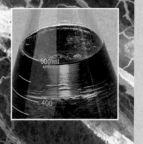

Safety

❖ Use caution in handling boiling hot water.
❖ Wash hands before handling food products.
❖ Clean all utensils after use.
❖ Use small paper cups for tasting.

Purpose

Iced tea is a popular beverage choice throughout the United States. However, people differ in their preference of how sweet it should be. Through testing and evaluation, you and your classmates will decide which molarity of sweetened ice tea is preferred by your class as a whole.

Equipment

electronic balance
1000-mL beaker
spoon

Supplies

sugar
freshly brewed tea
6 3-ounce paper cups per student

Procedure

1. Calculate the mass of one mole of table sugar or sucrose ($C_{12}H_{22}O_{11}$).
2. Measure 500 mL of unsweetened tea in the 1000-mL beaker.

3. Calculate and mass the moles of sugar needed for your assigned variation.

   Variation 1: Prepare a 0.30 M solution of sweetened tea.

   Variation 2: Prepare a 0.25 M solution of sweetened tea.

   Variation 3: Prepare a 0.20 M solution of sweetened tea.

   Variation 4: Prepare a 0.15 M solution of sweetened tea.

   Variation 5: Prepare a 0.10 M solution of sweetened tea.

   Variation 6: Prepare a 0.05 M solution of sweetened tea.

4. Use a spoon to stir the sugar into the tea until it is dissolved.
5. Taste a sample of each tea. Record your description of the flavor of each sample in a data table.
6. Select the molarity you liked best.
7. Record the preferences of everyone in the class.

Calculations

Use a bar graph to display the results.

Questions

1. Which of the molarities was preferred by the class as a whole?
2. Is there a relationship between sweetness preferred and any other factor you have observed?
3. How many teaspoons of sugar would you need in an 8-ounce glass of tea to equal the concentration of your personal variation preference?

Experiment 6B
Red Cabbage as an Acid-Base Indicator

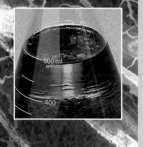

Safety

❖ Dispose of chemical solutions in the sink and flush all glassware with plenty of water.

❖ Wear splash goggles when titrating acids and bases.

❖ Do not taste the solutions.

Purpose

Before the twentieth century, if you wanted to know how acidic or basic a substance was, you would test it with natural indicators. In the scientific world, the most commonly used natural indicator is litmus. Many food products also have color pigments that make good indicators of acid and base levels. In this experiment, you will use red cabbage juice to make your own acid-base scale. You will use the red cabbage juice as a natural indicator to determine whether a variety of products commonly found in the home are acids or bases. Then you will confirm your results using pH indicator paper or a pH meter.

Equipment

2 burettes
burette stand
25 test tubes with lids or stoppers
wax pencil
test-tube rack
15-mL metric measuring spoon
pH indicator paper or pH meter

Supplies

1 *M* solution of sodium hydroxide (NaOH)
acetic acid
250 mL red cabbage juice
15 mL fruit juice

15 mL baking soda
15 mL buttermilk
15 mL milk
15 mL bleach
15 mL clear soda
15 mL egg white
15 mL dishwashing liquid
15 mL honey
15 mL lemon juice
15 mL milk of magnesia
15 mL tea
15 mL ammonia

Procedure
Part I

1. Use the wax pencil to number 12 test tubes from 1 to 12 and place them in a test-tube rack.

2. Dispense sodium hydroxide (NaOH) and acetic acid from burettes into the 12 numbered test tubes as specified in the following chart:

Test Tube Number	NaOH	Acetic Acid	Indicator
1		3 mL	10 mL
2		2 mL	10 mL
3		1 mL	10 mL
4		.5 mL	10 mL
5		1 drop	10 mL
6			10 mL
7	1 drop		10 mL
8	3 drops		10 mL
9	.5 mL		10 mL
10	1 mL		10 mL
11	2 mL		10 mL
12	3 mL		10 mL

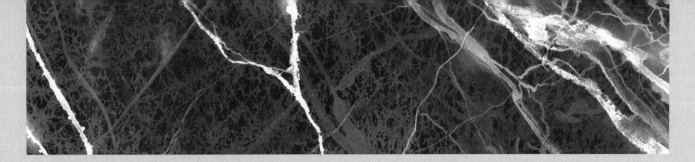

3. Measure 10 mL of the natural indicator (red cabbage juice) into each test tube.

4. Cover each test tube with a lid or stopper and shake gently 2 to 3 times to combine.

5. Record the color of each solution in your data chart.

6. Lay the test tubes in order on a sheet of white paper.

Part II

1. Use the wax pencil to label each of 13 clean test tubes with the name of one of the following substances: fruit juice, baking soda, buttermilk, milk, bleach, clear soda, egg white, dishwashing liquid, honey, lemon juice, milk of magnesia, tea, ammonia.

2. Measure 15 mL of each of the substances listed in Part II, step 1 into the appropriately labeled test tubes.

3. Add 10 mL of the natural indicator (red cabbage juice) to each test tube. Cover each test tube with a lid or stopper and shake gently to combine.

4. Match the color of the solution in each test tube to the color of the solution in the test tube prepared in Part I. Record the number of the test tube from Part I that is

closest in color in your data table in the appropriate row for each substance.

5. Test the pH of each of the solutions prepared in Part II with a 1- to 2-inch piece of indicator paper or a pH meter. Record the pH reading in the appropriate row of the data table.

6. Combine the lemon juice and the baking soda test tubes, match the color, and test with pH paper or a pH meter. Record your observations in your data table.

Questions

1. How accurate was the natural indicator compared to the pH paper or meter?

2. If other indicators were used, which was the easiest to work with?

3. What is the result of combining lemon juice and baking soda?

4. How can the information gained in this lab be applied to cooking foods that contain natural indicators? Removing stains on clothes? Dealing with accidental poisonings?

5. Rank substances from most acidic to most basic.

Experiment 6C
pH and Chemical Leavening in Muffins

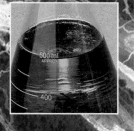

Safety

- ❖ Follow food preparation sanitation procedures.
- ❖ Wash hands before handling food products.
- ❖ Clean all utensils after use.
- ❖ Use hot pads to protect hands and counters.

Purpose

In this lab, you will compare the effects of four chemical leavening agents in a basic muffin recipe. You are to compare color, cell size, flavor, and texture of the muffins. It is crucial that mixing directions be followed exactly in order to limit outside variables that may affect the quality of the baked products.

Equipment

electronic balance
large mixing bowl
100-mL graduated cylinder
small mixing bowl
wooden spoon
muffin tin

Supplies

250 g all-purpose flour
65 g sugar
5 g salt
assigned leavening agent
1 egg
50 mL vegetable oil
250 mL milk
12 paper liners
50 mL distilled water

Procedure

1. Preheat the oven to 425°F.
2. Mass the flour, sugar, salt, and your assigned leavening agent. Combine these ingredients in a large mixing bowl.

   Variation 1: 7.0 g double-acting baking powder

   Variation 2: 3.5 g baking soda and 3.0 g cream of tartar

   Variation 3: 3.5 g baking soda and 30 mL vinegar, which should be added with the milk

   Variation 4: 3.5 g baking soda

3. Use the 100-mL graduated cylinder to measure the oil and milk. Combine these two ingredients with the egg (and vinegar in variation 3) in a small mixing bowl.
4. Make a well in the center of the dry ingredients.
5. Add the liquids all at once.
6. Stir the liquids into the dry ingredients with a wooden spoon until all the flour is moistened. *Do not beat; the batter will be lumpy.*
7. Spoon the batter into 12 paper-lined cups of a muffin tin. Fill each muffin cup two-thirds full.
8. Bake the muffins 18 to 20 minutes. Muffins are done if the tops spring back when gently pressed.
9. Remove muffins from the tin. With a serrated knife, cut the muffins in half from top to bottom. Place the muffins on a plate and label with the variation number.
10. Select one sample of each variation. Evaluate each sample for cell size, color, and shape before taste testing.
11. Crumble one-fourth of a muffin of your variation into 50 mL of distilled water. Mix to make a smooth paste. Measure and record the pH of the paste.

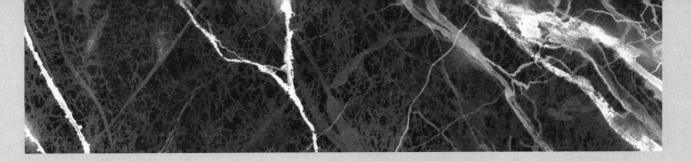

Questions

1. Which leavening agent produced the tallest muffins? Which produced the shortest?

2. Which leavening agent produced the best flavor?

3. Which, if any, of the variations have a bitter aftertaste?

4. Were there any differences in pH? If so, were the differences related to flavor or color differences?

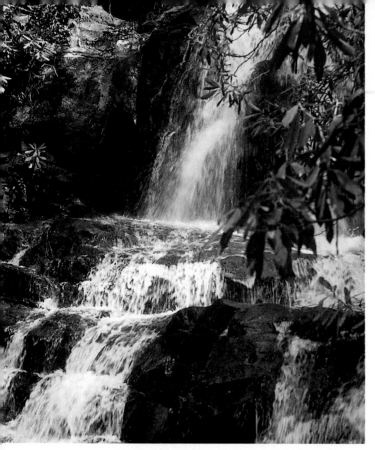

Water is a vital resource. It plays a tremendous role in everything from chemical reactions to food production and processing to health and nutrition.

Chapter 7

Water: The Universal Solvent

Objectives

After studying this chapter,
you will be able to

describe how the structure of a water molecule affects water's physical characteristics.

demonstrate a function of water in food preparation.

explain how the water content of a food affects how the food will react during preparation and storage processes.

identify four functions of water in the body.

list common contaminants in water.

Key Terms

nutrient

nonpolar covalent bond

polar covalent bond

hydrogen bond

intermolecular

surface tension

atmospheric pressure

impurity

free water

bound water

hydrate

anhydrous

water activity

hydrated

contaminant

pollutant

Few things necessary for life are as underrated and overlooked as water. It is the only substance in nature found in abundance in a solid, liquid, and gas state. People often marvel at the beauty of a snowflake and the diamond-like glitter of ice. However, few appreciate accumulations of snow that down power lines, close roads, and damage trees and property. People are seldom amazed by crop damage caused by freezing water in plant tissue, either.

Water is a nutrient. *Nutrients* are food components necessary to sustain life. There are six groups of nutrients. Besides water, the nutrient groups are carbohydrates, fats, proteins, vitamins, and minerals. You will study the chemistry of each of these nutrient groups in later chapters in this book.

Water is the main component of many foods. Water influences the texture, appearance, and taste of food. Nutritionally, it helps control your body's temperature. It also transports nutrients and wastes and provides the solution for hundreds of chemical reactions. It is an important heat medium in cooking and the main ingredient in beverages. Without water, cleanup and sanitation would be extremely difficult. It is critical to all forms of food preservation and its presence or absence determines a food's likelihood of spoilage. Where there is water, there is life.

The Structure of Water

Water is chemically composed of one oxygen atom and two hydrogen atoms. It is a relatively small compound held together by covalent bonds. Compounds such as methane

(CH_4) and ammonia (NH_3) are similar to water in size and atomic construction. However, the physical properties of water are quite different from these compounds. Water has higher melting and boiling points, more surface tension, a lower density, and a greater ability to conduct energy. These characteristics are caused by the nature of the molecule.

Types of Covalent Bonds

Water molecules are unique because of how the electrons are shared between the oxygen and hydrogen atoms. Covalent bonds share electrons in two ways: equally and unequally. Methane (CH_4), hydrogen (H_2), and oxygen (O_2) are examples of molecules that share electrons equally. The protons and electrons within the atoms have opposite electrical charges or *poles*. This is similar to the earth's opposite ends or poles. When the electrons are shared equally, these opposite charges balance or neutralize each other. As a whole, the molecule does not have an electrical charge. A *nonpolar covalent bond* is electrically neutral because the electrons are shared equally. That is, they spend the same amount of time orbiting the nucleus of each atom. See 7-1.

Nonpolar Covalent Bonds of a Hydrogen Molecule

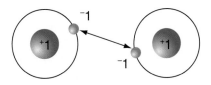

1. The electrons of two hydrogen atoms repel or push away from each other.

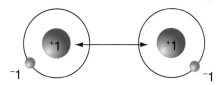

2. The protons of two hydrogen atoms also repel each other.

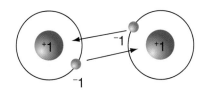

3. The proton of one atom attracts the electron of another atom. The outer orbital prefers to have two electrons.

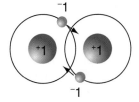

4. In covalent bonds, each electron travels in the orbitals around both nuclei.

7-1 A hydrogen molecule (H_2) is electrically neutral because the electrons are equally shared between the two hydrogen atoms.

The water molecule has a V shape with the angle between the two hydrogen atoms being 104.5°. This placement causes the electrons to be shared unequally. The larger oxygen nucleus tends to pull the shared electron toward the oxygen atom with greater frequency than the hydrogen atom. This *polarizes* the molecule, or causes it to develop regions of opposite electrical charge. The hydrogen end tends to be slightly positive and the oxygen end slightly negative. When a molecule with covalent bonds has a polar nature, its bonds are called **polar covalent bonds.** A polar covalent bond means there is an unequal sharing of electrons within the molecule. See 7-2.

Hydrogen Bonds

Like charges repel and opposite charges attract. Therefore, the positive end of one water molecule is pushed away from the positive ends of other water molecules. However, the positive hydrogen end of one water molecule is drawn toward the negative oxygen ends of other water molecules. This attraction is called a **hydrogen bond.** See 7-3.

Hydrogen bonds are *intermolecular,* or between molecules. Intermolecular bonds are much weaker than the covalent bonds within a molecule. You can think of two molecules of water as two people. Think of a hydrogen bond as the two people holding hands. Think of covalent bonds as the structure that holds

each person's arms to his or her torso. It is easy for the two people to separate by dropping their hands (breaking the hydrogen bond). It is much harder (and more dangerous!) to separate a person's arm from his or her body (breaking a covalent bond).

Surface Tension

Hydrogen bonds give water a greater surface tension than most compounds. *Surface tension* refers to the force between molecules at the outside edge of a substance. If you overfill a glass slowly, the water will form a convex surface that rises above the rim. The force of the hydrogen bonds keeps water from spilling. The water will spill over only when the force of gravity exceeds the force of the hydrogen bonds. It is impossible to observe this phenomenon with alcohol. Alcohol lacks the hydrogen bonds that would allow it to rise above the level of the container. This demonstration is also an example of the *cohesive* nature of water, or its ability to cling to itself.

The polar nature of water causes water to appear to climb the sides of a container. The water forms an upward curve or "smile" shape on its top surface. This curve of the top surface, as you learned in Chapter 2, is called

Polar Covalent Bond of a Water Molecule

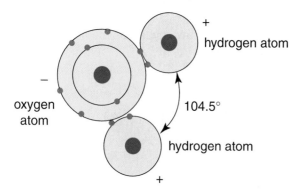

7-2 Because the oxygen and hydrogen atoms in a water molecule share the electrons unevenly, a division of charge is created. The oxygen end becomes negatively charged and the hydrogen end becomes positively charged.

Hydrogen Bonds Among Polar Molecules

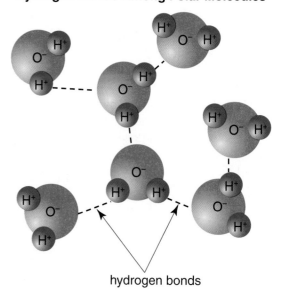

hydrogen bonds

7-3 The positively charged hydrogen end of one water molecule is attracted to the negatively charged oxygen end of another water molecule.

a *meniscus*. The meniscus is caused by water's adhesive property. An *adhesive* clings to something else as well as to itself. The curve forms because the adhesion between water and the container is stronger than the cohesion among water molecules. This characteristic of water is more obvious in narrow tubes like burets than it is in larger containers.

The increased surface tension of water accounts for its higher melting and boiling points as compared to other liquids. It takes more energy for polar molecules than for non-polar molecules to break free from a rigid solid like ice. It also takes more energy for a polar molecule to break out of a liquid. Water's great surface tension also explains why water freezes faster than it thaws. Hydrogen bonds can easily form and hold water molecules into a rigid structure. It is more difficult for hydrogen bonds to be broken so water molecules can slide by one another freely.

The push and pull among water molecules results in them forming a tetrahedral (four-sided pyramid) shape when ice is formed. This shape is a result of three-dimensional hydrogen bonding. Water molecules have greater space between them when frozen than when in liquid form. This is due to the repelling of like charges. The hydrogen bonding creates microscopic holes in ice much like air holes in foam. This is why water is unusual in its density. Most substances become more dense as they move from the liquid to solid state. Ice (solid water) becomes less dense than water (liquid). This is why ice cubes float in water. Water molecules are most dense at 3.98°C (39.16°F).

Hydrogen bonding can also occur between water and other polar molecules. Some food components that commonly form hydrogen bonds with water are sugars, starches, and proteins. Water's ability to hydrogen bond to other polar molecules helps substances like sugar dissolve and stay distributed in water. See 7-4.

Pressure, Temperature, and Phase Changes

Imagine you could see a tall column of atoms of air rising from the earth's surface.

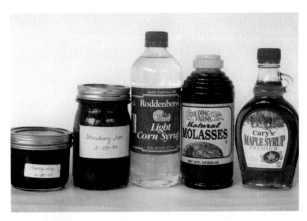

7-4 The sugars in jelly, jam, syrups, and molasses stay distributed due to hydrogen bonds with water molecules.

These atoms have a weight, which is determined by the pull of the earth's gravity. The force of this weight pressing down on a surface is called *atmospheric pressure* (atm).

Gases in the air are pressing against your body all the time. Therefore, you are not likely to be aware of atmospheric pressure. However, it is similar to the pressure that water puts on your body when you dive into a pool. The weight of the water pushes in on you all over your body. The deeper you go, the larger this force, or pressure, is on the surface area of your body.

Atmospheric pressure is measured based on the average pressure of the atmosphere on an object at sea level. At sea level with standard conditions, atmospheric pressure is measured as 1.0 atm, which equals 14.7 pounds per square inch. What will happen to atmospheric pressure as you drive into the mountains or take off in an airplane? As *altitude*, or height above the earth increases, the column of air above you becomes smaller. This means there is less atmospheric pressure. In Denver, Colorado, which is 1.61 km (1 mile) above sea level, the average pressure is 0.83 atm. Likewise, at locations below sea level, the column of air above you becomes larger and atmospheric pressure increases. At 0.09 km (282 feet) below sea level, Death Valley in California has an average pressure of 1.01 atm. See 7-5.

The *boiling point* of a substance is the point at which it changes from a liquid into a gas.

Atmospheric Pressure

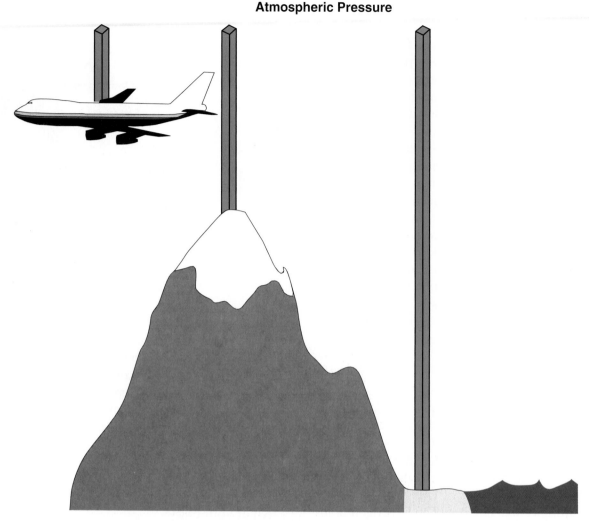

7-5 The column of atmosphere pressing down on a surface decreases as elevation above sea level increases.

When water reaches its boiling point, water molecules in the liquid are escaping into the air as steam.

As atmospheric pressure changes, the boiling point of water changes. When there is less atmospheric pressure on the water, the molecules need less energy to escape. When there is more atmospheric pressure on the water, the molecules need more energy to escape. Remember that temperature is a measure of energy. Therefore, at high altitudes, where the atmospheric pressure is lower, water will boil at lower temperatures. At low altitudes, where the atmospheric pressure is higher, water will boil at higher temperatures. At sea level, water boils at 100°C (212°F). At the top of Mount McKinley, which is 6,194 m (20,320 feet) above sea level, water boils at about 78°C (173°F). At

the Dead Sea, which is 392 m (1,286 feet) below sea level, water boils at about 101°C (214°F). See 7-6.

Understanding the effects of atmospheric pressure on the boiling point of water can benefit all cooks. These concepts explain how a pressure cooker works. Pressure cookers have a steam-tight seal. As steam is released inside the sealed cooker, pressure builds. The water in the cooker then has to have more energy, and thus a higher temperature, to boil. The higher temperatures cause foods inside a pressure cooker to cook faster. For instance, at 15 pounds of pressure above 1 atm, the boiling point of water will be 121°C (250°F). A 3-pound pot roast cooked at this pressure will be done in about 45 minutes. This roast would take two to three hours to cook conventionally.

High-Altitude Baking

Lower atmospheric pressure can affect cooking procedures for people who live 1,000 m (3,300 feet) or more above sea level. At this altitude, water boils at about 96°C (205°F). Therefore, foods simmered or boiled in water take longer to cook. This change in boiling point also has the following effects on baked goods:

❖ With less atmospheric pressure pushing down on the batter or dough, breads and cakes rise higher and have larger air cells. This can result in products that either become dried out and coarse in texture or collapse during baking.

❖ Liquids evaporate faster, resulting in dryer products or higher fat and sugar concentrations.

❖ Cakes can be underdone as a result of the lower boiling point.

To some extent, high-altitude baking requires trial and error. However, the following tips may help you convert standard recipes for use at high altitudes:

❖ Use 5% more flour. This will slow the leavening action.

❖ Use up to 20% more water. This helps balance the rapid evaporation and drying.

❖ Increase the oven temperature by 25°F and reduce baking time by about 20%. This will speed crust formation and help prevent overflow of batter.

❖ If increased oven temperatures will scorch the edges of the batter, try reducing sugar content by 30 to 45 mL (2 to 3 tablespoons) per cup. Cook products at the recommended temperatures.

❖ Bake yeast breads just before they double in size or reduce yeast by 20%.

❖ If a recipe calls for whipped egg whites to be folded in, beat the egg whites just to the soft peak stage. This allows for the extra expansion of the egg whites and will keep them from bursting.

❖ Reduce the leavening agent (baking soda or baking powder) by 15 to 60%, depending on your altitude.

7-6 Cooks need to make several adjustments when preparing foods at high altitudes.

Even if you do not have a pressure cooker, you can increase the boiling point of water. Placing a lid on a pot will increase the boiling point by as much as 5°C to 6°C (10°F to 12°F). The heavier the lid is, the greater the increase will be. The increase depends on the pressure needed to push up the lid.

The freezing point of water is also affected by atmospheric pressure. At sea level, water freezes at 0°C. The changes in freezing point are insignificant in most circumstances.

Impact of Impurities in Water

So far, you have looked at the characteristics and structure of pure water. It is important to remember that water's structure makes it an excellent solvent. Because so many substances dissolve in water, it is usually not in pure form. Anything that is added to water causes it to be impure. These *impurities,* or substances other than water, will affect the way water reacts.

Impurities are not necessarily unsafe. Salt and microorganisms are both impurities that could be found in water. Sharing a water glass with someone who has been eating potato chips would transfer a harmless amount of salt. However, sharing a glass with someone who is sick could transfer enough microorganisms to cause illness.

Substances present in or added to water can change water's physical and chemical characteristics. Impurities can change water's flavor, color, boiling point, freezing point, and hydrogen bonding. The amount of change will depend on the amount and kind of impurity.

Hot tap water may contain more impurities than cold tap water. The heat can cause impurities such as calcium and iron deposits in pipes and water heaters to dissolve into the water. These impurities can produce unpleasant flavors in foods and beverages. To avoid off-flavors in hot beverages, prepare them with cold tap water that you have heated.

Cooking Tip

Pasta put in cold water or cooked at low temperatures will begin to dissolve into the water before it is cooked. This causes the surface of the pasta to become sticky and mushy. This can especially be a problem when cooking pasta at high altitudes, where the boiling point is below 100°C (212°F). Adding 5 mL (1 teaspoon) salt per 1 L (1 quart) of cooking water will raise the boiling point 0.5°C to 1.0°C (1°F to 2°F). This higher temperature helps give pasta a desirable firm texture.

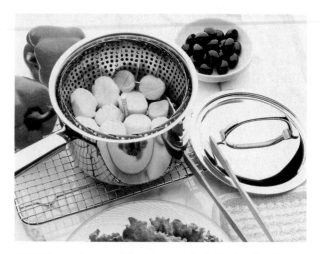

7-7 Steam from water is used to transfer the heat needed to cook these scallops.

Functions of Water in Food Preparation

Water serves two main functions in the preparation of food products. Water is an important medium for transferring heat. It is also a necessary ingredient for forming many food mixtures.

Heat Medium

Water, in both its liquid and gaseous states, is used to transfer heat energy into foods. See 7-7. When water is heated, energy is transferred from the heat source by both conduction and convection. Pieces of food suspended in water have little effect on the boiling point of water. As a result, water boils at a constant temperature. Gently boiling water has the same temperature as rapidly boiling water. However, energy is being transferred at a lower rate with the gentle boil.

Whether you choose a rapid or gentle boil will depend on the food you are cooking. Pasta, for example, needs a rapid boil. This will keep the pasta in motion and prevent the noodles from sticking together. Potatoes, on the other hand, need a gentle boil. A gentle boil keeps the potatoes from banging into each other in the cooking process. Potatoes that bang about in the pan may break apart and become mushy on the surface.

Cooking with Steam

To escape from the liquid to gaseous state, water molecules have to absorb much energy. Experiments have shown that 9.7 kilocalories of energy are needed to turn 1 mole H_2O at 100°C (212°F) into 1 mole of steam. In Chapter 5, you learned that this energy, called latent heat, does not change the temperature. Therefore, steam that is not under pressure will have the same temperature as boiling water.

It will actually take slightly longer to cook many foods in steam than boiling water. This is because steam is a poor conductor of heat. However, the steam can cook the food faster than boiling water if pressure is added. This is because the temperature of steam under pressure can be higher than the boiling point. Cooking occurs as latent heat is released into the food when the steam condenses on the cooler food surface.

Steam cooking has two main advantages. Steamed foods are more flavorful than boiled foods. Foods cooked in steam will also be more nutritious than foods cooked in water. This is especially true when the cooking liquid is discarded. Fewer flavor compounds and nutrients are dissolved into the steam than into boiling water.

Cooking Tip

Steam eggs for an alternative to poaching. Lightly coat a custard cup with nonstick cooking spray. Crack an egg into the custard cup, being careful not to break the yolk. Place the custard cup on a rack or steamer in a saucepan with gently boiling water in the bottom. Cover the saucepan and steam the egg for 4 minutes. Remove the lid and top the egg with a slice of low-fat cheese. Cover the saucepan and steam the egg for one minute longer. Serve the steamed egg on a toasted English muffin.

The Universal Solvent

Water is called the universal solvent because it can dissolve so many substances. Most substances in food other than fats and oils are dissolved in a water base. Beverages, candies, baked goods, soups, stews, casseroles, and sauces are all mixtures of substances dissolved in a water base, 7-8. Gases, liquids, and solids can all be found in water solutions. Understanding how water works in solutions is helpful when preparing many types of foods.

Gas-in-Water Solutions

Carbonated beverages are examples of gas-in-water solutions. Carbon dioxide is the gas solute dissolved in water. The first carbonated beverage was created by nature where underground water passed through limestone under pressure. This process is now copied in high-pressure tanks above ground. Every day, beverage manufacturers produce millions of liters of carbonated water for use in soft drinks.

Another gas that dissolves in water is oxygen. Hot water is able to hold less dissolved oxygen than cold water. When water is boiled, dissolved oxygen escapes into the

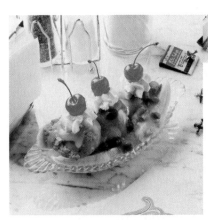

Item of Interest
Cooking with Steam

Place ½ cup water in a saucepan. Place vegetables on a steamer and then place the steamer in the saucepan. Cover with a lid and heat on high until steam begins to escape. (Starting the food on high heat will get the surface of the food to 100°C as quickly as possible.)

Wait two minutes and turn the heat down to low. (It takes about two minutes for the steam to push all the air out of the pan.) Time the cooking from this point. Do not lift the lid until cooking is done. When you lift the lid, cool air rushes in and the cooking will stop. The air has to be pushed out of the pan again before cooking can resume.

Once you have turned down the heat, all you have to do is maintain the temperature. This is where you save energy. At this point, high temperatures would force steam out of the pan. More water then has to be turned to steam whose energy is lost when it escapes. When the heat is turned down, only a little energy is needed to maintain the temperature of the trapped steam and boiling water.

Steam at 100°C has more energy than air at 100°C. This is because of the latent heat needed to turn boiling water into steam. Foods will cook faster if the heated air is forced out of the pan so only steam (vaporized water) remains. This means the food needs to be in a pan with a snug lid.

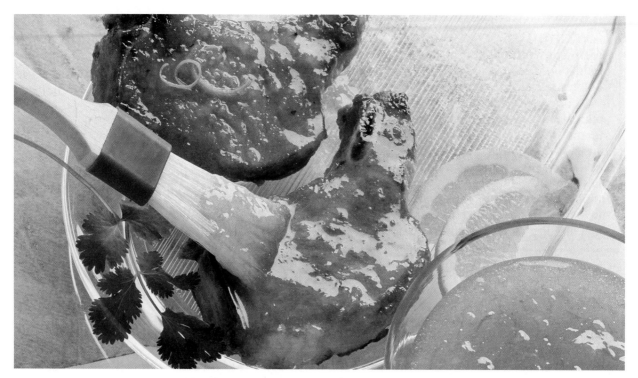

7-8 Sauces are among the many food products made from substances dissolved in a water base.

atmosphere. Water that has been boiled and allowed to cool will have a slightly flat taste. This flat taste is due to the lower dissolved oxygen levels.

Dissolved oxygen causes ice cubes to be cloudy. To create clear ice, boil water for several minutes, cool, and then freeze. Ice cubes made this way will also last slightly longer. This is because once the oxygen molecules have been boiled out, the water molecules can pack together more tightly. This creates denser ice cubes.

Cooking Tip
Freezing water does not cause it to lose its ability to dissolve substances. Freezing temperatures merely slow the ability of water to dissolve substances. Even the cleanest freezer will have a "freezer odor" that will dissolve into ice over time. The longer the ice stays in the freezer, the more obvious the taste change is. You can reduce this off-flavor by rinsing ice cubes in water for a few seconds before use. This will melt the outer layer where most of the odor has been dissolved into the ice.

Storage Tip
Carbon dioxide needs high pressure to stay dissolved or suspended in water. Soft drinks have to be sealed to keep the carbon dioxide dissolved in the water. You can squeeze excess air out of partially emptied plastic bottles and then replace the cap. This will increase the storage time before an opened soft drink goes flat.

Gas solutes such as carbon dioxide are released at faster rates as temperatures climb. Soft drinks stored at high temperatures will go flat faster. (This is especially true if the containers have been opened.) Therefore, you should avoid leaving soft drinks in your car on a hot summer day.

Liquid-in-Water Solutions

It is possible to have some liquid other than water dissolved or stirred into water. Most alcoholic beverages are examples of true liquid-in-water solutions. Another example is the solution of vinegar and water used to preserve pickled foods. See 7-9.

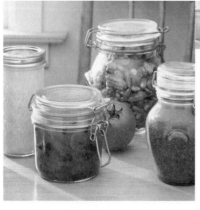

Historical Highlight
How Soft Drinks Got Started

Joseph Priestley was an English chemist. He wanted to imitate the bubbling water of mineral springs. He successfully dissolved carbon dioxide in water under pressure in 1772. This first artificial mineral water contained sodium salts (sodium bicarbonate or sodium carbonate). The carbonation was formed by adding acid to the sodium salts. The name "soda" came from sodium salts.

In 1806, the first artificial soda water in the United States was made and bottled. This was done by Benjamin Silliman, a chemistry professor at Yale.

Lemon-flavored soda water became popular after 1830. The flavors of ginger ale and root beer followed later. Cola flavored drinks are the result of medicinal syrups made from the Kola nut. These syrups were added to unflavored soda water to make them easier to swallow.

In the 1850s, soft drink companies sold bottled, flavored soda water. Most soda water was sold by "soda fountains." These food counters were usually located in the local drug store.

The name "soft drinks" was given to distinguish these beverages from "hard" alcoholic drinks. The name "pop" came about because of the noise the early bottles made when the lids were removed.

The average number of soft drinks consumed per person per year went from 12 in 1900 to about 585 in 1998. Today, carbonated beverages are the drink of choice for most people in the United States.

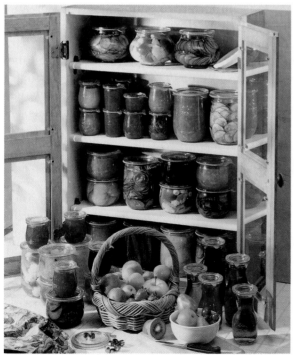

Glashaus, Inc.

7-9 The liquid used to pickle many of these foods is a solution of vinegar in water.

Many other liquid mixtures, such as fruit juice concentrates, are sold in water solutions. These are further diluted by adding more water.

Solid-in-Water Solutions

Water is frequently the solvent for many solids in food preparation. Whenever a substance is dissolved in water, the chemical properties of the solution will differ from those of pure water.

Salt and Sugar Solutions

The two most common solids used in a water solution are salt and sugar. Both substances cause water to freeze at a lower temperature and boil at a higher temperature than pure water. The more salt or sugar in the solution, the lower the freezing point and the higher the boiling point will be.

The addition of salt to ice is what makes homemade ice cream possible. Ice cream freezes at a lower temperature than pure water. Placing the ice cream solution in a container of ice will cause the solution to become cold. However, it will not freeze. Salt water also has a lower freezing point than pure water. When salt is sprinkled on the ice, two things happen. First, the ice melts and combines with the salt to form salt water. Second, heat energy is pulled from the ice cream solution and the ice, lowering the temperature. This transferred energy is needed for the salt crystals to break their bonds and dissolve in the water. The result is salt water with a temperature below 0°C (32°F) and frozen ice cream.

As salt and sugar concentrations increase, the boiling point increases. High salt levels are not desirable in most food products. Therefore, the amount of salt added will generally increase the boiling point by only a few degrees Celsius. Salt is often added at a ratio of no more than 5 grams per liter of water.

Sugar is used in food products in much higher concentrations than salt. Sugar in candy syrups can have a ratio as high as four parts sugar to one part water. This results in a wide range of possible boiling points for sugar and water solutions. As the concentration of sugar to water increases, so does the boiling point. The chemical interaction of sugar in water causes the temperature to climb as the solution is boiled. The next chapter will look at how important the boiling temperature of a sugar solution is to candy making. See 7-10.

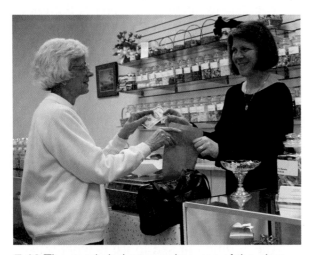

7-10 The candy industry makes use of the characteristics of sugar and water solutions to develop a wide range of sweet treats.

Tea and Coffee

Because water is a solvent, it will dissolve flavor compounds from tea leaves and coffee grounds. Changing the amount of tea leaves or coffee beans in proportion to the water varies the strength of tea or coffee. Increasing the brewing time will also increase the strength of the tea or coffee flavor. However, increasing the brewing time will allow more polyphenols to be dissolved in the water.

Some *polyphenols* are compounds that can create a bitter aftertaste in tea or coffee. These polyphenols can cause coffee prepared in a percolator to be more bitter than coffee prepared in a drip coffeemaker. This is because percolated coffee is brewed for 7 to 15 minutes, which allows more polyphenols to be extracted.

Polyphenols are also present when temperatures used to brew tea and coffee are higher than recommended. Proper brewing temperatures for tea and coffee allow maximum flavor extraction without the development of a bitter aftertaste. The ideal brewing temperature is just below the boiling point.

Water Content in Foods

It is important to understand water and how it reacts during food preparation and storage. This is because water is a major part of most foods. For instance, many fruits and vegetables are over 70% water. Even foods that are often considered dry contain water. Bread is 36% water, and popcorn contains 4% water. See 7-11.

Water in food becomes part of the structure of a food in three main ways. These are free, bound, and as a hydrate.

When you cut into a grapefruit and juice squirts on your face, you have been hit with free water. *Free water* is easily separated from food tissues. It can be pressed or squeezed from the food and often contains dissolved compounds. During processing, free water will easily boil or freeze. Free water also readily evaporates when foods are dried.

Bound water is tied to the structure of large molecules. Because of the small size and polar nature of water molecules, they slide into spaces between larger molecules. Water

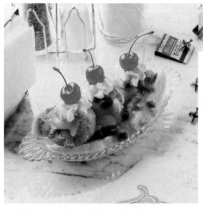

Item of Interest
The Solution to Brewing the Perfect Cup

Whether your preference is tea or coffee, the principles for successful brewing are similar. The goal is to get the right flavor compounds into the water and keep unpleasant ones out of the solution.

Drip coffeemakers release boiling water over coffee grounds. By the time the water hits the grounds, it has cooled to the ideal temperature range. The water picks up coffee flavor compounds as it pours over the grounds and drips to the pot below. The coffeepot sits on a warmer to maintain the temperature. Drink coffee immediately after brewing for best flavor. Coffee flavor compounds are extremely volatile and quickly escape from the pot. Extended warming causes coffee to develop bitter flavors.

For tea, pour the boiling water over the tea leaves or tea bags in a nonmetal teapot. (Tea reacts with some metals resulting in a metallic taste to the tea.) Cover the pot with a thick towel to help hold in the heat. Let the pot stand for 3 to 5 minutes. Maximum flavor is extracted in 5 minutes. Longer brewing pulls bitter polyphenols into the tea. To get a stronger tea, increase the amount of tea leaves *not* the brewing time.

Recommended brewing temperatures vary somewhat for different types of tea. Green tea is not fermented or aged. Oolong tea is aged for a short time, and black tea is aged for a longer period. As the tea leaves age, chemical changes occur. The different compounds present as a result of aging dissolve best at different temperatures.

Brewing Temperatures

Beverage	°C	(°F)
Coffee	85–96	(185–205)
Green teas	82–93	(180–200)
Oolong teas	91–99	(195–210)
Black teas	93–99	(200–210)

The Brewing Process

The Procedure	The Science
Start with cool water not hot tap water.	Hot water dissolves more metals and impurities from pipes and water heaters. This can increase off flavors from the water.
Use freshly boiled water.	Extended boiling or boiling, cooling, and then boiling again causes a loss of dissolved oxygen. Water that is heated repeatedly tastes flat.
Remove water from heat, then add coffee or tea.	The ideal brewing temperature is hot enough to extract the compounds responsible for coffee and tea flavor. If temperatures are too low, too few compounds are released to produce good beverage flavor. If temperatures are too high, bitter polyphenols are released into the brew.

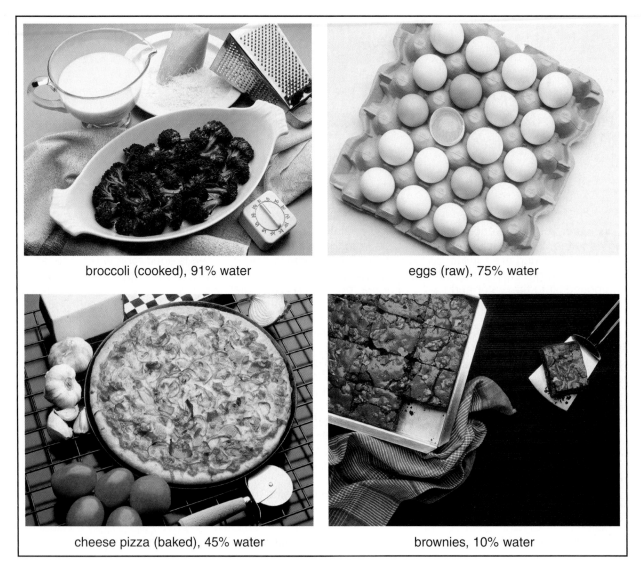

broccoli (cooked), 91% water

eggs (raw), 75% water

cheese pizza (baked), 45% water

brownies, 10% water

7-11 Water is a component of many food products.

molecules then form hydrogen bonds with the larger molecules, such as protein and starch molecules in fruits, meats, and vegetables. Bound water does not easily freeze or boil like free water. It chemically reacts as part of the larger molecule to which it is bound.

Much of the water in plant and animal tissue is inside the cells. Even when food tissue is cut or torn, the water does not flow out of the cells. This water is known as a hydrate. A *hydrate* is any chemical compound that is loosely bound with water. Hydrates can have one or more water molecules bound to the compound. For example, in its natural state, caffeine has one molecule of water attached to the caffeine molecule. The molecular formula for the hydrate of caffeine is written as follows:

$$C_8H_{10}N_4O_2 \bullet H_2O$$

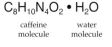

caffeine   water
molecule   molecule

hydrate of caffeine

The dot represents the hydrogen bonding between the two molecules. Hydrates can have more than one molecule of water attached to each molecule of the compound.

When the hydrate is heated, the water is driven off. Compounds that have the water driven off are **anhydrous**, or free of water.

Food scientists know there is a relationship between water content and food perishability. However, water content alone will not predict how perishable a food is. Water that is bound to other compounds is not as available to aid in food spoilage. Carrots and whole milk are both 88% water. You could safely eat a carrot that had been left at room temperature in a lunch bag. A large amount of the water in the carrot is bound to starch molecules. As a result, carrots are solid. Milk is a liquid with mostly free water. Therefore, an uninsulated container of milk in the same lunch bag would no longer be safe. Bacteria may have multiplied in the milk, causing it to spoil. The difference is related to water's interaction with other compounds.

The U.S. federal government regulations on good food manufacturing practices include water activity values. *Water activity* (A_w) is the measure of the partial water pressure over a food. This is compared to the vapor pressure (gaseous water) over pure water at a given temperature. Water activity takes into account the water available to support activity of enzymes and growth of microorganisms. Water activity is measured from 0 to 1. The higher the number is, the more perishable the food will be. Safe water activity levels have been identified for various processes, such as making concentrates and dehydrating fruits and vegetables. See 7-12.

Functions of Water in the Body

Water is necessary for many body functions. Maintaining body temperature is one main function of water. When your body temperature begins to rise, water is released to the surface of your skin. You perspire. To evaporate, water needs energy. The nearest source of energy is you. The extra heat energy is pulled into the water. As the water evaporates, it pulls the excess heat away from your body.

Transporting nutrients is a second function of water in the body. Minerals and water-soluble vitamins must first dissolve in water before they can be transported to where they are needed. Water also helps transport waste products out of the body.

A third function of water is to serve as a reactant in metabolism. *Metabolism* is the combination of chemical and physical processes that happen within the cells of the body. Chemical reactions are needed to produce, transfer, and store energy as well as to make new cells. Many of these chemical reactions require water as one of the reactants. For example, your body uses water to break down the energy nutrients during digestion.

Water Activity of Common Foods

A_w	Foods
1.0–0.95	Canned fruits, vegetables, meat, fish, milk, juices
0.95–0.91	Hard cheeses, cured meat, some fruit juice concentrates, foods with 55% sugar or 12% salt content
0.91–0.87	Salami, sponge cakes, dry cheeses, margarine, foods with 65% sugar or 15% salt content
0.87–0.80	Most fruit juice concentrates, sweetened condensed milk, chocolate syrup, maple syrup, flour, rice, fruitcake, country style ham, fondants (candy cream centers)
0.80–0.75	Jam, marmalade, marshmallows
0.75–0.65	Rolled oats, fudge, jelly, molasses, dried fruits, nuts
0.65–0.60	Dried fruits with 15–20% moisture, toffee, caramel, honey
0.50	Pasta, spices
0.40	Whole egg powder
0.30	Cookies, crackers, bread crusts
0.20	Whole milk powder, dried vegetables with 5% moisture, cornflakes

7-12 The water activity of a food affects the food's perishability. Foods with high water activity can better support enzyme activity and microorganism growth.

A fourth function of water is to become part of body tissue. The body is composed of about 60% water. The exact percentage depends on the ratio of bone, muscle, and fat. All body fluids are also largely composed of water.

Meeting Your Body's Water Needs

Most people know they need six to eight glasses of water a day. Many of you know that you can live much longer without food than without water. This may lead you to wonder how many people who "never" drink water can survive? Think back to what you read about water content in foods. Beverages are mostly water, as are soups and sauces. Your body can take water as well as nutrients and calories from the many foods you eat. Your body gets the water it needs from the foods you eat and the beverages you drink. Your body also gets water as a by-product of chemical reactions.

You should drink water rather than just getting water as a part of other foods for two main reasons. The first is that water by itself has no calories. If you drink four 12-ounce cans of regular soft drinks, you will have consumed about 600 calories worth of sugar. The drinks will make it harder for you to maintain a healthy weight. Their calories will replace calories from foods that provide all the other nutrients you need for good health. See 7-13.

Although diet soft drinks provide few if any calories, they are not a good substitute for water either. Carbonated soft drinks are a source of phosphorus. Too much phosphorus

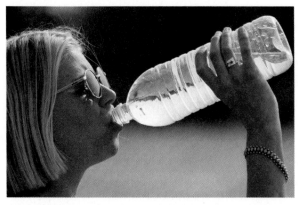

7-13 Plain water meets your body's fluid needs without providing calories.

in the diet can keep the body from absorbing some other nutrients, including calcium. Drinking plain water does not have such negative effects on your body's nutrient balance.

There is a second reason not to rely only on foods for water. Many foods that are high in water are also high in either sugar or salt. Most people in the United States consume too much sugar and salt. A diet high in these components is a risk factor for many diseases. These diseases include obesity, heart disease, high blood pressure, and diabetes.

The Role of Thirst

Thirst is the one way your body lets you know you need water. However, thirst is not an accurate warning system. Your body needs water before you feel thirsty and after your thirst appears to be quenched. It seems that thirst does not occur until water supplies are already short. There is a delay between the need for water and the feeling of thirst.

Water is critical to almost all body functions. A shortage of water can lower energy levels, reduce coordination, and begin to damage body tissue. It is best to consume water regularly throughout the day before thirst begins.

Ice water relieves thirst faster than warm water. Most of you know that ice water feels more refreshing. It is a faster thirst quencher because it cools the stomach. This causes the stomach to constrict and forces the water into the bloodstream at a faster rate.

Should you choose water or a sweetened beverage when thirsty? Water is better than soda or fruit drinks. This is especially true when you are taking part in moderate physical activity lasting less than an hour. In the next chapter, you will see how water is necessary to digest sugar. If you consume sweetened soft drinks, part of the water will be tied up digesting the sugar. This makes less fluid available for other uses. Your thirst will often return in as little as 30 minutes when you consume a sweetened soft drink.

If you will be physically active for more than an hour, you may wish to choose a sports drink. These drinks are specially designed to meet your body's fluid needs during extended physical activity. They provide smaller amounts of sugar than soda or fruit drinks.

This amount of sugar can be absorbed by the body and provide a source of energy during activity. Sports drinks also supply small amounts of sodium and potassium that your body loses through sweat. The sodium helps your body retain fluids, and the appealing taste of these beverages may encourage you to drink more.

You have learned that water has a lower boiling point at higher altitudes because of reduced atmospheric pressure. This reduced pressure also affects your water needs. More water evaporates from skin and through breath at high altitudes, where atmospheric pressure is lower. This affects water needs for airplane passengers as well as people in mountainous areas. The higher the altitude, the more water you will need to drink to stay *hydrated,* or full of water.

A Safe Water Supply

Water is the most valuable natural resource. All life depends on its availability and safety. Nature has been recycling water long before people named the concept. Rain washes and waters the earth. The rain becomes part of rivers, streams, and lakes or filters through the soil to the underground water table. Collected rainwater, groundwater from lakes and streams, and wells that tap underground water are plentiful in the United States. It is easy to forget that one person's wastewater later becomes another person's drinking water. See 7-14.

For years, people assumed they could dump waste in large bodies of water without any side effects. Following are some of the problems created by water that has been contaminated or polluted by this practice:

❖ Typhoid is caused by bacteria that spread from human and animal feces into water supplies. This disease is common in heavily populated areas without proper sanitation.

❖ The Mediterranean Sea along the Riviera is toxic to most life-forms due to factory and human wastes in the water.

❖ In the 1970s, dumping from factories caused mercury buildup in rivers and oceans. This endangered swordfish and tuna supplies.

Steps in Wastewater Treatment

1. Remove suspended solids in the water using filters and gravity to screen or settle out large particles.
2. Remove soluble organic matter by first allowing microbes to feed on the matter still present in the water.
3. Aerate the water. Adding oxygen kills some of the harmful bacteria.
4. Add a disinfectant to kill harmful bacteria. Common disinfectants are chlorine and fluorine.
5. Use advanced specialized treatments, such as adding activated carbon to absorb coloring agents, odors, herbicides, and pesticides. The carbon is periodically regenerated by heating to temperatures of 900°C (1652°F). These high temperatures vaporize all but the carbon.

7-14 Local communities in the United States carefully treat wastewater to make it safe for drinking.

❖ Fish in Lake Erie began to die as a result of factory and human waste disposal building to toxic levels. In the 1970s, the toxic buildup was so bad that some people declared Lake Erie to be "dead."

❖ On June 21, 1995, in North Carolina, dams holding 35 million gallons of hog sewage broke, polluting rivers and destroying fish populations.

A *contaminant* or *pollutant* can be anything that makes a substance impure or unsuitable. Anything that causes water to be unsafe for use is a water contaminant. Some of the more common sources of contaminants are animal and human wastes, chemicals, and garbage.

Biological Pollutants

Biological pollutants include bacteria, protozoa, viruses, and organic wastes. Many microbes that break down waste products are not harmful by themselves. In large volumes, however, their oxygen needs can deplete oxygen levels in rivers and lakes. This can cause fish to suffocate. Large volumes of decaying organic wastes will also reduce oxygen levels in water supplies. The main sources of organic wastes include human and animal sewage, wood and paper mills, and food processing plants. Another problem is organic wastes may leave particles in the water that can coat or clog machinery.

Chemical Contaminants in Water

There are three main kinds of chemical contaminants found in water: metal ions, acids, and toxic substances.

Metal Ions

A *temporary water hardness* is caused by the presence of calcium and magnesium ions. These ions dissolve in rainwater as it soaks into soil. The ions combine with bicarbonates in the water to form salts. These salts are easily removed through heating. However, they can coat pipes, valves, and cooking equipment. They can interfere with the transfer of heat and add to the difficulty of cleaning equipment. They provide a place for bacteria to multiply and reduce the effectiveness of soap. Hard water has also been found to toughen the textures of fruits and vegetables during processing.

When sulfur and chloride compounds combine with calcium and magnesium, water is called *permanently hard.* These ions must be removed through an ion exchange method. Permanently hard water is passed over material that contains loosely bound sodium and hydrogen cations. The exchanger, called a *water softener,* gives up the sodium and hydrogen and collects the calcium and magnesium compounds.

Acids

Acids that dissolve in the water supply can change the pH of water. Acid rain is an example of this kind of pollutant. Burned petroleum products give off carbon monoxide and carbon dioxide. Carbon monoxide is an example of a nonmetal pollutant. Carbon dioxide forms weak carbonic acid (H_2CO_3). The more carbon dioxide that dissolves in the rain, the lower the pH of the rainwater. Carbon dioxide is not the only source of acid rain. Other acids from manufactured sources include sulfur oxides (SO_2), nitrogen oxides (NO_2), and hydrochloric acid (HCl). Low (acidic) pH levels can kill plant and animal life.

Physical Contaminants in Water

An often overlooked source of pollution is garbage and litter. Many people thoughtlessly toss garbage when picnicking, boating, and fishing. People often drop soiled diapers, cans, bottles, and plastics with no thought of their potential harm. Fish have died because of swallowing plastics. Swimmers have been cut on discarded bottles and cans. Litter can harbor bacteria, cause physical harm, and break down into toxins that enter the water supply. See 7-15.

Water Contaminants and the Beverage Industry

Consumers expect a particular soft drink to taste the same whether they are in Tokyo, London, or New York City. Physical, biological, and chemical contaminants vary from one region to another. These contaminants can change the flavor of the water. Water processing plants generally remove only harmful contaminants. Therefore, most bottling companies have established water standards for their products. To make a uniform product, these companies treat water beyond the level of treatment provided by water processing plants. Beverage bottlers remove contaminants from their water sources that produce unwanted flavors before adding soft drink syrups.

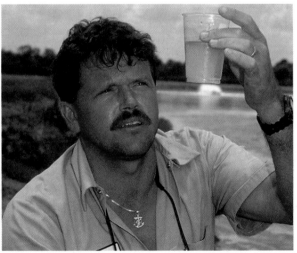

USDA

7-15 This worker is testing the contaminant levels of water to be sure the water will support the growth of shrimp.

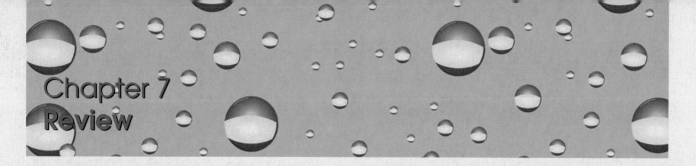

Chapter 7
Review

Summary

All areas of food science and food production require an understanding of water. The polar arrangement of the atoms in water molecules causes the molecules to form hydrogen bonds. This gives water a lot of surface tension. Surface tension affects the boiling and freezing points of water. Boiling and freezing points are also affected by atmospheric pressure and impurities in water.

Water plays two critical roles in food production. In both liquid and steam form, water serves as a heat medium for cooking. It also functions in many food products as a solvent of gases, liquids, and solids. A food's water content can affect how the food should be prepared and preserved.

Water serves many functions in the body. It moves nutrients, toxins, and other chemicals in, out, and around the body. Water also helps keep body temperature even and provides a medium for chemical reactions. This is why you must meet your daily water needs by drinking water and consuming foods and beverages that contain water. You cannot simply rely on your thirst to help you get all the water your body requires.

With all water does for humanity, it is important to keep the water supply safe. Biological, chemical, and physical pollutants can make water unsafe for use. Each person must do his or her part to maintain the quality of the water supply.

Check Your Understanding

1. List three functions of water in the body and three functions of water in the food supply.
2. How does the water molecule differ from other compounds of similar size?
3. Describe the structure of water.

4. Why does water form intermolecular hydrogen bonds with other molecules?
5. Explain why ice floats in water.
6. How are atmospheric pressure, temperature, and boiling point related?
7. Name two ways water can be used as a heat medium in cooking.
8. What are the advantages of steaming vegetables over boiling them?
9. Name three types of water-based solutions and give an example of each.
10. Define the three ways water becomes part of the structure of a food.
11. What does water activity measure and how is it related to food spoilage?
12. Why should you drink water before you feel thirsty?
13. List two examples of each of the three main types of contaminants that can be found in water.
14. Describe three problems that can be caused by hard water.

Critical Thinking

1. Explain why the polar nature of water makes it a good solvent.
2. Explain how a pressure cooker speeds cooking?
3. Why should you save water that you have used to cook vegetables? How can this water be used?

Explore Further

1. **Writing.** Write a short paper comparing and contrasting bottled spring water with distilled water. What are the advantages of each?

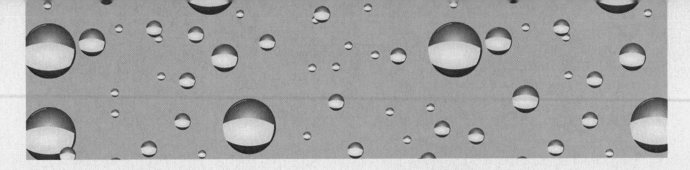

2. **Math.** How much salt does it take to change the boiling point of 1 liter of water 1°C? 1°F? What is the molarity of the salt water?

3. **Reading.** Research the most likely sources of water contamination in your community. What laws and regulations exist to reduce the risks of contamination? What contamination problems, if any, have occurred in your community in the last decade? Report your findings in class.

4. **Science.** Test your local water for pH, hardness, and physical or biological contaminants.

5. **Communication.** Debate a political issue related to water that is relevant to your community. Possible debate topics include the following:

❖ oil spills along coastlines

❖ elimination of swamplands due to urban development

❖ factory and city waste in and along a river

❖ hog sewage dams

❖ river water being diverted to another community

❖ mandatory water conservation during drought conditions

❖ buried industrial waste and/or tanks leaking into the water table

Experiment 7A
Thermometer Calibration

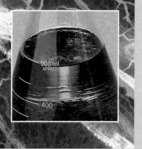

Purpose

You will need to be able to calibrate new thermometers to check their accuracy. You will also need to be able to recalibrate an instant-read thermometer each time it is dropped. Water is used as a standard for calibrating thermometers. You will use ice water and boiling water to calibrate an alcohol thermometer and boiling water to calibrate an instant-read or digital thermometer. Changes in atmospheric pressure can alter the boiling point of water-based solutions. This is a problem in the production of candies made from sugar-water solutions. This is why it is important that you calibrate a candy thermometer just before making a batch of many candies.

Equipment

2 400-mL beakers

glass stirring rod

alcohol thermometer

instant-read thermometer or digital
    thermometer

Supplies

water

ice cubes

Procedure

1. Pour 150 mL of cold tap water into one of the 400-mL beakers.
2. Add ice cubes until the water level reaches 300 mL.
3. Stir the ice water with a glass stirring rod until the melting of the ice cubes slows.
4. Insert the alcohol thermometer into the beaker. Wait one minute to allow time for the thermometer to stabilize. Record the temperature. Remove the thermometer from the ice water.
5. Pour 200 mL of tap water into the second beaker. Heat on medium-high until the water comes to a full rolling boil. Use this beaker of boiling water for steps 6, 7, and 8.
6. Insert the alcohol thermometer into the beaker of boiling water. Always position a thermometer so the bulb is just below the center point of the liquid. Wait until the temperature stops climbing, then record the temperature.
7. Insert the instant-read thermometer into the boiling water. Using a wrench, gently adjust the hexagonal nut under the dial until the pointer is pointing to 100°C.
8. If you have a digital thermometer, locate the tiny screws that are used to adjust or calibrate the thermometer. Insert the thermometer into the boiling water. Using a small screwdriver, adjust the screw until the readout is 100°C.

Calculations

Calibrate the alcohol thermometer by subtracting 100°C from the temperature recorded for boiling water. If the number is positive, add it to the temperature called for in a recipe. If the number is negative, substract it from the temperature called for in a recipe. For

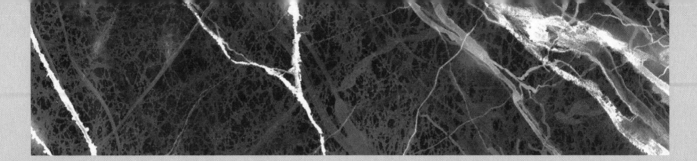

example, if your thermometer read 103°C in boiling water, you would add 3°C to the temperature specified in a recipe (103°C – 100°C = 3°C). Therefore, if a fudge recipe says to cook the mixture to 113°C, then you would cook it until your thermometer reads 116°C (113°C + 3°C = 116°C).

Questions

1. Which, if any, of the thermometers tested accurately?

2. How many degrees high or low was your alcohol thermometer?

3. Which type of thermometer required more calibration?

Experiment 7B
Water in Hot Dogs

Safety

❖ **Use a cutting board whenever you use a sharp knife.**

❖ **Clean all surfaces and equipment with hot soapy water after completing the lab.**

❖ **Handle the hot evaporating dish with test tube tongs or a hot pad.**

Purpose

Food manufacturers often add water to processed meats to increase the moisture and weight of the final product. In this experiment, you will be assessing the amount of water in various brands and its effect on flavor and texture.

Equipment

evaporating dish
electronic balance
utility or paring knife
cutting board

Supplies

$\frac{1}{2}$ hot dog of assigned variation

Procedure

Part I

1. Record the calories, fat grams, and protein in each hot dog variation from the nutrition labels on the packages. Get the cost of each brand from your teacher.

2. Tare a clean evaporating dish on an electronic balance.

3. Dice $\frac{1}{2}$ hot dog of your assigned variation and put the pieces in the evaporating dish.
   Variation 1: fat free
   Variation 2: lowfat

Variation 3: regular

Variations 4-6: can be a variety of hot dog brands of varying prices

4. Mass the hot dog.

5. Place the evaporating dish and hot dog in a food dehydrator at its highest setting. If you do not have a dehydrator, place the evaporating dish in an oven set between 175°F and 200°F. Leave the hot dog in the dehydrator or oven overnight.

6. Prepare the remaining hot dogs on a grill until plump and lightly browned.

7. Cut cooked hot dogs into enough pieces so all students can taste each variation.

8. Sample the cooked hot dogs and record your observations of flavor, texture, and appearance.

Part II

1. After 24 hours in the dehydrator or oven, carefully remove the hot evaporating dish. Mass the hot dog and the evaporating dish. Record the mass.

Calculations

1. Calculate the mass of water lost (mass of hot dog before dehydration minus the mass of hot dog after dehydration).

2. Calculate the percentage of water in the hot dog. Record the percentage in the class data table provided by your teacher.

Questions

1. Which type of hot dog had the highest and lowest water content?

2. What relationship, if any, was there between the water and fat content of the hot dogs?

3. What relationship, if any, was there between the water content and the cost of the hot dogs?

4. Which hot dogs had the best flavor and texture?

Experiment 7C
Water Purity

Purpose

In this lab, you will examine the effects of four water purification methods on stagnant water. One method you will test is the addition of chlorine, which is a step in many municipal water processing plants. You will also test filtering, boiling, and adding iodine, which is a method some backpackers use to purify water.

Equipment

beaker

wax pencil

5 test tubes with stoppers

25-mL graduated cylinder

test-tube rack

eyedropper

2 250-mL beakers

5 microscope slides with cover slips

microscope

Supplies

50 mL stagnant water

1 mL chlorine bleach

1 mL iodine tincture

2 coffee filters

100 mL boiling water

Procedure

1. Measure 50 mL of stagnant water from a pool cover, pond, or birdbath in a beaker.

2. Use a wax pencil to number five test tubes from 1 through 5. Pour 10 mL of the stagnant water into each of the test tubes.

3. Prepare the test tubes as follows:

   Test tube 1: Set aside in the test-tube rack for use as a control.

   Test tube 2: Use the eyedropper to add 5 drops chlorine bleach.

   Test tube 3: Clean the eyedropper and add 5 drops of iodine tincture.

   Test tube 4: Pour water through two coffee filters placed together in a 250-mL beaker. Return the filtered water to the test tube.

   Test tube 5: Place the test tube in a 250-mL beaker with 100 mL of boiling water. Heat the beaker until the water in the test tube boils. Boil for 2 minutes.

   Place a stopper in each test tube after you have finished preparing it and shake gently.

4. Clean the eyedropper. Then use it to place a few drops of the water from the control onto a microscope slide. Cover the slide with a cover slip.

5. Observe the water under a microscope. Note color, size, and shape of the particles. Record your observations and make sketches of the particles.

6. Repeat steps 4 and 5 with the solutions in each of the remaining test tubes. *Make sure you clean the eyedropper between each use to avoid cross-contamination.*

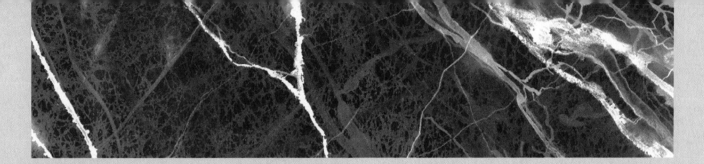

Questions

1. How were the particles you observed from each of the test tubes similar?

2. How were the particles you observed from each of the test tubes different?

3. What similarities did you find between the chemical and physical methods of purification?

4. Were all methods equally effective in removing contaminants? If not, which method was most effective? Explain your answer.

Large organic compounds make up the bulk or main mass of most foods. These compounds contain large chains or rings of carbon. Because of their comparatively large size and their importance in a nutritious diet, they can be called macronutrients. The macronutrients can all be used as energy sources by the body. They are divided into three categories based on similarities in their chemical structures. These categories are commonly known as carbohydrates, fats, and proteins.

Chapters 8 and 9 explore carbohydrates. The physical properties and functions of carbohydrates can be divided into two categories: simple and complex. Chapter 10 examines the category of compounds called fats. This category of organic compounds is referred to as lipids. The complex structure of proteins and their many functions are defined in Chapter 11. Chapter 12 analyzes enzymes, a category of proteins identified by their unique functions in food preparation, ripening, and spoilage.

Each chapter in this unit describes how the chemical structures of the macronutrients are related and defined. The relationship of each chemical structure to the compound's function in food preparation is analyzed. The last section of Chapters 8 through 11 evaluates the nutritional impact of the compound on your diet.

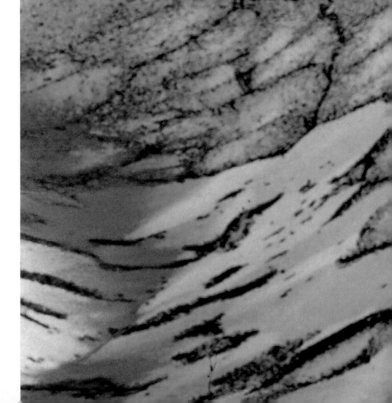

Unit III
Organic Chemistry: The Macronutrients

8 Sugar: The Simplest of Carbohydrates

9 The Complex Carbohydrates: Starches, Cellulose, Gums, and Pectins

10 Lipids: Nature's Flavor Enhancers

11 Proteins: Amino Acids and Peptides

12 Enzymes: The Protein Catalyst

This colorful image is a photomicrograph of valine, one of the amino acid building blocks of the macronutrient protein.

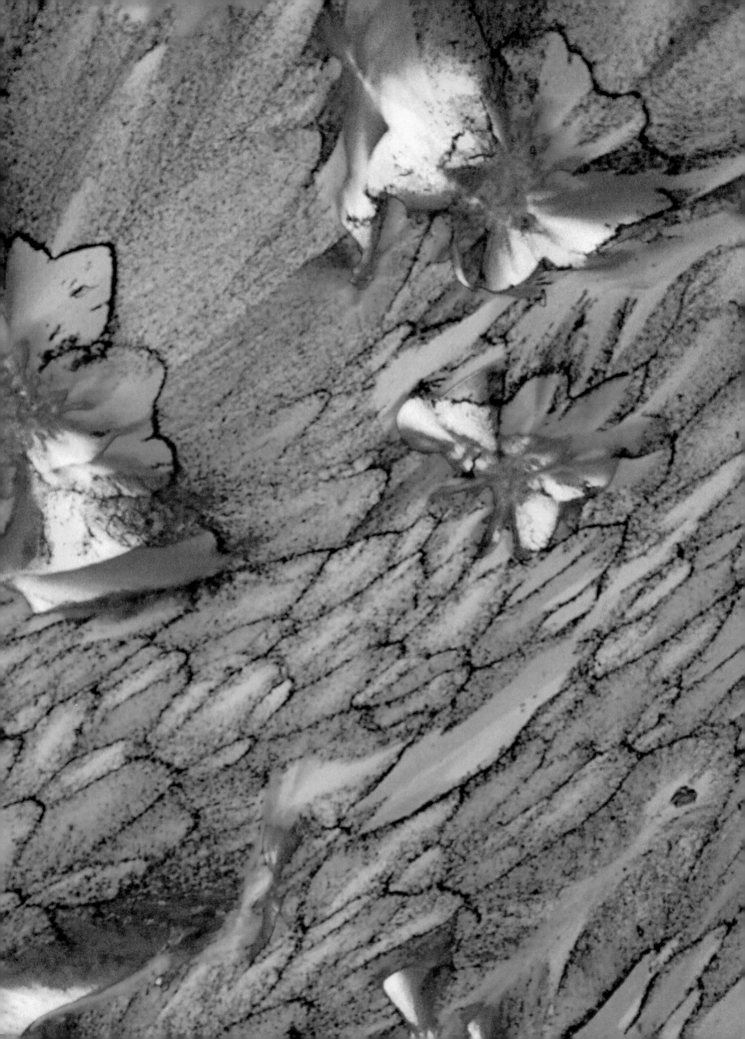

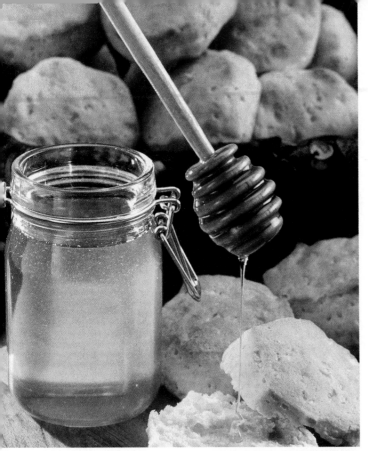

Agricultural Research Service, USDA

Honey has been used as a source of simple carbohydrates in food preparation for thousands of years.

Chapter 8

Sugar: The Simplest of Carbohydrates

Objectives

After studying this chapter,
you will be able to

summarize how carbohydrates are produced through the process of photosynthesis.

identify the monosaccharides that are combined to form each of the disaccharides.

explain the chemical process of hydrolysis.

name types of sugar used as food ingredients.

list the functions of sugar in food preparation.

evaluate the role of sugar in a nutritious diet.

Key Terms

carbohydrate
photosynthesis
saccharide
hydroxyl group
monosaccharide
fructose
glucose
mannose
galactose
ribose
ribonucleic acid
   (RNA)
disaccharide
sucrose
maltose

lactose
hydrolysis
invert sugar
alcohol
molasses
dextrose
solubility
supersaturated
interfering agent
agitation
ripening
caramelization
glycogen
diabetes mellitus
insulin

Scientists estimate that more than 50% of the earth's *biomass* is made up of carbohydrate compounds. (*Biomass* refers to the dry weight of all plants and animals.) About 75% of the dry mass of all land plants and seaweed are carbohydrates of some form. This includes the plants used to make such products as wood, paper, cotton, linen, and rayon.

Because of their abundance throughout nature, carbohydrates make up the bulk of the biomass in food. Carbohydrates are a major source of energy for humans, providing 55% to 80% of calorie needs. Compared with people in other countries, people in the United States have one of the lowest carbohydrate intakes. Even so, these organic compounds still provide the bulk of energy in the U.S. diet. See 8-1.

Carbohydrates provide a reserve energy store for all living things as well as forming the vital structure of living cells. Even DNA, which provides genetic information to all living things, is composed of a carbohydrate base.

Understanding the functions of carbohydrates is important to many areas of industry and research. However, it is vital to food science. You will rarely work with a food mixture that does not contain carbohydrates in some form.

You can group carbohydrates in food ingredients into three categories: sugars, starches, and fiber. In this chapter, you will examine the structures and functions of sugars. In Chapter 9, you will learn about starches and fiber.

Carbohydrate Production

All **carbohydrates** are compounds composed of the elements carbon, oxygen, and hydrogen. The name *carbohydrate* means a hydrate of carbon, or carbon that is loosely bound with water. This is because scientists originally felt the molecular structure was $C_6(H_2O)_6$. Although they quickly abandoned this view, the name carbohydrate has remained.

Carbohydrates are nature's means of storing solar energy. Through the process of **photosynthesis,** plants convert energy from the sun into the most common of the carbohydrates, glucose. Photosynthesis requires carbon dioxide, water, chlorophyll, and sunlight. Sunlight is the source of energy that powers the chemical reaction of photosynthesis. Chlorophyll is a green pigment found only in plants. It traps the radiant energy from the sun and turns it into chemical energy. All green plants use this process for growth as well as energy storage. The equation for photosynthesis is

$$6CO_2 + 6H_2O + \text{sunlight} \longrightarrow C_6H_{12}O_6 + 6O_2$$

carbon   water   energy   glucose   oxygen
dioxide   (simple sugar)

Initially, all carbohydrates are produced in the form of glucose. Plants can then convert glucose into whatever form of sugar, starch, or fiber they need at the time.

As the plant matures, it makes glucose into fiber to form the structure of the stems and leaves. As the plant reaches full size, it begins to transfer its energy into sugars and starches. These are storage forms of energy the plant uses for reproduction. As the seeds develop, the carbohydrates start mostly as sugars. Then they gradually change into more

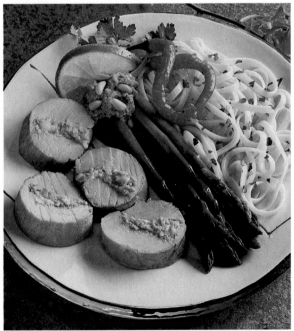

National Pork Producers Council

8-1 Most calories on the average plate and in the average diet should come from carbohydrate sources, such as pasta and vegetables.

complex starches. This is why baby corn and petite peas are sweeter than their full-sized counterparts. See 8-2.

Sugars

The simplest types of the carbohydrates are called *sugars*. In organic chemistry, the name **saccharide** has been given to all carbohydrates classified as sugars. *Sugar* was the common name used before organic chemists developed the naming system presently used to identify organic compounds.

Structure

Sugars are organic compounds. That simply means sugars contain carbon compounds. All living organisms are composed of organic, or carbon-based, compounds.

Organic compounds are grouped by their structure. For example, all carbohydrates contain hydroxyl groups. A *hydroxyl group* is an oxygen atom and a hydrogen atom bonded together. A hydroxyl group is represented by the chemical symbol -OH. As you know, oxygen atoms prefer to bond with two atoms. The second oxygen bond in a hydroxyl group is formed with a carbon atom, as represented in the following diagrams:

$$-\overset{|}{\underset{|}{C}}-O-H \quad or \quad -\overset{|}{\underset{|}{C}}-OH$$

Monosaccharides

A simple sugar is a molecule that cannot be broken down into a smaller molecule without changing its basic nature. The simple sugars are known as **monosaccharides**, or sugars that contain one basic molecule.

Examples of monosaccharides found widely in food products are fructose, glucose, galactose, and mannose. In organic chemistry, the names of saccharides end in *-ose*. *Fructose* is a monosaccharide found widely in fruits and honey. *Glucose* is the most abundant of the sugars, and it is people's basic energy source. It occurs naturally in blood, grapes, and corn, 8-3. The body converts all sugars and starches into glucose before using the glucose for energy. *Mannose* is found in eggs and

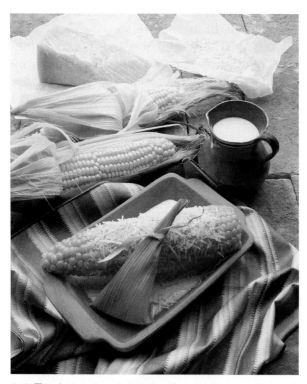

8-2 Tender, young kernels of corn are sweeter than mature kernels because they contain a higher percentage of sugars.

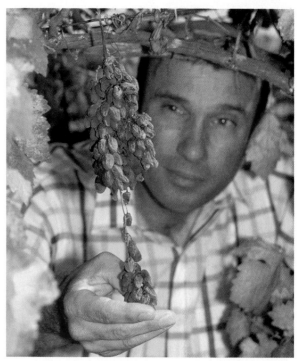

8-3 Glucose is one of the sugars found in grapes.

some plants and usually occurs as a component of long chains of sugars. *Galactose* can only be found in animals and humans and is one of the basic sugars found in milk. All these sugars have six carbon atoms, twelve hydrogen atoms, and six oxygen atoms.

Originally, scientists believed sugar molecules existed primarily in a linear form. The carbon atoms were thought to form a line. The hydrogen and oxygen atoms were believed to branch off the carbon atoms at different angles.

Scientists now know most simple sugars in nature have a central ring structure. Constructing three-dimensional models of sugars can give you a better idea of how the atoms align with each other. Fructose has a five-member ring. Glucose, mannose, and galactose have six-member rings.

When scientists create diagrams of any ring-shaped organic compound, they simplify the drawing. They use the junction of lines to represent the location of a carbon atom. They draw lines where hydrogen atoms are located, but they do not write the letter *H*. In the following example, the diagram on the left shows glucose as a ring with all the atoms represented by letters. The diagram on the right is the shorthand version of the same molecule.

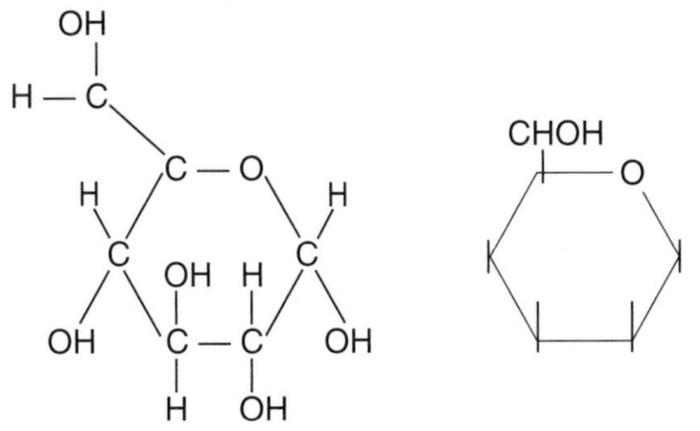

All monosaccharides occur most frequently in a ring structure that contains five carbon atoms and one oxygen atom. They differ in the way the hydrogen and oxygen atoms are arranged around the ring. The difference in position affects the characteristics of the sugar and how it will respond in food preparation.

To understand the importance of the arrangement of the atoms, look at two basic forms of glucose: α-D-glucose and β–D-glucose. As you can see from the following diagram,

the alpha (α) glucose and beta (β) glucose have only one difference. That is the position of the -OH group on the right side of the ring. This one change in position determines whether the body is able to digest the sugar. Alpha-glucose is the basic energy source for humans. Beta-glucose is the main component of dietary fiber that provides bulk for the digestive track. However, it provides no nutritive value because people cannot digest it.

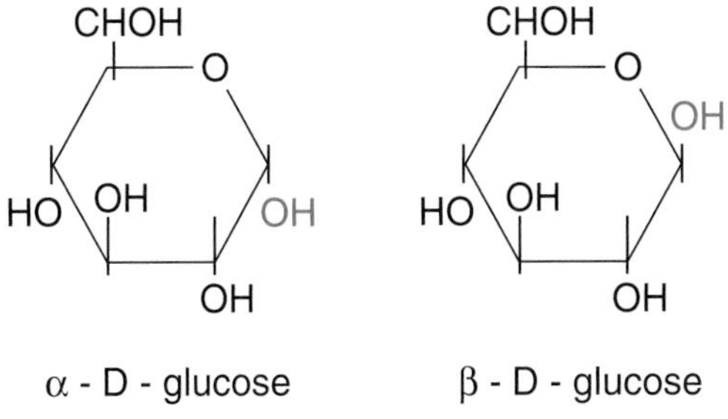

α - D - glucose   β - D - glucose

So far, the simple sugars described have a basic formula of $C_6H_{12}O_6$. There are also some sugars that contain only five carbon atoms. These are *riboses*. The body uses them as the basic building blocks for *ribonucleic acid (RNA)*. RNA carries the genetic code in the cells and is used for the production of DNA.

Disaccharides

Sugars found in nature do not normally occur as monosaccharides. The sugar molecule's structure enables it to readily combine with other sugars to form chains. A *disaccharide* is two joined monosaccharides. Most sugars consumed in the world are disaccharides. *Sucrose*, or table sugar, is a disaccharide that contains one glucose molecule and one fructose molecule. Other disaccharides found in the food supply are maltose and lactose. *Maltose* is commonly found in malted grains. It is made of two glucose molecules. This disaccharide is the least sweet. When in powder form, it is tan rather than clear or white like sucrose. *Lactose* is the sugar found in milk. It is composed of one glucose molecule and one galactose molecule. In pure form, it is white and contributes some of the color you associate with milk.

When two monosaccharides join, a hydroxyl group from one and a hydrogen atom from the other separate to form water. See 8-4.

Composition of Disaccharides

8-4 Two monosaccharide molecules combine to form one disaccharide molecule and one water molecule.

This process of molecules joining and releasing water is reversible. *Hydrolysis* occurs when a large molecule, such as sugar, is divided into smaller parts by adding water. If you hydrolyze a molecule of sucrose, you will get one molecule of fructose and one molecule of glucose. The body uses this hydrolysis process to digest the disaccharides in food. For hydrolysis to occur, water must be present. This is why sweetened drinks are not as thirst quenching as plain water. Part of the water is used to digest the sugar and is not available for other functions.

Three conditions can trigger hydrolysis. One condition is the presence of an enzyme to set off the reaction. A second condition is the addition of an acid. A third condition is the addition of heat. Digestion of sugar involves the addition of the enzyme sucrase. This enzyme is present in saliva. Thorough chewing of your food enables the enzyme to be mixed into the food so the enzyme can work

quickly. Lactose-free milk is produced by adding an enzyme to hydrolyze the sugar.

Each type of sugar requires a different enzyme for hydrolysis to occur. You can determine the names of the enzymes by simply changing the *-ose* ending of the sugar to *-ase*. For instance, sucrase hydrolyzes sucrose and lactase hydrolyzes lactose. Sucrase is also known as invertase. This is because the fructose and glucose mixture that results from the hydrolysis of sucrose is sometimes called *invert sugar.*

Alcohols

All organic compounds that contain at least one -OH group are called *alcohols.* Sugars are a related group of compounds that have multiple -OH groups plus an oxygen atom with a double bond. This similarity in chemical structure helps explain the high caloric content of most alcoholic (*ethanol*) beverages.

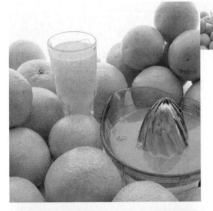

Nutrition News
Lactose Intolerance

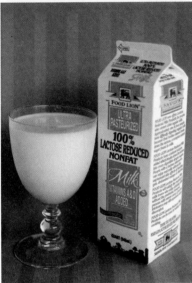

Lactose-reduced dairy products can be digested easily by people who experience lactose intolerance.

Lactase is an enzyme that is present in the small intestines. Its presence is necessary for the digestion of milk sugar. *Lactose intolerance* is an inherited inability to produce the lactase enzyme necessary to properly digest lactose or milk sugar. Most Asian, Native American, and African American adults experience this problem to some degree.

Symptoms of lactose intolerance include a sour aftertaste when drinking milk. Gas, bloating, nausea, diarrhea, and flulike stomach cramps followed by constipation are other symptoms.

People can buy lactase from most pharmacies in either pill or liquid form. Experimentation with dosages will help people determine how much of the enzyme they need to avoid symptoms when consuming milk products. The liquid lactase is usually added to milk and allowed to sit before drinking. The lactase will cause the milk to have a sweeter flavor. This is because the lactose has been broken down into glucose and galactose.

Dairy producers have developed a variety of lactose-free and lactose-reduced products. Examine the labels in the dairy case. Many stores stock milk that has 70% to 100% of the lactose removed. Some gourmet ice cream manufacturers are also making lactose-reduced ice creams.

Lactase is produced by *Lactobacillus acidophilus* bacteria, which normally live in the intestines. Antibiotics will kill these helpful bacteria as well as the bacteria that cause infections. Therefore, milk will sometimes be difficult to digest for several weeks after taking antibiotics. You can take care of this problem by eating a serving of yogurt shortly after finishing your antibiotic prescription. Be sure to choose yogurt that contains an active culture of *Lactobacillus acidophilus*.

Names of alcohols end in *-ol*. Examples include ethanol (ethyl alcohol), methanol (wood alcohol), and isopropanol (rubbing alcohol). All these alcohols are toxic if consumed in excess. Ethanol is the alcohol in alcoholic beverages. It can be made from any sugar or starch source. Small amounts of methanol in bad batches of "moonshine" have been know to cause permanent nerve damage, blindness, or death. Methanol is produced by burning wood without oxygen present. Isopropanol is derived from petroleum and is not safe to consume.

There are several commonly used additives that are "sweet" alcohols. These alcohols are glycerol, mannitol, sorbitol, and xylitol. One source of glycerol is animal fats. See 8-5.

The Sweet Alcohols

	Glycerol	Mannitol	Sorbitol	Xylitol
Structure	CH_2OH | $H—C—OH$ | CH_2OH	CH_2OH | $HO—C—H$ | $HO—C—H$ | $H—C—OH$ | $H—C—OH$ | CH_2OH	CH_2OH | $H—C—OH$ | $HO—C—H$ | $H—C—OH$ | $H—C—OH$ | CH_2OH	CH_2OH | $H—C—OH$ | $HO—C—H$ | $H—C—OH$ | CH_2OH
Sources	Exists in wine and beer By-product of soap manufacture	Extracted from seaweed	Fruits: apples, berries, pears, plums Seaweed and algae	Apples, berries, plums, and other foods
Description	Warm, sweet, oily liquid	Sweet, white, odorless crystalline solid	Sweet, white powder, flakes, or granules	Sweet, white, granules
Calories/ gram	2.0	1.6	2.6	2.4
Uses	Humectant[1] in candy Solvent for colors and flavors Used in beverages, baked goods, gelatin, chewing gum, meat products, and commercial hot fudge sauces	Texturizer[2] in gum and candy Sweetener in sugar-free products but does contain calories and carbohydrates	Texturizer, humectant, anticaking agent[3], diabetic sugar substitute	Texturizer, humectant, sugar subsitute Can be used in baking
Cautions	No limitations	May worsen kidney disease	Excess consumption may cause diarrhea	Excess consumption may cause diarrhea

[1]Humectants are additives that help products retain or hold onto moisture.
[2]Texturizers are additives that give food products a desired mouth feel.
[3]Anticaking agents are additives that keep powders or granules from lumping.

8-5 The sweet alcohols are used as additives to serve a variety of functions in food products.

Sources of Sugar

Sugars have a sweet flavor and provide 4 calories of energy per gram. Types of sugars commonly used as food ingredients are granulated, brown, and confectioner's sugars; honey; corn syrup; molasses; and maple syrup. Food companies often use several kinds of sweeteners in a single food product. This allows food scientists to optimize sweetness for each product and minimize product costs.

Each sweetener is listed separately in the ingredient list on product labels. Total carbohydrates are listed on the Nutrition Facts panel on a food label. Amounts of dietary fiber and sugars are identified under the figure for total carbohydrates. You can learn to recognize the names of sugars that may appear on food labels. This will help you be aware of the sugar content of products you consume. See 8-6.

Most sweeteners used today are extracted from plants that are high in sugar content.

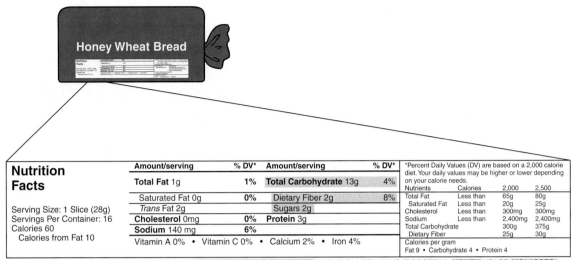

Nutrition Facts	Amount/serving	% DV*	Amount/serving	% DV*	*Percent Daily Values (DV) are based on a 2,000 calorie diet. Your daily values may be higher or lower depending on your calorie needs.

Serving Size: 1 Slice (28g)
Servings Per Container: 16
Calories 60
   Calories from Fat 10

	Amount/serving	% DV*	Amount/serving	% DV*
	Total Fat 1g	1%	Total Carbohydrate 13g	4%
	Saturated Fat 0g	0%	Dietary Fiber 2g	8%
	Trans Fat 2g		Sugars 2g	
	Cholesterol 0mg	0%	Protein 3g	
	Sodium 140 mg	6%		
	Vitamin A 0% • Vitamin C 0% • Calcium 2% • Iron 4%			

Nutrients	Calories	2,000	2,500
Total Fat	Less than	65g	80g
Saturated Fat	Less than	20g	25g
Cholesterol	Less than	300mg	300mg
Sodium	Less than	2,400mg	2,400mg
Total Carbohydrate		300g	375g
Dietary Fiber		25g	30g

Calories per gram
Fat 9 • Carbohydrate 4 • Protein 4

INGREDIENTS: WHOLE WHEAT FLOUR, WATER, HIGH-FRUCTOSE CORN SYRUP, WHEAT GLUTEN (WHEAT PROTEIN), HONEY, YEAST, MOLASSES, SOYBEAN OIL, SALT, DOUGH CONDITIONERS (MAY CONTAIN ONE OR MORE OF THE FOLLOWING: MONO- AND DIGLYCERIDES, SODIUM STEAROYL LACTYLATE, MALTED BARLEY FLOUR, AZODICARBONAMIDE, ASCORBIC ACID), YEAST NUTRIENTS (MONOCALCIUM PHOSPHATE AND AMMONIUM SULFATE), VINEGAR.

8-6 Reading Nutrition Facts panels and ingredient lists can help you become aware of the sugar content of food products.

Sweet syrups are extracted, the impurities are removed, and all or part of the water is removed. Sources of these sugars are sugar cane, sugar beets, maple trees, corn, and sorghum. One type of sweetener, honey, is manufactured by bees rather than being extracted from plants.

Sugar Cane

The Chinese were the first to discover the high concentration of sugar in sugar cane plants. They developed a process to extract sugar syrup from the cane.

The crude, boiled liquid pressed from sugar cane is known as *molasses.* The composition of molasses will vary with its degree of refinement. It contains 35% to 50% sucrose and 15% to 20% invert sugar. Molasses is 20% to 25% water and has a 2% to 5% mineral content. Popular foods containing large amounts of molasses are gingerbread cake, gingersnap cookies, and shoofly pie.

Brown sugar is cane sugar that has not been completely refined. Brown sugar is 85% to 92% sucrose. The brown color and characteristic flavor are due to the substances in sugar cane that form molasses when extracted. It is the molasses that gives brown sugar its moist texture and distinctive flavor. Brown sugar is

used in baking where the additional coloring and flavor are desirable.

Brown sugar must be stored in a sealed container to prevent loss of moisture. Brown sugar that is left open will become hard and crumbly. The moist texture can be regained by adding apple slices or a slice of fresh bread to the container. In time, the sugar will absorb enough moisture from the bread or apple to make the brown sugar moist again.

With further processing, all minerals, flavorings, and coloring agents can be removed from brown sugar. This leaves only the crystalline substance you know as *granulated sugar.*

The size of sugar crystals can be altered by grinding. *Confectioner's sugar* is granulated sugar that has been ground into a fine powder. Most confectioner's sugar has cornstarch added to help prevent caking during storage.

The number of Xs on the label of confectioner's sugar refers to how finely the sugar has been ground. The most common types are 4X, 6X, and 10X. The larger the number is, the finer the powder will be. Finer powdered sugars produce candies and icings with smoother textures. Type 4X sugar is used in the manufacture of cough drops and chewing gum. It is also the sugar of choice for marshmallows and chocolates. Type 6X sugar is used for cream fillings, uncooked fondants, and icings. It is also sprinkled on buns, pies, and pastries. Ultrafine, 10X, powdered sugar is used for the finest icings and fondant fillings.

Sugar Beets

Sucrose is also found in sugar beets. There is no difference in the performance of beet sugar and cane sugar. There is, however, usually a difference in cost. Sugar beets can be more economical to grow and process. See 8-7.

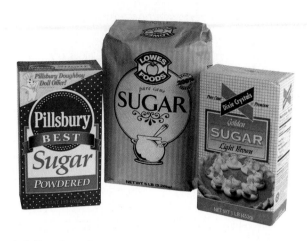

8-7 Powdered sugar, granulated sugar, and brown sugar are all made from sugar cane or sugar beets.

Health Tip

The source of granulated sugar is only important to a person who is allergic to the original plant source. Someone who is highly sensitive to beets may experience problems from consuming beet sugar due to plant residues in the sugar. Likewise, someone who is highly sensitive to sugar cane may experience problems from consuming cane sugar.

Maple Syrup

Maple syrup is the concentrated sap of sugar maple trees. It takes 40 gallons of tree sap, slowly simmered down, to make one gallon of maple syrup. Many people in the United States have never tasted true maple syrup. Because of the high cost of maple syrup, the food industry has developed substitutes. Most pancake syrups are only 2% maple syrup. The main ingredient in these syrups is corn syrup, another common sweetener in processed foods.

Corn Syrup

Corn syrup is processed by hydrolyzing cornstarch into glucose. Corn syrup is composed of varying amounts of dextrose, maltose, and dextrins or polysaccharides. (*Dextrose* is the name for glucose used by the confectionery trade.) A sweeter version of corn syrup, called *high-fructose corn syrup*, is used in many products. These products include soft drinks, pancake syrups, candies, and baked goods. It is produced by enzymatically converting some of the dextrose in corn syrup to fructose.

Technology has made it possible to use enzymes to convert starch from abundant corn supplies into sweet syrups. This has economic benefits because corn is a plentiful crop in the United States. Being able to use corn sweeteners makes it possible for food manufacturers to keep processed food prices stable.

Besides its availability and cost benefits, corn syrup has the advantage of being flexible in its properties. It is sometimes used to increase the viscosity, or thickness, of food products. Its sweetness can be varied by altering the hydrolysis process. This allows corn syrup to be used successfully for a wider variety of manufactured food products than sucrose.

Sorghum

Sorghum is a "grass" crop that resembles corn in the field. Sweet sorghum is grown in many areas for its sweet syrup, which resembles molasses. Sap is squeezed from the sorghum canes and then slowly boiled to evaporate away the excess water. In some rural areas, it is possible to watch farmers making sorghum syrup.

Honey

The first sweetener to be used in food preparation was honey. Bees extract an invert sugar syrup from the pollen of flowers and store it in their hives for future use. Honey is about 75% invert sugar and 15% to 20% water.

Bees are useful for the plant pollination

process as well as the production of honey. Honey producers construct hives that give the producers easy access to the honey stores. The honey producers place the hives near large fields of plants. These plants have sweet blossoms that will give a pleasant flavor to the honey. Orange blossom honey comes from hives near large commercial orange groves. Clover honey comes from growers whose hives are located near large fields of clover.

Isomalt

Isomalt is a mixture of one part mannitol, one part sorbitol, and two parts beet sugar. It is very popular among baking and pastry chefs because of its unique properties. It liquefies at 310°F. It does not form crystals, colors easily, and remains clear. Because it does not form crystals, it can be blown and spun into a wide variety of sugar creations.

Functions of Sugars in Food Preparation

Sugars from all sources have chemical structures that are similar but not identical. The similarities allow food manufacturers to use one sugar in place of another for some purposes. However, the unique aspects of each sugar structure determine which type of sugar is best suited for each function in foods.

Sugars have up to six functions they can perform in food products. They act as sweeteners, preservatives, and tenderizers. They also have a key role in the processes of crystallization, caramelization, and fermentation.

Sweeteners

Sugar's ability to sweeten is its major function in most food products. The ability to sweeten is connected to sugar's molecular structure. Sugars contain up to ten basic units of monosaccharides. Sensory evaluations have shown that most people rate the sweetness of sugars similarly. That is, most agree fructose is sweeter than sucrose and lactose is the least sweet of the three. Scientists have compared the structure of sugar molecules to the sweetness of the sugars. The scientists have found the sweeter the sugar is, the simpler the structure of the molecule is. The longer the sugar chain is, the less sweet the sugar will seem to be. See 8-8.

Recent research has revealed more information about sugar's ability to sweeten. Researchers have identified a triangular form on sugar molecules that bonds to taste buds for a short time. The nervous system registers this bond as a sweet flavor. The more of these bonding sites a molecule has, the sweeter the substance will seem to be. The perceived sweetness of the substance will also increase as the length of the bonding period increases.

Preservatives

Sugar helps prevent food spoilage. Water will be drawn to sugar molecules before it is drawn to bacteria. Therefore, most single-celled contaminants will dehydrate and die in concentrated sugar solutions. This is why sugar is the only preservative needed in most candies, jams, jellies, and syrups.

Sugar plays another preservative role in baked goods. It helps products such as cakes stay moist. Invert sugar has been found to maintain freshness of baked goods considerably longer than sucrose.

Tenderizers

When sugar is added to a dough, it will tenderize the product. You can observe the effects of this function by taste testing an

Relative Sweetness of Sugars	
Sugar	**Relative Sweetness**
Fructose	1.8
Sucrose	1.0
Glucose	0.8
Mannitol	0.7
Glycerol	0.6
Sorbitol	0.5
Galactose	0.3
Maltose	0.3
Lactose	0.2

8-8 The sweetness of sucrose, or table sugar, is the standard to which the sweetness levels of other sugars are compared.

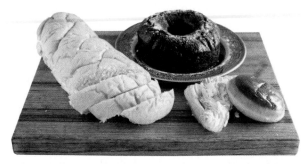

8-9 Sugar helps tenderize cakes, pastries, and doughnuts. The Italian bread on the left has a paler color and chewier texture because it does not contain any sugar.

Solubility of Sugar

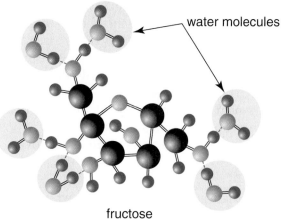

fructose

8-10 The polar OH groups in fructose are attracted to water molecules. For this reason, sugar will dissolve in water.

Italian hard roll that has no sugar added. Compare this with white bread that contains a small amount of sugar. Also test a sweet roll that has almost twice the sugar of white bread. Most of the difference in tenderness of the three products is due to the sugar in the dough. You can observe the same characteristic by comparing a bread-type muffin and a basic white or yellow cake. See 8-9.

The tenderizing effect of sugar also changes the viscosity or pourability of a batter. Sugar interferes with the flour's ability to form an elastic structure. This allows the batter to flow or pour more easily than the same mixture without sugar.

Crystallizing Agents

In candies, sugars function as crystallizing agents. This function is linked to the solubility of sugars in water. *Solubility* is the ability of a solute to dissolve in a solvent.

Sugar will dissolve in water because of its large number of hydroxyl groups. The position of the -OH causes the sugar molecule to have a polar nature near each hydroxyl group. These groups are then attracted to the polar water molecules, and hydrogen bonds are formed. These hydrogen bonds cause water molecules to surround the sugar molecules, suspending the sugar in a water solution. See 8-10.

Sugar's ability to dissolve in water increases as the temperature of the solution increases. The temperature of sugar solutions will steadily climb as heat is added. As the solution heats, water will evaporate. This changes the solute to solvent ratio, increasing the sugar concentration.

If a sugar solution has been heated to concentrate it and is then cooled, a supersaturated solution is created. Any solution that has been heated to dissolve more solute than the water would normally hold is called *supersaturated.*

Candy is made when sugar crystals separate from a supersaturated sugar solution during cooling. The entire candy industry revolves around understanding the concentrations of sugar to water at given temperatures. Candy producers know the optimum temperature for making each type of candy. See 8-11.

Sugar crystals form around particles that enter a sugar solution. These particles can be as tiny as lint or dust. However, the crystals that result may be large. Sugar crystals that form on the sides of the pan during cooking will also trigger further crystallization. This is why some candy recipes have you put a lid on the pan for two to five minutes. The steam trapped by the lid will wash sugar crystals from the sides of the pan.

Controlling the size of the sugar crystals is very important to the production of quality candy. In most cases, the finer the sugar crystals are, the higher the quality of the candy will be.

Boiling Point of Sugar Solutions

Boiling Point °C (°F)	Percentage of Sugar	Percentage of Water
100.4 (213)	10	90
101.0 (214)	30	70
102.0 (216)	50	50
106.5 (224)	70	30
107.3 (225)	75	25
114.9 (239)	85	15
117.7 (244)	87	13
120.8 (249)	89	11
122.6 (253)	90	10

Adapted from: Amendola J. & Lundberg *D. Understanding Baking,* 2nd ed., Van Nostrand Reinhold, 1992.

8-11 As the concentration of the solute increases, so does the boiling point of the solution.

Factors That Affect Crystal Formation

The following five factors affect sugar crystal formation:

❖ type of sugar
❖ use of interfering agents
❖ agitation of the sugar syrup
❖ cooling of the sugar syrup
❖ ripening of the finished product

Type of Sugar

The main sugar used by candy producers is sucrose. Sucrose crystallizes rapidly and can form large crystals. Candy producers add invert sugar when they need to slow the crystal formation. You read earlier that invert sugar occurs naturally in honey and molasses. Invert sugar is also produced commercially. This is done through the controlled addition of acids to sucrose, followed by a neutralization process.

Invert sugar helps prevent the crystallization and resulting graininess of candy caused by cane and beet sugar. This is because invert sugar is a mixture of two monosaccharides and cane and beet sugars are disaccharides. Monosaccharides are more soluble in water and therefore form smaller crystals. It takes skill to make homemade candy that has the fine texture that results from the use of commercial invert sugar.

Interfering Agents

Interfering agents are substances that can prevent or slow crystal growth. See 8-12. The most commonly used interfering agents are corn syrup, butter, and cream. Some recipes call for egg white, cream of tartar, or vinegar as interfering agents, too. Corn syrup is high

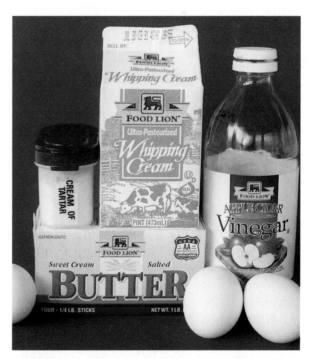

8-12 Each of these ingredients will interfere with the development of large sugar crystals in candy.

in the monosaccharide glucose. Glucose and fructose will consistently produce finer, smaller sugar crystals than sucrose. The fat molecules of butter and cream and the protein molecules of egg white help suspend and separate sugar crystals. This results in a smooth, creamy candy. Cream of tartar and vinegar are acids. Adding acids will hydrolyze the sucrose in a sugar solution. Hydrolysis results in increased levels of glucose and fructose.

Agitation

Agitation refers to the beating and stirring of a candy solution. The effects of agitation are directly related to the temperature of the candy solution. When the syrup is hot, even slight or occasional stirring increases the likelihood of crystal formation. Constant stirring of a cooled syrup prevents large crystals from forming and results in a smooth candy. This is why most fudge recipes specify letting the candy sit until it has cooled to 43°C (110°F). You are then to beat the candy vigorously until it begins to set. This helps prevent sugar crystals from forming into large clusters, which would feel grainy.

Cooling

Cooling times for candy are critical to crystal formation and should not be cut short. Stirring too early can cause a few crystals to come out of the slightly supersaturated mixture. This causes crystallization to occur slowly rather than rapidly. Crystals that form slowly are larger and give candy a grainy texture. Rapid crystallization creates small crystals, which give candy a high-quality, smooth texture. It can be difficult to wait patiently for candy to cool. However, this step is vital if the final texture is to be smooth.

Fondants and taffies are often cooled on a marble slab. The candy syrup is poured on the cool stone. Thinning out the candy syrup on marble results in fast, even cooling that produces lots of small crystals.

Ripening

Ripening is allowing candy to sit for a period in order to form a creamy, smooth texture. Fondant is a type of candy that should be allowed to ripen. It is wrapped securely and then allowed to sit for 12 to 24 hours. This

wait allows the time needed for smaller crystals to dissolve. The result is a smoother, moister fondant that kneads more easily. Some fondants have invertase added after cooking to cause further hydrolysis of disaccharides into invert sugar. The invert sugar results in a candy with a smooth, fine, even texture that is semisoft to liquid.

Tips for Successful Candy Making

Two factors must be carefully monitored when making candy. The first factor is the concentration of the sugar solution. The second factor is the size of the sugar crystals. Both of these factors are related to the temperature of the sugar solution. Therefore, it is important that your candy thermometer be calibrated every time you make candy. (You can review the calibration process by looking back at Chapter 5.)

The concentration of the sugar solution is directly related to temperature. If the solution is a few degrees too low, the sugar concentration will not be high enough. If you are making fudge, you will end up with a sticky sauce instead of a creamy candy. If the solution is a few degrees too high, the sugar concentration will be too high. This will turn your creamy fudge into a crumbly, grainy, dry product. When making caramels or suckers, a few degrees mean the difference between a delicious candy and an inedible, burnt one. See 8-13.

Keeping an eye on the candy thermometer is the easiest way to monitor the relative sugar-to-water concentration. However, remember that sugar tends to draw water. Therefore, a very humid day will change the sugar-water balance in candy as it cools. This is why some cookbooks will tell you never to make fudge on a rainy day. The high humidity may reduce the sugar concentration just enough to keep your fudge from setting. Candy manufacturers can prevent this problem by carefully monitoring and controlling the environment in the processing plant.

Caramelizing Agents

A fifth function of sugars in food products is to act as caramelizing agents. When sugar is subjected to high or prolonged heat, it

Candy Stages and Sugar Solution Temperatures

Stages*	Temperature Ranges °C (°F)	Candies
Thread	110–113 (230–235)	Candy creams or centers
Soft ball	113–118 (236–244)	Fondant, fudge, marshmallows
Ball	121–124 (250–255)	Caramel
Hard ball	127–130 (261–266)	Taffy, divinity
Soft crack	132–135 (270–275)	Butterscotch, popcorn balls
Crack	135–138 (275–280)	Nougat, toffee
Hard crack	140–157 (284–315)	Suckers, hard candy, peanut brittle, candied apples
Caramelized sugar	163–177 (325–351)	Coating for flan

* Stages refer to the physical characteristics of a small amount of syrup cooled quickly in a cup of ice water. This method of testing candy can be used if a thermometer is not available.

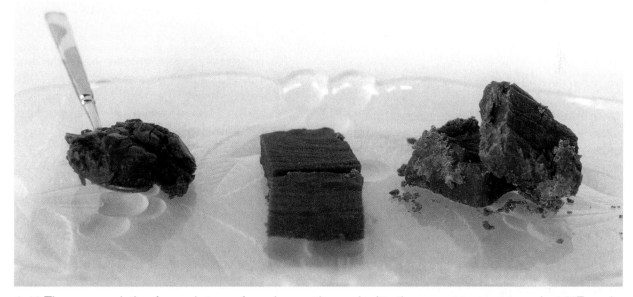

8-13 The sugar solution for each type of candy must be cooked to the correct temperature. Just 2°F made the difference between the soft fudge on the left and the creamy fudge in the middle. Another 2°F turned the creamy fudge into the dry, crumbly product on the right.

changes into a brown liquid. This is called *caramelization.* It is a complex chemical process that has not been completely identified. Researchers know that dehydration, or loss of water, is at least partially responsible for the browning and resulting flavor changes. Hydroxyl groups from some molecules and hydrogen atoms from others combine to form water that evaporates in the high heat. The sugar molecules recombine, having a higher carbon concentration. Commercially, sucrose is heated in solution with acids or acidic ammonium salts to produce caramel flavoring and coloring.

Caramelization is at least partially responsible for the brown crust on baked goods and toast. Caramelization also causes the beige color of evaporated milk and the distinctive color and flavor of caramel candy. *Flan,* a caramel custard, is a classic example of caramelization in cooking. Flan is made by browning sugar in a heavy pan until it liquefies and turns a golden brown color. This rich syrup is quickly poured into a custard cup or mold and swirled around to coat the bottom and sides. Custard is then poured into the cup or mold and baked. When the dessert is turned out of the cup or mold, the caramelized sugar syrup forms a flavorful coating for the custard.

Fermenting Agents

Sugar plays a major role in the fermentation process involved in the production of wines, beers, and yeast breads. Desired changes in these food products are caused by helpful microorganisms, such as yeast. Sugar fuels the fermentation process by serving as a food supply for the microorganisms. Alcohol is a by-product of this process, as illustrated by the following equation:

glucose + yeast → ethanol

(You will read more about fermentation in Chapter 17.)

The Nutritional Value of Sugar

All sugars produce 4 calories per gram when digested. The body uses this energy to move muscles and maintain body functions. Learning how the body accesses the energy in sugar will help you understand the role of sugar in the diet. You will also be able to recognize sugar's relation to several major health concerns.

Once simple sugars are absorbed into the bloodstream, they head to the liver. Fructose and galactose are changed into glucose in the liver. This extra step slows their availability to the body's cells and helps provide the steady supply of glucose the body needs. Glucose that is not needed immediately is changed into glycogen. *Glycogen* is multibranched chains of glucose.

The body stores two-thirds of its glycogen in the muscles and the remaining third in the liver. When the body needs energy, single glucose molecules can be broken off each branch of a glycogen molecule simultaneously. This enables large amounts of glucose to be available very quickly. During intense exercise, the body can use up to one-fifth of its total glycogen stores in 20 minutes. The body is constantly using and replenishing its glycogen stores. See 8-14.

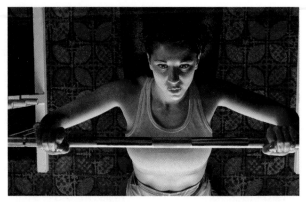

8-14 During physical activity, the body's muscles use stored glycogen as an energy source.

Studies have found the body needs sugars for proper digestion of fats and proteins. If there are no sugars present, toxins can build up in the blood that will eventually result in kidney damage.

A steady supply of glucose is needed for the brain to function. Sugars also increase the release of a brain chemical called *serotonin*. This chemical has a calming effect and acts as an antidepressant. After eating large amounts of sugar, people will become sleepy.

Although some monosaccharides are sweeter than others, it does not matter what form of sugar is eaten. Sugar is sugar as far as the body is concerned. The average U.S. diet provides about 18% of calories from sugars that are added to foods. Registered dietitians recommend that people reduce the percentage of calories consumed from added sugars to no more than 10%.

Health Concerns Related to Sugar Intake

Many people believe sugar causes tooth decay, aggravates diabetes, and causes weight gain. Although there is some truth to all these claims, there are also many misconceptions. According to an FDA report, sugar cannot be linked to any disease when consumed in moderate quantities.

Dental Caries

Dental caries, or tooth decay, is caused by acid damaging the enamel coating on teeth. Bacteria that live in the mouth feed on sugars and produce a sticky film called *plaque*. The sticky nature of plaque causes it to adhere to the teeth, creating an oxygen-deprived environment. When oxygen is reduced, the bacteria release lactic, pyruvic, and acetic acids. These acids will slowly dissolve tooth enamel.

Sugar can cause dental caries, but so can any food that contains carbohydrates. Bread or crackers are as likely to cause tooth decay as sugar. It is not so much the food you eat but how long it stays on your teeth that causes decay.

Many communities add fluoride to water supplies. Drinking fluoridated water helps increase the resistance of tooth enamel to decay. However, keeping your teeth clean is the best way to prevent tooth decay. Regular brushing with a fluoride toothpaste will help slow the production of plaque. Daily flossing will help remove plaque that is clinging to teeth. Seeing a dentist regularly is also an important part of caring for your teeth.

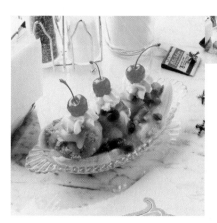

Item of Interest
Controlling Tooth Decay

❖ Brush your teeth after eating concentrated sources of sugars that can help dental caries develop. High-sugar foods include candies, syrups, soft drinks, and some breakfast cereals.

❖ Limit sticky foods. They are more of a problem than sweet ones. The stickiest

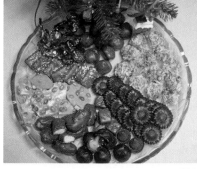

USDA

Candy is not the only culprit that can contribute to tooth decay. Any source of carbohydrate that stays on the teeth can promote dental caries.

carbohydrates are found in foods like crackers, cereals, and pretzels. Saliva washes sugars away fairly quickly. Complex carbohydrates can cling to the teeth where they are broken down into sugar.

❖ Limit how often you eat sugary foods. The amount of sugar you eat is not as great a factor as the frequency with which you eat it. Constant sucking on candy leads to increased tooth decay.

❖ Limit your consumption of acidic beverages. Acids eat away enamel, increasing tooth decay. All soft drinks are acidic. Sipping on diet sodas all day continually bathes the teeth in acid. Try sipping water instead.

❖ Chew a piece of sugarless gum for at least 10 minutes after eating if you cannot brush your teeth. Gum stimulates the flow of saliva, which

aids in clearing food particles from the teeth and neutralizes the acid. Sugared gum can be a problem if you chew one piece after another.

❖ Eat a small amount of aged cheeses in conjunction with or just after sugary foods. The cheese reduces acid levels in the mouth. Examples of aged cheeses include Cheddar, Monterey Jack, and Swiss.

❖ The American Dental Association recommends fluoride treatments as soon as teeth appear.

❖ Use fluoridated toothpaste. Dentists recommend fluoride supplements for children up to age 16 in areas where water is not fluoridated. Foods high in fluoride are tea and fish with edible bones.

Source: "Something to Sink Your Teeth Into," *Tufts University Diet & Nutrition Letter* Vol. 13, No. 3, May 1995.

Diabetes Mellitus

Diabetes mellitus is the body's inability to move glucose from the bloodstream to the cells. *Insulin* is a hormone produced by the pancreas. It allows glucose to move into the cells for use as energy. People who have diabetes either do not produce enough insulin, or their bodies fail to recognize its presence. Therefore, diabetics are unable to handle sudden large surges of sugar in their bloodstreams.

In the past, doctors recommended that diabetics eliminate sugar from their diets. Many believed excess sugar would cause diabetes. Research indicates the best diet for a diabetic is not much different from an ordinary healthful diet. In 1994, the American Diabetes Association concluded that there is no one right diet for diabetics. Guidelines need to be based on individual weight, cholesterol levels, and other health factors.

Diabetics must avoid sugar "spikes" in their diets. Health experts recommend a diet that will keep blood glucose levels fairly steady throughout the day. Diabetics can best

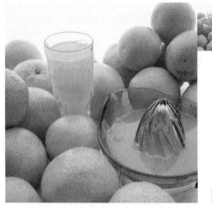

Nutrition News
Diabetic Diet Recommendations

These recommendations are for people who have adult-onset diabetes. However, the suggestions are good advice for most other people, too. Be sure to consult your doctor before making

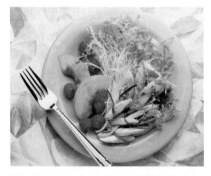

The fructose found naturally in fruits and vegetables is not a dietary concern for people with diabetes.

changes in your diet if you are diabetic.

Keep sucrose intake to less than 10% of total calories. Sugar can be eaten in small amounts. There is no difference in the way a diabetic handles any carbohydrates. Diabetics can eat sugar provided it replaces other high-carbohydrate foods and is part of a meal.

Limit foods containing high-fructose corn syrup. Fructose is okay when found in fruits and vegetables. The problem is the high level in high-fructose corn syrup, which is often used in drinks and cookies. Large amounts can raise blood sugar, cholesterol, and triglyceride levels.

Switch to monounsaturated fats. Three recent studies indicate that these fats are better for helping control blood sugar levels. Do not increase total fat intake! Good sources of monounsaturated fats (defined in Chapter 10) are olive oil, canola oil, some nuts, and avocados.

Watch your weight. Excess body fat interferes with the work of insulin. The more overweight a diabetic is, the more problems he or she is likely to have controlling blood sugar levels. Exercise and watch total calorie intake!

Increase vitamin C and E. High blood sugar levels increase cell-damaging free radicals. Recent studies indicate that neutralizing free radicals may reduce the risk of diabetic complications. Talk to your doctor about these findings.

Source: "The New Diabetic Diet," *University of California at Berkeley Wellness Letter* Volume 11, Issue 7, April 1995 p. 5

achieve this by eating nutritious foods in five to six small meals a day. This advice is probably the best preventive medicine for anyone with a family history of diabetes.

Weight Gain

Many people blame excess sugar in their diets for weight gain. However, the key to weight control is balancing calories going into the body with calories being burned by the body. All excess calories, whether from sugar, starch, fat, or protein, will be stored in the body as fat. Therefore, too much of any type of food can lead to weight gain.

It is possible to maintain a healthy weight and still enjoy foods that provide sugar. The important point to remember is to practice moderation. Many foods that are high in added sugar provide few other nutrients. Such foods should be consumed sparingly so they do not replace other sources of nutrients in the diet. For instance, you might enjoy a can of regular soft drink. If you are eating a nutritious diet, you can probably afford the 150 calories from sugar the soft drink provides. However, four cans of regular soft drink would provide about 600 calories from sugar and no other nutrients but water. This is 30% of the average woman's total daily calorie needs. Few people can get all the other nutrients their bodies need in the remaining 1,400 calories.

Recent research seems to indicate that the amount you eat is related more to the volume and mass of the food than its calorie content. The chart in 8-15 compares the volume, calorie content, and exercise needed to burn the extra calories in several foods. This chart shows how food intake, energy use, and body weight are related. A healthy weight requires knowledge about nutrition and exercise, moderation and balance in food choices, and learning to enjoy regular physical exercises.

Foods to Satisfy Your Sweet Tooth

Food (one cup portion)	Mass	Calories	Fat	Exercise*
Watermelon	154g	50	0	10 minutes
Apple	190g	70	0	14 minutes
Mandarin oranges	233g	110	0	22 minutes
Chocolate pudding	284g	310	6g	63 minutes
Chocolate chips	173g	830	51g	169 minutes

*Exercise needed is based on a 130-pound person hiking at a moderate rate.

8-15 Equivalent volumes of food can vary greatly in their weight and calorie content.

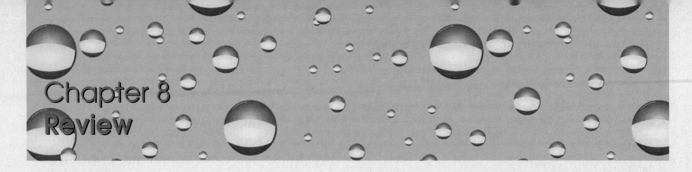

Chapter 8 Review

Summary

Carbohydrates are the main source of energy for people all over the world. This energy comes from the sun and is stored in plants as carbohydrates through photosynthesis. The simplest carbohydrates are called sugars. The most common sugars are the monosaccharides glucose, fructose, mannose, and galactose. Disaccharides are two joined monosaccharides. Examples are sucrose, lactose, and maltose. Disaccharides can be broken into two monosaccharides through hydrolysis. For hydrolysis to occur, there must be water and the addition of an enzyme, heat, or an acid. Alcohols are organic compounds that have chemical structures similar to sugars.

Most sweeteners used by the food industry have natural sources. Molasses, brown sugar, confectioner's sugar, and sucrose come from sugar cane. Sucrose also comes from sugar beets. Maple syrup comes from sugar maple trees. Corn syrup comes from corn. Sorghum is the syrup of a grass crop. Honey is produced by bees. Other names for sugar that may appear on food labels include invert sugar and dextrose.

The main function of sugar in food preparation is as a sweetener. Sugars also act as preservatives, and they help tenderize doughs. Sugar is a crystallizing agent, which makes it the key ingredient in most candies. Sugar's ability to caramelize is important in the browning of baked goods and in the production of caramel flavoring. Sugar also fuels the fermentation of many food products.

Understanding factors that affect sugar crystal formation is necessary in the production of cooked candies. Controlling the growth of sugar crystals in candy involves the type of sugar and the use of interfering agents. The timing of stirring, the cooling speed, and the ripening process also affect the growth of sugar crystals.

Sugars fit into a healthful diet. They provide energy and aid in the digestion of proteins. Sugars only become a problem when they are the source of too many total calories in the diet.

Check Your Understanding

1. What are the three categories of carbohydrates in food ingredients?
2. What elements make up all carbohydrates?
3. Name three monosaccharides and give a source of each.
4. Name the monosaccharides that make up each of the disaccharides and give a common food source of each disaccharide.
5. How are the molecular structures of sugars and alcohols similar? How do they differ?
6. What is the difference between brown sugar and granulated sugar?
7. Identify the six functions of sugars in food preparation and name a food in which sugar performs each function.
8. Name four interfering agents used to prevent crystal formation in candies and explain how one of them works.
9. How and where does the body store glucose that is not needed as an immediate source of energy?
10. How can sugar in the diet result in weight gain?

Critical Thinking

1. Why is the human body unable to convert the sun's energy into carbohydrates?
2. List all the sugars found in the ingredients list of your favorite ready-to-eat breakfast cereal.

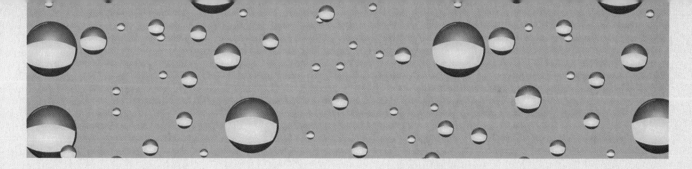

3. Why are members of a taste test panel likely to agree that sucrose is less sweet than fructose?

4. Although your friend carefully followed a recipe when making fudge, the fudge is too gooey to pick up. What are two possible reasons for this problem?

5. Which is more likely to cause dental caries: chewing sugared gum for 10 minutes every day or drinking a regular soft drink with each meal and snack? Explain your answer.

Explore Further

1. **Science.** Construct a model of each type of sugar molecule using a chemistry model kit or materials from home.

2. **Technology.** For one day, keep track of the amounts and types of food you eat. Enter the information into a computer nutrition analysis program. Compare the percentage of calories you get from sugar to the national average and to the recommendations of health experts.

3. **Science.** Select a favorite candy recipe that uses an interfering agent. Make a batch of the candy with and without the interfering agent. Conduct taste tests of the two batches and observe the candy's texture. Report your findings.

4. **Writing.** Write an article for your school newspaper on sugar and health.

5. **Math.** Create a bar graph comparing the sugar contents of the class's favorite breakfast cereals and candy bars.

Experiment 8A
Testing for Simple Sugars

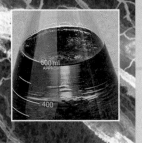

Purpose

In this lab, you will test two monosaccharides (glucose and fructose) and three disaccharides (sucrose, maltose, and lactose). These are common simple carbohydrates, or sugars, in foods. Starch is a common complex carbohydrate in foods. In this experiment, you will be testing substances with Benedict's solution. This solution changes color in the presence of mono- and disaccharides after heating. Starch will not cause a color change. After testing carbohydrate solutions, you will test several food products to determine whether monosaccharides or disaccharides are present.

Equipment

250- to 400-mL beaker
wax pencil
10 test tubes
10-mL graduated cylinder
safety glasses
test-tube tongs
test-tube rack

Supplies

105 mL water
50 mL Benedict's solution
5 mL fructose solution
5 mL glucose solution
5 mL sucrose solution
5 mL maltose solution
5 mL lactose solution
5 mL starch solution
5 mL each of 3 food sample solutions

Procedure

Part I

1. Pour 100 mL water into the beaker. Bring the water to a boil over medium heat on a range or hot plate.

2. Use a wax pencil to label seven test tubes 1 through 7.

3. Add 5 mL of Benedict's solution to each test tube.

4. Add 5 mL of water to test tube 1.

5. Add 5 mL of fructose solution to test tube 2. Rinse the graduated cylinder.

6. Add 5 mL of glucose solution to test tube 3. Rinse the graduated cylinder.

7. Add 5 mL of sucrose solution to test tube 4. Rinse the graduated cylinder.

8. Add 5 mL of maltose solution to test tube 5. Rinse the graduated cylinder.

9. Add 5 mL of lactose solution to test tube 6. Rinse the graduated cylinder.

10. Add 5 mL of starch solution to test tube 7. Rinse the graduated cylinder.

11. Place the test tubes in the beaker of hot water and heat for 5 minutes.

12. Use test-tube tongs to remove the test tubes to the rack. Observe the color and record the results in a data table.

Part II

1. Add 5 mL of Benedict's solution to each of the three remaining test tubes.

2. Add 5 mL of a different food sample solution provided by your teacher to each of the remaining test tubes. Rinse the graduated cylinder after measuring each solution.

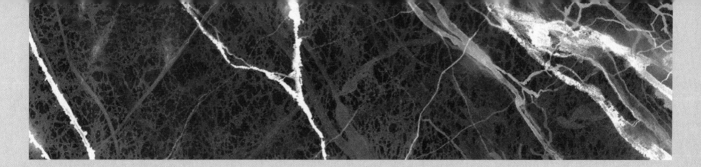

3. Label the test tubes with the types of food solutions added.

4. Place the test tubes in the beaker of hot water and heat for 5 minutes.

5. Use test-tube tongs to remove the test tubes to the rack. Observe the color and record the results in the data table.

Questions

1. Was there a difference between the reactions of mono- and disaccharides?

2. List the foods tested by decreasing sugar content.

Experiment 8B
Forming Sugar Crystals

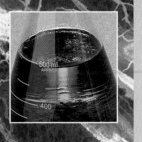

Purpose

In this lab, you will prepare rock candy and observe the growth of large sugar crystals. Large sugar crystals form from a supersaturated sugar solution that is allowed to cool undisturbed. The molecules in the solution will need an extended period for the formation of multiple layers of sugar molecules, which create the candy's crystalline structure.

Equipment

electronic balance

100-mL graduated cylinder

1½-quart saucepan

large spoon

thermometer with clamp or holder

Supplies

500 g granulated sugar

120 mL distilled water

1 250-mL (8-ounce) polystyrene cup per lab group member

1 seeded bamboo skewer per lab group member

plastic wrap

wax paper or aluminum foil

Procedure

Day 1

1. Mass sugar and measure distilled water. Combine sugar and distilled water in a 1½-quart saucepan.

2. Place the saucepan on a range over medium heat. Bring the sugar and water to a boil, stirring frequently with a large spoon.

3. Use a thermometer clamp or holder to position a calibrated thermometer so the bulb is suspended in the center of the boiling liquid.

4. Allow the mixture to boil without stirring until it reaches the appropriate temperature.

   Variation 1: 115°C

   Variation 2: 120°C

   Variation 3: 125°C

5. When the sugar syrup reaches the desired temperature, remove the pan from the heat and allow the syrup to cool to 100°C. Carefully pour the syrup into polystyrene cups. Fill the cups approximately two-thirds full.

6. Hold the seeded skewers in an upright position in the polystyrene cups while a lab partner carefully lowers plastic wrap over the skewers. The tops of the skewers should poke through the plastic wrap. The plastic wrap should cover the tops of the cups to protect the sugar syrup and hold the skewers in place.

7. Set the cups in the designated place overnight.

Day 2

1. Remove the plastic wrap from the cups and discard. If necessary, break the crust of sugar crystals at the top of each cup.

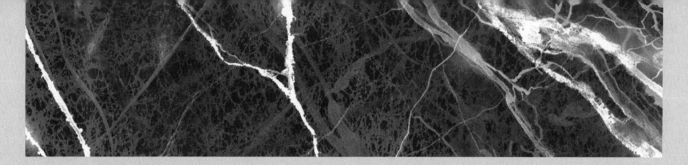

2. Drain off any liquid remaining in the cups. Then tear the cups off the sugar crystals attached to the skewers.

3. Rinse the sugar crystals briefly with cold water.

4. Examine the shape and size of the crystals. Record your observations.

Questions

1. Where did the crystals form?

2. How did changing the temperature of the sugar syrup change the crystal formation?

3. What was the function of the sugar crystals on the skewers?

Experiment 8C
Interferring with Crystal Formation

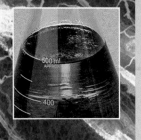

Purpose

In this experiment, you will examine the effect the fat content of the liquid ingredient in fudge has on the speed of sugar crystal growth. Quality candy is determined largely by the size of sugar crystals. Good rock candy has large crystals. Quality fudge has a smooth, creamy texture, which is a result of very small sugar crystals. Sugar crystals form as the candy cools. Ingredients can interfere with or encourage the growth of sugar crystals.

Equipment

1¹/₂-quart saucepan
100-mL graduated cylinder
metric measures
large metal or wooden spoon
candy thermometer
electric mixer
loaf pan
microscope slide
microscope

Supplies

butter
75 mL assigned liquid
28 g (1 square) chocolate
250 mL (1 cup) sugar
2 mL vanilla
1 drop glycerin

Procedure

Day 1

1. Butter the sides of a 1¹/₂-quart saucepan.
2. Measure 75 mL of the liquid for the variation your group is assigned from the list below.

   Variation 1: water
   Variation 2: fat free milk
   Variation 3: lowfat milk
   Variation 4: whole milk
   Variation 5: half-and-half
   Variation 6: whipping cream

   Combine the liquid, chocolate, and sugar in the saucepan.
3. Place a candy thermometer in the pan so the bulb does not touch the bottom or sides. Cook over medium heat until the mixture comes to a boil. Stir only as needed to prevent sticking. The mixture should boil gently over the surface. Continue cooking to 112°C or the soft ball stage.
4. Immediately remove from heat, leaving the candy thermometer in the pan.
5. Cool without stirring until the mixture reaches 48°C. Add the vanilla.
6. Beat vigorously with an electric mixer until the fudge becomes thick and just loses its gloss.
7. Immediately spread the fudge in a buttered loaf pan.

Day 2

1. Place a pinch of fudge on a microscope slide and add a drop of glycerin. Examine the sugar crystals under a microscope.
2. Note the differences in crystal size and shape.
3. Note any other substances that are visible under the microscope.
4. Taste a piece of each fudge variation and note the flavor, color, and texture.

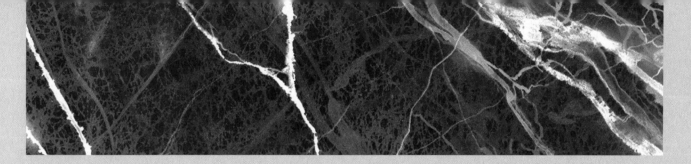

Questions

1. What relationship did you observe, if any, between the flavor of the fudge and the liquid used?

2. Was there a relationship between the color of the fudge and the liquid used?

3. Which, if any, variations have a texture other than the creamy texture typical of good fudge?

4. Which fudge had the largest sugar crystals? Which had the smallest sugar crystals?

5. Which variation made the best quality fudge?

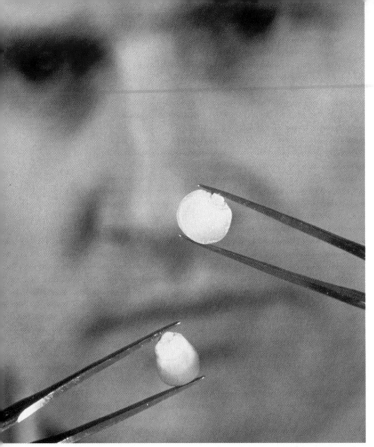

USDA

This researcher is comparing two varieties of corn. Both are sources of starch, a complex carbohydrate.

Chapter 9

The Complex Carbohydrates: Starches, Cellulose, Gums, and Pectins

Objectives

After studying this chapter,
you will be able to

describe characteristics of the four categories of complex carbohydrates.

identify the functions of complex carbohydrates in food preparation.

list five physical properties of starch and liquid mixtures that affect the selection of starches used in food products.

compare the advantages and disadvantages of the three main methods used to add starches to sauces.

analyze the role of starches in a nutritious diet.

Key Terms

polysaccharide
macromolecule
starch
polymer
amylose
amylopectin
granules
cellulose
carbohydrate gum
pectin
gelatinization
gelatinization point
slurry
sol
paste

gel
junction
retrogradation
syneresis
viscosity
stability
opacity
translucency
modified starch
cross-linked starch
cold water paste
buerre manie
roux
ketosis
ketone bodies

Breads, cereals, muffins, cakes, and cookies are well-liked foods in the typical U.S. diet. These foods are rich in carbohydrates. Some of the carbohydrates are simple carbohydrates, which you studied in Chapter 8. However, many of the carbohydrates in baked goods are complex carbohydrates, which are the focus of this chapter. See 9-1.

Complex carbohydrates are called *polysaccharides.* This is because they are made up of many sugar units, or saccharides. Another term used to describe polysaccharides is macromolecules. *Macromolecules* are very large molecules that contain hundreds or thousands of atoms each.

The Types of Complex Carbohydrates

Several types of complex carbohydrates are found in foods. These include starches, cellulose, gums, and pectins. These polysaccharides are abundant in grains, seeds, nuts, fruits, vegetables, and seaweed.

Starches

The most abundant complex carbohydrate in the diet is starch. Most *starches* consist of molecules of 100 to several thousand glucose units linked in chains. Because starches are made up of many sugar units, they are polymers of sugar. A *polymer* is a large molecule that consists of large numbers of small molecular units, which are linked. Starches are composed of glucose. Other polysaccharides

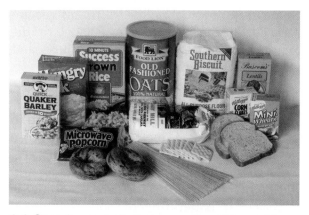

9-1 Complex carbohydrates are found in a wide variety of grains and grain-based products.

can consist of as many as six or seven types of sugars.

A main source of starch in the diet for most people in the United States is wheat flour. Wheat flour is used to make many types of baked goods and pasta. Starch is also found in rice, corn, potatoes, and oats. Any grain or seed is high in starch. Rye, soy, tapioca, and arrowroot are other less commonly used starch products in the U.S. food supply.

Starches have two basic structures. One is linear, and the other is branched. When the units are linked in a line (linear), they are called *amylose.* Starches that have a branched structure are called *amylopectin.* In most foods, starches occur as mixtures of amylose and amylopectin.

Starch is nature's reserve carbohydrate supply. Plants produce starch in packets called *granules.* Granules are not soluble in cold water. The size and shape of granules vary from plant to plant. Of the common food starches, rice has the smallest granules and potatoes have the largest. Starch granules are a mixture of amylose and amylopectin molecules. Amylose content can range from 25% to 85%. The varying amylose/amylopectin ratios within the granules cause each type of starch to perform differently in food mixtures.

Starches composed mainly of amylopectin are also called *waxy starches.* This is because of the appearance of the surface of the seeds from which the starches come. Waxy maize is a starch from corn that has more thickening power that regular cornstarch.

Cellulose

A second group of complex carbohydrates are called cellulose. *Cellulose* is a polysaccharide made from large amounts of β-D-glucose. Some animals, including cows and sheep, and insects such as termites can use cellulose as a food source. However, humans lack the digestive enzymes needed to break the bonds in cellulose molecules. Cellulose is among the complex carbohydrates that are known as fiber in the diet.

Cellulose forms the rigid structure of plants. The strings in celery and the membranes surrounding kernels of corn are made up largely of cellulose.

Carbohydrate Gums and Pectins

The last group of complex carbohydrates used in food preparation are not generally available to the home cook. These polysaccharides are called carbohydrate gums and pectins. *Carbohydrate gums* are polysaccharides that are soluble in water and extracted from plants. *Pectins* are complex carbohydrates that are found in plant cells and made of chemical derivatives of sugar called sugar acids.

Gums thicken and stabilize mixtures and trap color and flavor. The most common and widely used is gum arabic. It surrounds flavor particles, protecting them from moisture absorption, evaporation, or chemical oxidation. Other gums commonly used in foods include karaya gum, gum tragacanth, gum agar, carageenan, and algin. Gums provide stability and texture to such foods as salad dressings and gummy candies, 9-2.

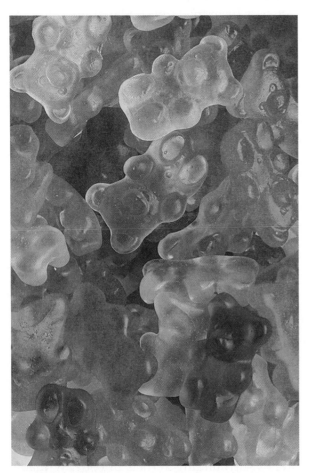

9-2 Gummy bears get much of their characteristic texture from carbohydrate gums.

Pectin is a complex carbohydrate that naturally occurs in fruits. It can produce a strong gel that will remain stable to near 100°C (212°F). In the presence of sugar, pectin molecules will dehydrate. Acid will cause hydrogen bonding to occur between negatively charged molecules, thus creating a thickened structure. These properties make pectin a key component in jams and jellies.

Functions of Complex Carbohydrates in Food Preparation

Complex carbohydrates serve a number of functions in food preparation. They provide structure, bind ingredients together, and act as absorbing agents or thickeners. All complex carbohydrates help stabilize food products by keeping ingredients evenly distributed throughout mixtures.

Provide Structure

Starch is the main component of wheat flour. Flour is the primary ingredient in most baked goods. Flour provides the majority of the bulk or structure of baked goods and many other food products. For instance, most ready-to-eat cereals retain their shape due to their starch content. The pieces are formed in a semiliquid state and remain shaped on drying.

Starch's ability to thicken when heated and gel when cooled enables foods containing starch to take and hold many shapes. Other complex carbohydrates also provide structure in foods. Cellulose forms the supporting framework or structure for fruits and vegetables. Pectins and gums are responsible for the texture of jams, jellies, ice cream products, and gummy-textured candies.

Bind

Binding agents are substances that tend to hold two other products together. Amylose molecules will work better than amylopectin molecules at holding batters to vegetables and meats during deep-frying. The binding is increased if batter-dipped foods set for 20 minutes before frying. This allows time for the chemical reactions needed to bind the batter to the food during cooking. See 9-3.

Carageenan is a gum used as a binding agent. It stabilizes the cocoa in chocolate milk so the cocoa does not settle out of the product. Carageenan is also used to stabilize ice cream and other dairy products.

Thicken

Starch can thicken liquids. This function is possible because of starch's chemical structure, the size of its molecules, and the way it reacts to heat. The molecules of starch are chemically altered as they swell and take up water.

Starches are usually combined with liquids in food preparation. Undamaged starch granules are not readily soluble in water nor do they absorb water. Starch must first be heated to break intermolecular bonds. This allows hydrogen bonds to form between the starch molecules and water.

When starch granules are suspended in water and then heated, gelatinization occurs. *Gelatinization* is the term food scientists use to describe thickening a liquid with starch. As the temperature increases, so does the swelling of the granule structure. The temperature at which maximum swelling occurs is the *gelatinization point.* This is the point at which the starch will hold the most water and have the greatest thickening power. The starch used in instant puddings has been pre-gelatinized. This allows it to *gel,* or set, at the temperature of cold milk. The starch in regular pudding mixes will not gelatinize until it is hot enough to boil. Then it will not gel until it is chilled.

Water is the main component of almost all liquids used in food preparation. Starch molecules are extremely large in comparison to water molecules. Not only are starch molecules large, but they have spaces between their sugar units. Imagine a tumbleweed rolling across a desert. The tumbleweed is a solid that has a ball shape. The ball is made of many branches with air spaces between them. If the tumbleweed rolls across a crumbled up piece of paper, the paper can become stuck between the branches. That piece of paper will now be carried along with the tumbleweed.

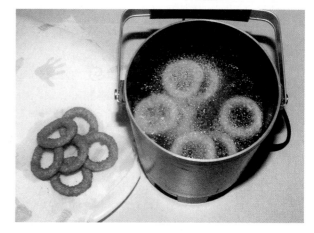

9-3 The starch in flour binds the batter to onion rings so it does not separate from the onions during frying.

That is similar to what happens as large starch granules roll around in water. The very small water molecules will slide between sugar units and be held in place by hydrogen bonding. The more water that "snuggles" into the starch molecule, the thicker the mixture will become. See 9-4.

Applying heat to a starch-water mixture causes it to thicken (gelatinization). As heat is added, starch opens up or stretches. This allows water molecules to slip down between the coils of the large molecule. The addition of heat increases the amount of water the molecule can trap in its coils and branches. The more water the molecule traps, the thicker the mixture will become.

Heat is needed to stretch starch molecules and increase their thickening power. However, too much heat will cause starch molecules to begin to hydrolyze or break apart. This will cause the starch to lose thickening ability and stability. Excess heat can result from using too high a temperature or too long a cooking time.

The presence of salt and sugar affects starch's thickening ability. Salt and sugar compete for water because they are also polar in nature. If a large amount of salt or sugar is present, it will interfere with the gelling ability of the starch. When sugar is combined with flour or any other starch, it will decrease the strength and viscosity of the gel. It will also increase the translucency of the paste. In most

Starch Molecule

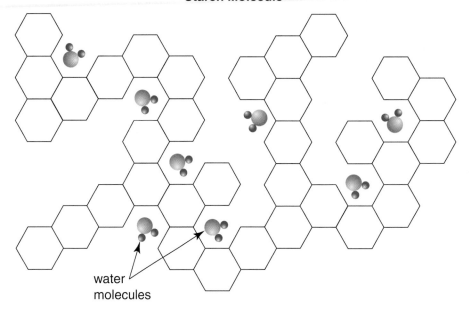

water
molecules

9-4 Starch thickens because of its ability to trap water molecules.

cases, low concentrations of salt have little effect on gelatinization or the ability to form a gel. Potato starch and some manufactured starches are exceptions. They are salt sensitive. Depending on the starch, salt can increase or decrease swelling.

Pectin is used to thicken jams and jellies. Some fruits, such as crabapples and gooseberries, can provide enough pectin to produce suitably thick jellied products. Other fruits require the addition of commercial pectin. Commercial pectin is made by extracting pectin from its fruit source. It may be dried into a powder or sold in a liquid form for home use. See 9-5.

The basic recipe for jams and jellies is 1% pectin and 60% to 65% sugar. The remaining 34% to 39% is made up mostly of crushed fruit or fruit juice. A little hot water may be added if needed for volume. Jams and jellies must have a pH of 2.0 to 3.5. If the fruit is not very acidic, lemon juice is added to achieve the desired pH level.

Pectin will bond with other pectin molecules and form a gel without sugar if calcium ions are present. This is how dietetic jams and jellies are made. Pectin plus calcium also firms canned tomatoes and pickled cucumbers.

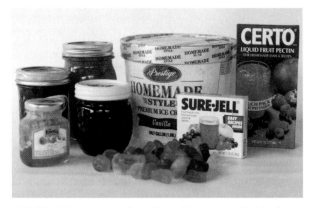

9-5 Liquid and powdered pectin are available for thickening homemade jams and jellies. Commercially, pectin is used as a thickener and stabilizer in such foods as ice cream and candy.

Alginates, a group of gums, thicken dressings and puddings. Xanthan gum may be used to help thicken instant puddings.

Physical Properties of Starch and Liquid Mixtures

Each starch has different physical properties. Therefore, food scientists must determine which starch source is best for a food product and the type of starch-liquid mixture. Scientists do this by examining how the starch works within a food mixture. The most important property to the consumer is usually flavor. For example, cornstarch does not taste the same as rye flour. However, wheat flour, cornstarch, and potato starch all thicken gravies and sauces without adding unpleasant flavors.

There are five properties that food scientists evaluate before selecting a starch. The properties they examine include: retrogradation, viscosity, stability, opacity versus translucency, and texture. Food manufacturers have to carefully evaluate all these characteristics of starches anytime they develop a new starch-thickened product.

Types of Starch and Liquid Mixtures

Starch and liquid combinations can be of four types: slurries, sols, pastes, and gels. *Slurries* are uncooked mixtures of water and starch. They are used in the processing and chemical alteration of starches. Acids and/or bases are added to the mixture to chemically alter the structure of the starch molecules.

Sols are thickened liquids. They are pourable. Examples of sols include pancake, waffle, and muffin batter. Cooked sols include white sauce and gravy.

Pastes are thickened mixtures of starch and liquid that have very little flow. However, they are thin enough to be spread easily. When making gravy, starch can be combined with water or milk to form a paste. The paste can then be stirred into hot broth without lumping, 9-6. This method works well when thickening soups and stews.

Gels are starch mixtures that are rigid. In a gel, molecules are bound together in a three-dimensional network. This network keeps molecules from shifting in comparison to one another. When two molecules of hydrogen bond together, a *junction* is formed. Short starch chains tend to form weaker junctions. This makes them unstable in heat. Long starch chains form firmer gels that are more stable in heat. Therefore, linear amylose starches will form more stable gels than branched amylopectins. By controlling the number and location of junctions, food scientists can vary the firmness and stability of gels.

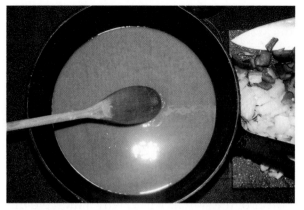

9-6 Combining flour with milk or water forms a starch paste, which can be added to broth to make a thick gravy.

Amylose molecules will set rapidly and form firm gels upon cooling. Amylopectin forms thinner gels or no gels at all. Amylose gels are also elastic, whereas amylopectin gels become rigid. This tendency of amylopectin starches to become rigid is a main cause of breads becoming stale. The rigidity is combined with moisture loss.

Retrogradation

Retrogradation is the firming of a gel during cooling and standing. It occurs because the starch granules are trying to return to the structure they had before cooking. Amylose will tend to hydrogen bond to other amylose molecules. These overlapping molecules will form crystalline structures that separate out of the gel. This is a problem with starch-thickened pie fillings or gravies that are frozen and then thawed.

Retrogradation is desirable when it causes a gel to thicken during cooling. It is undesirable if it continues to the point that cracks form in the gel. Gravy left uncovered in the refrigerator will develop these cracks after a couple days.

The changes of retrogradation are accompanied by water being squeezed from between the molecules of the gel. *Syneresis* is the term used for water leaking out of a gel in storage. The liquid that separates from many mustards is an example of syneresis. Stable gels will have little or no syneresis.

An important factor related to retrogradation is the serving temperature of a starch-thickened food product. A sauce will thicken as it cools. If you are planning to serve a sauce immediately, you should cook it to the desired thickness. This is not the case with most sweet sauces. They are often served at room temperature. Because they will thicken as they cool, they must be thinner than desired at the end of the cooking time.

Acids hydrolyze starch. Because acids break down starches, they will also weaken or break down gels. This reduces the thickening power of the starch. This is why lemon pie filling calls for more starch than coconut cream or chocolate cream pie filling. Lemon juice is added after the starch has thickened lemon pie filling. The filling is then cooled rapidly to minimize the thinning effect of the acid in lemon.

Viscosity

Viscosity is the resistance of a mixture to flow. When you spill a glass of water on the table, it spreads out in a large pool. If you spill a bowl of oatmeal, it will only flow a short distance before it stops. The difference between the water and the oatmeal is caused by the starch in the oatmeal.

Solids, including dry starches, hold their shape and stay where they are put. Liquids take the shape of their containers. If there is no container, liquids flow to the lowest point. When you mix solids and liquids, there are some particles trying to stay put and others trying to flow. The more solid that is present, the more resistance there will be to flow. Gels are more viscous than pastes, and pastes are more viscous than sols.

Food scientists run viscosity tests to measure how foods such as ketchup will flow. The scientists use line-spread sheets. A food scientist sets the cylinder in the center of the concentric circles of the line-spread sheet. He or she fills the cylinder with the mixture being measured. The scientist lifts the cylinder, which allows the mixture to flow as far as it will. Substances will rarely flow out in a perfect circle. Therefore, the food scientist takes readings at four equidistant points. He or she then averages the four readings to determine the viscosity. See 9-7.

Viscosity varies with molecular size, shape, and charge. Larger molecules are harder to move, and thus more viscous, than small molecules. Linear molecules are more viscous than branched molecules. This is because linear molecules will not roll over easily unless they are parallel to the direction of flow. Charged macromolecules will have more

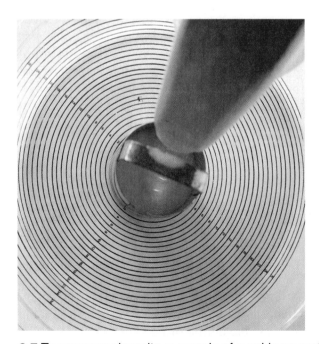
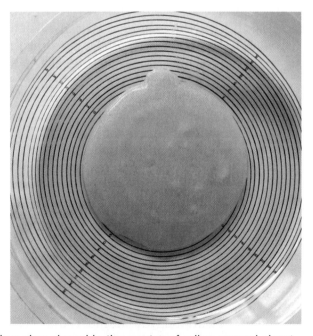

9-7 To measure viscosity, a sample of a sol is poured in a ring placed in the center of a line-spread sheet. After the ring is lifted and the sol is allowed to spread, readings are taken in at least four places.

resistance to flow than uncharged molecules. This is because of the resistance of opposite charges holding the molecules together. The main functions of starches in food products include providing viscosity, gelatinization, and structure. Therefore, linear starches, such as amylose, are generally more useful in forming gels.

Viscosity could be said to be a measure of a starch's thickening ability. Food scientists can use viscosity tests to rank the thickening ability of different starches. The scientists can determine the amount of each starch needed to thicken 1 cup of water to the same degree. Listing this information in a starch proportion chart creates a valuable tool for food product developers. They can use the chart to easily see how substituting one starch for another will affect a food product. For instance, changing the type of starch will change the flow of an uncooked batter. Commercial bakers have found they can substitute 30% of the flour in cookies with pure wheat starch. This starch has had protein removed. Protein molecules interact with one another, blocking the flow of a batter. Substituting pure wheat starch for flour will increase the spreading action of the batter. This helps achieve the evenly shaped cookies available in grocery stores.

Stability

Stability is the ability of a thickened mixture to remain constant over time and temperature changes. A stable sauce can be frozen and/or reheated. It will look and taste much the same as when it was first prepared. Waxy maize starch is an example of a starch that is stable when frozen or heated. It is a clear, soft paste that is as thick hot as cold.

Cornstarch has more thickening power than flour. It is smoother in texture and more translucent than white flour. However, cornstarch is not as stable in prolonged heat. Cornstarch makes an appetizing mushroom gravy to serve over beef tips. However, suppose you had to prepare the beef tips a day ahead of time. The cornstarch gravy would not thin out into a smooth sauce when reheated. Flour might be a better choice than cornstarch for thickening gravies that must be prepared in advance.

Opacity Versus Translucency

Opacity refers to how much an object blocks light. *Translucency* is a measure of how much light can pass through an object. An object with maximum opacity allows no light to pass through it. An object with maximum translucency blocks no light. Cornstarch, potato starch, and arrowroot produce gels that are more translucent than gels made with wheat starch. You can see through them to some extent. This makes these starches good choices for fruit sauces, fruit pie fillings, and glazes, which are translucent. Wheat flour is not used for most pie fillings because it becomes yellowish and stringy. However, wheat flour is suitable for use in chowders and white sauce, which are opaque. See 9-8.

Texture

The last property a food scientist looks at when choosing a starch is texture. Cornmeal will thicken a gravy, but most people would not like it. The gravy would feel gritty instead of smooth. Likewise, few people make a sauce or gravy from whole wheat flour because of its mouth feel.

Modified Starches

Food technologists can alter the structure of starch molecules to achieve special physical

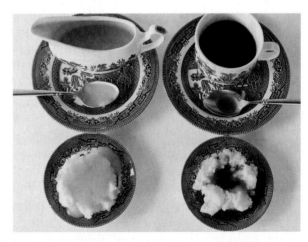

9-8 The opaque chicken gravy on the left is thickened with flour. The translucent beef gravy on the right is thickened with cornstarch. The patterns on the plate show through the beef gravy but not the chicken.

properties. Starches that have been changed structurally by chemical or mechanical means are called *modified starches.* FDA regulations do not require that labels identify the food product from which a modified starch originates. This can be a problem for those people who are sensitive or allergic to a specific grain product. Some of the most commonly used sources of modified starches are wheat, corn, and soy.

Most modified starches are altered by hydrolysis. They are allowed to set in a mixture or slurry of water and acids or water and enzymes. Starch modification can be controlled to produce various levels of sweetness and particle size. Viscosity, mouth feel, and appearance of starches can also be modified.

Cornstarch that has been modified is used in gum candies and confections as a stabilizer. In the 1970s, it became possible to hydrolyze cornstarch to form a low-cost sweetener. A slurry of cornstarch and acid was heated and combined with enzymes to promote a chemical reaction. The result was corn syrup. Corn syrup has quickly replaced 25% of the 23-billion pounds-per-year sucrose market in the United States. Many manufacturers of processed beverages, syrups, and confections now rely on corn syrup and high-fructose corn syrup. Besides low costs, these sweeteners have relatively reliable supplies.

Cross-linked starches are another type of modified starch. *Cross-linked starch* is changed chemically so cross-bonding or cross-linking takes place between starch molecules. The resulting molecular network is more resistant to acids and separation in the freezing and thawing process. Potato starch will break down if acid is added, but modified (cross-linked) potato starch will not. Cross-linked starches will not continue to thicken during storage and do not leak water on standing. They are used by food scientists to produce baby foods, salad dressings, cream-style corn, and fruit pie fillings.

Modified food starches can be made to the exact specifications needed for a food product. They have made many new food products possible. Many frozen entrees and instant, quick-mix foods would not be possible without modified food starches. Modified food starches are used to stabilize condiments, sauces, and relishes. They increase the shelf life of many foods thus reducing food costs. These manufactured starches also reduce processor's dependence on any one grain crop. This helps prevent shortages and keeps food prices more constant.

Thickening Sauces with Starch

Starch can be added to liquid to make a thickened sauce in three basic ways. In each method, starch granules are separated to prevent lumping. If starch granules combine into a lump, the outer granules will swell. This prevents water from reaching the granules in the center of the lump. The lump remains dry in the center, the starch loses thickening power, and the sauce becomes lumpy. The method used to prevent lumping depends on the dish, the desired flavor, and personal preference.

Cold Water Paste

One method for preventing lumps when thickening a sauce with starch is to form a *cold water paste.* This involves quickly stirring the starch while adding at least an equal amount of cold water. Continue stirring until a smooth paste is formed. Once the starch granules are evenly distributed, more liquid can be added and the sauce can be heated without lumping. This method can be used to thicken soup stock or milk gravy. It can also be used to make a gravy from broth.

Starch and Fat

A second method for preventing lumps in starch-thickened sauces is to separate the starch granules with melted fat. An equal amount of starch is added to heated fat. Once the starch is stirred into the fat, the liquid can be slowly added. Constant stirring is necessary to keep the sauce smooth. This method is used in making white sauce and gravy from meat drippings.

Professional chefs often thicken soups and sauces with prepared buerre manie. *Buerre manie* is a ball of equal amounts of solid fat and starch mixed together. These balls can be added to hot soups to thicken the broth. The heat of the broth melts the fat. This allows the starch granules to disperse into the broth with little risk of lumping. The French use this

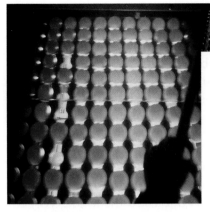

Technology Tidbit
Modified Corn Starches

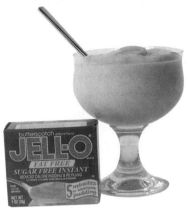

Instant pudding thickens without cooking because it contains pregelatinized starch.

To manufacture *pregelatinized starch,* a starch slurry is heated to above the gelatinization point. The slurry is carried in a trough between two heated horizontal rollers. The heated slurry dries to a thin film on the rollers. The dried starch film is scraped off as the rollers turn. The dried starch is then ground into a powder.

The starch in the powder has already been heated to its gelatinization point. Therefore, it will thicken within minutes of being rehydrated. This thickening without heating is used for instant puddings, pie fillings, and commercial cake frostings.

To manufacture *acid-modified starch,* a slurry of corn or waxy maize is mixed with HCl or sulfuric acid. The mixture sets for 6 to 24 hours at 25°C to 55°C (77°F to 131°F). The mixture is neutralized with soda ash or dilute NaOH. The mixture is then filtered and dried.

This type of starch is used to make gummy candies. The starch forms hot concentrated pastes that gel firmly on cooling. The cooled pastes are translucent and have a chewy texture that remains stable.

Source: Fennema, O. *Food Chemistry,* 2nd Ed, Rev. & Exp. Dekker, 1985 pp. 118-119.

---

method to make soups and sauces. The balls can be prepared ahead of time. They will keep in the refrigerator for several days or in the freezer for several months. See 9-9.

Cajun cooks who prepare foods from rural Southern Louisiana commonly use a roux to thicken sauces and gravies. A *roux* is a gravy that has had the starch heated in fat until it turns a rich red-brown. Toasting the flour adds a distinctive flavor to the gravy or sauce. A roux needs low heat and constant stirring during the browning process. This prevents uneven browning and reduces the likelihood of burning the flour. Extended heating will reduce a starch's thickening power. Therefore, a roux can have slightly more starch than fat (75 mL [1/3 cup] flour to 50 mL [1/4 cup] fat). It will also take more flour per cup of liquid to thicken the mixture. Continuous stirring after

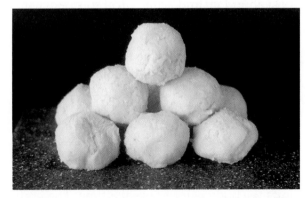

9-9 One way to thicken a stew or soup is to add a buerre manie. The ones pictured are made from 2 parts flour and 1 part shortening.

thickening will rupture starch cells in any thickened sauce and cause the sauce to become thinner.

Cooking Tip

If your sauce is too thick, add more liquid. If your sauce is too thin, add one or two buerre manie or add a cold water paste. If your sauce is lumpy, try a whisk to break up the lumps. A gravy stirrer with a spring-like end can also help eliminate lumps.

Starch and Sugar

The third method for avoiding lumps in sauces thickened with starch first requires thoroughly combining the starch and sugar. Then gradually add the liquid. If the liquid is added slowly with constant stirring, lumps will have little chance to form. This is because the sugar helps separate the starch granules and keep them from sticking together. This method of preventing lumping is used in most sweet sauces and puddings. The presence of sugar also helps reduce the viscosity of the liquid. The resulting gel will be tender and smooth rather than rigid.

Nutritional Impact of Complex Carbohydrates

Starches can be divided into two categories: digestible starches and indigestible fiber. Like sugar, digestible starches provide 4 calories of energy per gram. Starch is the most abundant and economical source of calories available to people. Carbohydrates should provide over half of your calories each day. Carbohydrates in the form of glucose are the only energy source the brain can use. The body is very efficient at changing starches and sugar to energy.

Excess carbohydrates are stored as glycogen. Glycogen is larger, heavier, and more branched than most amylopectins. The more branched the glycogen is, the more glucose units the body can release at a time. The body will usually use up glycogen stores in a little less than two hours of vigorous exercise. This is why it is so important to eat carbohydrates every 4 to 6 hours when you are awake. If you skip breakfast, your body will slow brain and organ functions to conserve the available glycogen. Students who skip breakfast will

have a harder time concentrating and will remember less of what they hear.

The size of glycogen stores depends on the amount of carbohydrates consumed and how frequently you exercise. Muscles that use up glycogen stores in exercise will increase their future storing ability. The more you exercise, the more energy the muscles will store. The less you exercise, the less glycogen will be available when you need it.

Glycogen is stored in two locations. The liver stores about one-third the total glycogen. It is readily available to the brain and other organs when blood glucose levels drop too low. The muscles store the other two-thirds of the glycogen for times of physical exertion. Suppose your body does not need carbohydrates for immediate energy and your glycogen stores are full. In this case, your body will turn the excess carbohydrates into fat.

If excess starch becomes fat, why not eat a high-fat diet? One reason has to do with the differences in the way the human body uses starches and fats. The body does not need fat to properly use starch. However, carbohydrates must be present to combine with fat fragments for the body to use fat for energy. If carbohydrates are not present, the body goes into ketosis. *Ketosis* is the process of burning fat without carbohydrates. This process produces **ketone bodies** as a by-product. High levels of ketones over an extended period will damage the kidneys and interfere with the body's normal acid-base balance. High levels of ketones during pregnancy can cause brain damage and irreversible mental retardation in the fetus.

Fiber, Bran, and Bulk

Much has been written about how people in the United States need to increase the fiber in their diets. *Fiber, bran,* and *bulk* are all terms used on labels and in advertising that refer to indigestible carbohydrates. As you read in Chapter 8, the type of glucose determines the digestibility of the starch. A molecule composed of beta-glucose is indigestible and is known as cellulose.

Cellulose provides bulk in the diet. It helps you feel full and aids in digestion and elimination. Many dietary polysaccharides, mainly from the cellulose components of cell walls, are insoluble and indigestible. The sources of fiber in your diet are vegetables, fruits, and grains, 9-10. Cellulose gives crispness and mouth feel to many foods. Some commercial bakers add cellulose to bread products to improve the water-binding ability of the flour. This slows the staling rate of bread and has been found to improve loaf volume in preparation.

Nutritional Functions of Starches

The main function of carbohydrates is to provide energy for bodily functions. In addition to energy, carbohydrates

❖ provide bulk for the digestive processes

❖ tie up bile acids, decreasing their reabsorption

❖ lower cholesterol levels in the blood, retarding atherosclerosis

❖ promote the utilization of fat

Carbohydrates are so important that their main food sources represent the largest portion of the USDA's MyPyramid symbol. The Dietary Guidelines recommend choosing fiber-rich fruits, vegetables, and whole grains often. Six ounce-equivalents of grains, two cups of fruit, and two and one half cups of vegetables per day are recommended for a 2,000-calorie food plan.

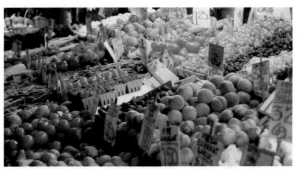

9-10 Fresh fruits and vegetables are excellent sources of dietary fiber.

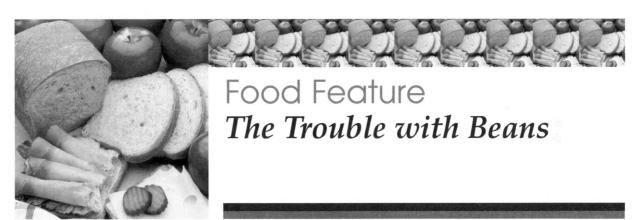

Food Feature
The Trouble with Beans

Dried peas and beans, which are called legumes, are excellent sources of many nutrients. However, some people avoid eating these nutritious foods due to concerns about gas. Beans contain the fiber tetrasaccharide stachyose. Like other types of fiber in the diet, tetrasaccharide stachyose is undigested when it reaches the large intestine. Once in the large intestine, multiflora work to attack and break down fiber. (*Multiflora* are bacteria that naturally live in the intestines.) By-products of this process

include acetic and lactic acids. If present in large enough quantities, these acids can have a laxative effect. Another by-product of the multiflora attack is gas. Excess gas produces flatulence, or unwelcome noise and odor.

One way to minimize problems from eating beans is to take a special digestive enzyme. The enzyme product is now available in many grocery stores and pharmacies. It works by breaking up the stachyose in the stomach and small intestine. This prevents the high levels of acids and gas

from developing. A drawback to the enzyme product is that it reduces the positive effects of fiber in the body. Use of this product also increases the caloric value of beans.

Another way to avoid problems from eating beans is to maintain a consistent intake of high-fiber foods. This promotes the growth of bacteria that will digest fiber with minimal distress. Eating yogurt also helps promote growth of beneficial bacteria.

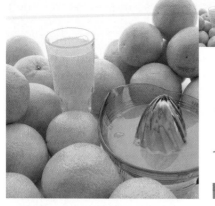

Nutrition News
Carbohydrates and the Athlete

Research indicates that diets high in complex carbohydrates will improve an athlete's performance. This kind of diet is known as carbohydrate loading. A classic study compared three groups of runners eating varying amounts of carbohydrates. Members of one group consumed 55% of their calories from carbohydrates. A second group ate 83% of their calories from carbohydrates. The third group had 94% of their calories from carbohydrates.

First and most importantly, athletes need nutrient-dense foods. These are foods that are high in vitamins and minerals for the energy provided. Athletes should choose highly processed foods with care because processing often removes nutrients. Reading the Nutrition Facts panel can help athletes choose products that are nutrient dense.

Eat for energy. The more you exercise, the higher your calorie needs. If you compete for 90 or more minutes at a time, heed the following recommendations:

❖ Eat a high carbohydrate diet during training.

❖ Never restrict complex carbohydrates.

❖ Increase exercise intensity *without* restricting carbohydrates.

❖ During the week before competition, gradually cut back on exercise.

❖ Eat a very high carbohydrate diet for several days before competition.

❖ Rest the day before competition.

Athletes who compete for less than 90 minutes at a time need only a high-carbohydrate diet every day.

Tips

❖ Drink at least 8 glasses of water a day.

❖ Choose a pregame meal that is light and easy to digest. This meal should provide 300 to 1,000 calories. It should provide fluids, plenty of carbohydrates, and little fiber. Carbohydrates are easily digested. Fiber absorbs water and can cause digestive discomfort. The best food choices are breads, potatoes, pasta, and fruit juice.

❖ Finish eating 3 to 4 hours before competition to keep digestion from interfering with muscle performance.

❖ Eat a high-carbohydrate meal within two hours after exercise to increase glycogen storage by as much as 300%.

❖ During extended periods of exercise, consider consuming a sports drink instead of water. Such drinks are designed to replace electrolytes and fluids while restoring glucose levels for energy.

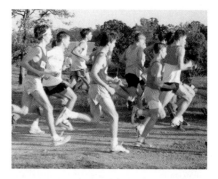

A high carbohydrate diet is especially important for cross country runners.

Types of Energy Foods	Maximum Endurance Times
55% carbohydrates, 45% fat and protein	57 minutes
83% carbohydrates, 17% fat and protein	114 minutes
94% carbohydrates, 6% fat and protein	167 minutes

Source: Sizer, Frances and Whitney, Eleanor, *Nutrition: Concepts and Controversies,* 1997, pp. 383-384.

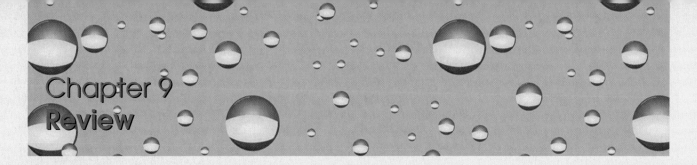

Chapter 9
Review

Summary

Complex carbohydrates are polysaccharides—complex molecules of thousands of linked sugar units. The different types of complex carbohydrates include starches, cellulose, gums, and pectins. Complex carbohydrates serve several functions in food preparation.

Starch and liquid mixtures are classified by their physical properties. These characteristics are evaluated by food scientists anytime they develop a new starch-thickened product. Modified food starches and cross-linked starches are manufactured. The wide variety of manufactured starches has greatly increased the number of food products available to the consumer.

When used as thickeners, starches can be added in three different ways to prevent lumping. All three methods work by separating starch granules.

Carbohydrates should be your main source of energy. The body is designed to work best from the energy derived from sugars and starches. You need a new supply of carbohydrates every four to six hours when you are awake. As with all other nutrients, your body will function best with the proper balance of nutrients.

Check Your Understanding

1. Name the two basic structures of starches and describe their shape.
2. Explain the difference between starch granules, cellulose, and gums and pectins.
3. List the three functions of complex carbohydrates in food preparation and give an example of each.
4. Describe how starches thicken a liquid mixture.
5. List three factors food scientists evaluate before selecting a starch for thickening.
6. Identify and define the four types of starch and liquid mixtures.
7. How are retrogradation and syneresis related?
8. List the four types of starch and liquid mixtures from least to most viscous.
9. Which starch would you use to make a translucent sauce? To make an opaque sauce?
10. How are modified starches produced?
11. Describe three methods used to add starch to a liquid without lumps forming.
12. List the nutritional functions of starch in the diet.

Critical Thinking

1. Why must jelly have a pH of 2.0 to 3.5 in order to gel?
2. Describe how instant pudding mixes can thicken without cooking.
3. Why is it possible to refresh a slice of stale bread by sprinkling water on it and heating it briefly?
4. Name a favorite food prepared using each of the three methods of adding starch without forming lumps.
5. Why is carbohydrate loading important to athletes, but not recommended for others?

Explore Further

1. **Technology.** Use a nutrition analysis program to compare the nutritive values of cornmeal, rye flour, wheat flour, buckwheat, and tapioca.

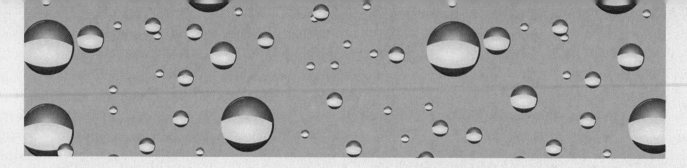

2. **Math.** Construct a bar graph showing the fiber content of eight types of bread available at a local grocery store.

3. **Communication.** Write an article for your school newspaper that explains the advantages and disadvantages of whole grain versus white bread products.

4. **Reading.** Research the procedure for making cornmeal mush and polenta. What starch principle is important in the production of these foods?

5. **Foods and Nutrition.** Examine several gravy and sauce recipes. What proportions of flour to liquid are used? What proportions of cornstarch to liquid are used?

Experiment 9A
Characteristics of Starch

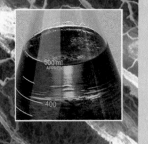

Purpose

Starches found in grocery and health food stores include wheat flour, arrowroot powder, cornstarch, potato starch, rice flour, and tapioca starch. Understanding the physical and chemical characteristics of each starch will help cooks know which starches can be substituted in a recipe. How will you decide which thickener is best for a particular type of food?

Equipment

mortar and pestle
2 slides
microscope
electronic balance
100-mL graduated cylinder
400-mL beaker
glass rod
glass pie plate
viscosity ring
beaker tongs
rubber scraper
thermometer

Supplies

11 g assigned starch
250 mL water plus 1 or 2 drops
line-spread sheet
2 foil muffin papers

Procedure

Part I

1. Crush the assigned starch with a pestle in a mortar until very fine.

   Variation 1: arrowroot powder

   Variation 2: cornstarch

   Variation 3: potato starch

   Variation 4: rice flour

   Variation 5: tapioca

   Variation 6: wheat flour

2. Place a small amount of starch on a slide and examine under the microscope. Record the physical characteristics you observe.

3. Add a drop of water to starch on a second slide and examine under the microscope. Record your observations in a data table.

Part II

1. Mass 10 g of the assigned starch.

2. Combine the starch and 50 mL of water in a 400-mL beaker.

3. Add 200 mL more water and stir with a glass rod.

4. Heat on a range over moderate heat until the mixture comes to a boil that cannot be stirred down.

5. Place a glass pie plate over a line-spread sheet. Place a viscosity ring in the center of the pie plate. Use beaker tongs to remove the beaker from the range and fill the ring with the hot starch mixture.

6. Lift the ring, allowing the starch mixture to flow for 1 minute.

7. Record the number of circles covered by the mixture at each of four points on the sheet. Average the four readings. Record the average in a data table.

8. Scrape the starch mixture back into the beaker. Insert a thermometer into the mixture and allow it to cool to 25°C.

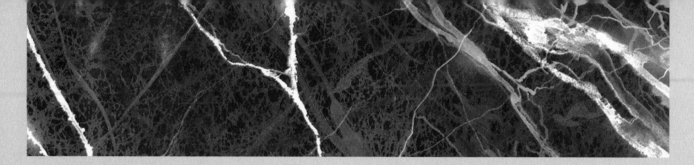

9. While your starch mixture is cooling, note the appearance of the gel and record a description in the data table.

10. View the other groups' dry and wet starches from Part I under the microscope. Record the physical characteristics of each in the data table.

11. Wash the pie plate. Then repeat the viscosity test with the cooled starch mixture.

12. Label two foil muffin papers with the name of your assigned starch. Fill each of the muffin papers with half of the cooled starch mixture. Refrigerate one and freeze the other overnight.

Next Day

1. Thaw the frozen sample. Examine the thawed and refrigerated samples for retrogradation and syneresis.

2. Record your data on a class data chart on an overhead projector. Copy the data from the other lab groups into your data table for Part II.

Lab Extension

Repeat steps 1 through 11 with 20 g of starch.

Questions

1. Which starch has the smallest particles?
2. Which starch has the greatest thickening power in a hot liquid?
3. Which starch has the greatest thickening power at room temperature?
4. Which starches produce a transluscent gel?
5. Which starches maintain a gel after refrigeration?
6. Which starches maintain a gel after freezing and thawing?
7. Which starches experienced syneresis after refrigeration? Which experienced syneresis after freezing and thawing?
8. Give an example of a food that could be thickened effectively with each type of starch tested.

Experiment 9B
Which Fruits Contain Pectin?

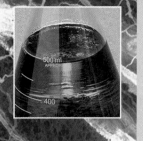

Purpose

Pectin, sugar, and acid must be present in combination for jellies and jams to set up in a gel. The sugar bonds with the fruit juice molecules and the acid alters the pectin. This allows a three-dimensional network of linked pectin molecules to develop. Although fruit contains pectin, sugar, and acid, many types of fruit do not have enough pectin to easily form a gel. If heated fruit juice contains pectin, adding Epsom salts and sugar will cause a semisolid mass to form. Adding ethanol to fruit juice will also cause pectin to form a solid mass if it is present in large enough amounts.

Equipment

paring knife
blender
400-mL beaker
strainer
100-mL graduated cylinder
2 150-mL beakers
wax pencil
metric measuring spoons
glass rod

Supplies

1 medium piece of fruit or 250 mL (1 cup) grapes or berries
10 mL (2 teaspoons) sugar
15 mL (1 tablespoon) Epsom salts
30 mL (2 tablespoons) ethanol (ethyl alcohol)

Procedure

1. Wash your assigned fruit. The apple and pear should be cored. The pit should be removed from the peach. Cut fruit into chunks before pureeing in a blender.

   Variation 1: apple

   Variation 2: peach

   Variation 3: pear

   Variation 4: 250 mL (1 cup) grapes

   Variation 5: 250 mL (1 cup) berries

2. Pour pureed fruit into a 400-mL beaker and place on a range over medium heat. If necessary, add water to prevent sticking. (The fruit should not float in the water.)

3. Simmer the fruit 10 minutes then strain it to separate the juice from the pulp.

4. Pour 30 mL (2 tablespoons) of fruit juice into each of two 150-mL beakers. Use a wax pencil to label one beaker *A* and the other *B*.

5. Add the sugar and Epsom salts to the fruit juice in beaker A. Stir the mixture with a glass rod until the sugar and Epsom salts are dissolved.

6. Wash the glass rod and let the mixture stand 20 minutes. Record your observations.

7. While beaker A is standing, add the ethanol to the fruit juice in beaker B. Stir the mixture with a glass rod. Record your observations.

8. Compare your results to those of other lab groups.

9. Dispose of juice mixtures by flushing them one at a time down the sink with hot water.

Questions

1. Which fruits contain the most pectin?

2. Which fruits contain the least pectin?

3. What procedures will help low-pectin fruits form jams and jellies?

Experiment 9C
Comparing Thickeners in Fruit Sauce

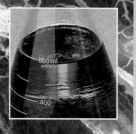

Purpose

One of the many uses of starch in food preparation is as a thickener. The addition of acids, sugar, and other substances, such as fruit, can alter a starch's ability to thicken. As you learned in Experiment 9A, different starches have different thickening ability. Viscosity tests help food scientists compare the thickening power of one starch to the thickening power of another. In this experiment, you will determine how much cornstarch is needed to equal the thickening ability of a given amount of flour in a fruit sauce.

Equipment

metric measuring spoons
400-mL beaker or 1-quart saucepan
100-mL graduated cylinder
3 small bowls
wooden spoon
glass pie plate
viscosity ring

Supplies

45 mL (3 tablespoons) sugar
   assigned starch
125 mL (½ cup) water
125 mL (½ cup) berries
   line-spread sheet

Procedure

1. Combine the sugar and the assigned starch in a 400-mL beaker or a 1-quart saucepan.

   Control: 30 mL (2 tablespoons) flour

   Variation 1: 15 mL (1 tablespoon) cornstarch

   Variation 2: 30 mL (2 tablespoons) cornstarch

   Variation 3: 45 mL (3 tablespoons) cornstarch

2. Measure 125 mL (½ cup) of water into a small bowl. Heat the water on high power in a microwave oven for 30 seconds.

3. Slowly add the hot water to the sugar and starch mixture while stirring constantly with a wooden spoon.

4. Cook the sauce on a range over medium heat, stirring constantly until the sauce comes to a boil.

5. Add the berries and bring the sauce back to a full boil, stirring constantly.

6. When the sauce begins to boil again, remove it from the heat.

7. Center a glass pie plate on a line-spread sheet. Place the viscosity ring in the center of the pie plate.

8. Fill the viscosity ring with the hot sauce.

9. Lift the ring and let the sauce flow for 1 minute.

10. Record the number of circles covered by the sauce at each of four points on the sheet. Add the four readings together and divide by 4 to get an average. Record the average in a data table.

11. Let the sauce cool to room temperature and repeat steps 7 through 10.

12. Divide the remaining sauce among three small bowls and deliver a portion to each lab group.

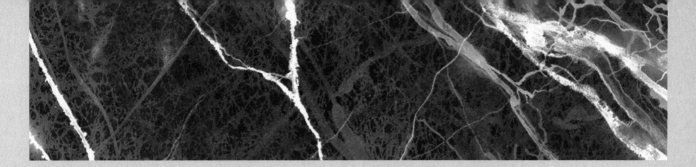

13. Sample each variation of sauce and record observations on the appearance and flavor of each.

Calculations

Determine the relative proportion of cornstarch that is needed to match the thickening power of flour.

1 part flour to _____ part(s) cornstarch

Questions

1. Which starch has the most thickening power, cornstarch or flour?
2. Describe any differences in the flavors of the sauces.
3. Describe any difference in mouthfeel between the sauces prepared with cornstarch and the control.
4. Describe any differences in appearance.
5. Which starch makes the best fruit sauce? Why?

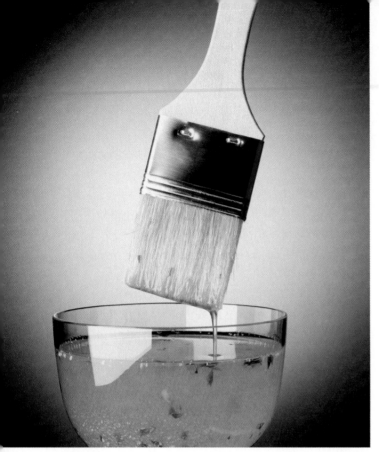

Fats and oils, which are known as lipids, serve many important functions in food preparation.

Chapter 10

Lipids: Nature's Flavor Enhancers

Objectives

After studying this chapter,
you will be able to

describe the molecular structure of glyc-erides, phospholipids, and sterols.

define saturated, monounsaturated, and polyunsaturated fatty acids.

list categories of lipids based on physical state and dietary sources.

relate physical characteristics of lipids to their performance in foods.

examine the functions of lipids in food preparation.

analyze the nutritional impact of lipids in the diet.

Key Terms

lipid
glyceride
fatty acid
carboxyl group
monoglyceride
diglyceride
triglyceride
nonpolar
phospholipid
sterol
saturated
unsaturated
monounsaturated
polyunsaturated
fat

oil
melting point
hydrogenation
marbling
solidification point
auto-oxidation
rancidity
antioxidant
smoke point
flash point
essential fatty acid
omega-3 fatty acid
plaque
atherosclerosis
lipoprotein

In today's society, much is written about the dangers of fat in the diet. Many weight-loss plans recommend cutting fat and counting fat grams. It is true that too much fat can be harmful. However, fat plays an important role both in food preparation and general health.

In this chapter, you will examine the structure of fat. You will learn how it functions in food preparation and why it is a vital part of a healthful diet. As you study this chapter, it is important to remember that fat *does* have a place in a healthful diet. The key is to keep everything in balance.

Chemical Structure of Lipids

Lipids are a category of organic compounds that are insoluble in water and have a greasy feel. *Fats, oils, shortening, grease, phospholipids, sterols*, and *cholesterol* are all terms used for lipids and their related compounds.

Lipids, like carbohydrates, contain carbon, hydrogen, and oxygen. However, lipids differ from carbohydrates in several ways. Lipids are not polymers, they do not provide structure to food products, and they cannot be dissolved in water.

There are three general types of lipids in foods and the human body. These are triglycerides, phospholipids, and sterols. Each of these types has a unique chemical structure.

The Glycerides

Most lipid molecules found in foods and the body have two basic parts. The base or core of these lipids is a glycerol molecule. Molecules that have a glycerol base are called *glycerides.* Glycerol has three hydroxyl groups that will react easily with other compounds. See 10-1.

The second part of most lipid molecules is called a fatty acid. *Fatty acids* are organic molecules that consist of a carbon chain with a carboxyl group at one end. A *carboxyl group* is a carbon atom, two oxygen atoms, and a hydrogen atom. See 10-2. The carboxyl group of a fatty acid will readily react with a hydroxyl group of glycerol. The products of this reaction are a lipid and water.

Glycerol Molecule

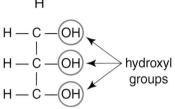

10-1 A glycerol molecule forms the base of most lipids found in foods and the body.

Carboxyl Group

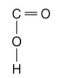

10-2 The carboxyl group found at one end of a fatty acid molecule allows the molecule to bond readily with glycerol.

Because glycerol has three hydroxyl groups, it can join with one, two, or three fatty acids. A *monoglyceride* is a glycerol with one fatty acid attached at the site of a hydroxyl group. A *diglyceride* is a glycerol with two fatty acids attached. *Triglycerides* have a fatty acid joined at each of the three hydroxyl sites. See 10-3.

Fatty acid chains vary in length from 4 to 24 carbon atoms. There are 20 fatty acids that can combine with glycerol to form lipids.

Most of the lipids found in foods and in the body are triglycerides. Triglycerides can have three different fatty acids attached to the glycerol base. It is also possible for triglycerides to have two or three fatty acids that are identical. With 20 fatty acids to choose from, many combinations of triglycerides are possible. These options create triglyceride molecules with different characteristics. The chemical variations lead to differences in cooking performance, shelf life, and nutritional value. See 10-4.

Fatty acids and glycerol are polar molecules. The bodies of fatty acid are nonpolar. However, the carboxyl groups on fatty acids are slightly positive. The hydroxyl groups on glycerol are slightly negative. When fatty acids are mixed with glycerol, the polar ends

Formation of a Triglyceride

Reactants: glycerol and
3 fatty acids

Products: 1 triglyceride and
3 water molecules

10-3 This chemical formula shows how fatty acids and glycerol combine to form lipids and water. R_1, R_2, and R_3 represent the carbon chains that make up the center of the fatty acids.

combine. The newly formed lipids have two ends that are *nonpolar*, or neutral in nature. Because fat molecules are nonpolar, they will not dissolve in water.

Mono- and diglycerides are partially soluble in water because of their hydroxyl groups. Their fatty acids also make these molecules soluble in fat. This dual solubility gives mono- and diglycerides an important function in the food industry. They are often added to processed foods to keep mixtures of water and fats stable. Butter and margarine are examples of foods to which mono- and diglycerides are often added.

Phospholipids

A second basic type of lipids is the phospholipids. A *phospholipid* is a glycerol base with two fatty acids and a phosphorus-containing acid attached. The fatty acids are soluble in fats. The phosphorus-containing acid is soluble in water. This allows phospholipids to mix with both water-based and fat-based substances.

Phospholipids play important roles in the body and in food products. In the body, cell membranes contain lipids, but the fluids on both sides of the membranes are water based. Phospholipids help carry fats back and forth across cell membranes into the water-based fluids. In food products, phospholipids help fats stay mixed in water-based solutions. Phospholipids keep foods like mayonnaise from separating.

Sterols

The third general type of lipids is the sterols. The *sterols* are complicated molecules derived or made from lipids. They include cholesterol, vitamin D, and the steroid hormones, including sex hormones. The most familiar sterol, cholesterol, is a part of every cell in the human body. See 10-5.

Categories of Lipids

You need to understand the ways lipids are categorized before you can understand the effects of lipids in food mixtures. Lipids are grouped according to molecular structure, physical state, and dietary sources.

Categories Based on Molecular Structure

One way to categorize lipids, or more specifically fatty acids, is by how saturated their carbon chains are with hydrogen atoms. In Chapter 4, you learned that each carbon atom is capable of forming four bonds. If two carbon and six hydrogen atoms combine, all the resulting bonds will be single bonds.

Common Fatty Acids

Abbreviation*	Name	Structural Formula	Melting Point (°C)	Food Sources
Saturated Fatty Acids				
4:0	Butyric	$CH_3(CH_2)_2COOH$	-4.2	butter
6:0	Caproic	$CH_3(CH_2)_4COOH$	-3	milk fats, coconut
8:0	Caprylic	$CH_3(CH_2)_6COOH$	16–16.5	
10:0	Capric	$CH_3(CH_2)_8COOH$	31–32	
12:0	Laurie	$CH_3(CH_2)_{10}COOH$	44	palm and coconut oils
14:0	Myristic	$CH_3(CH_2)_{12}COOH$	54	nutmeg
16:0	Palmitic	$CH_3(CH_2)_{14}COOH$	63	milk
18:0	Stearic	$CH_3(CH_2)_{16}COOH$	70	milk, beef
20:0	Eicosanoic	$CH_3(CH_2)_{18}COOH$	74–76	
Monounsaturated Fatty Acids				
18:1	Oleic	$CH_3(CH_2)_7CH=CH(CH_2)_7COOH$	14	milk, corn, cottonseed, peanuts, olives, sesame seeds, sunflowers, canola oil, almonds, walnuts
22:1	Erucic	$CH_3(CH_2)_7CH=$ $CH(CH_2)_{11}COOH$		canola oil
Polyunsaturated Fatty Acids				
18:2	Linoleic	$CH_3(CH_2)_4CH=CHCH_2CH=$ $CH(CH_2)_7COOH$	-5	corn, cottonseed, olives, peanuts, sesame seeds, sunflowers
18:3	Linolenic	$CH_3(CH_2)_2CHCH_2CH=$ $CHCH_2CH=CH(CH_2)_7COOH$	-11	soybeans, wheat germ
20:4	Arachidonic	$CH_3(CH_2)_4CH=CHCH_2CH=$ $CHCH_2CH=CHCH_2CH=$ $CH(CH_2)_3COOH$	-49.5	

*Abbreviation: This column is a shorthand description of the fatty acid chains. The first number is the number of carbons in the fatty acid. The second number is the number of double bonds.

10-4 These fatty acids commonly combine with glycerol to form a variety of triglyceride molecules.

What happens if only four hydrogen atoms are available? The carbon atoms are still looking to form four bonds. A carbon atom can bond twice to another carbon atom. This will result in the carbon atoms sharing two electrons. When two atoms form two bonds with each other, the bond is called a *double bond*.

double bond

In the following examples, the carbon chain on the left contains the maximum number of hydrogen atoms. The one on the right does not. Notice that each double bond reduces the total number of hydrogen atoms by two.

Fatty acids can be grouped by the number of double bonds in their carbon chains. Fatty acids will have zero, one, or multiple double bonds. The number of double bonds determines how close the carbon chain is to containing the maximum number of hydrogen atoms.

The first group of fatty acids has no double bonds present in the carbon chain. This means the carbon chain contains the maximum number of hydrogen atoms. When fatty acids have the maximum number of hydrogen atoms, they are described as *saturated.*

Butyric acid is a saturated fatty acid found in butter. Stearic acid is a saturated fatty acid that is a major component of beef fat. Notice these examples of saturated fatty acids are found in animal sources. Generally, lipids found in animal sources are high in saturated fatty acids. See 10-6.

If a fatty acid does not contain all the hydrogen atoms it could contain, it is *unsaturated.*

Fatty acids that have one double bond in the carbon chain are called *monounsaturated.* Foods that are high in monounsaturated fatty acids include olive oil, almonds, walnuts, and canola oil.

Polyunsaturated fatty acids have two or more double bonds in the carbon chain. Each double bond bends the fatty acid chain. The bends make it difficult for the molecules to pack together tightly. Safflower, sunflower, and corn oils are all high in polyunsaturated fatty acids.

A single triglyceride molecule can be made of one saturated, one monounsaturated, and one polyunsaturated fatty acid. This molecule would have characteristics of all three types of saturation.

Most lipids contain a combination of saturated, monounsaturated, and polyunsaturated fatty acids. The type of fatty acid present in the largest amounts has the greatest effect on the characteristics of the lipid. See 10-7.

Categories Based on Physical State

One of the easiest ways to categorize lipids is by their physical state at room temperature. Lipids that are solid at room temperature are commonly called *fats.* If lipids

Cholesterol

10-5 Cholesterol, like other sterols, is a complex lipid molecule.

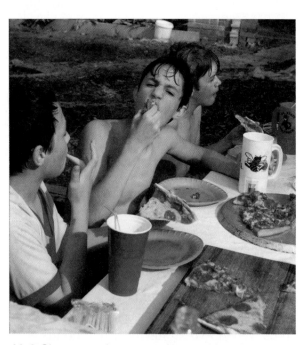

10-6 Cheese and pepperoni can make pizza a food that is high in saturated fat.

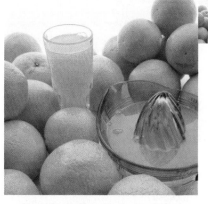

Nutrition News
What Are Trans-Fatty Acids?

Research has indicated that trans-fatty acids might be as harmful to your health as highly-saturated butterfat. Trans-fatty acids are found in many margarines. Until more research is done, some health experts have recommended eating solid margarines in moderation.

What is at the heart of the concern is the shape of unsaturated fatty acids at the double bond site. One of two things can happen when a double bond forms in a fatty acid. As seen in the figure to the right, cis-isomers bend or kink at the bond. The trans-isomers take a fairly linear shape. *Isomers* are two molecules that have the same molecular formula, but the atoms are arranged in different patterns.

Most unsaturated vegetable oils in nature have the

cis- formation. The bends and kinks make it difficult for the molecules to move close together and solidify. Trans-fatty acids will solidify at lower temperatures because they are linear. Trans-fatty acids are a product of hydrogenating vegetable oil. Originally it was thought that trans-unsaturated fatty acids

would be nutritionally identical to the cis-unsaturated fatty acids. Evidence indicates that the body may not be able to effectively digest the trans- form. These fatty acids could build up in blood vessels, increasing the risk of atherosclerosis. More study needs to be done to understand how the body reacts to trans-fatty acids.

Cis–

Trans–

are liquid at room temperature, they are called *oils.*

The numbers of hydrogen and carbon atoms on a fatty acid chain determine the temperature at which lipids liquefy. Double bonds in the fatty acid chain lower the temperature at which a lipid will be liquid rather than solid. Lipids that are liquid at room temperature have one or more double bonds in the carbon chain of the fatty acids. Polyunsaturated fatty acids become liquid at lower temperatures than saturated and monounsaturated fatty acids. This characteristic is due to the bent shape of the chain and the lower number of hydrogen atoms.

Fats contain mostly saturated fatty acids. Oils contain more monounsaturated and polyunsaturated fatty acids. This means fats have more hydrogen atoms than oils. Therefore, fats are denser and require more energy to liquefy. This causes the melting point of fats to be higher than the melting point of oils. *Melting point* is the temperature at which a lipid is completely liquid. Although oils are liquid at room temperature, they will solidify if chilled to a low enough temperature.

Different types of fats and oils are saturated to different degrees. Therefore, each type of fat or oil has a different melting point. For

Fatty Acids in Common Fats and Oils

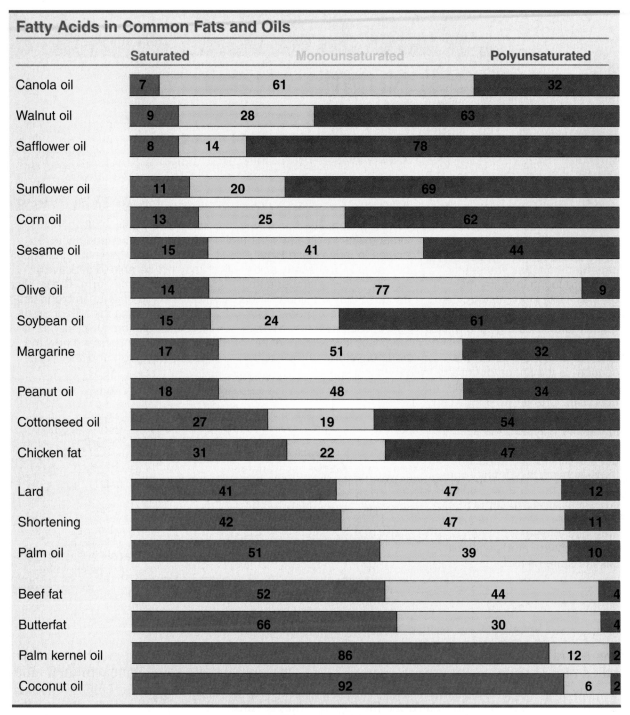

	Saturated	Monounsaturated	Polyunsaturated
Canola oil	7	61	32
Walnut oil	9	28	63
Safflower oil	8	14	78
Sunflower oil	11	20	69
Corn oil	13	25	62
Sesame oil	15	41	44
Olive oil	14	77	9
Soybean oil	15	24	61
Margarine	17	51	32
Peanut oil	18	48	34
Cottonseed oil	27	19	54
Chicken fat	31	22	47
Lard	41	47	12
Shortening	42	47	11
Palm oil	51	39	10
Beef fat	52	44	4
Butterfat	66	30	4
Palm kernel oil	86	12	2
Coconut oil	92	6	2

10-7 The way fats and oils perform in cooking and food products is determined by the types of fatty acids they contain.

instance, oils high in polyunsaturated fatty acids will have lower melting points than oils high in monounsaturated fatty acids.

Oleic acid has one double bond in its carbon chain and is therefore monounsaturated. It is used extensively in the production of margarine. Remember that double bonds lower the melting point of lipids. Therefore, margarines with high oleic acid content will be softer than butter, which contains more saturated fatty acids. These margarines will also melt at lower temperatures than butter. Margarines have been developed with a wide range of melting points. Squeeze margarines stay fluid in the refrigerator. Baker's margarine, which is designed for making puff pastry, melts completely at 57°C (135°F). Butter melts at body temperature of 37°C (98°F).

Fats and oils usually come from different sources. Fats usually come from animal sources. Examples include butterfat from milk, lard from pigs, and tallow (used in candles) from animals such as sheep and cattle. Most oils come from plant sources. Examples include corn, soybean, peanut, canola, and olive oils. See 10-8.

Hydrogenated Vegetable Oils

Hydrogenation is the process of adding hydrogen atoms to an unsaturated lipid to increase its saturation level. This process is used to make some oils solid at room temperature. The result is a product that has a higher melting point than the oils. An example is margarine made from 100% corn oil. Solid vegetable shortening is also made from hydrogenated vegetable oils.

Hydrogenation is done by bubbling hydrogen through liquid oil in the presence of a nickel catalyst. The double bonds in the fatty acid chains of the oil break. The chains pick up extra hydrogen atoms, becoming more saturated. The process can be stopped at any point. If oils were to be completely saturated, they would become too brittle for most uses of solid fats.

The most commonly hydrogenated oil is soybean. Cottonseed and palm oils are often added in small amounts.

Advantages of hydrogenated vegetable oils include

❖ longer shelf life than oil or lard

❖ greater stability than lard

❖ lower production costs than lard

❖ faster dissolving and setting properties in chocolate production

Categories Based on Dietary Sources

Another way to group lipids is based on the food sources from which they come. Triglycerides come from seven main groups of dietary sources. Each group of triglycerides has a similar molecular structure and physical characteristics.

Milkfats come from the milk of cows, goats, and other mammals. Milkfats are high in palmitic, oleic, and stearic acids. The main difference between milkfats and fats such as lard or tallow is the length of the fatty acid chains. Most fatty acids in milk are shorter chains of 4 to 12 carbon atoms.

Lauric acids are the main component of a group of lipids found in palms such as coconut. Lauric acid makes up 40% to 50% of all the fatty acids in this lipid group. Lauric acid has a low melting point. These lipids are the most saturated of the oils found in plants.

Vegetable butters come from the seeds of tropical plants. These lipids have at least one unsaturated and one saturated fatty acid on every molecule. Because the molecular arrangements are so similar, these lipids have a very narrow melting range. The most

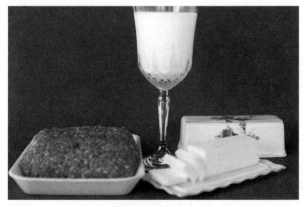
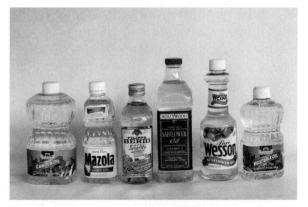

10-8 Hamburger, milk, and butter are sources of animal fats in a typical U.S. diet. Sources of vegetable oils include rapeseeds (canola oil), corn, olives, safflowers, sunflowers, and soybeans.

important member of this group is cocoa butter, which is used frequently in candies.

Oleic-linoleic acids come from corn, peanuts, sunflowers, olives, cottonseeds, and sesame seeds. These lipids make up the largest group of triglycerides. They contain less than 20% saturated fatty acids.

Linolenic acid is found in large amounts in soybeans and wheat germ. Wheat germ needs to be refrigerated after opening. This is because linolenic acid reacts easily with oxygen during storage. This reaction causes flavor changes that are often undesirable. Refrigeration will help prevent these unwanted flavor changes.

Animal fats are found in meats and poultry. They contain large amounts of fully saturated fatty acids. This gives them high melting points. Animal fats are present as visible fat deposits as well as specks and streaks scattered throughout muscle fibers. The specks or streaks of fat in muscle tissue are called *marbling.* Marbling is an indicator of flavor and tenderness. The more marbling a meat cut has, the more flavorful and tender it will be. However, marbling also indicates a higher fat content.

Marine oils come from fish. These oils contain large amounts of long-chain polyunsaturated fatty acids. These fatty acids have as many as six double bonds each. The high degree of unsaturation makes these oils spoil or develop off flavors and odors very quickly. This is why fish must be eaten or frozen within 24 hours. See 10-9.

Physical Characteristics of Lipids

Three physical characteristics impact the way lipids perform in food products. One is the melting and solidification points of lipids. The second is the nonpolar nature of lipid molecules. The third physical characteristic is the tendency of lipids to react with oxygen.

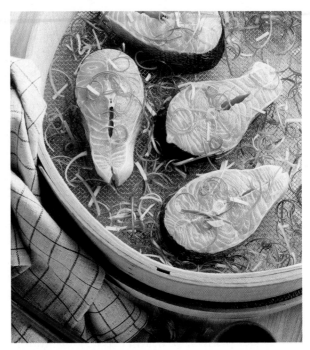

10-9 Fish is a source of marine oils, which are highly unsaturated.

Differing Melting and Solidification Points

Ice melts at 0°C. Water freezes at 0°C. The melting and freezing points of water are the same temperature. Unlike water, lipids do not have a specific melting point. This is because most lipids are mixtures of different kinds of fatty acids. Because each fatty acid has a different melting point, the lipids in a mixture will melt at different temperatures.

The lipids in a mixture will also become solid at different temperatures. This results in a temperature range between the point at which all lipids are solid and all lipids are liquid. Lipids within this range are a mix of solid and liquid. The temperature at which all lipids in a mixture are in a solid state is called the *solidification point.* (Lipids are said to solidify rather than freeze.) The solidification point for lipids is lower than the melting point. This is illustrated by the following diagram.

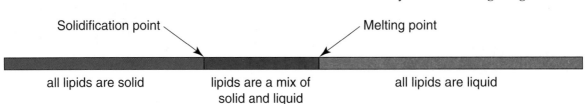

Solidification point → | all lipids are solid | lipids are a mix of solid and liquid | all lipids are liquid | ← Melting point

Lipids containing mostly saturated fatty acids have a higher melting point than lipids containing mostly unsaturated fatty acids. This is because the number of hydrogen atoms per carbon atom affects the melting point. The number of carbon atoms in the fatty acid chain also affects the melting point. The shorter the chain of carbon atoms in the fatty acid is, the lower the melting point will be. For example, butter has high levels of butyric acid, which contains 4 carbon atoms. Butter melts at a lower temperature than beef fat. Beef fat is high in stearic acid, which contains 18 carbon atoms. Both butyric and stearic acids are saturated. However, stearic acid's longer chain of carbon atoms results in a higher melting point than butyric acid.

You may have noticed that vegetable oil becomes cloudy when you refrigerate it. This is because some of the triglycerides have a solidification point that is higher than the temperature in most refrigerators. The oils used in salad dressing have been processed to prevent solidification at refrigerated temperatures. The vegetable oil is chilled until solidification of the higher-melting triglycerides occurs. The oil is then filtered to remove the solid fat crystals. This is why commercial salad dressings are easier to pour after chilling than homemade ones.

Nonpolar Molecules

As you recall from Chapter 7, water molecules are polar. This means they have an unequal sharing of electrons. Lipid molecules have an equal or balanced sharing of electrons. This causes lipid molecules to be nonpolar. Substances that are nonpolar dissolve or readily mix with other substances that are nonpolar. Polar compounds dissolve in or readily mix with other polar compounds. However, polar and nonpolar molecules are not attracted to each other. Therefore, water and oil will not mix.

Lipids are very large molecules. The variety and shape of fatty acid chains create spaces between the parts of the molecules. These spaces cause lipids to be less dense than water. These spaces also prevent lipid molecules from packing together tightly. Because lipids are nonpolar, polar water molecules will not slip in and fill the spaces between lipid molecules. This results in the low density of lipids compared to water-based compounds. This is why oil floats on water.

You can demonstrate this physical characteristic of lipids by combining vinegar and oil. The oil will rise to the top. For vinegar and oil to stay mixed in salad dressings, another substance, called an emulsifier, must be added. This substance must have polar and nonpolar portions. See 10-10.

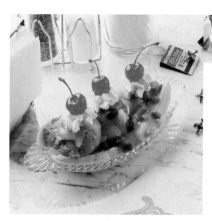

Item of Interest
Melt in Your Mouth...

The next time you eat a piece of chocolate, savor the flavor by letting it *melt in your mouth*. The reason chocolate melts in your mouth is that fat in chocolate has a very narrow melting range. This is because most of the lipids in chocolate have the same chemical structure. The melting point of these lipids is close to body temperature. As the fats melt, they release the chocolate flavor. The melting fat also gives chocolate candies their smooth mouth feel.

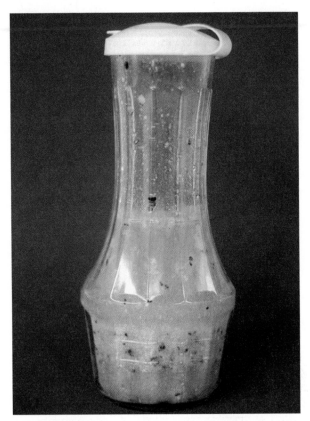

10-10 Oil and vinegar dressing separates because the fat molecules in oil are nonpolar and the vinegar molecules are polar in nature.

Tendency to Deteriorate

An important characteristic of lipids is their tendency to react with oxygen. *Auto-oxidation* is a complex chain reaction that starts when lipids are exposed to oxygen. The oxygen will bind to the lipid molecules and then to other compounds. Once started, auto-oxidation is like knocking over dominoes. It is hard to stop and spreads quickly.

Auto-oxidation causes lipids to deteriorate. When oxygen is added to lipids, new compounds are formed. These compounds have an unpleasant flavor and odor that is described as rancid. *Rancidity* is a form of food spoilage, but it poses no short-term health risks. The main problem is the color and flavor changes.

Unsaturated oils are more susceptible to auto-oxidation than saturated fats. This is because unsaturated oils contain double bonds, which are weaker than single bonds. Oxygen can readily bind with lipid molecules at the sites of the double bonds.

Another type of deterioration occurs when triglycerides are hydrolyzed. You recall from Chapter 8 that hydrolysis occurs when a large molecule is divided into smaller parts by adding water. When water is added to lipid molecules, the molecules break apart into free fatty acids and glycerol. The shorter the carbon chains are, the more likely the fatty acids are to become rancid and develop off flavors. Butyric and caproic acids are short-chain fatty acids in butter. They are responsible for the unpleasant odor and flavor that develops when butter becomes rancid. Long-chain fatty acids like stearic, palmitic, and oleic usually do not develop off flavors unless auto-oxidation occurs also.

Oxygen exposure can cause high-fat foods to become rancid. To minimize oxygen exposure, some products are vacuum sealed or flushed with nitrogen gas. Rancidity can also be prevented or slowed by adding antioxidants to lipids. *Antioxidants* are compounds that will quickly react with oxygen to form new substances. Antioxidants will react with the oxygen before lipids do. Important dietary antioxidants are vitamins A, C, and E.

> ### Storage Tip
> **Store high-fat foods in a dark, oxygen-free environment. This will slow the development of rancid flavors.**

Functions of Lipids in Food Preparation

The structures and characteristics of the various types of fatty acids affect how they perform in food products. Lipids serve six main functions in cooking. Lipids act as heat mediums, tenderizers, aerators, flavor enhancers, lubricants, and as liquids in emulsions.

Transfer Heat

Lipids are an excellent heat medium. They transfer heat from cooking utensils to food quickly, evenly, and at very high temperatures. At normal air pressure, water boils at 100°C and will not get any hotter no matter how long you heat it. The temperature of lipids will continue to increase as heat is added. Because of this characteristic, lipids will get hot enough to brown food. The exterior of the food will also develop a crisp texture.

Heat cannot be added to lipids indefinitely. Every lipid has a temperature at which the fatty acids begin to break apart and produce smoke. This temperature is called the *smoke point*. As the fatty acids break down, they combine with oxygen to form new compounds. These compounds have strong, unpleasant flavors. Once oil begins to smoke, breakdown has occurred and the oil should be discarded. It will no longer fry food successfully without creating undesirable flavor and color changes in the food. See 10-11.

Lard has a smoke point of 185°C (365° F). This is the same as the recommended temperature for deep frying. This means you have to heat lard to its smoke point when using it for deep frying. Therefore, you can use it for deep frying only one time for a short period.

If oil is heated long enough, it will become hot enough to burn. The *flash point* is the temperature at which lipids will flame. If oil is heated without close monitoring, the temperature will rise until small flames appear across the surface. This occurs at around 315°C (600°F).

Successful deep frying requires a hot enough temperature to cook the food all the way through without burning the outside. If food is fried at temperatures below 175°C (350°F), the exterior does not brown fast enough. Excess oil will soak into the food. The result will be pale, soggy food that is extremely high in fat content. If the oil reaches 205°C (400°F), the exterior of the food will begin to burn before the interior is done. The result will be very dark colored food with a raw center.

Using an electric deep fryer can make successful deep frying easier and safer. These appliances are thermostatically controlled. The fryer will automatically turn off the heat when the oil reaches the set temperature. This reduces the risk of starting a kitchen fire.

When cooking at home, you may wish to use a number of guidelines food scientists follow for successful deep frying. Cut foods for deep frying into small even pieces to decrease cooking time. Remove excess moisture from foods to reduce splattering. Cook only a small

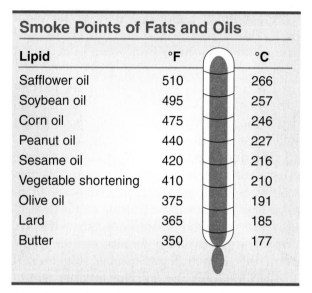

Smoke Points of Fats and Oils		
Lipid	**°F**	**°C**
Safflower oil	510	266
Soybean oil	495	257
Corn oil	475	246
Peanut oil	440	227
Sesame oil	420	216
Vegetable shortening	410	210
Olive oil	375	191
Lard	365	185
Butter	350	177

10-11 Each time oil or fat is heated, the smoke point drops. The higher the smoke point is, the more the oil or fat can be reused.

amount of food at a time. The more food that is added to the hot oil, the more the temperature of the oil will drop. If the oil drops below 175°C (350°F), the food will become soggy.

After coating foods in batter for deep frying, let them sit for 20 to 30 minutes. (This allows the starch in the batter to bind to the food.) Fewer pieces of the batter will break off into the oil and burn.

Do not salt food until after deep frying. Salt pulls water to the surface of the food. This will cause increased splattering when the food is placed in hot oil. Salt also lowers the smoke point of the oil and will, therefore, reduce the time the oil can be used.

Tenderize

Fats are used to tenderize baked products. Flour makes up the structure of most baked goods. The protein in flour has the tendency to form long strands. The longer the strands are, the tougher and chewier the food will become. Fat tenderizes by shortening these long strands. (This is why the solid white fat sold for baking is called *shortening*.) Solid fats coat the flour particles, making the dough slippery. This prevents long protein strands from forming.

The fat to flour ratio of a dough will determine how flaky a baked product is. Biscuits have a ratio of about one part fat for eight parts flour. This is just enough fat to give biscuits the ability to pull apart in sheets of moist bread.

Pie crust recipes call for about one part fat for every four parts flour. Too much fat will cause the pie crust to fall apart. Too little fat will cause the pie crust to be tough.

The first step in preparing biscuits and pie crust is cutting the fat into the flour. This step continues until the mixture resembles small peas or coarse crumbs. Cutting in fat distributes it evenly throughout the dough. Overmixing will cause the fat to soften to the point that it will begin to cling together. If worked too long, the fat-flour mixture would form a greasy ball. The dough would no longer be suitable for biscuits or crust.

Puff pastry has a mixture of fat and flour layered between thin sheets of yeast dough. The dough is kneaded to develop its structure, then it is rolled into a thin rectangle. A mixture of two parts fat to one part flour is rolled between waxed paper and chilled. Once this mixture has solidified, it is placed on top of the yeast dough. The dough is then folded, sealed, and rolled thin. The dough is folded and rolled until there are as many as fifty layers of dough and fat. The flakiness of puff pastry, croissants, and Danish result from the thin layers of fat melting during cooking. The dough browns and separates into the characteristic thin, tender, flaky sheets. See 10-12.

In each of these food products, tenderizing is a result of the fat separating but not soaking into the flour. The lipids that work best for this function are the solid fats. The higher the melting point of the fat is, the longer the mixture can be worked without the fat melting into the flour. Butter, regular margarines, lard, and shortenings give the best performance. Whipped and liquid margarines will not work because of their high air and water contents.

Lipids tenderize other baked goods, including cakes, pancakes, muffins, and waffles. Fats aid in giving these products a fluffy, moist texture. The separating of the flour keeps the products tender. Oil can be used instead of fat when the batter is a quick mix type. This type of batter combines the liquids in one bowl and the dry ingredients in another. The two mixtures are then blended.

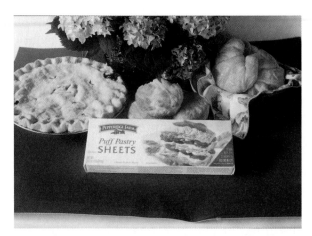

10-12 Pie crust, biscuits, croissants, and pastries made from puff pastry are flaky and tender because of the solid fat in the dough.

Aerate

Aeration is the addition of air into a batter. Saturated fats allow tiny air pockets to form when batters are sufficiently beaten. In order for aeration to occur, the fat must be able to hold its shape around the air pockets. This is why oils cannot be successfully substituted for fat in most cake recipes. Because oils are not solid at room temperature, they cannot provide the structure needed to trap air. The oil will start to separate from the mixture before cooking can stabilize the nonpolar molecules throughout the batter. The result is a grainier textured cake.

Most conventional cake recipes call for the fat and sugar to be creamed (beaten together). The purpose of this step is to aerate the fat. The creaming process requires a fat that will soften but not melt when beaten. Butter remains workable between 18°C and 21°C (65°F and 70°F). At higher temperatures, the fat in butter becomes too liquid to support trapped air cells.

Timing the creaming step is important. Because beating increases friction, it increases the batter temperature. If the temperature goes too high, the fat will melt and the trapped air will be lost. This results in a crumbly, grainy texture.

Another example of aeration in lipids is whipped margarines. Whipped margarine and butter products are made more spreadable by adding air. The fat is beaten until tiny air pockets are trapped throughout.

Unwhipped butter and margarine are often packaged as four quarter-pound sticks. Whipped butter and margarines come six sticks to a pound. The extra volume in the whipped products is due to trapped air. That is why one stick of whipped butter cannot be substituted in recipes for one stick of butter. Whipped products can help lower fat in the diet. They make it seem as if you are using more butter on your food than you really are.

Enhance Flavor

An important function of fat in foods is providing flavor. Much of the flavor in food comes from salt, sugar, and fats. Because they want more flavor, most people in the United States get too much of these three ingredients.

Some of the fats in your diet are used as seasonings to flavor foods. People spread butter and margarine on bread and rolls mainly for flavor. Cooks add bacon fat to beans, soups, and sauces for the distinctive flavor it will give the finished product. Chefs cook onions, garlic, celery, and peppers in fat as a first step in preparing many sauces, soups, and casseroles, 10-13. Fat dissolves and disperses the flavor compounds from the vegetables. The flavor will be stronger than if the vegetables were just simmered in a broth base. Olive oil provides flavor to salad dressings, and sesame oil enhances the taste of many Asian dishes.

There are times when you want to taste the flavor of the main food product and not the fat. When this is the case, it is best to use oils that have little or no flavor of their own. Cottonseed oil is one of the most flavorless of the oils. This is one reason why it is a favorite of potato chip manufacturers. Vegetable shortening, soybean oil, and canola oil are other relatively flavorless fats and oils.

Lubricate

Lipids lubricate food components, making it easier for them to slide over one another. This characteristic makes meat easier to chew as the fat content increases. Meat that is marbled has small flecks of fat evenly distributed throughout the muscle fibers. The even distribution of the fat creates a pleasant mouth feel.

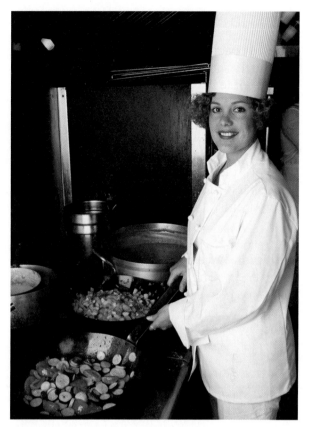

10-13 Sautéing vegetables in fat brings out their flavors.

Because lipids have a greasy texture, they feel slick or smooth to the tongue and palate. This characteristic causes many foods to seem moister. This is one reason why butter, margarine, and mayonnaise are popular spreads for breads and rolls. These spreads add to the feeling of moistness without making the bread soggy.

Serve as Liquids in Emulsions

Lipids are usually one of the two liquids in an emulsion. An *emulsion* is a mixture that contains a lipid and a water-based liquid. This mixture will not stay mixed together unless a compound is added that has a polar and a nonpolar end. Examples of common fat-based emulsions in food are mayonnaise, butter, milk, and bottled salad dressings. Phospholipids are compounds that help create emulsions. You will read more about the chemistry, application, and characteristics of emulsions in Chapter 11.

Lipids in Your Diet

Most people in the United States consume too much saturated fat. On the other hand, some people try to eliminate all fats from their diets. See 10-14. Because lipids are an important part of a healthful diet, it is important to find a balance. To correctly monitor lipids in your diet, you need to understand the functions of lipids in your body. You also need to understand the role of cholesterol and its relation to lipids.

Functions of Lipids in the Body

Lipids have four important functions in your body. The first is as a concentrated source of energy. Lipids have 9 Calories per gram. That is more than twice the energy provided by a gram of sugars or starches. Lipids take longer to digest than carbohydrates and give a feeling of fullness longer. They help provide a steady supply of energy to your body between meals.

Your body stores fat not needed for energy in fat cells. Triglycerides are the body's storage form of fats. There are two kinds of fat cells: white fat cells and brown fat cells. White fat cells are mainly composed of one large droplet of fat. The body tends to hold onto these reserves. The cell expands as fat is added and shrinks when fat is used. The brown fat cells contain many mitochondria. This is the part of the cell in which the body produces energy.

Two other functions of fats in the body are cell production and temperature regulation. A diet that is 100% fat free for extended periods is dangerous. Cell walls are made from a

---

Fat Consumption Trends in the United States (1977–1997)

Food Source	Annual Increase per Person	Food Source	Annual Decrease per Person
Baking and frying fats	5.8 lbs	Table spreads	2.3 lbs
Salad and cooking oils	8.8 lbs	Margarine	2.2 lbs
Cheese	17 lbs	Cottage cheese	2 lbs
Fat free milk	2.7 gal	Whole milk	11 gal
Poultry	31 lbs	Beef, pork, and lamb	21 lbs
Fish	3 lbs	Eggs	72

Overall Changes

❖ People have decreased their total fat consumption by 8% of total calories.

❖ People are drinking 23% less milk and eating 2.5 times more cheese.

❖ Annual per capita consumption of red meat has decreased by 21 pounds. However, total meat consumption has increased by 13 pounds per person annually.

❖ Calories consumed when eating out has almost doubled. The percentage of those calories from fat has decreased by 4%. The percentage of calories from fat is over 6% higher than that of home-prepared foods.

❖ The percentage of calories from fat in foods prepared at home has decreased by over 10%. However, this percentage is still 1.5% above the goal of 30% of total calories from fat.

Sanford, Scott and Allshouse, Jane. "Have We Turned the Corner on Fat Consumption?" *Food Review*, Sept.–Dec. 1998, pp. 12–18.

10-14 Health and nutrition findings toward the end of the twentieth century encouraged many people to change their fat consumption patterns.

combination of lipids and protein. The body also deposits fatty tissue around the vital organs to protect them from injury. Fatty tissue under the skin has two functions: to insulate and to provide a reserve energy supply. Fat helps maintain your body temperature by acting as an insulator that holds in body warmth. Fat reserves in the body provide energy when you consume too few calories or deplete your glycogen stores through exercise.

The last function of fat is to help transport vitamins. Some vitamins are fat-soluble. They need to combine with fat to be transported to where they are needed in the body.

Essential Fatty Acids

Fatty acids that cannot be produced by the human body are called *essential fatty acids.*

The only two fatty acids the body cannot make are linoleic acid and linolenic acid. Both of these fatty acids are polyunsaturated and are found in most plant and fish oils. They are essential for growth and development. Linoleic acid is found in large amounts in corn, cottonseed, and soybean oils. Chicken is another good source of linoleic acid. Linolenic acid is found in canola oil, soybean oil, walnuts, and fish.

Omega-3 Fatty Acids

Studies have been done on Greenlanders and Inuits. Researchers have tried to find out why these groups have low rates of heart disease in spite of high-fat diets. Most of the fat in their diets has been found to come from fish. Fish are very high in the omega-3 fatty acids.

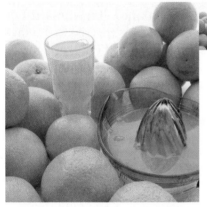

Nutrition News
Carbohydrates vs Fats

Question: Which is more fattening, 100 calories of carbohydrates or 100 calories of fat?

Recent research with rats has revealed that people may gain more weight from fat calories than from carbohydrate calories.

The toast on the left has 100 calories worth of fat from butter. The toast on the right has 100 calories worth of carbohydrates from jam.

This is because fats require less energy than carbohydrates require to be converted for storage in the body.

When 100 calories of fat is digested, the triglycerides break into fatty acids and glycerol. These parts pass through the intestinal wall into the bloodstream, where they can quickly recombine. The recombined fat goes into fat storage cells if it is not needed for energy. It takes 3 of the 100 calories to digest the fat and then store it.

Carbohydrates that are not needed for energy can also be stored as fat in the body. However, to change 100 calories of carbohydrates from starch into

fat, the body must first break down the starch. Once the starch is broken into individual sugar molecules, the sugar is dismantled. Then it must be assembled into fatty acid chains. The fatty acids join to a glycerol and then are stored as fat. This process uses 23 of the 100 calories.

If you eat 100 calories of fat you do not need, 97 calories are stored as fat. If you eat 100 calories of carbohydrates you do not need, the body will first store it as glycogen. If glycogen stores are full, the carbohydrate is changed to fat. Only 77 calories are left to be stored as fat.

Answer: Fat calories are more fattening!

Omega-3 fatty acids have a double bond between the third and fourth carbon atoms from the end with the methyl group (CH_3).

Further study is needed to understand how omega-3 fatty acids work in reducing heart disease. However, research indicates these fatty acids help lower triglyceride levels in the blood and slow the growth of plaque in the arteries.

Fatty fish are high in two kinds of omega-3 fatty acids, eicosapentaenoic acid (EPA), and docosahexaenoic acid (DHA). Recent research on fatty acids from fish sources seems to indicate that EPA and DHA strengthen brain-cell membranes improving cell-to-cell communication. They may also reduce joint inflammation and prevent heartbeat irregularities and mental decline.

Researchers are now recommending two to four meals (eight ounces) of fatty fish per week. Fish that have pink or red flesh are higher in omega-3 fatty acids than fish with white flesh. Albacore tuna, salmon, lake trout, and sardines are good sources, 10-15. Canola oil, flaxseed, and walnuts are good sources of alpha-linolenic acid that can become omega-3 fatty acid in the body.

The Role of Cholesterol

Cholesterol is used to build cell membranes. Up to 25% of all cell walls are cholesterol. Cholesterol is a rigid molecule that helps solidify cell walls. Because cholesterol

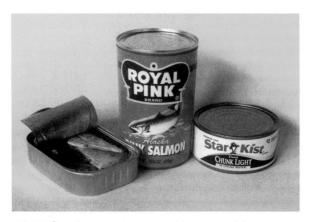

10-15 Sardines, salmon, and tuna provide omega-3 fatty acids.

is insoluble in water, it adds stability to the cell's structure. The body makes cholesterol from lipids.

Too much cholesterol in the blood results in lipids and cholesterol being deposited on artery walls. These deposits are called *plaque.* Because cholesterol is rigid and insoluble in water, these deposits reduce the elasticity of artery walls. This hardening of the arteries is known as **atherosclerosis.** Blood pressure climbs as the heart works harder to force blood through the narrowing arteries. This disease is the leading cause of heart attacks and stroke.

Cholesterol is transported throughout the body by lipoproteins. *Lipoproteins* are clusters of lipid and protein molecules. *Low-density lipoproteins (LDL)* carry cholesterol from the liver. *High-density lipoproteins (HDL)* find unneeded cholesterol and return it to the liver. HDL and LDL work together to keep cholesterol levels in balance. Too much LDL can clog arteries, increasing the risk for heart attack or stroke. High levels of HDL appear to protect against heart attack. An optimal level for LDL is less than 100 mg/dL and greater than 40 mg/dL for HDL.

The average adult consumes 300 mg of cholesterol a day. The liver makes another 1,000 mg from fats. Although high cholesterol intake is not wise, it is not the only problem. A higher level of LDL means a higher risk of developing atherosclerosis. To a small degree, you can lower LDL through your diet. However, the most successful means of changing HDL and LDL levels appears to be regular exercise and maintaining a healthy weight.

A number of tips can help people limit the fats and cholesterol in their diets. It is important to monitor overall fat intake, not just cholesterol. This is because saturated fats increase the liver's production of LDLs. High-fat diets can cause buildups of plaque to begin during the teen years.

Choosing lowfat and fat free foods is one way to limit fat intake. Food scientists have been busy developing hundreds of new products. The scientists are trying to meet the consumer demand for lowfat versions of high-fat favorites.

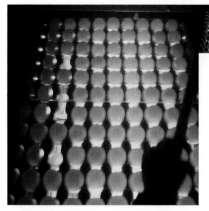

Technology Tidbit
Measuring Fat Content

Sandra E. Kays, a research chemist for the USDA in Athens, Georgia, her graduate student Laura L. Vines, and her colleagues have developed a way to measure fat content in cereal products with near infrared reflectance readings. Traditional methods of measuring fat content require 10 hours and the use of chemical solvents. When perfected, this method will require 10 minutes and a spectrometer with a spectral resolution of 10 nm. The FDA and Food Safety and Inspection Service must certify the technique, and near-IR-reflectance models will have to be developed for each application.

Some vegetable oils have "cholesterol free" on their labels. Such labels are intended to make products appear more healthful. However, all vegetable oils are cholesterol free. Cholesterol is found only in animal sources, such as meats, dairy products, and egg yolks.

Keep in mind that many cholesterol-free foods are high in fat. Remember the body can change fat into cholesterol. Beware of foods whose label reads "pure vegetable oil." Many of these foods contain high levels of coconut and palm oils. These tropical oils are more economical than other vegetable oils, but they are highly saturated. This makes them as likely to raise blood cholesterol levels as animal fats.

> ## Health Tip
> **A high-fiber diet can help trap dietary cholesterol and move it through the body. This keeps the digestive tract from absorbing some of the cholesterol from foods.**

Unsaturated Oils

Heart disease has been found to be low among people in the Mediterranean region. Their diets are not low in fat. However, most of the fat consumed is from olive oil. The very low levels of saturated fatty acids in olive oil are an important factor. The most important factor, however, appears to be the high number of monounsaturated fatty acids.

Polyunsaturated oils lower LDL however, they also lower the beneficial HDL. Monounsaturated oils lower LDL without lowering HDL. This is why some health professionals recommend olive and canola oils as the preferred oils in a healthful diet.

Olive oil has two disadvantages. It has a distinctive flavor that is popular in salads but may not be suitable in all foods. It also has a low smoke point. This makes it a poor choice for deep frying. However, it can be used successfully for stir-frying because of the short cooking time.

Dietary Recommendations

What is the balance when it comes to fat in the diet? The recommended guidelines are 20%-35% of calories should come from fat. Children and adolescents typically require the higher percentage of calories in their diets from fat. Adults whose body mass index (BMI) is in the low to mid 20's should stay under 30% of their calories from fat. People who are overweight should keep their fat intake around 20%. Most fats in the diet should come from sources of polyunsaturated and monounsaturated fatty acids. A fat-free diet does not provide the essential fatty acids needed for new cell growth and other body functions.

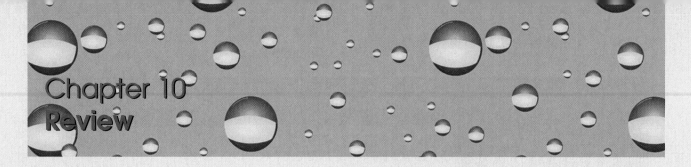

Chapter 10
Review

Summary

Lipids are a category of organic compounds that are insoluble in water and have a greasy feel. The three general types of lipids in food and the human body are glycerides, phospholipids, and sterols. Each of the three types has a unique chemical structure. Most of the lipids in foods and the body are triglycerides.

Lipids are grouped according to molecular structure, physical state, and dietary sources. The number of double bonds present in the carbon chain determine if a fatty acid is saturated, monounsaturated, or polyunsaturated. Lipids can be either solid or liquid at room temperature. The numbers of hydrogen and carbon atoms on a fatty acid chain determine the temperature at which lipids liquefy.

Triglycerides come from seven main groups of dietary sources. Each group has a similar molecular structure and physical characteristics. The physical characteristics of lipids impact the way they perform in food products.

Lipids are an important part of a healthful diet because they perform important functions in the body. Essential fatty acids cannot be produced by the body. Because cholesterol is made from fat in the body, it is important to monitor both fat and cholesterol consumption. Understanding the roles of lipids in the body and reading labels can help you develop healthful eating habits.

Check Your Understanding

1. Describe three ways lipids differ from carbohydrates
2. Name the two parts of a lipid molecule.
3. What are glycerides and how are they categorized?
4. Define three categories of fatty acids based on molecular structure.
5. Explain two ways in which fats and oils differ.
6. List the seven main groups of triglycerides and a dietary source of each.
7. Identify three physical characteristics of lipids that affect the way lipids perform in food products.
8. List five functions of lipids in cooking.
9. List the nutritional functions of lipids.
10. How are cholesterol, HDL, and LDL used by the body?
11. Name two foods that have been found to reduce the risk of heart disease.

Critical Thinking

1. Calculate the maximum recommended number of fat grams a person who consumes 2000 calories per day should eat. Round to the nearest gram.
2. Find examples of foods you enjoy that contain monoglycerides and diglycerides as additives.
3. Would you recommend restaurants to change the oil they use for frying periodically? Why or why not?
4. Create a day's menu that meets the medical guidelines for patients with high cholesterol. These people should consume 17 grams or less of saturated fatty acids per day.
5. Explain the advantages and disadvantages of using fat as a heat medium.

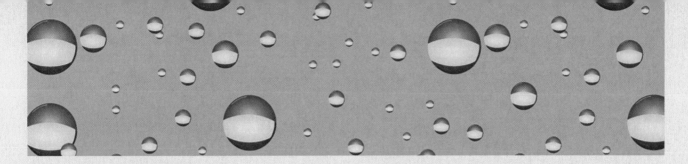

Explore Further

1. **Chemistry.** Construct a fat molecule that contains a saturated, monounsaturated and polyunsaturated fatty acid.

2. **Reading/Communication.** Explore recent studies on trans-fatty acids, their sources, and health risks. Report your findings to the class.

3. **Communication.** Write an editorial for your high school newspaper entitled *Cholesterol: Good or Bad?*

4. **Technology.** Use nutrition analysis software to determine the percentage of calories in your diet that come from fat.

5. **Math.** Calorie density is a simple way to examine the ratio of calories to the weight of food. Some research indicates that people will eat until they have consumed a certain mass or volume of food. Calorie density is calculated by dividing the total weight of the food by the total calories the food provides. Select five of your favorite foods at home that have a nutrition label. Calculate their calorie density. Rank them from lowest to highest calorie density. As a class, compare and discuss your results.

Experiment 10A
Testing Vegetable Oils for Frying

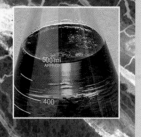

Safety

❖ Wash hands before handling food.

❖ Make sure French fries are not covered with ice.

❖ Do not drop fries into hot oil from more than 2 to 3 inches above the oil.

❖ Following the experiment, clean all work surfaces and utensils with hot, soapy water.

Purpose

The physical characteristics and chemical makeup of vegetable oils affect the flavor of foods cooked in the oils. The smoke point of an oil also determines how well it will hold up when deep-frying foods like French fries. In this experiment, you will test six types of vegetable oil with frozen French fries.

Equipment

1000-mL graduated cylinder

2-quart saucepan or small deep fryer

thermometer

slotted spoon or tongs

Supplies

30 French fries

400 to 500 mL assigned oil

paper towel

Procedure

1. Measure 400 to 500 mL of your assigned oil and pour it into a 2-quart saucepan or deep fryer.

    Variation 1: soybean oil

    Variation 2: corn oil

    Variation 3: canola oil

    Variation 4: peanut oil

    Variation 5: olive oil

    Variation 6: safflower or sunflower oil

2. Place the saucepan on a range and heat the oil on medium-high heat until the temperature reaches 190°C. If using a deep fryer, set the thermostat to 375°F.

3. Make sure the French fries are similar in size. When the oil has reached the appropriate temperature, add the French fries to the oil all at once.

4. Cook the fries for the time suggested on the package. Shoestring fries take less time than crinkle-cut or steak fries. Stir occasionally to keep the fries from sticking together.

5. Remove the French fries with a slotted spoon or tongs to a paper towel. Remove the oil from the heat.

6. Taste one French fry cooked in each type of oil. Record your observations in a data table. Make sure to rinse your mouth with warm water after tasting each French fry.

7. Dispose of the cooled oil according to your teacher's instructions. Clean all equipment and your workstation with hot, soapy water.

Questions

1. Which, if any, of the French fries have a flavor different from typical French fries?

2. Which French fries were the crispest?

3. Which, if any, fries were soggy?

4. Which, if any, of the oils start to smoke during cooking?

5. Which, if any, of the oils change color after heating?

6. Which oil produced the best French fries?

Experiment 10B
Fat in Ground Meat Products

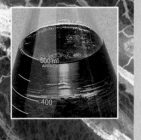

Safety

❖ Wear safety glasses when heating glass beakers.

❖ Use a separate cutting board for each type of raw meat product.

❖ Wash all surfaces contaminated by raw meat products with hot, soapy water.

❖ Wash hands with hot, soapy water for 20 seconds before and after handling raw meat products.

Purpose

In this experiment, you will evaluate the fat content of different types of ground meat products. Fat will be rendered from the meat products by cooking them in water for 15 minutes. The fat will rise to the surface and harden during cooling for easy removal. If time and supplies allow, you can also compare taste and juiciness of burgers panbroiled from each ground product.

Equipment

electronic balance

400-mL beaker

310-mL graduated cylinder

glass rod

beaker tongs

hot pad

skillet

bent-edged spatula

instant-read thermometer

Supplies

454 g (l pound) assigned ground meat product

100 mL water

waxed paper

Procedure

Part I

1. In a data table, record the price per pound of all the ground meat products, as provided by your teacher.

2. Mass 100 g of your assigned ground meat product and place it in the 400-mL beaker.

   Variation 1: ground beef

   Variation 2: ground chuck

   Variation 3: ground round

   Variation 4: extra lean ground beef

   Variation 5: ground turkey

   Variation 6: vegetable burger mix

3. Add 100 mL of water to the beaker.

4. Place the beaker on a hot plate or range and heat until the water comes to a boil. Reduce heat and simmer for 15 minutes, stirring occasionally.

5. Remove the beaker from the heat with beaker tongs. Place it on a hot pad in the refrigerator overnight.

6. While the ground meat product is simmering, divide the remaining 354 g of ground meat product into equal portions, one for each lab group. Shape the product into patties.

7. Place the patties in a skillet over medium heat and cook until the product reaches an internal temperature of 74°C (165°F), approximately 5 minutes per side.

8. Taste a bite of each type of ground meat product. Record your observations of the taste, texture, and appearance of each variation.

Part II

1. The next day, carefully lift the hardened fat off the top of the water and ground meat product.

2. Tare a sheet of waxed paper to use as weighing paper.

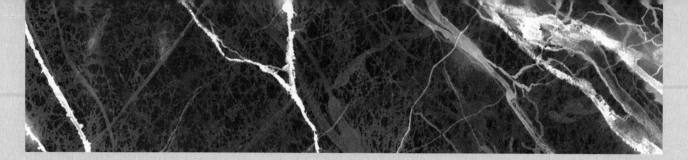

3. Mass the fat. Record the mass in a data table. Also record the masses of fat for the other variations.

4. Calculate the percent fat content for each variation and record it in the data table. Percent equals part (mass of the fat) divided by the whole (mass of the ground meat product before cooking).

Questions

1. What relationship exists between the percent fat content and the price per pound of each variation?

2. Compare and contrast the taste, texture, and appearance of the patties with the highest and lowest percent fat content. Which had the best flavor? Which was the juiciest?

3. When might you render fat when preparing foods at home? When might fat rendering be used in commercial food production?

Experiment 10C
Fats in Dropped Cookies

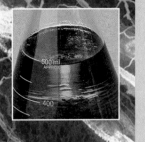

Safety

- ❖ **Wash hands before beginning the lab.**
- ❖ **Clean all work surfaces before beginning.**
- ❖ *Do not taste uncooked dough.* **Eggs used in the dough may be contaminated with bacteria.**
- ❖ **Use hot pads to remove pans from oven. Place pans on cooling racks.**

Purpose

Changing fat types may not only change the nutritive value of cookies but their sensory characteristics as well. In this experiment, you will observe the effects changing the type of fat in the cookie dough has on chocolate chip cookies.

Equipment

2 mixing bowls
electronic balance
metric measuring spoons
metric measuring cups
electric mixer
wooden spoon
teaspoon
cookie sheet
bent-edged spatula
cooling racks
hot pads

Supplies

150 g flour
2 mL (¹/₂ teaspoon) baking soda
2 mL (¹/₂ teaspoon) salt
125 mL (¹/₂ cup) assigned fat

100 g brown sugar
90 g granulated sugar
1 large egg
2 mL (¹/₂ teaspoon) vanilla
185 g chocolate chips

Procedure

1. Combine the flour, baking soda, and salt in a mixing bowl.
2. Cream your assigned fat with the brown sugar and granulated sugar in another mixing bowl. Beat with an electric mixer on medium speed for 1 minute.

   Variation 1: vegetable shortening

   Variation 2: vegetable oil

   Variation 3: butter

   Variation 4: stick margarine

   Variation 5: tub margarine

   Variation 6: lard
3. Add the egg and vanilla and mix on low speed until blended.
4. With a wooden spoon, stir in the flour mixture until all flour has been moistened.
5. Stir in the chocolate chips.
6. Drop the batter by teaspoonfuls onto an ungreased cookie sheet.
7. Bake at 375°F for 12 minutes.
8. Remove cookies to a cooling rack.
9. Sample one cookie from each variation to evaluate the flavor, color, and texture. Record your observations in a data table.
10. Use the nutrition labels to record the calories from fat and grams of total and saturated fat for each fat variation.

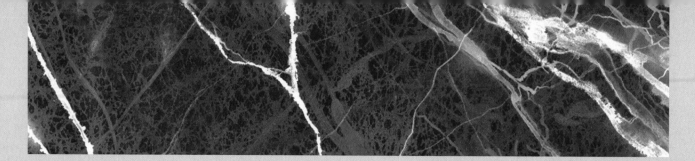

Questions

1. Which cookie variation do you think had the best flavor?

2. Describe any difference in color from one variation to another.

3. Which variation made the crispest cookie? Which variation made the chewiest cookie? Which variation made the moistest cookie?

4. Based on the information gathered in step 10, which variation is the most nutritious? Explain your choice.

5. Which variation of chocolate chip cookies is your favorite? Explain your choice.

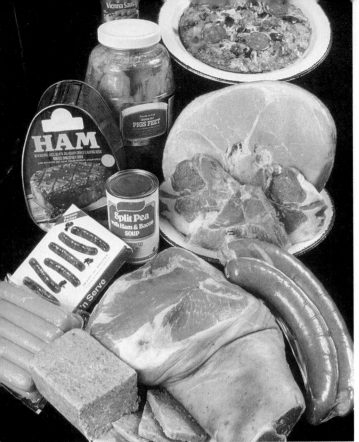

USDA

Meat products such as these are common sources of proteins in the diet.

Proteins: Amino Acids and Peptides

Objectives

After studying this chapter,
you will be able to

identify amino acid classifications based on nutritional use and chemical properties of the side chains.

describe the primary, secondary, and tertiary structures of proteins.

list at least six factors that denature proteins.

state the functions of protein in food production.

apply basic principles of the chemistry of protein to cooking eggs, milk, and meat products.

compare the nutritional functions of proteins with the functions of carbohydrates and fats.

Key Terms

amino acid

amine group

peptide bond

polypeptide

essential amino acid

complete protein

incomplete protein

disulfide cross-link

hydrophobic

casein

whey

myoglobin

oxidation

reduction

denaturation

coagulation

gluten

protein gel

albumin

collagen

aldehydes

Maillard reaction

Proteins are complex molecules that make up as much as 50% of the dry weight of living cells. Proteins have a diverse nature. This makes it possible for them to play many roles in living organisms as well as in food products.

The primary sources of dietary protein are eggs, dairy products, meat, poultry, and fish. Specific cooking principles must be followed when preparing these foods due to their high protein content. These foods provide the body with an important nutrient that serves many functions.

The Structure of Protein

Proteins are largely composed of the same elements as carbohydrates and fats—carbon, hydrogen, and oxygen. In addition, proteins contain nitrogen and usually sulfur. Some proteins also contain iron, copper, phosphorus, or zinc. Like carbohydrates, protein molecules are made up of subunits. These subunits are organic acids—acids that contain carbon atoms. All organic acids, like fatty acids, contain carboxyl groups (–COOH).

Amino Acids

The organic acids in proteins are called *amino acids.* Amino acids have three basic parts to their structure. They have a side chain of carbon and hydrogen atoms, a carboxyl group, and an amine group. The *amine group* is one nitrogen and two hydrogen atoms bonded to a carbon atom. It can be represented by –NH$_2$ or as the following chemical formula.

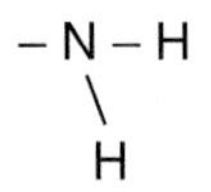

$$- N - H \atop \backslash H$$

There are 20 amino acids in the human body. As many as 150 more amino acids have been isolated in animals, plants, and single-celled organisms. Generally, the amine and carboxyl groups in an amino acid are bonded to the same carbon atom. Chemists use the letter *R* to represent the various carbon side chains. Therefore, most amino acids can be represented by the following formula:

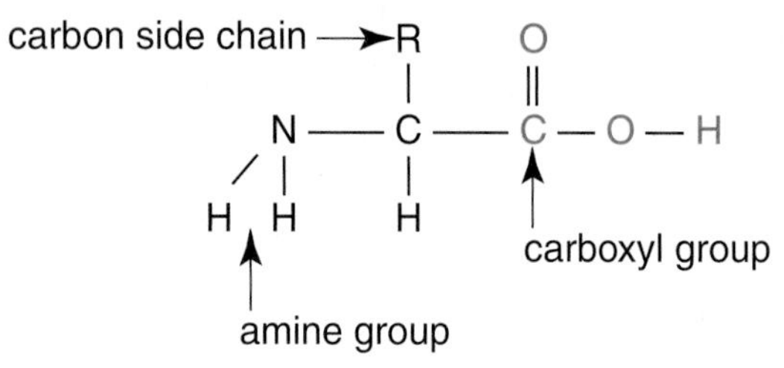

Because of its polar nature, the carboxyl group acts as an acid and the amine group as a base. The amine group from one amino acid will readily combine with the carboxyl group of another. When two amino acids combine, a water molecule is released. The bond formed between the two amino acids is called a *peptide bond.*

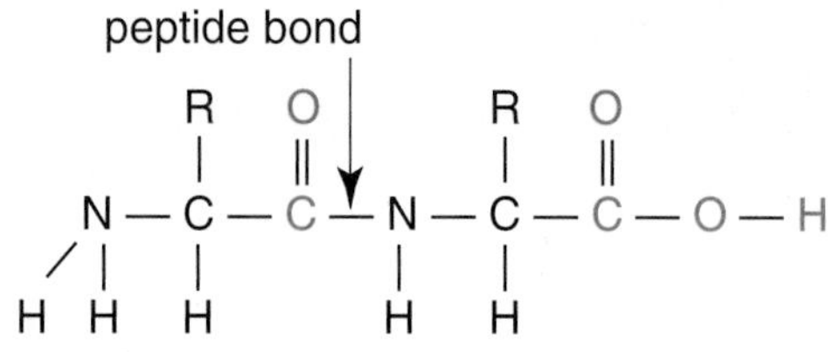

The new *dipeptide* is a protein molecule made from two amino acids. It also has an amine group on one end and a carboxyl group on the other.

Proteins are chains of many amino acids bonded together. The shortest known protein is a chain of 20 amino acids. Most proteins have from 100 to 500 amino acids. Because of the many peptide bonds, proteins are also called polypeptides. *Polypeptides* are molecules with many peptide bonds.

Amino Acids Essential for Good Nutrition

There are two ways to classify amino acids. Amino acids can be classified based on nutritional use. They can also be classified as to the chemical nature of their side chains.

The 20 amino acids used in the human body are necessary for growth and body functions. The body can make many of these amino acids as they are needed. It is not essential for them to be provided by the diet. However, 8 of the amino acids cannot be produced by the body. They are leucine, isoleucine, lysine, methionine, phenylalanine, threonine, tryptophan, and valine. These amino acids are classified as essential amino acids. *Essential amino acids* are amino acids that must be supplied by foods in the diet. The body cannot grow new tissue or maintain health without these 8 amino acids. See 11-1.

A ninth amino acid, histidine, is also essential for infants and toddlers. The body cannot make enough histidine to meet the demands of the rapid growth that occurs in early childhood. Extra histidine from complete proteins is needed daily.

Foods that contain all 8 essential amino acids are called *complete proteins.* Most complete

Essential Amino Acids

Amino Acid	Symbol	Structure of Side Chain
Isoleucine	I	$-CH-CH_2-CH_3$ $\quad\mid$ $\quad CH_3$
Leucine	L	$-CH_2-CH-CH_3$ $\qquad\mid$ $\qquad CH_3$
Lysine	K	$-CH_2-CH_2-CH_2-CH_2-NH_2$
Methionine	M	$-CH_2-CH_2-S-CH_3$
Phenylalanine	F	$-CH_2-\bigcirc$
Threonine	T	$-CH-OH$ $\quad\mid$ $\quad CH_3$
Tryptophan	W	$-CH-$ (indole ring with N-H)
Valine	V	$-CH-CH_3$ $\quad\mid$ $\quad CH_3$

11-1 Your diet must provide the essential amino acids to support growth and maintenance of body tissues. Scientists use symbols for the amino acids to diagram protein molecules.

proteins come from animal sources and include eggs, milk, fish, poultry, and meats. One plant source of protein—soybeans—is also known for being quite high in quality. Before soybeans can support growth, they must be heat processed for several hours. This destroys toxic compounds that prevent use of the essential amino acid trypsin. Soybeans are low in methionine, and most soy products have methionine added to improve the quality of the amino acids.

Other plant sources of protein come from grains and vegetables. These proteins tend to be lower in quality and are called incomplete proteins. *Incomplete proteins* are short of one or more of the essential amino acids needed for human growth. The amino acids that are short are called *limiting amino acids*. For instance, lysine is often the limiting amino acid in cereal grains. Tryptophan and threonine are also limiting amino acids in some cases.

Vegetarians must choose plant foods carefully to receive all 8 essential amino acids necessary for good health. Vegetarians can combine some sources of incomplete protein to form a complete source. Combining legumes with grains, nuts, or seeds will generally create a complete source of protein. See 11-2. Some combinations that contain adequate amounts of all 8 essential amino acids are

❖ whole wheat bread and peanut butter

❖ rice and red beans

❖ refried beans and corn tortillas

❖ hummus—a dip made with chickpeas and sesame seeds

Classification of Amino Acids by Side Chains

The second method for classifying amino acids is based on the chemical properties of the side chains. The way the protein molecule

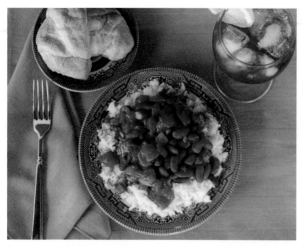

11-2 Although this meal does not include meat, the combination of red beans and rice provides all the essential amino acids.

is shaped and how it functions depend on the polarity of the side chains. Side chains can be nonpolar, uncharged polar, positively charged, or negatively charged.

Alanine, tryptophan, and leucine are examples of amino acids with nonpolar side chains. Nonpolar side chains are less soluble in water. However, because they are nonpolar, they are attracted to other nonpolar compounds, such as lipids and cholesterol. For instance, you read in Chapter 10 about lipoproteins, which are clusters of lipid and protein molecules. Some lipoproteins transport cholesterol in the blood. They are able to do this because the protein molecules in the lipoprotein clusters have nonpolar side chains. These side chains are positioned toward the outsides of the molecules, allowing them to attract cholesterol molecules.

A second group of amino acids has neutral polar side chains that will form hydrogen bonds. These side chains are attracted to other polar molecules, such as water. The hydroxyl group causes such a polar nature on serine, threonine, and tyrosine. The hydrogen bonding can also form between sections of the protein molecule. These hydrogen bonds are partially responsible for the shape a molecule will take. They are also partially responsible for some of the protein's physical properties and how proteins function in food preparation.

A third group of amino acids has side chains that have a positive or negative charge.

Positively charged amino acids, such as lysine and arginine, have a second amine group on the molecule. Negatively charged amino acids are aspartic and glutamic acid. The presence of positively and negatively charged side chains enables some proteins to act as buffers.

Protein Structures

The number of possible protein structures is endless. However, all protein molecules are complex. This is due to the number of amino acids and the order in which they combine. It is also due to the interaction between the side chains.

Primary Structure

The *primary structure* of a protein molecule is the order the amino acids occur in the chain. Food scientists have "maps" of food proteins, such as casein from milk. These maps identify the order of the amino acids. The primary structure is a result of the chain of peptide bonds formed in making the protein molecule.

Secondary Structure

The *secondary structure* of a protein molecule refers to the shape of sections of the amino acid chain. The secondary structure is due to hydrogen bonding between amino acids. These bonds cause bending of the molecule. The peptide bonds change direction based on the types of amino acids that are joined. Secondary structures of protein occur in three patterns: helix, random coil, and pleated sheet.

A *helix* structure is a repeating coil. Think of the shape of a Slinky or a telephone cord. That is a helix shape. The amino acid side chains are on the outside of the helix. As the amino acids twist around a central axis, hydrogen bonds form between amino acids on the chain. These hydrogen bonds increase the stability of the molecule.

A *random coil* shape forms when some of the side chains prevent the setting up of a helix. If you have ever played with a Slinky, you have probably had it eventually tangle. One of the sections would become twisted backwards. This is similar to what happens with random coils. It is like grasping and balling up a string. The string becomes twisted and turned and folded in on itself with no set pattern.

The third shape common in protein molecules is the *pleated sheet*. This shape is much like the paper fans you may have made as a child. Side chains can be located both above and below the pleated sheet. This enables side chains of one molecule to bond to side chains in protein molecules above and below.

Tertiary Structure

The *tertiary structure* of a protein molecule refers to the three-dimensional structure of an entire amino acid chain. Think of the primary structure as the individual fibers in a piece of yarn. The secondary structure would be like the fibers twisted together into a ply of yarn. The tertiary structure is like a balled up strand of yarn. The main tertiary structures are globular (balled up) and fibrous (strands). See 11-3.

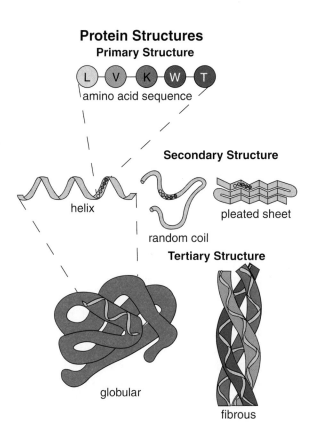

Protein Structures
Primary Structure

amino acid sequence

Secondary Structure

helix   random coil   pleated sheet

Tertiary Structure

globular   fibrous

11-3 Peptide bonds link amino acids into a chain, forming the primary structure of a protein molecule. Hydrogen bonds between the C=O and N–H groups of a peptide chain cause the chain to fold into a secondary structure. Hydrogen bonding among sections of the side chains result in the formation of the tertiary structure.

Globular proteins do not tend to form links that will create a protein network. Hemoglobin, which carries oxygen in the blood, and lipoproteins, which carry cholesterol in the bloodstream, are globular proteins. Casein in milk and albumin in egg white are other examples of globular proteins.

Fibrous proteins are usually made from helix-shaped strands. They are strong and are part of connective tissues. Collagen, elastin, keratin, and myosin are examples of fibrous protein. These proteins are found in muscle fibers, ligaments, tendons, fingernails, and hair. Fibrous proteins tend to link to form a network of tissue.

Molecular Interactions of Proteins

As you have read, proteins have a complex nature, large size, and various side chains. These factors allow many interactions within protein molecules and with other compounds. Understanding these interactions will help you understand the many ways proteins can function in food preparation.

A hydrogen bond can occur between the hydrogen atom of one side chain and the hydroxyl group of another. A hydrogen bond can also occur between the oxygen atom in one peptide bond and the hydrogen atom of another peptide bond. The formation of hydrogen bonds is basic to the stability of the secondary and tertiary structures of protein molecules. Polar groups on the outside of protein molecules also allow protein molecules to hydrogen bond with water. This is why some proteins are water soluble. Albumin, the protein found in egg white, readily dissolves in water. Water that is hydrogen bonded to protein is an example of bound water.

hydrogen bond between two peptide bonds

A second interaction that occurs between protein molecules is disulfide cross-links. *Disulfide cross-links* are covalent bonds that form between two protein molecules at side chains that contain sulfur. The more disulfide cross-links that are formed, the more stable the protein will become.

A third molecular interaction of proteins is between nonpolar side chains. These interactions are called *hydrophobic,* or water repelling. These interactions occur between side chains with carbon rings.

Remember, nonpolar side chains are not water soluble. They do not form covalent bonds. However, nonpolar side chains can react with lipids. Hydrophobic side chains enable proteins to form lipoproteins, which are an important part of cell walls. Proteins that are water soluble tend to have the hydrophobic side chains facing into the center of the protein molecule.

An example of a hydrophobic protein is *casein* found in milk. This protein is vital to the forming of curds in cheese making. When a mixture of rennin, salts, and acids are added to milk, the globular casein untangles. The nonpolar side chains of the casein bind with milkfat, calcium, and one another to form curds. See 11-4.

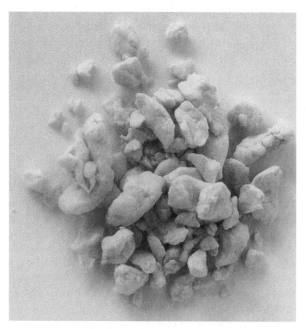

11-4 These cheese curds were formed when globular casein molecules untangled, allowing nonpolar side chains to bind with milkfat and one another.

A by-product of cheese production is whey. *Whey* looks like a watery milk and is mainly composed of a group of water-soluble proteins, lactose, and minerals. It is used as an additive in many commercially processed foods. The water-soluble proteins in milk are called whey proteins. They form hydrogen bonds with water. Whey protein molecules do not change their shape in reaction to rennin, salts, and acids the way casein molecules do.

Color Changes of Protein Pigments

Understanding color changes in protein pigments helps food scientists control color changes in meat during storage and processing. This is important because consumers believe that bright red color means meat is fresh. *Myoglobin* is the iron-containing protein pigment in muscle tissue that provides the color. Myoglobin stores or holds onto oxygen in live animal tissue. When an oxygen molecule is attached, myoglobin is a bright cherry-red color. When oxygen is not present, the tissue becomes purplish in color. After prolonged exposure to oxygen, the myoglobin changes to metmyoglobin which has a brown color. The process of adding oxygen is a reversible chemical reaction. This reversible process of adding and removing oxygen to a compound is called *oxidation* and *reduction.* Oxidation adds oxygen and reduction removes it. Hemoglobin is the other protein that uses the oxidation/reduction process to distribute oxygen in the body. Hemoglobin is found in the blood and myoglobin is found in muscle tissue.

Once meat is bright red, it can be quickly wrapped in packaging that limits exposure to more oxygen. Although the bright red color does not guarantee freshness as compared to a purplish or brown color, consumers will choose the bright red meat over other colors. Consumers commonly mistake red juice from meat as blood. Red juice that pools around meat cuts is water with dissolved myoglobin, not blood that contains hemoglobin.

Nitrites are added during curing processes to preserve meats. They also maintain a pink or red color and are very stable. Nitrite combines with myoglobin to form nitric oxide myoglobin. When cooked, this is converted to nitrosohemochrome causing the pink or red of cooked ham and bacon. When fresh or cured meats develop green or yellow discolorations, it is a sign of bacterial growth.

Denaturation of Proteins

Protein is unique in that its shape can be changed without changing the primary structure of the molecule. The secondary and tertiary structures of protein are fragile. They can be changed by physical or chemical means. Any change of the shape of a protein molecule without breaking peptide bonds is called *denaturation.* Denaturation usually results in a loosening or unfolding of the protein molecule.

Denaturation is sometimes reversible. If the denaturation is slight, the protein will tend to return to its original shape. Protein will also tend to return to its original shape if the denaturation involves only hydrogen bond interactions. You can see an example of this by beating egg whites until frothy or foamy. If you allow the egg whites to sit, they will return to their liquid state.

Denaturation of proteins is usually not reversible. This is the case when denatured proteins interact with other proteins while unfolded. Breaking disulfide cross-links is also irreversible denaturation.

Another type of permanent denaturation is coagulation. *Coagulation* results when a liquid or semiliquid protein forms solid or semisoft clots. One example of coagulation is milk curdling to form cheese. Cooked eggs are another example of coagulation due to permanent changes in disulfide links. Eggs are liquid before they are heated. After heating causes eggs to begin coagulating, they will not return to their liquid state. See 11-5. Gelatin, on the other hand, solidifies as it chills due to the formation of hydrogen bonds. When the gelatin is heated, the proteins return to a liquid state.

Denaturation will change many of the physical characteristics of a protein. If hydrophobic side chains are exposed through denaturation, a protein's water solubility can be reduced. This can lead to proteins forming precipitates (solids) that can be separated from a mixture.

Denaturation can alter the ability of a protein to bind water. Cooking meat causes the proteins to shrink, releasing water-based fluids and reducing the ability to hold water. Some cooking is needed to kill bacteria and develop flavors. However, too much cooking causes too much coagulation. This results in protein foods that are dry, tough, and rubbery.

Denaturing protein can also interfere with the biological reactions of enzymes. You will read more about this in Chapter 12.

Methods of Denaturing Protein

Proteins can be denatured by a number of physical and chemical methods. Physical factors that denature proteins are hot and cold temperatures, mechanical actions, sound waves (including ultrasound), pressure, and irradiation. Chemical factors that denature proteins are pH changes (acid or alkali) and mineral salts. Because each protein is unique, the rate of the denaturing will vary greatly. The amount of denaturing that occurs also varies.

Temperature Changes

Heat is the most common method of denaturing proteins in food production. The amount of denaturation will depend on the temperature. Most chemical reactions double their rate with every 10°C increase in temperature. The rate of increase for protein denaturation is 600

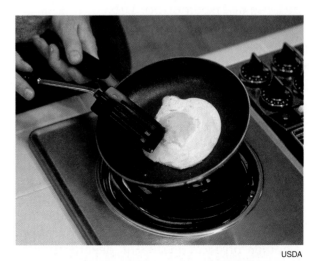

11-5 When eggs are denatured by heating, they will permanently coagulate into a solid state.

times for every 10°C increase in temperature. This is because it does not take very much energy to break the hydrogen bonds.

Denaturation will occur at a faster rate when the protein is wet, as in food mixtures. This is because of interactions between the water molecules and the broken hydrogen bond sites.

Cold temperatures can also alter protein structures. This most often happens when foods are frozen. Milk that is frozen and then thawed will have a curdled look due to the denaturation of the milk proteins. Soy proteins and eggs are also likely to denature in freezing temperatures.

Mechanical Actions

Mechanical actions such as beating, rolling, and kneading can disrupt protein structures. Vigorous or prolonged actions will cause proteins to lock into new positions with other molecules. When bread dough is kneaded, proteins react with water and each other. They realign to form a viscoelastic (thick and stretchy) structure.

The network of elastic protein strands that give bread dough its structure is called *gluten.* The protein in wheat flour is responsible for this elasticity. Gluten changes its shape and strengthens during the kneading process. Gluten enables yeast breads to rise without tearing the dough. Gluten also enables breads to solidify during baking to form the main structure of the bread. This is why bread flours need a higher protein content than all-purpose or cake flour. See 11-6.

In some food products, care must be taken to avoid denaturing the protein too much. When beaten, egg whites will trap air and become light and fluffy. If overbeaten, overcoagulation occurs and unattractive clumps form.

Other Physical Methods of Denaturation

Several other physical methods can be used to denature protein. One of these methods involves the use of sound waves. It takes prolonged exposure to sound waves at high volumes to cause permanent denaturation. Another physical means of denaturation is irradiation. This will be discussed in detail in Chapter 21.

Chemical Methods of Denaturation

Some of the methods used to denature proteins involve chemical factors. One such method is a change in pH. Exposure to acids or alkalis can cause proteins to unfold. The pH needed to denature proteins will vary. Each type of protein has a pH range in which it is stable.

It is important for food scientists to know what pH range results in denaturation for each protein. The scientists can then put this information to use in developing food products. For example, soy proteins will dissolve into a sticky liquid in alkali. By forcing this liquid through tiny holes into an acid bath, the protein will coagulate into stringy fibers. These fibers resemble the texture of meat. The denatured soy protein is then used to make simulated meat products.

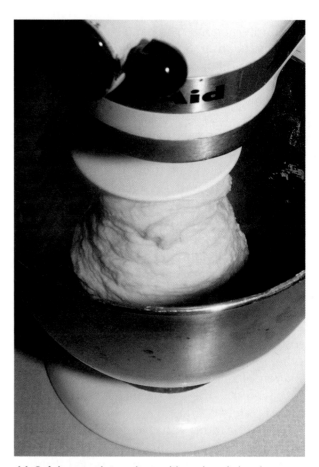

11-6 A heavy-duty mixer with a dough hook can knead bread dough to develop the gluten needed to give bread its structure.

Add vinegar or lemon juice to milk and note the coagulation and curdling caused by the low pH. Many dairy products, such as sour cream, buttermilk, and yogurt, are the result of acids denaturing the milk proteins.

Poached eggs are best when cooked in water with a little vinegar added. The vinegar (acetic acid) coagulates the egg protein, which helps keep the egg compact. Try poaching eggs with and without vinegar and note the shape of the cooked eggs.

Another chemical method of denaturing proteins is exposing proteins to mineral salts or metals. Sodium and potassium salts will react to some extent with proteins, causing denaturation to occur. This is why adding salt early in the cooking process of high-protein legumes can cause some toughening of the product. Metals such as copper, iron, magnesium, and calcium will readily react with proteins. The presence of calcium is important in the curdling process in cheese production.

Functions of Protein in Food

A full understanding of all the interactions of protein in food production is not possible. The combination of so many complex proteins in equally complex food mixtures makes identifying all the interactions and reactions difficult. However, it is possible to study the proteins involved in some simpler food mixtures. It is also possible to examine types of functions proteins perform in foods. Some of these involve proteins being used as gelling agents, texturizers, emulsifiers, and foaming agents. Protein is also important in dough formation in baked products.

To determine how effectively proteins will work in a given food product, food scientists analyze some important physical characteristics. Proteins have varying degrees of water absorption, solubility, and viscosity (ability to flow when poured). Each protein's viscosity and reaction to water can be altered through denaturation.

Form Gels

In Chapter 9, you studied the ability of starches to form gels. You learned that gels can be produced by cooking amylose in liquid to the gelatinization point to make sauces. Gels can also be made by combining pectin, sugar, and acid as in jellies. Proteins have the ability to form gels, too. This is what happens when the protein gelatin is heated in water and then cooled. It is also what happens when a mixture of eggs, milk, and sugar is heated to make custard.

A *protein gel* is a mixture of mostly fluids locked in a tangled three-dimensional mesh. This mesh is made of denatured and coagulated proteins. Protein gels contain long, thin, chainlike polymers of amino acids. The molecules are cross-linked randomly to produce gels that behave like a rigid solid. Protein gels have two parts: the three dimensional molecular structure and the liquid that is attracted to the proteins. The liquid keeps the proteins from collapsing, and the proteins keep the liquid from flowing away.

Unlike starch gels, gelatin has a narrow melting and solidifying temperature range. Starches begin to gelatinize as they are cooked and form gels as they cool. Some protein gels are very liquid when hot and thicken when they cool. The coagulation process is gradual and requires lower temperatures than starch gels. Like most starch gels, gelatin is softened by acids and may develop syneresis (leakage) if cooked or stored too long.

To make a protein gel, plain gelatin is first dissolved in cold water. If hot water is added first, it will cause the gelatin to clump, making it difficult to dissolve. The cold water causes the gelatin molecules to swell. Boiling water is then added to disperse the gelatin. Dispersion occurs at 35°C (95°F). The gel forms when the mixture is cooled to between 10°C (50°F) and 16°C (61°F). See 11-7.

Gelatin dessert mixes are prepared by first adding boiling water to dissolve the gelatin. Boiling water does not cause clumping because the gelatin particles in dessert mixes are separated by sugar and flavoring.

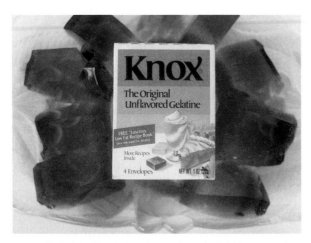

11-7 Gelatin dessert mixes are available in a rainbow of colors. Unflavored gelatin can be used to create your own flavor combinations.

Stiffness of protein gels increases with standing at cool temperatures. Gelatin will set quickly when ice cubes are added to lower the temperature of the dispersed mixture. However, a gelatin that is set quickly will melt more quickly at room temperature than a gel that sets slowly.

Once gelatin is rehydrated, it must be kept refrigerated. Gelatin will lose its rigid structure and become runny at room temperature. It will also be susceptible to bacterial growth.

Protein gels are strengthened by several factors. The more gelatin a mixture contains, the firmer the gel will be. However, too much gelatin causes the product to become gummy. Mineral salts will add strength to the gel by helping to establish the cross-linkages in the structure. Because of this, hard water or milk will produce a firmer gel than distilled or softened water.

Gels are weakened by acid, sugar, and fruit or vegetable pieces in the mixture. Gelatin can have up to 30 mL (2 tablespoons) of lemon juice added per 250 mL (1 cup) of liquid. This amount of acid will not keep a gel from forming. Sugar slows the gelling process as well as preventing some cross-linkages from forming. This results in a weaker structure. Most gelatin mixes carefully balance the gelatin and sugar. Pieces of fruits or vegetables break the flow of the three-dimensional

gel structure. This mechanically interferes with the gelling process. If too much fruit is added, then gelatin concentrations must be increased to compensate.

You probably are familiar with gelatin as a jiggly, cool, easy-to-prepare dessert or salad. However, gelatin is also used as an additive in food products for the following reasons:

❖ to provide structure and support
❖ to stabilize the foam in whipped products
❖ to thicken puddings and pies
❖ to control crystal growth in frozen foods

A protein gel can also be formed from muscle tissue. Salt is added to destabilize some of the proteins. The meat or meat pieces are then massaged or tumbled. The salt pulls some proteins into solution. The agitation ruptures some cells, increasing the protein available for gelatinization to occur. This process is used on some hams, chicken hot dogs, bologna-type sausages, and a Japanese fish sausage.

Texturize

The texture or feel of protein can be changed from globular to fibrous by denaturation. Most globular proteins can be spun into fibers if there are few nonprotein compounds present. You have briefly read about this with reference to soy proteins being texturized for use as simulated meat products.

Another method of texturizing soy protein for use as meat substitutes involves heat-coagulation under pressure. High-protein soy flours are mixed with water, heated under pressure, and then *extruded*. Extrusion involves pushing the mixture through openings that shape the product. Flavoring and coloring are added to make the product more closely resemble meat. These texturized proteins can be mixed with meat to extend or stretch its volume. Hamburgers made with these texturized-protein extenders are lower in cost and fat content.

Protein texturization is also used in developing process cheeses. Different natural cheeses are mixed and then melted together by heating to about 71°C (160°F). The mixing and heating denature the proteins in cheese.

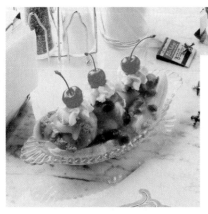

Item of Interest
The "Bare Bone" Facts About Gelatin

The protein, *gelatin*, is made from collagen extracted from the bones and hides of animals. *Collagen* is a protein in connective tissue. It is extracted from the raw material, mixed with water, and processed to form gelatin. The gelatin is then purified, refined, and dried.

Pure gelatin is nearly flavorless and odorless. It may be packaged and sold as unflavored gelatin. It can also be combined with artificial flavors, colors, and sugar and sold as flavored gelatin.

Gelatin is used to thicken chilled pies, gelatin desserts, and ice cream. Only 15 mL (1 tablespoon) of gelatin is needed to thicken 250 mL (1 cup) of liquid.

Gelatin is a rather insignificant source of nutrients. It provides only low-quality protein because it lacks the essential amino acid tryptophan. Most of the nutritional value of gelatin salads and desserts comes from added ingredients, such as fruits and vegetables.

When cooled, the process cheese has a smoother texture than the natural cheeses used in its production.

Emulsify

An *emulsion* is a stable mixture of a fat and a water-based liquid. Most stable emulsions have three parts. One part is a nonpolar substance, like fat. A second part is a polar liquid, like water. The third part of an emulsion is an emulsifier, which can be a denatured protein. An *emulsifier* is a molecule that has a polar end and a nonpolar end, 11-8. Emulsions usually require heat or mechanical action, such as beating, to denature the protein and then form the emulsion. Temporary emulsions of a fat and polar liquid usually are created by beating or shaking without an emulsifier present.

Egg yolk is an excellent protein emulsifier. It is often used in home recipes for ice cream and mayonnaise to keep the mixtures stable.

Other food product emulsions in which proteins act to keep the fats and liquids dispersed include milk, cream, butter, and cheese. The casein in milk, with its loose random coil structure, serves as a protein emulsifier in these foods. Homogenized milk is a stable emulsion for two reasons. Homogenization forces milk through screens under high pressure. This ruptures the membranes around the fat globules, reducing the size of the globules in the milk. The pressure used in the homogenization process also changes the structure of the casein molecules. This structure change makes the casein better able to bond to the fat.

Protein's ability to form emulsions can sometimes be a problem. For instance, soy, sunflower, and canola oil production involve separating protein and oil emulsions with minimal damage to either by-product. However, grain proteins can make it difficult to fully extract the oils from the grain kernels.

Form Foams

In a *foam*, gas is suspended in a liquid or semisolid. The gas is usually air or carbon dioxide surrounded by a film or bubble containing protein. In food production, foams are made in three main ways: bubbling gas through a mixture, whipping or beating, and depressurization.

Emulsifier

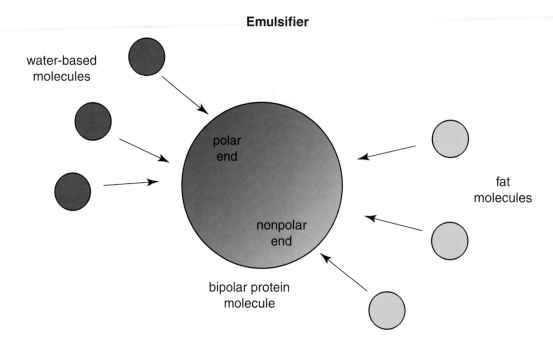

11-8 Protein emulsifiers are bipolar molecules. They stabilize mixtures by attracting water-based molecules to the polar end and fat molecules to the nonpolar end.

As a child, you probably practiced the first method of forming foams. You would have done this by inserting a straw into a glass of cold milk and blowing. The bubbles that resulted were a foam formed by bubbling gas through a mixture. The elasticity of the protein molecules in milk makes this foaming action possible. This method can create very large foam volumes.

The second and most common method of forming foams is whipping or beating the protein mixture. Whipping gives a more uniform dispersion of gas than blowing air through a mixture. Small uniform bubbles tend to be more stable. Stiffly beaten egg whites are an excellent example of this method of making a foam.

The third method of forming foams uses a sudden release in pressure, as in aerosol cans. The release in pressure causes air spaces to rapidly expand. Dissolved air and liquid are released as a foam. Whipped cream in cans is the main example of this method. Another example of this method can be seen by opening a warm 2-liter bottle of root beer.

Food foams include meringue, foam cakes, marshmallows, whipped cream, whipped toppings, ice cream, soufflés, and bread, 11-9. All these products have a light texture due to gas being trapped within their structures. One protein that is a good foaming agent is *albumin,* which is found in egg whites and milk. Some caseins, whey, gelatin, glutenin, and soy protein are also good foaming agents. You will read about factors that affect the stability of food foams in Chapter 22.

Develop Gluten

Another main function of protein in food products is the development of gluten in baked goods. Gluten is a strongly cohesive and elastic protein. It is formed when wheat flour is combined with moisture and stirred or kneaded. The strength of gluten is partially a result of disulfide cross-links that form during mixing. As carbon dioxide is released in the dough, it forms tiny air pockets or bubbles. This causes the gluten structure to stretch. When baked, the gluten coagulates, forming the light airy texture of bread and other baked products.

The ability to form cohesive and elastic gluten is not present in other grains, such as rye and corn. This is why breads made with rye flour or cornmeal have a denser, heavier texture. Recipes for such breads usually

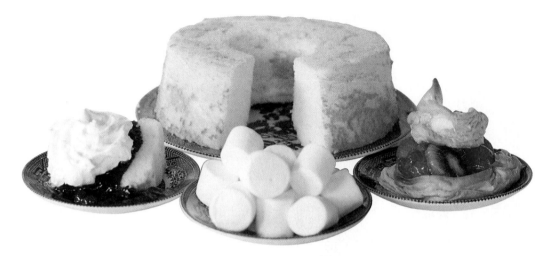

11-9 Whipped topping, angel food cake, marshmallows, and fruit-filled meringue are examples of protein foams.

require at least as much wheat flour as flour or meal from other grains.

The addition of other proteins to bread doughs can increase the nutritional value. However, other proteins can also interfere with the development of the gluten network. Cold milk contains globular proteins that will interfere with gluten formation. Scalded milk has been denatured and does not interfere with the gluten structure. This is why most yeast bread recipes with milk call for scalded milk.

Cooking High-Protein Foods

High-protein foods include eggs, milk products, meat, poultry, and fish. All these foods are damaged by cooking temperatures that are too high or cooking periods that are too long. This is because of the rapid denaturation of protein when heated. The protein molecules tend to shrink and lose water. Too much heat will result in a dry, rubbery, tough product.

Principles of Storing and Cooking Eggs

Two factors cause the deterioration of eggs in storage. The first is the loss of carbon dioxide through the eggshell. As carbon dioxide moves through the shell, the pH of the egg changes from neutral to basic. This causes the proteins to break apart.

The second factor that causes the deterioration of eggs in storage is part of the water moving into the egg yolk. This stretches and weakens the membrane surrounding the yolk. This is why it is harder to separate older eggs. It is also harder to turn a fried egg without breaking the yolk if the egg is not fresh.

Many egg producers apply a special spray to eggs to reduce the loss of carbon dioxide and moisture through the shell. This spray helps eggs maintain quality for a prolonged shelf life. See 11-10.

Lengthy storage is not the only factor that will affect the outcome of cooked eggs. Egg whites are composed of protein, water, riboflavin, niacin, magnesium, and potassium. Albumin, the protein in egg white, is easily denatured by heat. If eggs are heated at high temperatures or for long periods, the coagulation will be more extensive. This will result in a firm to tough egg white. Low temperatures and short cooking times will allow the egg white to coagulate while remaining soft and tender.

Principles of Cooking Milk

Milk-based products include white sauces, cheese sauces, puddings, and cream soups. Two common problems can occur when preparing such products. The first problem is curdling. *Curdling* occurs when acid causes

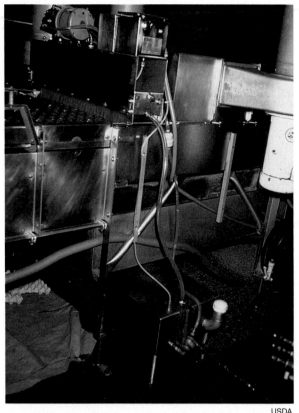

USDA

11-10 This equipment is used to dry and then oil eggs. The oil slows the loss of carbon dioxide and preserves the quality of protein in the egg white.

the globular casein protein molecules in milk to unfold and stick together. Curdling can be avoided by combining the acid with starch before the milk is added. Cream of tomato soup is an example.

The second common problem that can occur when cooking with milk is scorching. *Scorching* occurs when the protein clumps formed by the heat sink and burn to the pan. Whey proteins will begin to coagulate at 66°C (150°F). Constant stirring helps prevent scorching by keeping the whey proteins from sinking. Scorching can also be prevented by cooking milk-based products in a double boiler. A double boiler suspends the product over boiling water and steam. This keeps the temperature of the product lower than if it were in a pan in direct contact with the heat source. The lower temperature will help prevent the milk proteins from sticking and burning to the pan.

Casein will not coagulate unless concentrations are high or certain salts or acids are present. Pretreatment is necessary to prevent coagulation of casein in evaporated milk. Preheating alters the calcium salts that trigger coagulation. Stabilizers are then added just before concentration.

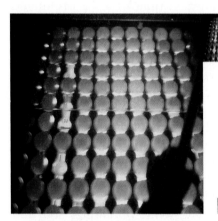

Technology Tidbit
"Eggs"actly Stable

Hens lay fewer eggs during the winter months than they do during other times of the year. To help stabilize the egg supply throughout the year, the food industry uses cold storage technology to slow egg deterioration.

Before eggs are placed in cold storage, they are dipped in a thin coating of mineral oil. This is done within 12 hours of laying. The coating reduces the loss of moisture and carbon dioxide through the porous eggshell. This helps stabilize the pH of the egg and maintain freshness.

The coated eggs are placed in a controlled atmosphere of carbon dioxide or ozone. This atmosphere must have 85% to 90% humidity and be at -1.5°C to 0°C (29°F to 32°F). This atmosphere will maintain egg freshness for up to 6 months.

Commercial cold storage costs money. This accounts for the rise in egg prices seen in some areas each year between Christmas and Easter.

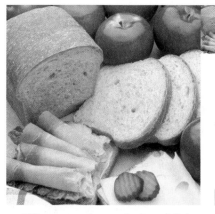

Food Feature
Is My Chicken Done?

When you see a dark reddish stain near a chicken bone, you may wonder if the chicken is thoroughly cooked. The only reliable way to test the doneness of cooked poultry is with a meat thermometer. Insert the probe of the thermometer into the thickest part of the thigh of a whole bird. Insert the probe into the thickest part of individual poultry pieces. Make sure the probe does not touch bone. Whole birds and thighs should reach an internal temperature of 80°C (180°F). Breast pieces should reach an internal temperature of 75°C (170°F).

When eating out, you are not likely to have the opportunity to check cooked poultry with a meat thermometer. If you are in doubt about the doneness of poultry in such a situation, check the color of the meat juices. Press the poultry gently. If the juices from the meat are clear, the poultry is done. A light pink color on the outside portions of poultry is usually from a chemical reaction caused by smoking the meat. However, if the inner meat and meat juices have a pink tinge, the poultry may be undercooked. You can request further cooking.

Even poultry that is thoroughly cooked according to a meat thermometer may have a dark reddish stain near a bone. This is caused by hemoglobin (blood protein) seeping out of the bone marrow during cooking. A dark reddish stain is more likely to happen in poultry that has been frozen. Such stains may also occur in poultry from very young birds. However, the stain is not related to doneness.

Cooking Tip
Baked custard is a sweetened milk and egg mixture that will curdle if overheated. You can use a technique that applies a principle similar to a double boiler to keep baked custard smooth. In the oven, place the pan filled with custard into another pan, which is partially filled with water. Water maintains a temperature of 100°C during heating. Therefore, it will protect the custard from the hotter temperatures of the oven.

Principles of Cooking Meat

Most meats contain three categories of proteins: muscle fibers, connective tissue, and myoglobin (deep red pigment). One of the goals in cooking meat is to soften the connective tissue to make the meat more tender. *Collagen* is a protein in connective tissue. It begins to soften and break down into gelatin when cooked in moist heat. Collagen in connective tissue of young animals (veal, lamb, and pork) does not begin to soften until it reaches 50°C (122°F). Collagen of older animals (beef and mutton) does not begin to soften until it reaches 60°C (140°F). Unfortunately, as the internal temperature of meat reaches 50°C (122°F) during cooking, muscle fibers will start to toughen. This means the heat needed to soften connective tissue toughens muscle fibers.

Roasts with much connective tissue need to be well done to allow enough time to soften connective tissue. Cooking a roast in 60°C (140°F) liquid would require five to six hours of cooking to soften connective tissue. This time and temperature combination makes the meat vulnerable to bacterial contamination. Boiling the roast for one hour will soften connective tissue without risk of bacterial contamination. However, muscle fibers will toughen considerably. The best balance seems to be simmering the roast in 86°C to 93°C

(180°F to 200°F) liquid for at least two to three hours. This time and temperature combination provides enough heat to soften connective tissue without excessive toughening of the muscle fiber. (Cuts of meat larger than 3 to 4 kg [7 to 9 pounds] will take longer.) Foodborne illness is not a risk if the meat is kept hot (above 60°C [140°F]) until it is served.

Meat with little connective tissue can be prepared with dry heat and shorter cooking times. Cooking time with dry heat methods is determined by the internal temperature of the meat. See 11-11.

The Maillard Reaction

When amino acids in grains and meats are heated at high temperatures, a three-phase chemical reaction occurs that causes a change in color and flavor. One step in this process is the oxidation or dehydrogenation of alcohols to compounds known as aldehydes. An *aldehyde* is an alcohol that has been dehydrogenated.

$$CH_3CH_2OH \xrightarrow{[O]} CH_3CH\overset{O}{\underset{\parallel}{}}$$

The reaction between proteins and carbohydrates that causes food to brown when cooked is called the *Maillard reaction.* The chemist Louis Maillard first identified this reaction.

The Nutritional Contributions of Proteins

Protein is one of the energy nutrients. However, this is not its most important function. Protein is needed for growth and repair of body tissue. Protein is also needed for fighting disease, fluid and electrolyte balance, pH balance, and regulating body functions. See 11-12.

Support Growth and Repair

The most important function of protein in the body is to provide nitrogen and amino acids for growth and repair. Every cell in the body contains protein. As many as 10,000 proteins have been identified in a single human

Recommended Temperatures for Cooking Meat and Poultry

Product	Internal Temperature
Beef and Lamb	
Ground beef or lamb	71°C (160°F)
Medium rare	63°C (145°F)
Medium	71°C (160°F)
Well done	77°C (170°F)
Pork	
Fresh, medium	71°C (160°F)
Fresh, well done	77°C (170°F)
Ground pork	71°C (160°F)
Ham, fresh	71°C (160°F)
Ham, precooked	60°C (140°F)
Poultry	
Chicken	82°C (180°F)
Ground poultry	74°C (165°F)
Turkey	82°C (180°F)

11-11 Checking internal temperatures with a food thermometer will ensure that meat and poultry are cooked to the desired degree of doneness.

Daily Protein Needs

Age	mg/kg Body Weight
Infants (0 to 6 months)	2,000
Infants (6 to 12 months)	1,500
Children (1 through 6 years)	1,200
Children (7 through 14 years)	1,000
Adolescents (15 through 18 years)	
males	900
females	800
Adults (19 years and over)	800

Pregnant women need an extra 10 g of protein per day, and lactating women need an extra 15 g.

11-12 People in every age group need high-quality proteins from animal sources or complementary plant sources.

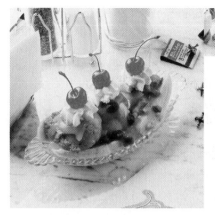

Item of Interest
What Causes Light and Dark Meat?

Myoglobin is a protein that holds oxygen in muscle tissue. Myoglobin gives meat its color. It is also responsible for the color changes that take place in meat during cooking. Fresh meat has a red color because myoglobin is red when exposed to oxygen. Pork is lighter than beef because it contains less myoglobin. When meat is cooked, the heat causes myoglobin molecules to lose an electron. The result is a color change to brown.

Have you ever wondered why some pieces of chicken are white meat and some are dark? The color of chicken and turkey meat is related to the type of muscle

fibers in the meat. The type of muscle fiber is based on the energy source used most often by those muscles. Breast and wing muscle fibers are designed for rapid sudden use. They burn glycogen for energy, which does not require oxygen. Legs and thighs have muscles designed for duration, or slow steady use. These muscles burn fat as well as glycogen. Oxygen must be present for fat to be turned into energy.

Like beef and pork, chicken and turkey meat contain the protein myoglobin. Myoglobin holds oxygen and is brown to red in color, depending on the amount

of oxygen present. Because breast and wing muscles do not require oxygen to produce energy, breast and wing meat are light in color. Because leg and thigh muscles need oxygen to turn fat into energy, leg and thigh meat have a darker color. Fat stored in these muscle tissues also gives dark meat a higher fat content than white meat.

Duck and goose meat is all dark because these birds fly for long distances at a time during migration. This requires the fat and oxygen stores of dark meat. This is why duck and goose are fattier than chicken and turkey.

---

cell. Protein is used to make muscle fibers, connective tissue, cell walls, and red and white blood cells. Hair cells and nails also contain large amounts of protein. Whenever the body is injured, under stress, or ill, the need for protein increases.

Most body cells are replaced within a seven-year period. Cells lining the intestinal tract must be replaced every three days. Blood cells must be replaced every three to four months. Therefore, even adults need a daily supply of protein to replace worn out cells.

Fight Disease

A second key function of protein in the body is to help fight disease. *Antibodies* are proteins designed to attack foreign substances that enter the body. Whenever the body is

exposed to germs, it manufactures antibodies designed to destroy those specific germs. Amazingly, the body remembers and produces more of those antibodies the next time it is exposed to the same germs.

Maintain Fluid and Mineral Balance

Another function of proteins in the body is performed by proteins in cell walls. These proteins help control the movement of water and minerals in and out of the cells. Too much fluid in the cells will cause cells to rupture. If cells contain too little fluid, they will die. Maintaining the right mineral balance is important for the nerves, brain, and muscles to function properly.

Maintain pH Balance

Proteins in the blood perform another important function in the body. Normal body processes result in the production of acids and bases. The blood must carry these acids and bases to the liver and kidneys to be processed or excreted. The pH of the blood must be maintained between a pH of 7.4 and 7.6. If the blood pH changes too much, it can cause coma or death.

Proteins in the blood control this important pH balance. These proteins are buffers that pick up acids or bases when there are too many. These proteins can also release acids and bases when the blood level drops too low. The polar side chains of the amino acids make this possible. The carboxyl group on an amino acid acts as an acid and the amine group acts as a base.

Control Bodily Functions

Proteins play a role in controlling many bodily functions. They do this by being a part of *hormones* and *enzymes*. Hormones are an important part of many body processes. For instance, the hormone insulin is involved in regulating glucose levels in the blood. Hormones control growth, regulate the reproductive system, and maintain other critical body functions. Enzymes are a necessary part of the many chemical reactions that occur within the body. Chapter 12 discusses the importance of these proteins.

Provide Energy

The body does not store extra protein or turn it into muscle. (This is contrary to what you might read in some ads for body-building protein and amino acid supplements.) When you consume more protein than your body needs, your body can change the amino acids into an energy source. Your body does this by removing the NH_2 and $C=O$. The NH_2 is turned into ammonia. The $C=O$ becomes part of a compound known as *ketones*.

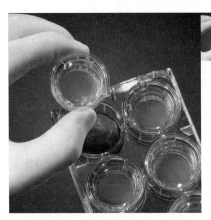

Recent Research
Browned Foods and Carcinogens

A new health concern in the news is the formation of possible carcinogens in baked and grilled protein-based foods. One of the compounds is called *acrylamide.* Acrylamide is a compound formed from glucose, fructose, and the amino acid asparagines. It is formed from the Maillard browning reaction. It forms in foods that are cooked at high temperatures. For example, the browner the crust on toast or French fries, the greater the acrylamide content.

It was first identified in food in April 2002 by a group of Swedish scientists. So far scientists have learned that it is harmful to the reproductive and development processes of rats and mice. More research is needed to determine if the low levels in the food supply are harmful to humans.

Recommendations are to maintain a balanced diet and

❖ avoid overcooking or using extremely high temperatures in cooking,

❖ fry foods to a light rather than dark golden brown,

❖ scrape dark crumbs off toast and baked items,

❖ soak and rinse potatoes before making homemade French fries.

"Acrylamide: Putting the Current Findings into Perspective," *Food Insight: Current Topics in Food Safety and Nutrition,* IFIC Foundation, May/June 2004

Both ammonia and ketones put a strain on the kidneys. A person must consume large volumes of water to flush these substances from the body. This is why high-protein, low-carbohydrate diets can be dangerous.

Future Protein Needs

When researchers compare present food production to world population projections, they predict there will be food shortages in the future. New sources of protein must be found if there is to be enough for everyone. Food scientists worldwide are working on several solutions to meet future protein needs.

One area of research is developing grains that yield higher levels of protein. *Triticale* is a cross of wheat and rye that has more protein than any variety of wheat. Triticale has improved cereal production in many developing countries. *Amaranth* is a traditional Aztec grain with high-quality protein. It has been found to grow in areas with very low rainfall. See 11-13. More work is needed to find tasty, high-protein grains that will grow without irrigation or fertilization.

Another area of research that may increase high-protein grain sources is biotechnology. Researchers are working at altering the genetic structure of plants. They hope to change incomplete protein sources to complete proteins. Care must be taken and extensive testing done to ensure that unwanted changes do not occur as well.

Health Concerns

Food allergies are the immune system's reaction to a protein in food that is mistaken for a harmful substance. Allergies to nearly 175 different foods have been documented. Symptoms can occur within seconds or may take as much as 72 hours to occur. Symptoms can vary dramatically from one person to another and one food to the next. Symptoms include but are not limited to hives, itching, tingling, swelling, red and watery eyes, sinus drainage, edema, swollen joints, vomiting, diarrhea, coughing, wheezing, dizziness, and anaphylaxis. Anaphylaxis is a severe life-threatening allergic reaction where swelling closes air passages, suffocating the victim. As little as one-fifth teaspoon of an allergen can

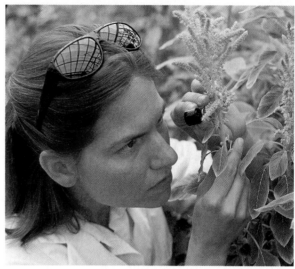

Agricultural Research Service, USDA

11-13 Food scientists are studying the protein value of amaranth and other grains in an effort to address the world hunger problem.

cause death. The most common food allergens are peanuts, tree nuts, dairy, soy, wheat, eggs, fish, and shellfish.

Food sensitivities are allergic-like responses to nonprotein substances in food. They can be just as dangerous to the person who is susceptible and can have the same symptoms as a true allergy. Reactions to the additives sodium nitrite and nitrate are a common example.

Concerns for the food industry include accurate ingredient labeling to alert consumers of allergens, sharing equipment in the manufacturing process that can result in undeclared residues of allergens, and the use of processed ingredients that come from common allergens. For example, hydrolyzed vegetable protein could come from soy or wheat that are common food allergens.

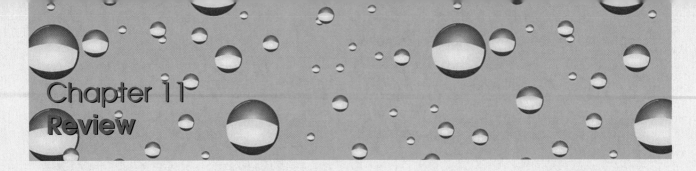

Chapter 11 Review

Summary

Proteins are complex molecules built of many organic acids called amino acids. The amino acids are bound together with peptide bonds. The chemical nature of side chains in amino acids impacts both the shape and function of proteins in food. The variety of shape and chemical properties gives proteins many functions in food preparation.

Unique to protein is its ability to denature, or unfold without breaking peptide bonds. This characteristic allows proteins to form new relationships in food mixtures. Proteins can be denatured by a number of methods, both physical and chemical. Because of this, high-protein foods must be cooked carefully at lower cooking temperatures or shorter cooking times.

Dietary protein needs can be met through a wide range of foods. Like other nutrients, protein serves many functions in the body. However, too much protein can be harmful. In addition, researchers predict that there will be food shortages in the future. Food scientists are working now to find ways of meeting the protein needs of the future.

Check Your Understanding

1. What is the basic molecular structure of amino acids?
2. Describe how amino acids combine to form proteins.
3. What is the difference between the structures of complete and incomplete proteins?
4. List four types of carbon side chains found in protein molecules.
5. Explain the difference between the primary, secondary, and tertiary structures of protein.
6. Identify three common interactions of protein molecules with other molecules.
7. Name two types of denaturation that are not reversible.
8. What can cause a protein molecule to denature?
9. Identify the functions of protein in food and give an example of each.
10. Describe what happens when protein foods are cooked at high temperatures for too long.
11. Why do milk products require frequent stirring during preparation?
12. Describe the nutritional contributions of protein.

Critical Thinking

1. Describe how a protein-based gel develops.
2. Create a one-day menu for a vegetarian who will eat egg and dairy products.
3. Explain why protein molecules can act as emulsifiers.
4. Why are most protein foods cooked at low temperatures or high temperatures for a very short period?

Explore Further

1. **Science.** Construct models of the three structures of protein molecules—helix, random coil, and pleated sheet.
2. **Foods and Nutrition/Math.** Plan a lacto-ovo vegetarian diet for one day that provides 10 to 15 percent of the calories from protein.
3. **Technology.** Use nutrition analysis software to determine the percentage of calories in your diet that come from fat.

Experiment 11A
Working with Egg White Foams

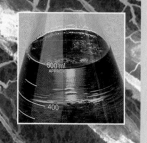

Purpose

One function of protein in cooking is forming foams. Foams are bubbles of air surrounded by a protein film. Egg whites will form a foam when beaten. Factors such as temperature, pH, and additives can help or hinder the formation of the foam. Sugar can help stabilize an egg foam. In this experiment, you will examine the best time to add sugar to an egg white foam. You will also determine which types of foods will interfere with the formation of an egg foam.

Equipment

electronic balance

small mixing bowl

metric measuring spoons

portable electric mixer

rubber scraper

2 funnels

ruler

2 10- or 25-mL graduated cylinders

Supplies

25 g sugar

2 egg whites

plastic wrap

2 mL (½ teaspoon) assigned additive

Procedure

Part I

1. Mass 25 g of sugar.

2. Separate one egg white from the yolk. Place the egg white in a small mixing bowl.

3. Begin beating the egg white, sprinkling the sugar over the egg white at the point indicated in your assigned variation. Record the length of time the egg white is beaten before and after adding sugar.

   Variation 1: Add the sugar before beating.

   Variation 2: Beat the egg white until foamy (like the froth on root beer) then add the sugar.

   Variation 3: Beat the egg white until the foam has turned white but does not form a peak when the mixer is lifted out then add the sugar.

   Variation 4: Beat the egg white until it forms soft peaks (when the mixer is lifted, a peak will form and bend over at the top) then add the sugar.

   Variation 5: Beat the egg white until it forms a stiff peak (a peak that stands straight up when the mixer is lifted) then add the sugar.

   Variation 6: Do not add any sugar.

4. Beat the egg white at high speed until the sugar is dissolved in the foam. Rub a small amount of the foam between your thumb and index finger. If you feel any grittiness, the sugar is not dissolved. Beat variation 6 until stiff peaks are formed.

5. Use a rubber scraper to push the foam into a funnel. Level the foam. Hold the base of the funnel beside the top edge of a counter or lab table. Stand a ruler upright on the counter or table beside the

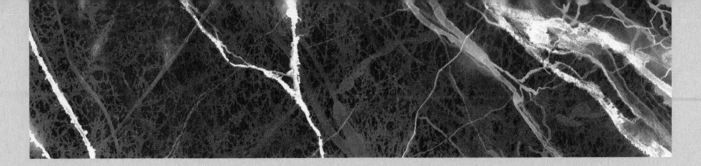

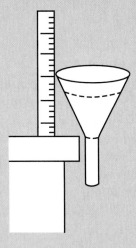

3. Beat the egg white with the assigned additive until the foam is stiff enough to hold a soft peak. Record the length of time the egg white was beaten.

4. Use a rubber scraper to push the foam into a funnel and level. Measure the height of the foam.

5. Cover the funnel with plastic wrap and sit it in a graduated cylinder for 20 minutes.

6. Record the volume of any leakage found in the graduated cylinder after 10 minutes and again after 20 minutes.

funnel and measure the height of the foam. (See the sketch.) Record the measurement. Cover the top of the funnel with plastic wrap.

6. Place the funnel in a graduated cylinder and allow it to sit for 20 minutes.

7. Record the volume of any leakage found in the graduated cylinder after 10 minutes and again after 20 minutes.

Part II

1. While the egg foam in Part I is sitting for 20 minutes, separate a second egg.

2. Place the egg white in a clean, dry mixing bowl. Put in 2 mL (½ teaspoon) of the assigned additive.

   Variation 1: cream of tartar

   Variation 2: salt

   Variation 3: egg yolk

   Variation 4: water

   Variation 5: lemon juice

   Variation 6: cream

Questions

1. At what point in beating should you add sugar to get the maximum volume in an egg white foam?

2. At what point in beating should you add the sugar to get the most stable foam?

3. What types of ingredients can be added before beating egg whites that will not interfere with foam formation?

4. What types of ingredients will increase egg white foam volume when added before beating? (Compare foam heights in Part II with Variation 6 in Part I)

5. How can this information be applied to the production of meringues and foam cakes?

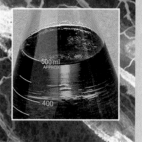

Experiment 11B
Making Gluten Balls

Purpose

Varieties of wheat that are used in food production are hard, soft, summer, winter, white, red, and durum. These wheats have different compositions. Flour producers mix the different types of wheat according to the protein level needed for a particular type of flour. Wheat flours that are available in most grocery stores include whole wheat, all-purpose, self-rising, cake, and bread flours. These wheat flours form varying amounts of gluten when they are moistened and stirred or kneaded for a period. Flours from other grains do not form cohesive, elastic gluten. In this experiment, you will evaluate the effectiveness of different types of flour on the production of gluten.

Equipment

electronic balance
100-mL graduated cylinder
small mixing bowl
electric mixer
large spoon

Supplies

150 g assigned flour
100 mL warm water

Procedure

1. Mass 75 g of your assigned flour and combine it with 100 mL of water in a small mixing bowl.

   Variation 1: whole wheat flour

   Variation 2: all-purpose flour

   Variation 3: cake flour

   Variation 4: bread flour

   Variation 5: masa (corn flour)

   Variation 6: rye flour

2. Beat the flour and water with an electric mixer for 2 minutes.

3. Mass another 75 g of your assigned flour and add it to the mixture. Stir with a spoon until the flour is absorbed and the dough forms a ball.

4. Gently knead the dough on a lightly floured surface for 10 minutes. Do not add flour unless the dough begins to stick to the work surface.

5. Shape the dough into a ball. Record your observations about the appearance and texture of the dough in a data table.

6. Grasp the ball of dough in both hands so your fingers and thumbs meet around the center of the ball. Gently stretch the ball until the dough begins to tear. (Small sections of the dough will separate.)

7. Measure the length of the dough from one end to the other. Record the measurement in your data table.

8. Record your data in a class data chart on an overhead projector. Copy the data from other lab groups into your data table.

Questions

1. Which dough ball stretched the farthest?

2. Which dough ball stretched the least?

3. Which flours will form the most gluten?

4. How can you apply this information to bread production?

Experiment 11C
Proteins, pH, and Coagulation

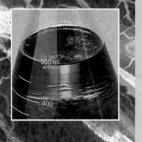

Purpose

One of the challenges of cooking with protein-based foods is the coagulation that occurs in the presence of acids. This is desirable when poached eggs are cooked in water with a small amount of vinegar. Coagulation or *curdling* of milk proteins is not desirable in cream of tomato soup. In this experiment, you will determine what cooking procedure will minimize curdling and result in the best textured cream soup.

Equipment

paring knife
2-quart saucepan
tongs
blender
1½-quart saucepan
wooden spoon or whisk
plastic spoons for tasting

Supplies

1 large tomato
15 mL (½ tablespoon) flour
125 mL (½ cup) milk
salt and pepper

Procedure

1. With a paring knife, cut an X-shaped slit through the skin of the tomato at the blossom end.
2. Fill a 2-quart saucepan half full of water. Bring the water to a boil.
3. Completely submerge the tomato in the water and blanch it (cook in boiling water) for 30 seconds.
4. Use tongs to remove the tomato from the boiling water and hold it under cold running water for a few seconds. Peel the skin off the tomato.
5. Cut the tomato in half and scoop out as many seeds as possible.
6. Puree the tomato in a blender.
7. Prepare your assigned variation in a 1½-quart saucepan.

   Variation 1: Add the flour to the tomato puree. Stir in the milk. Bring to a boil then reduce heat and simmer 2 minutes. Add salt and pepper to taste.

   Variation 2: Add the flour to the milk. Stir in the tomato puree. Bring to a boil then reduce heat and simmer 2 minutes. Add salt and pepper to taste.

   Variation 3: Add flour to the tomato puree. Bring to a boil then reduce heat and simmer 2 minutes. Slowly stir in the milk. Heat until steaming. Add salt and pepper to taste.

   Variation 4: Add flour to the milk. Bring to a boil then reduce heat and simmer 2 minutes. Slowly stir in the tomato puree. Heat until steaming. Add salt and pepper to taste.

   Variation 5: Combine tomato puree and milk. Bring to a boil then reduce heat and simmer 2 minutes. Omit flour from this variation. Add salt and pepper to taste.

8. Record your observations of the appearance, texture, and taste of each variation.

Questions

1. Which variations have the most curdling?
2. Which variations have the least curdling?
3. What are the functions of the flour in the soup?
4. How can this information be applied in other food preparation?

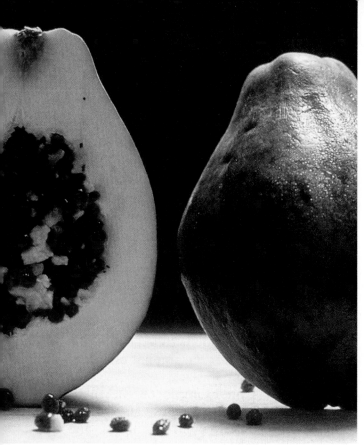

USDA

Papayas are a source of natural enzymes that are used in meat tenderizers because they break down proteins.

Chapter 12

Enzymes: The Protein Catalyst

Objectives

After studying this chapter,
you will be able to

describe the relationship between a substrate and an active site in enzymatic reactions.

identify the role of coenzymes in enzymatic reactions.

list factors that affect enzymatic activity.

explain how some foods are developed as a result of enzymatic activity.

demonstrate how to prevent enzymatic browning of foods.

Key Terms

enzyme
catalyst
activation energy
substrate
active site
coenzyme
nomenclature

blanching
electrolyte
enzyme inhibitor
marinate
oxidase
enzymatic browning

Eating meat, eggs, beans, and cheese will provide the body with protein needed to build tissue. However, the body does not use all protein to build tissue. A second function of protein is to provide the amino acids needed to build enzymes. *Enzymes* are proteins that start chemical reactions without being changed by the chemical reaction. Most body processes involve chemical reactions. Practically all biochemical reactions (chemical reactions that occur in living cells) involve the use of specialized proteins called enzymes. There are thousands of enzymes in a single cell. Each enzyme is involved in a specific chemical reaction.

Understanding the function of enzymes is necessary for the food scientist. This is because many enzymatic reactions are involved in the development of food products such as beverages and cheeses.

Enzymes Are Specialized Catalysts

A *catalyst* is a substance that starts a reaction between substances without being affected by the reaction. Enzymes are a group of proteins that act as catalysts. Enzymes participate in chemical reactions but are not the reactants or the products. Because enzymes are not changed with use, cells can contain thousands of different enzymes in very low concentrations.

You can demonstrate this with two small pieces of steak and meat tenderizer. Sprinkle one piece of meat with the tenderizer and then refrigerate it for one hour. If you remove the meat from the refrigerator and gently rub it, the surface will crumble. This is because the enzymes in the meat tenderizer are breaking up the protein in the meat. Now lay the second

piece of meat on top of the piece with the tenderizer. Place both pieces in the refrigerator. After another hour, remove the meat from the refrigerator. Gently rub the side of the second piece that was placed on top of the tenderizer. The second piece of meat will also begin to crumble. This demonstrates that the enzymes were not changed in the chemical reaction. They can be used repeatedly. See 12-1.

How Enzymes Work

You learned earlier that the rate of chemical reactions can be increased by adding energy. Most chemical reactions in the body cannot occur unless energy is added. The energy needed to start a reaction is called *activation energy*. Enzymes lower the amount of energy needed for a reaction to start.

Digestion is an example of enzymatic chemical reactions (reactions started by enzymes). Unless carbohydrates, lipids, and proteins are broken down, their nutritive value is not available for your body to use. Most of the chemical reactions in digestion require much heat energy. The amount of heat needed would destroy body tissue before the energy level became high enough to start digestion. Digestive enzymes allow the chemical reactions to occur without the use of as

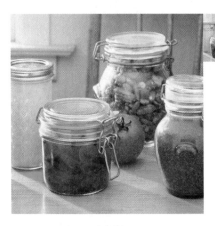

Historical Highlight
Enzymes and Insulin Production

In 1955, a team of chemists made a breakthrough for diabetics who need insulin injections. The team identified the order of amino acids in the protein insulin. This team was led by the English chemist Frederick Sanger. He studied insulin's chemical makeup

in different species of animals. This allowed him to determine the structure of insulin.

Sanger's work led to the development of a method to mass-produce insulin. The gene that produces the enzyme that makes insulin can be inserted

into single-celled organisms. The organisms multiply rapidly and produce large volumes of pure insulin. This insulin is cheaper to produce and easier to obtain than the previous sources, which were oxen, sheep, and pigs.

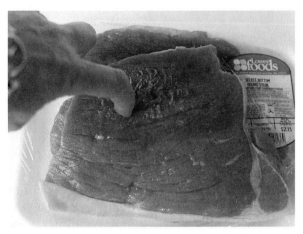

12-1 Meat tenderizer was allowed to set on this steak for 35 minutes. Notice how the surface of the meat crumbles apart when rubbed.

much heat energy. With enzymes, the body can completely break down protein in 4 hours. Without enzymes, breaking down protein would require much more time and energy. The protein would need to be boiled for 24 hours in a 20% hydrochloric acid (HCl) solution.

Think about skiing down a mountain as a chemical reaction. Enzymes are like the ski lift. To ski down a mountain, a skier must first climb to the top. If the mountain is very big, the skier is out of time and energy after only one round trip. When a ski lift is present, the

skier gets a boost. The skier can get in place to ski many times in one day. One ski lift can also lift many skiers a day. Therefore, more skiers go down the mountain more often. Enzymes, like the ski lift, give chemical reactions a boost. When enzymes are present, more chemical reactions can occur more often.

Enzymes are very specific as to the compounds with which they will react. For example, sucrase is an enzyme that breaks sucrose into glucose and fructose molecules. Sucrase cannot break a lactose molecule into glucose and galactose. Conversely, the enzyme lactase can break the chemical bond between glucose and galactose, but it has no effect on sucrose. Although sucrose and lactose are both sugars, they each require a different enzyme for digestion.

Working Models

When trying to understand complex or microscopic reactions, it helps to compare them to familiar concepts. There are two models or pictures that will help you see how enzymes can start chemical reactions.

The first model used to illustrate enzymatic reactions was the *lock-and-key model*. In this model, the enzyme is compared to the key of a lock. Without the key, the lock cannot be opened without a great deal of difficulty. With the key, the lock opens easily. However, the

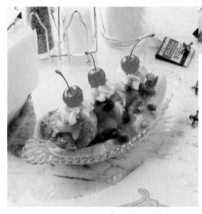

Item of Interest
Enzymes Keep Going and Going. . .

The hydrochloric acid (HCl) in the stomach is one of the strongest acids known. It would take 10 to 20 tons of this acid to digest the protein in 2 tons of

egg white. This colossal digestion task would require 24 to 48 hours to complete. One ounce of the enzyme pepsin will do the same job in a few hours. This is

because most enzymes break down substrates at the rate of 1,000 to 500,000 molecules per minute.

key must be inserted into the right spot in the right way. The lock represents the substance being changed. In enzymatic reactions, the substance on which the enzyme acts is known as the *substrate.* The keyhole is called the active site. The *active site* is the location where the substrate attaches to the enzyme. See 12-2.

This model falls short at the point of turning the key. Substrates do not turn when inserted into the active site. Research has revealed that an enzyme is not a perfect match to the substrate.

The second model of enzymatic reactions was developed as a result of this research. This model is called the *induced-fit model.* The induced-fit model also has a substrate, an enzyme, and an active site. The difference is in the fit of the substrate at the active site. In the induced-fit model, the enzyme is not quite the right size. The enzyme's presence adds force or pressure that causes the substrate to break apart. See 12-3.

All enzymatic reactions can be described as following the same basic process. The enzyme and the substrate are the reactants that combine to form an enzyme-substrate complex. The enzyme-substrate complex is unstable and quickly breaks apart. The product of the reaction includes the enzyme, which

Lock-and-Key Model

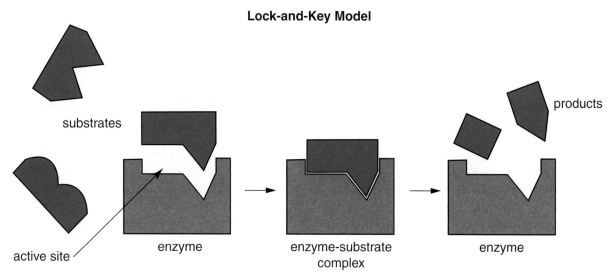

12-2 In the lock-and-key model, the active site on an enzyme is the exact size and shape needed to fit a particular substrate.

Induced-Fit Model

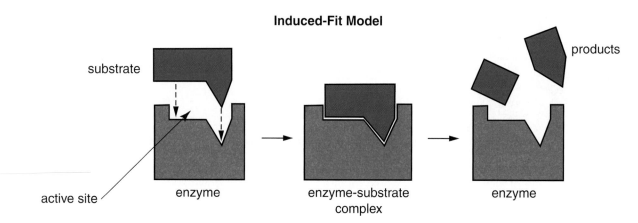

12-3 In the induced-fit model, the active site on an enzyme is not an exact match for the substrate. However, as the substrate is drawn to the enzyme, the enzyme takes on the appropriate shape.

is free to act again on another substrate. This can be represented by the following chemical formula:

$$substrate + enzyme \rightarrow$$
$$enzyme\text{-}substrate\ complex \rightarrow product + enzyme$$
$$(S + E \rightarrow ES \rightarrow P + E)$$

Coenzymes

Many enzymatic reactions require a fourth factor known as a coenzyme. A *coenzyme* is a substance that must be present for an enzymatic reaction to occur. Coenzymes work in one of three ways. One way a coenzyme works is to attach to the enzyme so the combined shape can react with the substrate. The coenzyme changes the shape of the enzyme so the substrate will fit in the active site. See 12-4.

A second way a coenzyme works is to attach to the substrate. When the coenzyme is present, the shape of the substrate is changed. Now the substrate will fit the active site of the enzyme. In both types of reactions, the coenzyme loosely bonds to either the enzyme or the substrate.

In the third type of reaction, the coenzyme is a transfer agent. It accepts an atom or molecular group that is broken off the substrate. The coenzyme then transfers the atom or molecular group to another compound. If the coenzyme were not present, the atom or compound could simply reattach itself to the substrate. The enzyme would just keep breaking the same substrate apart.

A coenzyme can be as small as an electron or as large as a complex molecule. Two types of coenzymes that are of interest in the study of food are minerals and vitamins. They have

been found to be important coenzymes that are necessary for many body functions. All the B vitamins act as coenzymes or part of coenzymes. Calcium (Ca^{2+}), magnesium (Mg^{2+}), and zinc (Zn^{2+}) are metal ions that function as coenzymes.

Naming Enzymes

The *nomenclature*, or naming system, for organic chemistry was not established until the twentieth century. As researchers discovered a growing number of enzymes, they realized they needed some system for naming the enzymes. In 1956, the International Union of Biochemistry established a commission to work on the problem. The commission presented and received acceptance for their recommendation in 1961. They recommended a naming system based on the names of the substrates on which enzymes acted.

Enzymes are named for the types of reactions or the substances for which they are the catalysts. For example, lactase is the enzyme that causes lactose to break down into glucose and galactose. The root name for the enzyme (*lact-*) is the same as the root name for the substance digested. You have learned that the ending *-ose* denotes a sugar. The *-ase* ending represents an enzyme. Therefore, lactase is the enzyme that works on the sugar lactose.

Plants and animals produce enzymes to assist in digesting foods. Plants and animals also produce enzymes as catalysts for chemical reactions within cells. These enzymes are involved in such functions as rebuilding body tissue and producing energy.

Many of the enzymes studied by food scientists are digestive enzymes. Digestive

Coenzyme Reaction

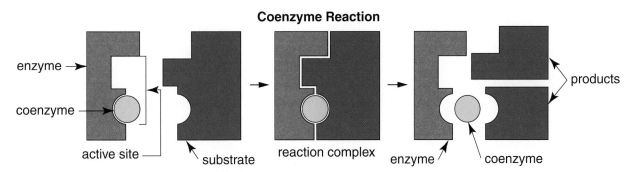

12-4 In one type of coenzyme reaction, a coenzyme attaches to an enzyme to change the shape of the active site.

enzymes are divided into three main categories. Enzymes that break apart proteins are proteases. Enzymes that work on lipids are lipases. Enzymes that break apart carbohydrates are carbohydrases.

Enzymes cause catalytic reactions, which are reactions started by a catalyst. Catalase is an example of an enzyme named for the type of reaction it creates. Catalase is found in the liver and throughout body cells. It catalyzes hydrogen peroxide (H_2O_2), which is toxic, into water and oxygen, which can be "recycled" by the body. Hydrogen peroxide is a by-product of chemical reactions within cells. Catalase is one of the fastest-acting enzymes in the body. A single catalase molecule can break down as many as five million H_2O_2 molecules per minute.

$$2H_2O_2 + \text{catalase} \longrightarrow 2H_2O + O_2 + \text{catalase}$$

Some enzymes that work on proteins had already been identified and named before the current naming system was adopted. One example is rennin. This enzyme is used to curdle milk in cheese production. Rennin and many other proteases are still known by the names given to them before the new nomenclature. See 12-5.

Some enzymes are commonly known by more than one name. Sucrase is an example. This enzyme breaks sucrose down into glucose and fructose. This mixture of glucose and fructose is often called invert sugar in the food industry. Therefore, sucrase is also known as invertase.

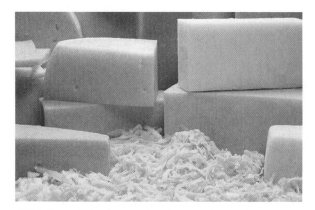

12-5 Rennin is the name of an enzyme that breaks down the proteins in milk as part of the process of making cheese.

Factors That Affect Enzyme Activity

The first factor that affects enzyme activity is the availability of water. This is because enzymatic reactions, like most chemical reactions, occur in solution. Any chemical reaction is also affected by the concentration of the reactants. The more reactants there are, the more reaction or change that can occur.

Enzymes work because of their shape. If the shape of an enzyme or substrate is changed, the substrate cannot attach itself to the active site. The specific reaction involving that enzyme will stop. Any factor that affects the structure of proteins will have an effect on enzyme activity. The factors that affect the shape of enzymes (proteins) include heat, pH, and electrolytes.

Water Availability

Water must be available to act as a reactant as well as a solvent in enzymatic reactions. If there is not enough water present, enzymatic reactions will be slowed or stopped. Enzyme reactions will not occur in dry products. Therefore, drying is often used to preserve products such as milk and wheat flour.

In your study of carbohydrates, lipids, and proteins, you read that water is released whenever macromolecules are made. When two sugars are joined, a water molecule is formed. When a fatty acid bonds to glycerol, a water molecule is a product of the reaction. For each peptide bond formed in a protein molecule, a water molecule is released.

To reverse these reactions and break down carbohydrates, lipids, and proteins, a water molecule must be present. The H^+ and OH^- ions from water join to the two parts of the substrate. For instance, a triglyceride molecule can be broken down into three fatty acids and glycerol. Three water molecules must be present for this reaction to take place. The three H^+ ions bond to each of the three hydroxyl groups of the glycerol molecule. The three OH^- ions bond to the three carboxyl groups on the fatty acids. If water is not present, the two parts of the substrate—the glycerol and fatty acids—can simply rejoin. There will be no net reaction or change. See 12-6.

The Hydrolysis of Maltose

maltose   water   glucose   glucose

12-6 Water must be present to break down substrates. This model shows the roles water and the enzyme maltase play in the breakdown of the disaccharide maltose.

Concentration of the Solution

The more substrate there is in a solution, the greater the rate of reaction will be. The enzymes will have more material with which to react. It will take less time to come in contact with a substrate. A mixture of sucrase and 50% sucrose will have a rapid rate of reaction. A mixture of sucrase and a 10% sucrose solution will have a much slower rate of reaction.

The rate of enzymatic reaction in a solution will increase as the concentration increases, up to the saturation point. You can demonstrate this by setting up a simple experiment using two concentrations of hydrogen peroxide.

Factors That Denature Enzymes

Remember that enzymes are proteins. You learned in the last chapter that denaturation is a process that changes the shape of protein molecules. Any factor that will change the molecular shape of an enzyme will stop enzymatic activity. This is because enzymes are shape specific. If the shape changes, the substrate will no longer fit into the active site of the enzyme.

Heat

Like the rates of most chemical reactions, enzymatic reaction rates increase as the temperature increases. For all enzymes there is a point at which additional heat slows and eventually stops all enzymatic activity. Most animal enzymes will rapidly denature at temperatures above 40°C (104°F). This is one of

the main reasons a body temperature above 106°F (41°C) can be deadly.

Heating is one way to prevent undesirable enzymatic reactions. This principle is applied when freezing vegetables. Freezing merely slows enzymatic activity; it does not stop it. Active enzymes can cause vegetables to develop "haylike" flavors and odors during freezer storage. To halt enzyme activity, vegetables are blanched before freezing. *Blanching* is briefly plunging food in boiling water to stop enzyme activity. After blanching, food is quickly submerged in ice water to stop the cooking action. The heat of blanching changes the shape, or denatures, the enzymes in vegetables. This keeps the enzymes from affecting the vegetables' fresh flavors during freezer storage.

Enzymes have varying degrees of sensitivity to heat. One of the more heat-resistant enzymes in plant tissues is catalase. Food scientists know if catalase has been inactivated, most other flavor- and texture-altering enzymes in vegetables have been inactivated, too.

You can observe catalase activity by pouring a small amount of hydrogen peroxide over a piece of freshly peeled potato. The fizzing you see results from the catalase in the potato breaking down the hydrogen peroxide into water and oxygen, 12-7. If you blanch a potato for one minute and then pour hydrogen peroxide over it, you will still see fizzing. This tells you that the catalase is still active. Try repeating this test after two, three, four, and

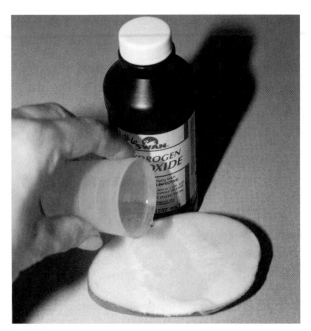

12-7 Hydrogen peroxide fizzes when poured on a raw potato because of the catalase naturally found in potatoes.

five minutes of blanching. This will allow you to identify the point at which the catalase has been denatured.

Food scientists have used similar tests in a laboratory to develop blanching charts. These charts tell food processors and homemakers how long to blanch different foods before freezing to maintain top quality.

Meat tenderizers are another example of heat treatment stopping enzymatic activity. Instructions on meat tenderizer packages tell consumers how long to allow the product to be on the meat before cooking. Once the meat is heated, the enzymes in the tenderizer are denatured. The meat tenderizer will cease to work.

Acids and Bases

Two more factors that denature enzymes are acids and bases. Enzymes are most reactive at certain pH ranges. Each enzyme has an optimum pH at which it will react rapidly. Each enzyme also has a pH at which it denatures. Pepsin is an enzyme that works on protein. It is one of the proteases found in the stomach, which has a pH of 1.5 to 1.7. The amylases, proteases, and lipases that work in the intestines need a pH of about 7.

Most enzymes will denature if the pH is too high or too low. Rennin is used in cheese production. Rennin needs a pH of no more than 5.8 to work. Milk normally has a pH of around 6. For the rennin to coagulate milk proteins, the milk must first have an acid added to lower the pH. Homemade cheeses usually have buttermilk added to lower the pH to rennin's optimum pH range. Lowering the pH of the milk speeds up the curdling process in cheese making.

By changing the pH, it is possible to speed up, slow down, or stop enzymatic reactions. Adding lemon juice to freshly cut apples and bananas is an example of slowing enzymatic reaction by changing the pH. The lemon juice will slow down, but not prevent, an enzymatic reaction from eventually turning the fruit brown.

Electrolytes

Another factor that affects enzymes is electrolytes. *Electrolytes* are positively and negatively charged ions in solution. The most common electrolyte used in food production is salt, or sodium chloride. Salt binds to the enzymes in foods that cause spoilage. This prevents the enzymes from reacting with the substrate.

High concentrations of *anions* (negatively charged ions) or *cations* (positively charged ions) can either hinder or promote enzymatic activity. For example, mercury (Hg^{2+}) and lead (Pb^{2+}) are poisonous because they stop important enzymatic activity. On the other hand, iron (Fe^{2+}), calcium (Ca^{2+}), and potassium (K^+) are cations that work as coenzymes. They must be present to activate enzymes that are responsible for such bodily functions as transporting oxygen and contracting muscles.

Enzyme Inhibitors

Another factor that affects enzymatic activity is enzyme inhibitors. An *enzyme inhibitor* is any substance that will prevent the enzyme-substrate complex from forming. Enzyme inhibitors can bind with and change the shape of either the substrate or the enzyme. When the shape of the substrate or the enzyme is changed, the enzymatic reactions are stopped or slowed.

Enzyme inhibitors occur naturally in many food products. They act as natural preservatives by stopping the action of invading "germs" or by slowing the spoilage process. Enzyme inhibitors are found in animal foods, such as egg white, milk, and meat. Two examples of enzyme inhibitors are found in egg white. One enzyme inhibitor binds with biotin (a vitamin) and interferes with the growth of bacteria that require this vitamin. Another enzyme inhibitor in egg white is *conalbumin*. It combines with iron to form a stable compound. Bacteria and yeast require the presence of free iron for growth. When iron combines with conalbumin, it is no longer available to support the growth of bacteria or yeast. Conalbumin does not stop the spoilage of egg white, but it does slow the process.

Enzyme inhibitors have also been found in plant foods. Many of the enzyme inhibitors in foods may help stop or slow the growth of molds and bacteria. Single-celled organisms, such as molds and bacteria, release digestive enzymes. Then these organisms absorb the products of the enzyme reaction through their cell walls. If this action is stopped, the bacteria or mold dies. One of the functions of enzyme inhibitors in plants is as a defense mechanism. Foods that have enzyme inhibitors include grains, such as corn, wheat, and barley; olives; onions; garlic; and tomatoes. For example, tomatoes contain the enzyme inhibitor tomatin. This substance blocks enzyme activity, which results in the death of fungi and bacteria that cause spoilage. See 12-8.

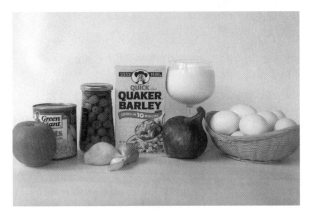

12-8 These foods contain natural enzyme inhibitors, which can be inactivated by cooking.

Enzymes and the Food Supply

Enzymes can produce both desirable and undesirable qualities in foods. Therefore, enzymes can be considered positive or negative.

The food industry uses enzymes in three basic ways to help develop food products.

❖ Enzymes help convert one food product into another. An example is the use of enzymes to convert milk into cheese. This is one of the main uses of enzymes in the food industry.

❖ Enzymes are used to extract food components from food systems. For instance, pectinase speeds up the separation of juice from insoluble residues. This results in a clearer juice and a maximum yield from the fruit.

❖ Enzymes play key roles in developing new foods and food ingredients. Lipases are used to convert palm oils into a cocoa butter equivalent and to produce oleic acid from beef fat. Oleic acid is used to make margarine.

The volumes of enzymes needed in commercially produced foods are quite large. Therefore, scientists have developed ways to mass-produce enzymes. Enzymes are commercially produced and sold to food manufacturers. The enzymes produced vary depending on the demands of the food industry.

Changes Produced by Enzymes

The changes produced by enzymes are almost as varied as the number of enzymes. Enzymatic reactions can produce positive and negative changes. Some of the positive effects used in food production are

❖ to make food easier to eat, such as putting meat tenderizer on a steak

❖ to preserve food, such as changing milk into cheese

❖ to improve the flavor, quality, or appearance of a food, such as adding lactase to produce lactose-free dairy products

Enzymes also play a major role in the fermentation of various food products. (You will read about this process in Chapter 17.) See 12-9.

Uses of Enzymes in Food Production

Enzyme	Food	Function of the Enzyme
Amylases	Baked goods	Releases sugar to feed yeast for leavening
	Beer and ale	Releases sugar to feed the yeast for fermentation
	Cereals	Changes starch to dextrins (starch fragments that can be further broken into sugars)
	Confections	Recovers sugar from candy scraps
	Corn syrup	Converts cornstarch to dextrins
	Syrups and sugars	Converts starches to dextrins and dextrose
Amyloglucosidase	Corn syrup	Converts dextrins to glucose
	Light beer	Converts dextrins normally in beer to glucose, which is used by the yeast during brewing
Catalase	Milk	Destroys hydrogen peroxide formed during cold pasteurization methods
Cellulase	Coffee	Breaks down cellulose during the drying process
Invertase	Artificial honey	Converts sucrose to glucose and fructose
	Candies	Produces a soft cream center in chocolate-coated candies
Lactase	Ice cream	Prevents crystallization of lactose
	Milk	Stabilizes milk proteins in frozen milk by removing the lactose and reduces or eliminates lactose to produce milk products for the lactose intolerant
Narginase	Citrus fruits	Breaks down bitter flavor compounds
Pectic enzymes	Coffee	Breaks down the gelatin coating on the beans during processing
	Fruit juices	Increases the release of juice, prevents cloudiness, and improves the concentration process
	Olives	Aids in extraction of oil
	Wine	Helps clarify wine
Proteases	Baked goods	Softens the dough, reduces mixing time, increases loaf volume, and improves grain texture
	Beer and ale	Aids in developing body, flavor, and nutrient content as well as filtering and clarifying the brew
	Cereals	Increases the drying rate and aids in handling characteristics
	Eggs	Improves drying
	Meat and fish	Aids in tenderizing, recovering protein from bones and fish scraps, and freezing oils
	Other products	Aids in production of soy sauce, tartar sauce, bouillon, dehydrated soups, gravy mixes, and processed meats
Rennin	Cheeses	Coagulates the casein to form cheese curds

12-9 Enzymes are used in the production of a wide range of food products.

Enzyme action is not always considered positive. For example, enzymes are responsible for rotting action in foods. This process breaks down the structure of foods, turning them soft and mushy. Enzymes can cause flavor changes that are unpleasant. An example of this is fat turning rancid in prolonged storage. Enzymes can cause unpleasant flavors and odors to develop in raw vegetables that are stored in the freezer. You have probably noticed that apple slices will turn brown if allowed to sit for very long. In each case, undesirable changes in texture, flavor, and/or color occur because of enzyme activity.

Carbohydrases in Food Production

Carbohydrases are a large group of enzymes that react with sugars and starches. Amylases are enzymes that react with amylose-type starches. Cellulase will hydrolyze cellulose. Lactase and invertase are other carbohydrases that react with sugars.

Amylases are enzymes involved in the breakdown of carbohydrates. Some of the commercial uses of amylases are

- manufacturing corn syrup and high-fructose corn syrup
- clarifying fruit juices
- fermenting wine and beers
- stabilizing chocolate syrup
- aiding salvage and reuse of scraps of candy from candy manufacturing
- clarifying vegetable canning liquid

One of the largest consumers of amylases is the baking industry. Amylases increase the sugar available for yeast and impact the leavening of breads and baked goods. Wheat flour naturally contains α–amylase, but the amount varies. Standardized levels of α–amylase are needed for consistent quality of bakery items. Yeast releases an amylase to break the starch in bread dough into glucose molecules. The yeast then utilizes the glucose for energy.

Cellulase works on indigestible cellulose. It is used to clarify citrus juices and to aid in extracting essential oils for flavorings. Cellulase can also improve the nutritive value of foods by freeing the sugars bound in cellulose. Cellulase breaks down the cellulose structure, freeing compounds that would otherwise be unavailable for humans to digest.

Another important enzyme in the breakdown of sugars is lactase. Lactase is used to make powdered milk easier to dissolve. Lactase hydrolyzes lactose into glucose and galactose. This increases the speed with which the milk powder will dissolve in water. Lactose is also used to reduce calories in some products. Lactose is not as soluble or as sweet as the glucose and galactose molecules it contains. Because glucose and galactose are sweeter, products that have lactase added will need fewer sweeteners added. This results in lower-calorie products. Many dairy products have lactase added to make lactose-reduced or lactose-free foods. These foods can be used by people who cannot digest lactose.

Invertase is used to convert solid sucrose mixtures to more fluid mixtures of fructose and glucose. Invertase is used in the production of chocolate-covered candies that have fluid centers.

Lipases in Food Production

Lipases are used to extract unwanted egg yolk from egg white to improve the whipping properties of the egg white. Lipases are also used to improve the flavor and texture of cheeses, ice cream, margarine, and butter. They can be used to improve the flavor of many baked goods, too.

Proteases in Food Production

A common use of proteases in food production is as meat tenderizers. Meat tenderizers work by breaking long protein fibers into shorter pieces that are easier to chew. Two popular proteases used as meat tenderizers are bromelain and papain. Bromelain is an enzyme found in pineapple; papain is found in papaya. These enzymes help protect fruit from bacterial invasion by breaking down the protein structure of the cell walls of bacteria. Bromelain and papain can also break down other protein structures, including the proteins in meat. They are commercially extracted from their fruit sources and sold in dry form as meat tenderizers. See 12-10.

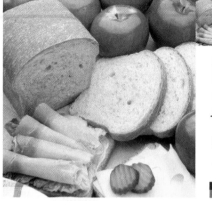

Food Feature
How Do They Make the Cherry Centers?

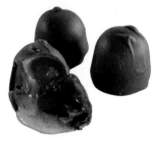

The fluid center of a chocolate-covered cherry is the result of an enzymatic reaction.

To make chocolate-covered cherries, maraschino cherries are wrapped with a sucrose paste that contains the enzyme invertase. These paste-covered cherries are covered with chocolate and allowed to stand. They will become the centers of the finished candy.

Because the water content in the sucrose paste is low, the enzymatic reaction of the invertase takes a while. As the candy sits, the invertase breaks down the sucrose into fructose and glucose. A water molecule is released into the sucrose paste as a by-product of this reaction. This causes the paste to liquefy. Fructose and glucose crystals are also more soluble in water than sucrose crystals. The result is a candy with a firm chocolate outside and a fluid center.

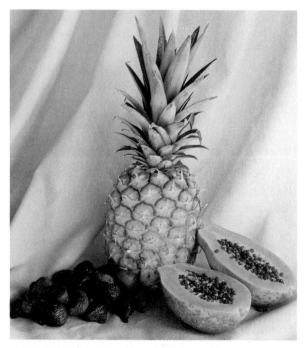

12-10 Figs contain the protease ficin, pineapple contains bromelain, and papaya contains papain. These proteases are extracted and dried for use in meat tenderizers.

The instructions for using meat tenderizers give recommended time limits for use. This is because enzymes can be used repeatedly. What would happen if you left meat tenderizers on uncooked meat too long?

Besides using commercial tenderizers, meats dishes can be tenderized with several hours of marination. Meats that are *marinated* are soaked in a flavorful solution. Many marinades are made with a food acid, such as vinegar, wine, or tomato juice. These marinades rely on the acid to denature the proteins in meat. However, other marinades rely on natural enzymes to tenderize the meat. A marinade made with pineapple juice is an example.

Commercial use of proteases is found in the brewing industry. Proteases are added in the finishing steps of beer and ale production. These enzymes reduce the size of the proteins extracted from the malt and grains. The smaller particle size results in a clearer beverage. It also prevents the liquid from forming an undesirable haze or clouding during cooling.

Another commercial use of proteases is in the baking industry. Doughs that have proteases added do not need as much mixing. These doughs are also more pliable, easier to use in mass production machinery, and will have a larger loaf volume. The proteases hydrolyze the gluten, enabling the dough to rise higher. Reducing the elasticity of the gluten also results in a softer texture.

Proteases can be used to change a food into a different product. An example of this is the use of rennin in milk to make cheese. In the early days of cheese production, rennin was obtained from the stomach linings of animals such as calves. However, the rennin used in most cheese factories today is manufactured. The enzymatic action of the rennin causes the proteins in milk to coagulate or clot. The liquid that separates from the cheese curds is called *whey*. Whey has an unpleasant flavor due to the high concentration of lactose. Lactase may be added to the whey to improve its flavor. With new technology, the lactose is usually separated from the whey mechanically.

> ## Cooking Tip
> **Gelatin is a protein. Gelatin salads often have fresh fruit added during the gelling process. Fruits that contain proteases, such as pineapple and papaya, will keep the gelatin from forming a gel. Heating these fruits before adding them to gelatin will denature the enzymes and allow the gelatin to set.**

Controlling Enzymatic Reactions

In some cases, whether the work of enzymes is positive or negative is a matter of degree. For example, enzymes that break down pectin help ripen a fruit so its texture is soft and its flavor sweet. If the enzymes are not stopped, however, the fruit will eventually become mushy. The continued breakdown allows oxygen, mold, and bacteria to enter the fruit and cause spoilage.

Enzymes are a factor food processors have to consider when determining how to best preserve food for future use. For instance, researchers look for ways to inhibit enzyme reactions once fruits and vegetables are ripe. The researchers want to reduce waste and increase the shelf life of the produce. Their goal is to slow spoilage and make a wider variety of foods available.

Produce handlers control some enzymatic reactions by storing fruits in an oxygen-free environment before sending them to market. Oxygen in the storage facility may be replaced by carbon dioxide or nitrogen. This prevents deterioration of produce caused by oxidases. *Oxidases* are enzymes that react only in the presence of oxygen. These enzymes cause darkening or browning on cut or bruised surfaces of many fruits and vegetables. The enzyme reactions involved in ripening can continue once exposed to oxygen.

Enzymatic Browning

When sliced apples and pears sit out, they begin to turn brown. White grapes that are left in the sun to dry turn into dark brown raisins. These are both examples of enzymatic browning. *Enzymatic browning* occurs when the enzyme polyphenol oxidase (phenolase) reacts with oxygen. This chemical reaction produces brown pigments called *melanins*.

The results of enzymatic browning may or may not be desirable. Enzymatic browning causes desirable color changes in the production of raisins, figs, and dates. However, many delicate fruits, such as apples, peaches, and pears, can be destroyed. Bruising or injury to fruits that contain phenolase allows oxygen to reach the enzyme. This sets off the enzymatic reaction, which is one step in the spoiling process. Besides creating color changes, the reaction creates structural changes that cause the produce to become mushy.

Enzymatic browning can be controlled by preventing oxygen from reaching the phenolase or by denaturing the enzyme. This browning process occurs most rapidly at room temperature when the pH is between 5 and 7. Most delicate fruits are kept in cold storage after sorting. This slows any enzymatic browning that might result from bruising or injury during harvest.

There are several substances that the food industry uses to help prevent browning of cut fruit. They are sulfites, ascorbic acid

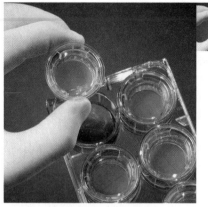

Recent Research
Enzyme-Producing Gene

Sato and Theologis are researchers with the United States Department of Agriculture (USDA). They work at the Agricultural Research Service (ARS) lab in

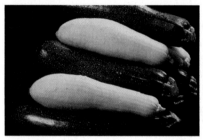

USDA

Research with zucchini may lead to the manufacture of an enzyme that produces ethylene. Ethylene, which has a broad range of uses, is currently made from limited petroleum resources.

California. They have isolated and cloned a gene in zucchini that produces the enzyme ACC synthase. This enzyme stimulates the production of ethylene (C_2H_4). Ethylene is a hormone in plants that triggers the ripening process.

According to estimates, almost half of all produce harvested in the United States each year is lost to spoilage. Gene technology could be used to develop a way to block ACC synthase from working until produce arrives in stores. Produce could then be placed in an ethylene chamber to trigger the ripening process. The goal would be to reduce waste and stabilize fresh produce prices for the consumer.

Some produce that is shipped long distances is already stored

in a controlled atmosphere to slow ripening. When it reaches warehouses near the point of sale, it is exposed to C_2H_4 to complete the ripening process.

A second use of Sato and Theologis's research would be to develop bacteria that contained the ACC synthase gene. Ethylene could then be biologically produced at a lower cost than present sources. Currently, more than 50 million pounds of C_2H_4 are produced each year from petroleum. Besides food applications, C_2H_4 is used to make plastics, antifreeze, and high-tech fibers. The importance of such research is great when you look at the shrinking reserves of petroleum.

(vitamin C), citric acid, and acetic acid. *Sulfites* or sulfite ions (usually added as sodium bisulfite) inhibit or prevent the melanin pigments from forming. These sulfiting agents are classified as preservatives. Sulfites will be discussed in more detail in Chapter 16.

Ascorbic acid acts as an enzyme inhibitor. The oxygen will react with the ascorbic acid before it will react with phenolase. Browning cannot occur until the oxygen has reacted with all the ascorbic acid.

Citric and acetic acids slow the enzymatic browning by changing the pH. If the pH is lowered to below 3.0, the phenolase is denatured. Citric acid will also tie up copper ions that act as coenzymes to speed up enzymatic browning. The presence of either iron or copper can increase the rate of browning. This is why you should avoid slicing fruit with a rusty knife or storing cut fruit in copper bowls. Use a knife with a stainless steel blade to cut fruit. If you are using a knife with a steel blade, be sure to clean it before cutting fruit. Avoid using copper bowls and cast iron skillets and pots when enzymatic browning is a problem.

Researchers are working to develop compounds from other sources, such as soy, that will inhibit browning of cut fruit. See 12-11. USDA researchers have found two new compounds that inhibit enzymatic browning. The first, ascorbic acid-2-phosphates, is related to vitamin C but is more stable. Like ascorbic acid, this compound will prevent oxygen from reacting with phenolase. As long as the compound is present, enzymatic browning will not occur.

The second new compound that inhibits enzymatic browning is a cyclodextrin. This compound works as an enzyme inhibitor by tying up the substrate. Cyclodextrins are shaped like donuts. The inside is nonpolar like the substrates that are responsible for the browning action. When the cyclodextrins are present, the substrate slides into the "donut holes." The substrate can then be filtered out of the solution. Cyclodextrins, which are already mass-produced, provide an economical way to make clear apple juice that resists browning indefinitely.

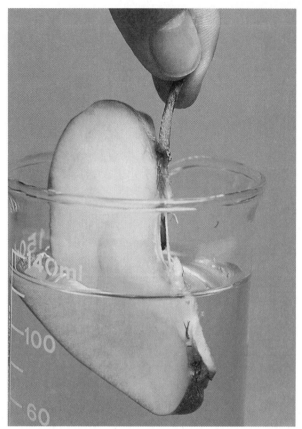

USDA

12-11 This apple is being dipped in a soy protein solution to protect it from enzymatic browning.

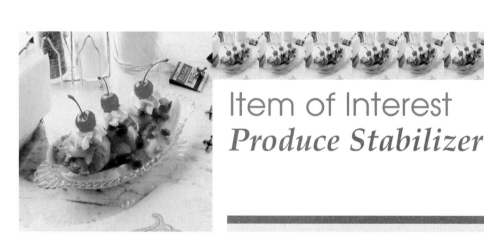

Item of Interest
Produce Stabilizer

Astaris LLC has a produce stabilizer on the market called Snow Fresh® that is a blend of sodium acid pyrophosphate (SAPP), calcium chloride, ascorbic acid, and citric acid. This product carries GRAS status and is sulfite free. Snow Fresh is tasteless and odorless and dissolves in water. Most freshly cut produce when dipped in a 1% concentration of Snow Fresh for three minutes, sealed, and then chilled, will maintain its color, texture, and quality for a minimum of five days. Potatoes and pears require a 4.5% solution. The SAPP binds trace metals to prevent discoloration. The calcium chloride slows enzyme activity and helps to maintain the crisp texture by preventing release of moisture from the surface.

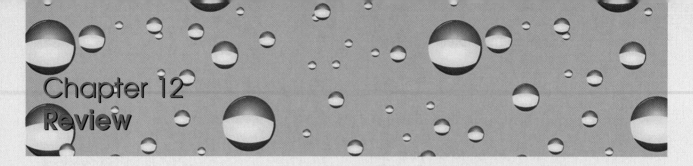

Chapter 12 Review

Summary

Enzymes are an important group of proteins in understanding food production, processing, and preservation. They initiate numerous chemical reactions, but are never used up. They remain free to act again repeatedly. Enzymes enable many chemical reactions to occur at lower temperatures than would be needed if the enzymes were not present.

Scientists use two models to understand how enzymes work. The lock-and-key model illustrates how the enzyme, active site, and substrate work together. The induced-fit model provides an updated explanation of the reaction. Sometimes an enzyme needs a helper, called a coenzyme, to start a chemical reaction.

Enzymes are added to foods to develop new products. An example of a new product is the development of a margarine component from beef fat. Enzymes are also added to help extract food components or change the quality of products. Meat tenderizers, for example, change the texture of meat to make it easier to chew.

Controlling enzyme activity in food processing is absolutely necessary. Control is accomplished by adjusting factors that affect enzyme activity—water availability, concentration of the enzyme or substrate, temperature, pH, and electrolytes. These factors can slow or stop enzyme activity by changing the enzyme's shape or by interfering with the enzyme reaction. Enzyme inhibitors also act as control agents by reacting with either the substrate or enzyme before the reaction can occur.

Inhibitors can be used to slow or stop the food spoilage caused by enzyme reactions. Enzymatic browning is one such cause. Enzymatic browning requires oxygen, but several substances will help prevent oxygen from triggering the enzymatic browning process.

Check Your Understanding

1. How are enzymes and activation energy related?
2. Describe the induced-fit model of enzyme reactions.
3. List three ways coenzymes work.
4. What is the method used for naming enzymes?
5. Name one of the fastest enzymes in the body, the substrate it breaks down, and the resulting products.
6. How can enzyme activity be stopped?
7. Why are vegetables blanched before freezing?
8. Name three foods that naturally contain enzyme inhibitors.
9. List three ways enzymes are used in food production.
10. List three important enzymes used in food production to break down carbohydrates.
11. Name three popular proteases used as meat tenderizers and identify their sources.
12. What causes enzymatic browning?
13. List four substances that can be used to prevent enzymatic browning.

Critical Thinking

1. Predict the effects of lipase on celery.
2. Identify three ways you could prevent a fruit salad of apples, bananas, and pears from turning brown.
3. What is the principle reason that a box of nonfat dry milk remains unspoiled much longer than a gallon of fat free milk?
4. Explain why protein-free fruits like pineapple, papaya, and figs contain proteases.

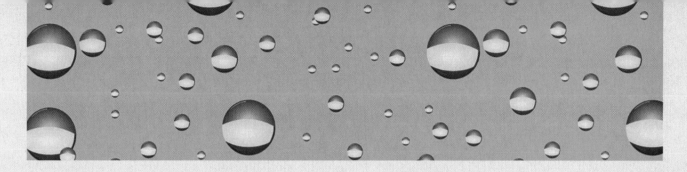

5. Which of the following shiny new coins would promote enzymatic browning: a quarter, dime, or penny? Explain your answer.

Explore Further

1. **Reading.** Research the parts of the body that produce digestive enzymes, the names of the enzymes produced, the location of each enzyme's work, and the ideal pH range for each.

2. **Writing.** Write an article for your school newspaper on the problems associated with lactose intolerance, the benefits of lactase, and some food products that contain the enzyme.

3. **Food and Nutrition.** Develop a meat recipe that takes advantage of naturally occurring proteases as tenderizers.

Experiment 12A
Catalase in Potatoes

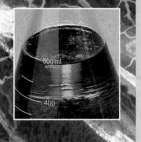

Safety

❖ **Wear safety glasses when heating beakers.**

❖ **Use beaker tongs to move hot glassware.**

❖ **Do not taste the potatoes.**

Purpose

Potatoes are a food that is high in the enzyme catalase. Catalase is one of the more heat-resistant enzymes in vegetables. However, it can be inactivated if temperatures are sufficiently high. If catalase has been inactivated in a vegetable, most other enzymes in the vegetable would also have been inactivated. This includes the enzymes that cause enzymatic browning. In this experiment, you will determine the temperature required to inactivate catalase in potatoes.

Equipment

wax pencil
7 50-mL beakers, custard cups, or paper cups
vegetable peeler
utility knife
100-mL graduated cylinder
blender or food processor
10-mL graduated cylinder
400-mL beaker
thermometer

Supplies

1 medium potato
100 mL water
35 mL hydrogen peroxide

Procedure

1. Use a wax pencil to label seven small containers as follows: *uncooked, 30°C, 35°C, 40°C, 45°C, 50°C,* and *55°C.*

2. Wash, peel, and quarter a medium potato.

3. Place the potato and 100 mL of water in a blender or food processor with a knife blade. Process until the potato is in tiny chunks.

4. Place 25 to 30 mL of the potato mixture in the small container labeled *uncooked.*

5. Pour 5 mL of hydrogen peroxide over the uncooked potato mixture. Record your observations.

6. Pour the remainder of the potato mixture into a 400-mL beaker. Insert a thermometer into the mixture and place over medium heat.

7. Heat the potato mixture until the temperature reaches 30°C. Pour 25 to 30 mL of the heated potato mixture into the appropriate small container.

8. Pour 5 mL of hydrogen peroxide over the heated potato mixture. Record your observations.

9. Repeat steps 7 and 8 five times, increasing the temperature of the potato mixture by 5°C each time. Note the point at which there is no visible reaction when the hydrogen peroxide is added.

Lab Extension

How would you determine how long 2- to 3-cm cubes of potatoes should be blanched in boiling water? Test your procedure.

Questions

1. What happened to the potato mixture that was not heated?

2. How did you determine when the catalase was inactivated?

3. What changes, if any, occurred to the first couple potato mixtures after heating?

4. How would you determine the exact temperature at which catalase is inactivated?

Experiment 12B
Enzymatic Browning

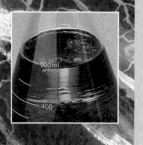

Purpose

Enzymes act as catalysts that trigger chemical reactions. In food production, this can be beneficial or harmful, depending on the enzyme and the food product. For example, the enzyme rennin is used to curdle milk for cheese production. In this experiment, you will look at polyphenol oxidase. This is the enzyme that causes enzymatic browning in many fruits and vegetables. You will examine five methods to determine how effectively they will inactivate the enzyme.

Equipment

wax pencil

5 small beakers or dishes

paring knife

tongs or spoon

cutting board

Supplies

assigned fruit or vegetable

25 mL ascorbic acid solution

25 mL lemon juice

25 mL white vinegar

25 mL sugar solution

25 mL water

paper towel or plate

Procedure

1. Use a wax pencil to label five small beakers or dishes as follows: *ascorbic acid, lemon juice, vinegar, sugar,* and *water.*

2. Fill each beaker with 25 mL of the appropriate solution.

3. Cut your assigned fruit or vegetable into six pieces of equal size.

   Variation 1: apple

   Variation 2: banana

   Variation 3: peach

   Variation 4: pear

   Variation 5: potato

   Variation 6: turnip

4. Place one fruit or vegetable piece into each solution so it is completely covered. Let the samples soak three minutes.

5. While the samples are soaking, use a pen or marker to divide a paper towel or plate into six segments. Label the first segment *control* and place the sixth fruit or vegetable piece in that segment. Label the other five segments with the names of the five solutions.

6. After the samples have soaked three minutes, remove them from the solutions and place them in the appropriate segments of the paper towel or plate.

7. Note the extent of browning on the surface of each sample after 5, 10, and 20 minutes. Record your observations in a data table. Also make observations of the samples from each of the other lab groups.

Questions

1. What was the purpose of the various solutions?

2. Which solution did the best job of preventing enzymatic browning?

3. When might each of these solutions be used in food preparation?

Experiment 12C
Proteolytic Enzymes in Fruit

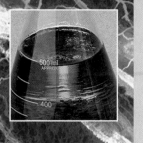

Purpose

Proteolytic enzymes trigger the chemical reactions that hydrolyze proteins into amino acids. Many of these enzymes are found in fruits. For instance, papain, the enzyme in many meat tenderizers, is found in the tropical fruit papaya. Ficin is produced by fruits in the fig family. Bromelain is found in pineapple. In this experiment, you will examine the effects of proteolytic enzymes from papayas, figs, and pineapple on the protein in unflavored gelatin.

Equipment

glass mixing bowl

100-mL graduated cylinder

large spoon

4 petri dishes

cutting board

paring knife

2 saucers

glass rod

wax pencil

2 50-mL beakers

50-mL dry measuring cup

Supplies

1 package unflavored gelatin

120 mL water

figs, papaya, or pineapple

meat tenderizer

Procedure

Part I

1. In a glass mixing bowl, combine one package of unflavored gelatin with 60 mL of water. Stir 1 minute with a large spoon.

2. Heat the gelatin mixture in a microwave oven on high power for 40 seconds. Stir for 1 to 2 minutes or until all the gelatin is dissolved.

3. Add 60 mL cool water.

4. Fill each of four petri dishes half full of the gelatin mixture and chill in the freezer until the gel sets. This will take about 20 minutes. Set aside the remaining gelatin for use in Part II.

5. Cut two thin slices from the assigned fruit. Microwave one slice on a saucer for 1 minute. Let it cool to room temperature.

6. When the petri dishes have gelled, prepare them as follows:

   Dish 1: Control.

   Dish 2: Sprinkle the gelatin with meat tenderizer.

   Dish 3: Lay the slice of uncooked fruit on top of the gelatin.

   Dish 4: Lay the cooled cooked fruit on top of the gelatin.

7. Observe the gelatin in each petri dish after 5 minutes and again after 10 minutes. Note any changes in the gelatin. Gently poke the gelatin with a glass rod. Record your observations in a data table.

Part II

1. Use a wax pencil to label a 50-mL beaker *uncooked*. Label a second beaker *cooked*. Divide the gelatin mixture remaining from Part I equally into the two beakers.

2. Finely chop 50 mL of the assigned fruit.

3. Stir half of the chopped fruit into the beaker labeled *uncooked*.

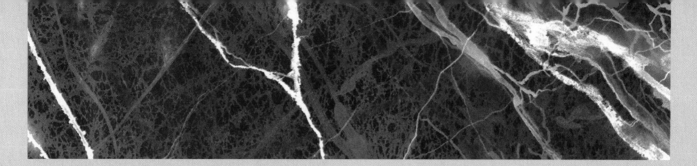

4. Place the remaining half of the chopped fruit on a saucer and heat in the microwave oven for 1 minute or until steaming hot. Stir the hot fruit into the second beaker.

5. Place both beakers in the refrigerator.

6. Remove the beakers from the refrigerator after 20 minutes and note any changes in the thickness of the gelatin. Record your observations in a data table.

7. Return the beakers to the refrigerator overnight. Check them again during the next class period. Record your observations.

Questions

1. What effect did the meat tenderizer have on the gelatin in the petri dish?

2. What effect, if any, did the raw fruit have on the gelatin in the petri dish? What effect, if any, did the raw fruit have on the gelatin in the beaker chilled overnight?

3. Was there a difference in the way the cooked fruit reacted with the gelatin in the petri dish? Was there a difference in the way the cooked fruit reacted with the gelatin in the beaker?

4. What similarities did you observe between the gelatin with fruit added and the gelatin sprinkled with meat tenderizer?

5. What recommendations can you make about adding fruit to gelatin salads?

6. What recommendations can you make regarding the use of meat tenderizers before and during cooking and grilling?

You have already read about the molecular properties of several nutrients found in foods. In Unit II, you learned about the first and most abundant nutrient—water. In Unit III, you examined three other major categories of nutrients—carbohydrates, fats, and proteins. Together, these four categories of nutrients make up most of the mass of all food products.

The two other groups of nutrients—vitamins and minerals—are found in foods in small amounts. However, they are very important for good health and normal development. In Chapter 13, you will study vitamins and minerals and their roles in food quality.

Some compounds in foods do not fit into any of the six categories of nutrients. These compounds are called phytochemicals. They have only recently received attention as to their possible nutritive value. You will read about phytochemicals in Chapter 14.

Chapter 15 examines a group of compounds called food analogs. These compounds are developed by food scientists to provide the appearance, flavor, and texture of naturally occurring substances. Chapter 15 looks at analogs commonly used in place of sugars, fats, and salts.

Another group of substances found in foods is additives. These are substances that are not normally found in foods. However, they are added to improve the characteristics of food products. Many additives affect the nutritive value of foods. Chapter 16 explores this last group of compounds, which is commonly found in processed foods.

This photomicrograph shows phenethyl isothiocyanate. It is one of a group of compounds called phytochemicals, which are found in plant foods and are active in the body.

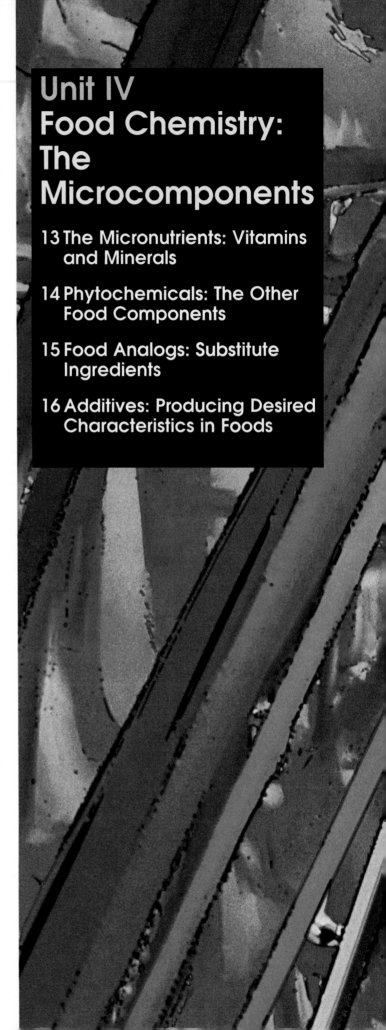

Unit IV
Food Chemistry: The Microcomponents

13 The Micronutrients: Vitamins and Minerals

14 Phytochemicals: The Other Food Components

15 Food Analogs: Substitute Ingredients

16 Additives: Producing Desired Characteristics in Foods

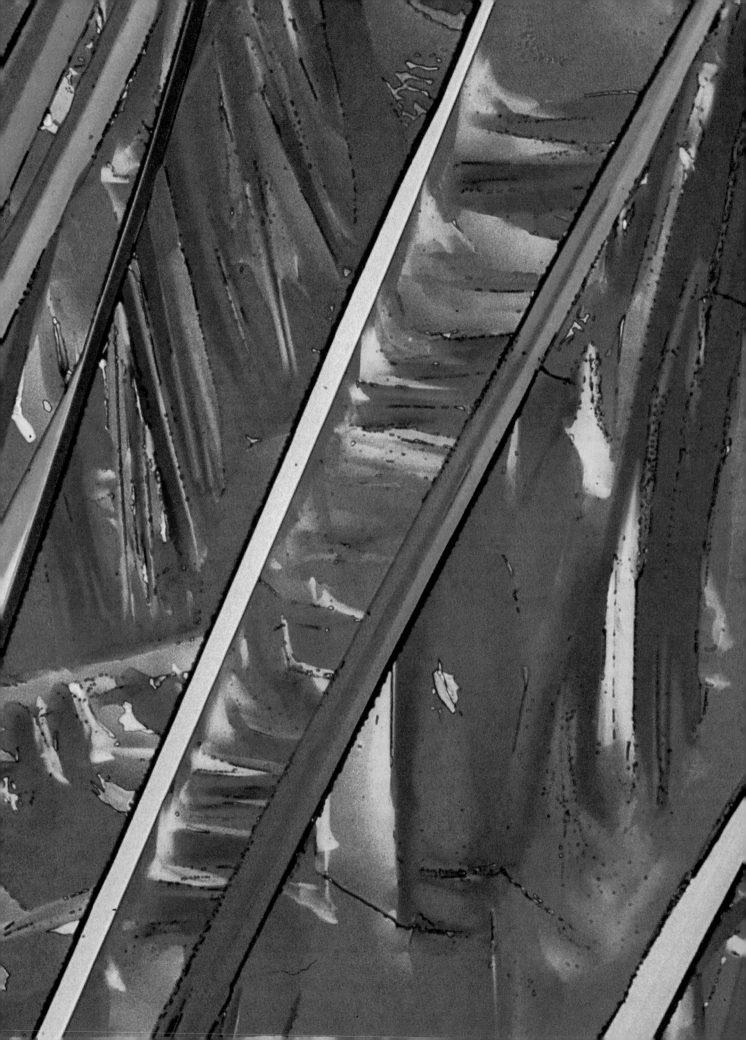

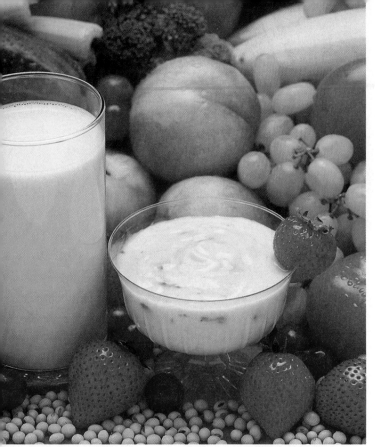

Agricultural Research Service, USDA

Vitamins and minerals are abundant in fresh foods.

Chapter 13

The Micronutrients: Vitamins and Minerals

Objectives

After studying this chapter,
you will be able to

differentiate between fat-soluble vitamins and water-soluble vitamins.

list functions and sources of major minerals and trace minerals.

explain the impact food processing and preservation methods have on the nutritive value of food.

identify non-nutritive functions of vitamins and minerals used as additives in food products.

describe how to reduce vitamin and mineral losses during home food storage and preparation.

Key Terms

vitamins

fat-soluble vitamins

water-soluble
   vitamins

retinol

precursors

beta-carotene
   (β-carotene)

major minerals

trace minerals

enrichment

fortification

fortificant

food vehicle

bioavailability

When food is processed, packaged, and preserved, changes occur. Many of the changes make food easier to eat or enable the food to be stored for later use. Sometimes the changes damage the nutrients found in the food. To protect these valuable nutrients, food scientists must know what nutrients are present and how the body uses them. Food scientists must also know what happens to nutrients in processing and how they interact in mixtures.

This chapter will look at the properties of vitamins and minerals. Most knowledge of these nutrients has come from research conducted in the last 50 years. There is so much information that it is impossible to cover it all in one chapter. You will, however, be able to examine the general characteristics of each category of vitamins and minerals. You will also study how these characteristics can affect the quality of food.

Vitamins

Vitamins are organic compounds that are needed in small amounts in the diet. They are not sources of energy. Vitamins help regulate body processes. They are necessary to maintain health. The main role of vitamins is to work as components in enzyme systems. When vitamins are missing from the diet, enzyme reactions are slowed or stopped and body processes are impaired.

Vitamins are needed in such small amounts that it took a long time for scientists to isolate and identify them. The first vitamin to be identified was vitamin A in 1915. Between 1915 and 1950, scientists isolated and identified 12 more vitamins.

As vitamins were discovered, they were given names. Many were also given letters. As different chemical forms of some vitamins were discovered, numbers were used with the letters to identify vitamins. For example, vitamin B_1 is also called thiamin.

Vitamins fall into two main categories: those that dissolve in water and those that dissolve in fat. *Fat-soluble vitamins* have a nonpolar molecular structure and dissolve in fats and oils. *Water-soluble vitamins* have a polar molecular structure and dissolve in water and water-based liquids.

Fat-Soluble Vitamins

Vitamins A, D, E, and K are fat soluble. These vitamins are generally found in the fats and oils in foods. They require bile from the liver for digestion. Fat-soluble vitamins, once absorbed by the body, cannot be easily excreted. Any excesses are stored in the liver or fatty tissues for future use. The body can easily survive for weeks without foods containing these vitamins if there are surpluses stored. The ability to store fat-soluble vitamins has a negative side. Large doses of these vitamins can build up in the body to poisonous levels. See 13-1.

Vitamin A

Vitamin A has a large number of roles in the body. One of the first functions identified is aiding in night vision. Vitamin A must be present in the retina. Otherwise, the cells at the back of the eye cannot react when stimulated by light. Vitamin A is involved in maintaining healthy skin and the internal linings of the lungs and digestive tract. The body needs vitamin A to ensure proper function of the immune system and production and regulation of hormones. Growing children need vitamin A to break down formed bone. This allows for the reshaping and forming of larger new bone tissue as growth occurs. Vitamin A works in conjunction with folic acid, protein, and iron to form red blood cells. Research indicates there may also be a link between vitamin A and the risk of skin, lung, and bladder cancers.

Vitamin A is found in two basic forms in foods. The first, *retinol,* is the active form of vitamin A needed for use by the human body. It is yellow and is found in foods from animal sources, such as liver, butter, egg yolks, milk, and cheese. Retinol is just one of a group of related compounds called *retinoids* or *preformed* vitamin A.

The second form of vitamin A found in foods is a precursor. *Precursors,* which are also called *provitamins,* are chemical compounds the body changes into the active forms of vitamins. The precursor for retinol is *beta-carotene (β-carotene).* When beta-carotene is converted to retinol, losses occur. It takes about three units of beta-carotene to make one unit of retinol. Beta-carotene is bright orange and is found in foods from plant sources. Plant foods high in beta-carotene can usually be identified by their color. Bright orange foods high in beta-carotene are carrots, sweet potatoes, pumpkins, cantaloupe, and apricots. Carotene and chlorophyll combine in other foods to create a dark green color. Dark

Fat-Soluble Vitamins

Vitamin and Chemical Names	Sources	Functions
A (Retinol)	Butter, cheese, cream, eggs, fortified milk, liver	❖ Aids in night vision ❖ Maintains skin and mucous membranes ❖ Promotes bone and tooth growth ❖ Aids in reproduction ❖ Helps synthesize and regulate hormones ❖ Protects against some forms of cancer
Beta-carotene	Apricots, broccoli, cantaloupe, carrots, collard greens, kale, pumpkin, spinach, squash, sweet potatoes, tomatoes	
D (Calciferol)	Eggs, fortified milk and margarine, liver, sardines	❖ Aids in bone formation ❖ Increases absorption of calcium and phosphorus
Cholesterol (body's precursor)	Synthesized when exposed to sunlight	
E (Tocopherol)	Leafy green vegetables, margarine, nuts, plant oils, salad dressings, seeds, wheat germ, whole grain products	❖ Serves as an antioxidant ❖ Protects vitamin A ❖ Stabilizes cell membranes ❖ Regulates oxidation reactions
K (Phylloquinone)	Cabbage, leafy green vegetables, liver, milk Produced by bacteria in intestines	❖ Aids in the blood-clotting process

13-1 Excess fat-soluble vitamins are stored by the body.

green foods that are good vitamin A sources include spinach, collard greens, kale, and broccoli. See 13-2.

Vitamin D

Vitamin D is unique in that the body can make all it needs. When the skin is exposed to sunlight, a cholesterol compound in the skin is changed to a vitamin D precursor. The precursor is absorbed and turned into vitamin D by the liver and kidneys. The body will only convert the precursor to vitamin D as needed.

Vitamin D teams with other nutrients, including calcium, to maintain blood calcium levels and to develop bones and teeth. Vitamin D must be present to make calcium available to form bone. A similar but slower process involves vitamin D in the formation of teeth.

The few foods that naturally contain vitamin D are butter, cream, egg yolks, and liver. Because of the teamwork between vitamin D, phosphorus, and calcium, vitamin D is added

to milk in the United States. This helps the many people who do not get enough exposure to the sun to meet their vitamin D needs.

Vitamin E

Many food components and body tissues are permanently damaged by oxidation. Oxidation is the chemical reaction between oxygen and other compounds. Vitamin E prevents oxidation by acting as an antioxidant in the body. It quickly reacts with oxygen, so the oxygen is no longer available to damage tissues.

Good sources of vitamin E are wheat germ oil, whole grains, green plants, nuts, and seeds. Vitamin E is not stable at high temperatures. Therefore, foods that are fried or highly processed have little vitamin E remaining.

Vitamin K

Vitamin K is necessary for the production of two proteins involved in blood clotting. Like vitamin D, some vitamin K is provided

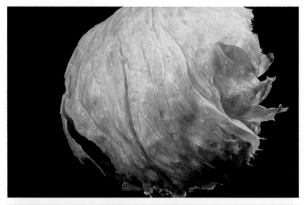

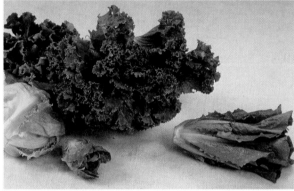

USDA

13-2 Although iceberg lettuce is popular in the United States, the light green color indicates it is low in vitamin A. Dark leafy greens are much richer sources of this vitamin.

from a nonfood source. Certain bacteria that normally live in the intestines produce vitamin K as a waste product. Recent studies indicate the bacteria in your intestines meet half of your vitamin K needs. The other half comes mainly from dark green leafy vegetables.

Health Tip

Many antibiotics will destroy the bacteria in your intestines that help meet your body's need for vitamin K. You can reduce the risk of a vitamin K deficiency by adding yogurt with active cultures to your diet. Yogurt with active cultures contains some of the bacteria that produce vitamin K. Wait until several days after completing the antibiotics prescribed before eating the yogurt.

Water-Soluble Vitamins

The B vitamins and vitamin C are water soluble. Because these vitamins are water soluble, most excesses leave the body in the urine. It is not possible to receive toxic doses of water-soluble vitamins from the food you eat. See 13-3.

The B-Complex Vitamin Group

Most B vitamins act as coenzymes in reactions all over the body. B vitamins are involved in the production of new cells, including red blood cells. They are also involved in releasing energy, making genetic material in the cells, and building proteins.

The vitamins in the B-complex group are found in whole grains, molasses, organ meats, and brewer's yeast. See 13-4. Vitamin B_1, *thiamin*, is also found in nuts, egg yolks, legumes, pork, poultry, and fish. Vitamin B_2, *riboflavin*, is found in dairy products, egg yolks, and nuts. Beans, green vegetables, rice bran, nuts, fish, dairy products, poultry, lean meats, and milk are good sources of *niacin*. The chemical name for vitamin B_6 is *pyridoxine*. Good vegetable sources of pyridoxine include cabbage, cantaloupe, legumes, peas, prunes, and leafy green vegetables. Animal sources of vitamin B_6 include beef liver and chicken. Vitamin B_{12}, *cobalamin*, is found in dairy products, eggs, and fish. *Folate* is found in leafy green vegetables, chicken liver, and legumes. It is also added to breads, cereals, pasta, and rice. Folate helps lower homocysteine levels, a blood component that contributes to clogged arteries. Egg yolks, orange juice, legumes, mushrooms, and salmon are good sources of *pantothenic acid.* B vitamins are absorbed better and work best when taken together.

Vitamin C

Vitamin C is also called ascorbic acid. Vitamin C helps to produce the connective tissue collagen and protect the body against infections. Vitamin C helps the body absorb iron. During times of stress, vitamin C assists in the release of adrenaline. Ascorbic acid is needed for the series of chemical reactions involved in the formation of bones and teeth.

Vitamin C also works as an antioxidant in the same way as vitamin E. Ascorbic acid will react with oxygen before many other compounds will react. This prevents these other

Water-Soluble Vitamins

Vitamin and/or Chemical Name	Sources	Functions
B_1 (Thiamin)	Bacon, ham, legumes, liver, nuts, pork, whole grains	❖ Serves as part of a coenzyme in energy metabolism ❖ Helps maintain appetite ❖ Supports nervous system
B_2 (Riboflavin)	Cottage cheese, leafy green vegetables, meat, milk, whole grain and enriched breads and cereals, yogurt	❖ Serves as part of a coenzyme in energy metabolism ❖ Supports normal vision ❖ Supports skin health
B_3 (Niacin) Precursor: dietary tryptophan	Eggs, fish, meat, milk, nuts, poultry, whole grain and enriched breads and cereals	❖ Serves as part of a coenzyme in energy metabolism ❖ Supports skin health ❖ Supports nervous system ❖ Supports digestive system
B_6 (Pyridoxine)	Fish, fruits, leafy green vegetables, legumes, meats, poultry, shellfish, whole grains	❖ Serves as part of a coenzyme in protein and fat metabolism ❖ Helps convert tryptophan to niacin ❖ Aids in red blood cell formation
Folate, folic acid, folacin	Leafy green vegetables, legumes, liver, meats, seeds	❖ Serves as part of a coenzyme in new cell formation
B_{12} (Cyanocobalamin)	Cheese, eggs, fish, meat, milk, poultry, shellfish	❖ Serves as part of a coenzyme in new cell synthesis ❖ Helps maintain nerve cells
Pantothenic acid	Widespread in food	❖ Serves as part of a coenzyme in new cell synthesis ❖ Helps maintain nerve cells
Biotin	Widespread in food	❖ Serves as part of a coenzyme in energy and protein metabolism ❖ Serves as part of a coenzyme in fat and glycogen synthesis
C (Ascorbic acid)	Cabbage, cantaloupe, citrus fruits, dark green vegetables, mangos, papayas, peppers, potatoes, strawberries, tomatoes	❖ Aids in collagen synthesis ❖ Serves as an antioxidant ❖ Aids in resistance to infection ❖ Aids in iron absorption ❖ Aids in amino acid metabolism

13-3 You need to consume good sources of water-soluble vitamins daily.

compounds from being destroyed by oxidation. As long as there is ascorbic acid present, body tissue is protected from excessive exposure to oxygen.

Because vitamin C is water soluble and easily oxidized, it needs to be replaced in the body daily. Many fresh fruits and vegetables are high in vitamin C. Some of the best sources are citrus, kiwi, strawberries, tomatoes, cabbage, spinach, bell pepper, and broccoli.

Choline

Even though people can synthesize choline in small amounts, it must be consumed in the diet to maintain good health. In 1998 choline, a

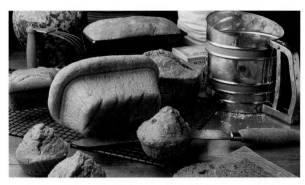

13-4 Breads made with whole grains or enriched flour are good sources of many of the B vitamins.

bioactive compound, was added to the essential nutrient list and assigned recommended intakes.

Choline is categorized as a phospholipid. It is part of cell membranes and the myelin sheath that coats nerve fibers. A choline compound is an important neurotransmitter and necessary for lipoprotein production in the liver. Choline deficiencies can cause liver damage, impair memory, and alter the development of nervous tissue in fetal development. Sources of choline include liver, eggs, steak, cauliflower, lettuce, and peanuts.

Minerals

Minerals have the simplest chemical structure of any group of nutrients. This is because minerals are elements. Minerals make up about 2.3 kg of the average adult's mass. Registered dietitians divide minerals into two categories: major minerals and trace minerals.

Major Minerals

Major minerals are needed in the diet in amounts of 100 mg or more each day. They include calcium, phosphorus, potassium, sulfur, chloride, and magnesium. See 13-5.

Calcium and Phosphorus

About 99% of the body's calcium is found in bones and teeth. The remaining 1% plays major roles in the body. Calcium (Ca) regulates the movement of ions across cell membranes. It is important in the sending of messages along nerve fibers. Calcium helps maintain the body's blood pressure. It must be present before muscles, including the heart muscle, can contract and then relax. Calcium is also a catalyst in one of the steps of the blood clotting process.

Milk is considered the best source of calcium. One glass of milk or 250 mL (1 cup) of yogurt contains about 300 mg of calcium. A similar amount of calcium is contained in 500 mL (2 cups) of cottage cheese or 42 g (1.5 ounces) of cheese. Sardines and canned salmon are high in calcium because they contain edible bones. Good vegetable sources are broccoli, collards, kale, mustard greens, watercress, parsley, and seaweed.

Although most of the body's phosphorus (Ph) is in bone tissue, it plays other roles that are critical to life. Phosphorus works as a salt buffer in the body's acid-base balance. It functions as part of the genetic material of every cell. Phosphorous is found in compounds that extract energy from nutrients. It also works with lipids to form cell membranes.

Fortunately, phosphorus is found in most foods, including most soft drinks. Deficiencies are not known to occur.

> ### Cooking Tip
> A good source of calcium is soup stocks made from cracked meat or poultry bones. This stock can contain as much as 100 mg of calcium per tablespoon. The bones are soaked in vinegar and then boiled. The acetic acid in the vinegar draws the calcium from the bones into the broth. The boiling removes most of the vinegar flavor.

Sodium, Potassium, and Chloride

Sodium (Na^+) and chloride (Cl^-) are the main positive and negative ions in maintaining the body's fluid balance. Sodium is the primary mineral in sweat and, along with potassium, helps regulate body temperature. Chloride ions are used by the stomach to produce hydrochloric acid, which promotes the digestion of proteins.

Sodium is the main positively charged ion *outside* the cells. Potassium is the main positively charged ion *inside* the cells. Like sodium, potassium helps regulate the balance of fluid inside and outside cells. Potassium also plays a critical role in maintaining the heartbeat. Recent studies show that when in the form of potassium citrate, it helps to reduce bone loss and prevent kidney stones. Processing often affects the potassium content of foods. However, this mineral is found in all fresh foods, such as meats, milk, fruits, vegetables, and grains.

About 10% of the sodium in your diet occurs naturally in the foods you eat. The rest comes from salt (NaCl). Most people use some salt in cooking or at the table. However, about 75% of the salt in the average U.S. diet is found in processed foods. Besides being the major source of sodium, salt is the primary source of chloride in the diet. Chloride is found in some vegetables, too.

Researchers have found a link between high blood pressure and salt intake. It is not known whether sodium or chloride is the source of this link. High levels of salt have not been proven to cause high blood pressure. However, medical studies have shown that salt-sensitive people with high blood pressure

Major Minerals

Name and Chemical Symbol	Sources	Functions
Calcium (Ca)	Fish eaten with small bones, greens, legumes, milk, milk products, tofu	❖ Forms part of bones and teeth ❖ Acts in muscle contraction and relaxation ❖ Aids in blood clotting ❖ Helps maintain blood pressure and immune function
Chloride (Cl)	Processed foods, salt, soy sauce	❖ Serves as part of digestive acids in stomach
Magnesium (Mg)	Chocolate, cocoa, dark green vegetables, legumes, nuts, seafood, whole grains	❖ Aids in bone formation ❖ Helps in protein synthesis ❖ Plays a role in enzyme actions ❖ Helps muscles contract ❖ Aids in transmission of nerve impulses ❖ Aids in maintaining teeth
Phosphorus (Ph)	All animal tissue	❖ Forms parts of bones and teeth ❖ Forms part of cells' genetic material ❖ Forms part of cell membranes ❖ Aids in energy transfer ❖ Works in buffering systems
Potassium (K)	Fresh fruits, grains, legumes, meats, milk, and vegetables	❖ Aids in making protein ❖ Helps maintain fluid and electrolyte balance ❖ Assists in transmission of nerve impulses and contraction of muscles
Sodium (Na)	Processed foods, salt, soy sauce	❖ Helps maintain fluid balance in cells ❖ Aids in acid-base balance ❖ Aids in nerve impulse transmission ❖ Helps regulate body temperature through sweating
Sulfur (S)	All foods containing protein	❖ Becomes a component of some amino acids ❖ Becomes part of biotin and thiamin ❖ Becomes part of the hormone insulin ❖ Stabilizes shape of protein molecules

13-5 The major minerals are those needed by the body in larger amounts.

benefit from a low-salt diet. The estimated minimum requirement of sodium to maintain good health is 500 mg per day for adults. The recommended maximum intake is 6 g of salt or 2,400 mg of sodium. The average U.S. diet provides at least two to three times the estimated minimum requirement for sodium. See 13-6.

Magnesium and Sulfur

Magnesium is found in small amounts in the body. However, this small amount has many uses. Magnesium is involved in hundreds of enzymatic reactions. It is necessary

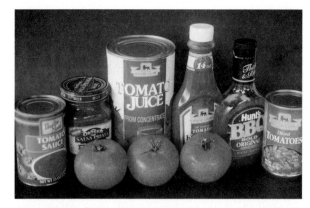

13-6 Although fresh tomatoes contain very little sodium, many processed tomato products provide large amounts of this mineral.

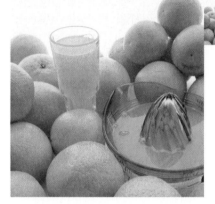

Nutrition News
Conserving Calcium

Calcium is one of the nutrients that is in short supply in many teen diets. Nutrition experts are concerned this may lead to an

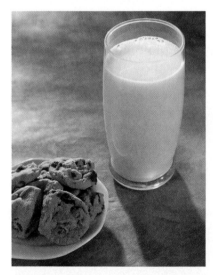

Choosing milk in place of or in addition to soft drinks can help boost calcium intake.

increase in osteoporosis in the future. If the diet does not provide enough calcium, the body will take the calcium it needs from the bones. If teens do not increase their calcium intakes through early adulthood, their bones may become less dense as they age. This could result in an increase in fractures and related complications.

Several factors may be contributing to a low calcium intake among teens. One factor is an increase in soft drink consumption. Many teens drink soft drinks instead of milk, which is rich in calcium. Soft drinks provide no calcium. However, many soft drinks contain phosphorus, which can inhibit calcium absorption when consumed in excess. Many soft drinks also contain caffeine. Caffeine increases the loss of calcium through urination.

Another factor may be contributing to a lack of calcium in

some teen diets. Teens who choose some nondairy sources of calcium may be disappointed to learn how little calcium these foods provide. Some foods, such as spinach and rhubarb, appear to be high in calcium but have little or no calcium availability. These foods contain compounds that bind the calcium so the body cannot absorb it. These foods are excellent sources of other nutrients, such as vitamin A, iron, and riboflavin. However, people cannot count them as sources of calcium.

Following a few simple tips can help teens increase their calcium intakes. Teens who drink soft drinks need to make a point of drinking milk, too. One glass of milk for every two soft drinks will help offset calcium losses. Other dairy foods, such as yogurt and some cheeses, are also rich in calcium.

for the use of vitamin D, potassium, and calcium. Magnesium must be available before energy can be released for muscle contractions. It is also used to help maintain the ability of nerves to send messages. Calcium and magnesium need to be balanced in a 2:1 ratio. It is best to distribute the dose throughout the day since the body excretes any excess. Legumes, whole grains, and dark green vegetables are all good sources of magnesium.

Sulfur has no major function of its own. However, it is an important part of protein molecules and other compounds. Sulfur is found in any protein-rich food.

Trace Minerals

Trace minerals are needed in the diet in amounts less than 100 mg per day. Trace minerals include iron, iodine, zinc, and fluoride. Very small amounts of boron, copper, manganese, chromium, and selenium are also needed by the body. Some minerals are present in such small amounts that researchers have had trouble studying the minerals' roles in nutrition. What researchers know is a result of carefully controlled diets in laboratory animals. Understanding about trace minerals is rapidly expanding and the need for trained researchers in this area is increasing.

Iron

Iron is an important element in the production of red blood cells. Iron is part of the protein in hemoglobin and myoglobin. *Hemoglobin* is the protein compound in red blood cells. The iron in hemoglobin holds oxygen and transports it from the lungs throughout the body. *Myoglobin* is the compound that holds oxygen in muscle tissue until it is needed.

Iron deficiency results in a condition called *anemia.* A lack of iron causes too little oxygen to be available for energy metabolism. An estimated 50% of all people in low-income inner city and rural areas suffer from mild iron deficiency. In the United States and Canada, 20% of women and 3% of men have no iron stores in their bodies. Early signs of iron deficiency include low energy levels, inability to concentrate, and irritability. Lack of iron poses the greatest risks for children, teens, and menstruating and pregnant women.

You need to know more than just good sources of iron. You also need to know factors that can hinder or help the absorption of iron. One cause of iron deficiency is poor absorption of the iron in the diet. A number of foods seem to interfere with the body's ability to absorb iron. These include tea, coffee, soy protein, wheat bran, and fiber. High doses of calcium also interfere with iron absorption.

Vitamin C helps the body absorb iron. Therefore, eating a hamburger with a slice of tomato will help the body absorb more iron from the hamburger. Legumes are high in iron, but they need the help of vitamin C to make the iron more absorbable. Adding tomatoes to red beans and rice increases the amount of iron the body will be able to absorb.

Another factor that can increase iron absorption is the kind of pan used. Some foods cooked in cast iron will increase in iron content by absorbing some iron from the cookware, 13-7.

Foods high in iron include meats, organ meats, and leafy green vegetables. Other iron-rich foods include asparagus, bananas, beans, broccoli, chard, dates, lentils, molasses, nuts, okra, peas, plums, prune juice, rice bran, squash, strawberries, and whole grains. Some sources of iron are easier for the body to absorb. The body seems able to absorb almost three times more of the iron available from meats than from vegetables. The color of a meat source indicates how much iron is present. Red meat contains more iron than white meats, such as fish and poultry.

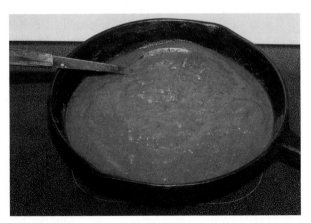

13-7 Cooking acidic foods, like spaghetti sauce, in cast iron pans can increase the iron content of the food from two to nine times.

Iodine

Iodine is needed for mainly one reason, the production of the hormone *thyroxine.* Thyroxine is responsible for regulating the body's use of energy. This hormone is produced by the thyroid gland, which is in the neck.

One of the best sources of iodine is seafood. This is because iodine is found in large amounts in the ocean. However, sea salt is not a good source. This is because the iodine becomes a gas and escapes during the process of separating the salt from the water. A readily available source of iodine is iodized salt. Iodine, like chloride, readily combines with sodium. An iodide salt added to sodium chloride has helped reduce iodine deficiency in the United States. Other sources of iodine are seaweed, kelp, and plants grown in iodine-rich soil.

Zinc

Zinc is necessary for the function of many enzymes. A number of these enzymes are involved in the body's use of carbohydrates and proteins. Zinc is necessary for wound healing and proper immune function.

Meat, fish, and poultry are the best sources of zinc. Nonmeat sources are some legumes and whole grains. Fair sources of zinc include milk, cheese, spinach, broccoli, and green peas.

Fluoride

Because of toothpaste commercials, you may know that fluoride (F⁻) is related to healthy teeth. Fluoride causes the crystals in bones and teeth to be larger and more regular in form. The result is stronger, healthier bones and teeth.

The main source of fluoride in many communities is the drinking water. Fluoride is commonly added at the rate of one part per million to public water supplies.

Other Trace Minerals

Many other trace minerals are found in your body and your diet. Research is constantly revealing new information about the ways these nutrients interact with one another. See 13-8. The following trace minerals are examples:

Boron. Boron, which is found in dark green leafy vegetables, has been found to help the body hold onto calcium.

Copper. Copper aids in the production of red blood cells and the use of iron. It has been noted that zinc and copper must be balanced for healthy heart tissue.

Manganese. Manganese seems to activate the enzymatic reactions involved in the breakdown of carbohydrates, proteins, and fats.

Chromium. Chromium is necessary for proper insulin action. When there is not enough chromium, diabetes-like symptoms occur.

Selenium. Selenium works with vitamin E to protect body tissue from oxidation. Selenium is widely distributed in meats and produce grown in selenium-rich soil.

Other trace minerals found in the body include aluminum, arsenic, barium, cadmium, lead, lithium, mercury, silver, tin, and vanadium. There is still much to learn about the roles of these minerals and their interaction with other nutrients. A nutritious diet will usually provide all the trace minerals needed for good health.

Health Tip

Drugs and nutrients are chemicals, and chemicals can and do interact. Drugs can interfere with the absorption of nutrients. Some nutrients can interfere with the function or absorption of drugs. This is true for both over-the-counter and prescription drugs. For example

❖ Antacids reduce absorption of iron and increase excretion of calcium.

❖ Antibiotics reduce absorption of calcium, magnesium, and zinc.

❖ Aspirin increases excretion of vitamin C, thiamin, and vitamin K.

❖ Caffeine increases excretion of calcium and magnesium.

❖ Laxatives reduce absorption of fat-soluble vitamins and calcium.

❖ Oral contraceptives reduce absorption of folic acid.

To prevent harmful interactions, carefully read labels for instructions on consumption of food with drugs. Ask your doctor or pharmacist about what foods, if any, should be avoided or increased with prescription drugs.

Trace Minerals

Name and Chemical Symbol	Sources	Functions
Chromium (Ch)	Whole grains	❖ Aids in proper insulin action ❖ Aids in hemoglobin production
Copper (Cu)	Chocolate, currants, dried legumes, liver, mushrooms, nuts, oysters	❖ Helps form hemoglobin and collagen ❖ Becomes part of many enzymes
Fluoride (Fl)	Fluoridated drinking water, seafood	❖ Aids in formation of bones and teeth
Iodine (I)	Iodized salt, seafood	❖ Becomes part of the thyroid hormone that regulates growth and metabolic rate
Iron (Fe)	Dried fruits, eggs, fish, legumes, poultry, red meat, shellfish	❖ Becomes part of hemoglobin, which carries oxygen throughout the body ❖ Becomes part of myoglobin, which moves oxygen into the cells
Manganese (Mn)	All animal tissue	❖ Activates enzymatic reactions in energy metabolism
Molybdenum (Mo)	Cooked spinach, strawberries, whole milk	❖ Activates several enzymes ❖ Aids in formation of blood, bone, and cartilage
Selenium (Se)	Widely distributed in animal foods	❖ Works with vitamin E to protect the body from oxidation
Zinc (Zn)	Fish, grains, meats, poultry, vegetables	❖ Becomes part of the hormone insulin ❖ Aids in production of genetic material ❖ Aids in immune functions ❖ Plays a role in taste perception ❖ Helps heal wounds ❖ Plays a role in sperm production

13-8 Small amounts of trace minerals in your diet play big roles in your health.

Effects of Processing and Preservation

Whenever a portion of a natural food product is removed in processing, the nutritive value of the food is changed. Exposure to heat, oxygen, or moisture during processing can also affect a food's nutrient content. Sometimes processing improves the availability of certain nutrients. Interactions between components in food mixtures can reduce or limit the body's ability to absorb some nutrients. Food scientists must carefully examine all these factors when developing and monitoring the nutritive value of food products. In many cases, nutrients are restored or added to processed foods.

Enrichment and Fortification

Two general processes are used to add nutrients to food products. The first is enrichment. *Enrichment* involves restoring some of the nutrients removed from refined grain products during processing.

Many B-vitamin deficiencies are connected to the staple grain of a population group. This is especially true if the grain is processed in a way that removes nutritional factors. For instance, in the 1800s, people in the Far East ate polished rice as their staple grain. The polishing process removes the part of the rice grain that supplies B vitamins. As a result, many people in the Far East developed the thiamin deficiency disease beriberi. See 13-9.

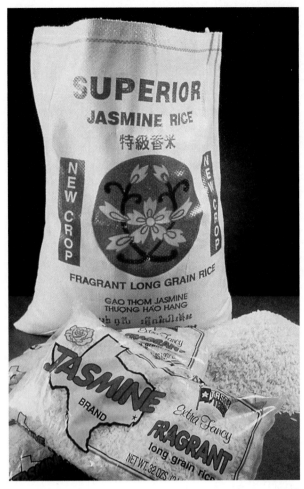

USDA

13-9 The brown bran layer that naturally covers each kernel of rice contains iron, niacin, riboflavin, and thiamin. Many of these nutrients are lost when the bran layer is removed to produce white rice.

In Europe and the United States, white flour used to be a status symbol. It was a sign of wealth because it was harder to make and had a lighter texture in baked goods. People who could not afford white flour made breads from whole wheat and rye flours. These breads were darker in color and had a heavy, chewy texture.

Unfortunately, the processing needed to make white flour removes most of the niacin, thiamin, riboflavin, and iron found in wheat. Legislation was passed in the 1930s to protect people in the United States from deficiencies of these nutrients. All processed flour now has niacin, thiamin, riboflavin, and iron added to it after processing. Voluntary enrichment

began in 1938. Mandatory enrichment went into effect in 1942.

In October 1993, the FDA proposed that a fourth B vitamin be added to refined grain products. Research showed a direct connection between several severe birth defects and the B vitamin folic acid, or folate. This B vitamin is involved in the manufacture of all new cells. In February 1996, the FDA announced regulations for the mandatory enrichment of most grain and cereal products with folic acid.

The second method of adding nutrients to processed foods is fortification. *Fortification* is the process of adding nutrients to food to correct a nutritional deficiency in a population. A *fortificant* is the nutrient that is being added to the food. Fortificants may or may not normally be contained in the food. The *food vehicle* is the specific food to which a fortificant is added. The most common fortificants are iron; iodine; calcium; and vitamins A, C, and D.

The first fortified food in the United States was iodized salt, which was introduced in Michigan in 1924. Fortification of salt by manufacturers is voluntary. However, 78% of all salt consumed in the United States is iodized. Adding iodine to table salt has practically eliminated the widespread iodine deficiency disease called *goiter*.

Food fortification usually results from research showing a sizable risk of a nutrient deficiency disease in a large population. Ideally, a fortified food will

❖ be commonly used by the target population

❖ be regularly consumed by the bulk of the population without risk of excess fortificant consumption

❖ remain stable in storage

❖ be relatively low in cost

❖ have no known negative interactions between the fortificant and the food vehicle

❖ be available to all consumers, regardless of socioeconomic status

Fortification is usually used when foodstuffs cannot naturally provide essential nutrients to the target population. Fortified foods need to be carefully evaluated and adjusted to ensure that needs of the target population are being met. See 13-10.

Fortificants and Common Food Vehicles

Fortificants	Food Vehicles	Target Populations
B-complex vitamins	Grains, cereals, baked goods	Vegetarians, people who use large amounts of highly refined foods, populations in transition from rural to urban areas
Calcium	Orange juice	People who are lactose intolerant, people who consume large amounts of soft drinks, people with small body frames who are at risk for osteoporosis
Iodine	Salt	People living in areas with low iodine levels in soil, people who do not eat or have easy economical access to seafood
Iron	Cereal, milk products, sugar, curry powder, soy sauce, cookies	People who consume diets low in meat or high in refined grain products
Vitamin A	Sugar	Central American populations with low vitamin A consumption
Vitamin C	Fruit juices, fruit drinks, fruit-flavored beverages, dairy products, some breakfast cereals	People who consume diets low in fresh fruits and vegetables
Vitamin D	Margarine, vegetable oils, dairy products	Children under 3, older adults, populations where cultural practice or climate limit exposure to sunlight
Vitamin E	Fats and oils	People who consume large amounts of highly refined foods

13-10 Fortification is done to address the nutritional needs of specific population groups. However, fortified foods can be excellent sources of nutrients for all people.

When evaluating a fortified food, food scientists review literature to learn about the bioavailability of the added nutrient. *Bioavailability* refers to the body's ability to absorb and use a nutrient in the form consumed. For instance, food scientists can choose from 20 forms of iron to add to food products. Scientists often choose iron sulfate because it is highly soluble. This gives the iron a high degree of bioavailability. Food scientists might also add vitamin C to an iron-fortified food. The vitamin C will increase the bioavailability of the iron by helping the body absorb more of it. On the other hand, food scientists might choose not to add iron to a food that contains polyphenols or calcium. These substances can reduce the bioavailability of iron by hindering the body's ability to absorb it.

Factors Affecting Nutrient Stability

The stability of fortificants is another factor food scientists must think about when developing fortified foods. Several factors can affect nutrient stability. These include heat, oxygen, and water activity level.

Most B-complex vitamins have no problems related to processing. Thiamin is an exception. Thiamin has low stability in heat. This requires thiamin to be added after all heat treatment of a product is completed. Heat stability is also a problem with vitamins A, C, and E.

The reactivity of some nutrients with oxygen can affect the presence of the nutrient in a finished food product. Vitamins C and E and β-carotene are damaged when exposed to oxygen. Vitamin C is especially unstable when the presence of oxygen is coupled with a high moisture

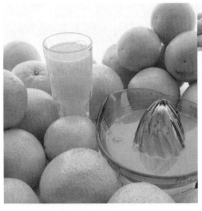

Nutrition News
MyPyramid

MyPyramid is the interactive food guidance system and symbol the USDA released in 2005 to replace the Food Guide Pyramid. The MyPyramid symbol was designed to represent activity, moderation, personalization, proportionality, variety, and gradual improvement:

❖   The person climbing the steps is a reminder that daily physical *activity* is a necessary part of any healthy lifestyle. You need to be physically active for at least 30 minutes most days.

❖   The bands vary in width from top to bottom because every category has choices that are more or less nutrient dense. For example, an apple is nutrient dense and located at the bottom of the red band. Sweetened applesauce is in the middle due to the added sugar. Because apple pie has added fat and sugar, it is found at the top of the red band. *Moderation* encourages selection of more foods from the lower parts of the bands.

❖   The person climbing the side of MyPyramid represents *personalization.* MyPyramid offers 12 food plans and helps you select the one that is right for you based on your age, gender, and level of physical activity.

❖   The bands vary in width to show *proportionality.* Although you need foods from each category daily, you should eat more of some foods than others. For example, you should eat more fruits than oils.

❖   Each of the six bands is a different color to represent the five food groups and oils. The bands are rainbow colored to emphasize the need for a *variety* of foods from each band daily for good health.

❖   The phrase "Steps to a Healthier You" encourages taking small steps to improve your lifestyle each day. Making many dramatic changes all at once often leads to failure. Setting small, achievable goals can result in *gradual improvement.*

The MyPyramid Web site offers tips for making healthier food choices and a nutrition analysis tool that helps you track your diet and exercise. This information will help you choose goals and track progress over time. Visit MyPyramid.gov to find more useful tools and information.

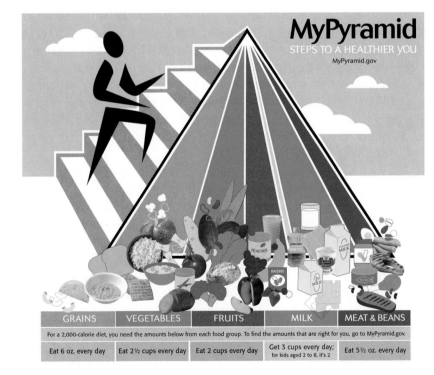

GRAINS	VEGETABLES	FRUITS	MILK	MEAT & BEANS
Eat 6 oz. every day	Eat 2½ cups every day	Eat 2 cups every day	Get 3 cups every day; for kids aged 2 to 8, it's 2	Eat 5½ oz. every day

For a 2,000-calorie diet, you need the amounts below from each food group. To find the amounts that are right for you, go to MyPyramid.gov.

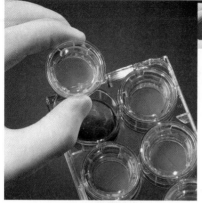

Recent Research
Tea with Lemon Please!

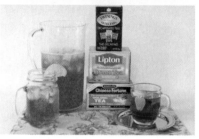

Tea interferes with the body's ability to absorb calcium and iron from food.

Black, green, and instant teas have been studied to see if they affect the bioavailability of calcium and iron. The answer is yes; teas interfere with the absorption of these minerals by the body. The degree of impact depends on the kind of tea. In all cases, adding lemon juice to the tea helped increase the absorption of iron and, to some extent, calcium.

More study is needed to understand how teas interfere with mineral absorption. In time, such study may lead to the development of teas that overcome this problem. In the meantime, if you drink tea with meals, add a slice of lemon. (The benefits of drinking tea are covered in Chapter 14.)

---

level. Oxidation can increase in the presence of copper, iron, brass, or bronze. Therefore, these metals are seldom used in commercial food processing equipment. Some food formulations may also include additives to keep these metals from affecting nutrient content.

Water activity levels affect the stability of vitamins A and C. Moisture levels over 7% to 8% reduce the stability of vitamin C. Vitamin A losses are greater in dehydrated foods because water activity levels are low.

Vitamins and Minerals as Food Additives

The vitamin and mineral levels in foods can be increased as a result of processing. This usually occurs when a vitamin, mineral, or nutrient compound is added to a food for non-nutritive reasons.

Some foods contain calcium salts as a result of processing. Tofu, for example, will not develop its characteristic texture until calcium salts are added. Calcium salts, such as calcium chloride, help vegetables hold their shapes during canning. (Aluminum and magnesium salts are also used as firming agents in vegetables.) Other foods that contain calcium salts include self-rising flours, stone ground flours, and molasses. The addition of calcium salts increases the calcium content of all these foods.

Salt, or sodium chloride, is used widely in processed foods. It is an economical flavor enhancer. Potassium chloride is also a salt that will enhance flavors. Manufacturers that wish to reduce the sodium levels of food products often replace sodium chloride with potassium chloride. The potassium levels of these foods are increased as a result of reducing sodium levels.

Iodine is used as a dough conditioner in the bakery industry. It is also used as a disinfectant and medicine in the dairy industry.

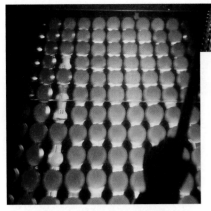

Technology Tidbit
Packaging May Decrease Vitamin Loss

Some vitamins are easily destroyed by factors such as light

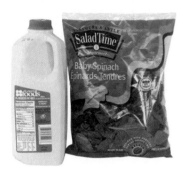

Translucent milk bottles and vented vegetable bags are just two examples of packaging technology designed to decrease vitamin losses.

and heat. Food scientists are working to design packaging that will help reduce such nutrient losses. For example, milk is a good source of the B vitamin riboflavin. However, riboflavin is very sensitive to light. Within a few hours, store lighting can destroy most of the riboflavin in milk sold in transparent containers. This is why most milk is sold in opaque cartons or translucent plastic containers. These containers help block the light rays that destroy the riboflavin.

Another example of packaging that helps decrease nutrient losses is the bags used to hold precut vegetables. Dr. Margaret Barth is a food scientist at the University of Kentucky. She

compared the vitamin content of bagged and loose vegetables. She discovered precut and bagged vegetables have more β-carotene and vitamin C than whole, unbagged vegetables. This is because the high-tech bags contain a mini-environment of nitrogen, oxygen, and carbon dioxide. This gas mixture helps preserve vitamins.

Dr. Barth recommends that you store unused vegetables in the same bag in which they are sold, even after opening. Store unpackaged vegetables in resealable vegetable bags. The tiny vents in these bags slow spoiling by maintaining the right amount of moisture.

This increases the iodine content of many baked goods and dairy products. The use of iodized salt as a flavoring agent in any processed food will also increase iodine levels.

Ascorbic acid is often used to prevent browning (oxidation) of cut fruits such as apples, bananas, and pears. Foods containing added ascorbic acid have higher levels of vitamin C.

When food scientists use fortified ingredients in a food mixture, the nutrient content of the finished product is increased. Scientists must analyze this factor when determining the appropriate levels of fortificants to add to the product. Unless scientists examine all possible sources of consumption, they cannot accurately predict total nutrient

levels consumed over time. It is important that enrichment and fortification not result in possible toxic levels of a nutrient.

Preserving Vitamins and Minerals at Home

Some of the foods consumers eat are not produced and monitored commercially. It is important for the average consumer to understand which vitamins are easily destroyed during cooking and processing. Any water-soluble nutrient can move from the food product to the cooking water. Vitamin C leaches into cooking water and is destroyed by heat. Folic acid can also be lost during cooking.

The amount of nutrients lost will vary from vitamin to vitamin and from one food to another. However, the way you cook your food determines how much damage is done to its nutritional value. The same factors that affect the nutrient values of commercially processed foods can affect foods prepared in the home. Ways to reduce nutrient losses include

❖ Eat some fruits and vegetables raw or uncooked, 13-11.

❖ Save water used for cooking vegetables to add to soups and gravies.

❖ Cook fruits and vegetables in large pieces, using short cooking times and as little water as possible.

❖ Serve fruits and vegetables as soon as possible after cooking.

❖ Choose stainless steel, glass, and aluminum cookware for foods high in easily oxidized nutrients.

❖ Read labels to monitor nutritional value of foods.

❖ Eat a wide variety of foods to increase the chances of meeting all nutrient needs.

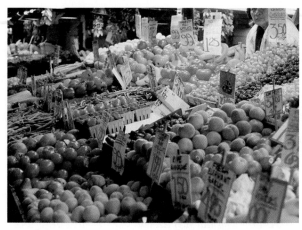

13-11 Eat fresh fruits and vegetables as soon as possible to avoid nutrient losses that occur during storage.

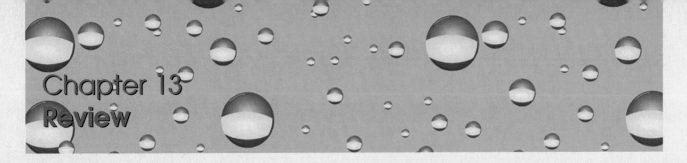

Summary

Though small in volume, vitamins and minerals are very important for maintaining good health. Some vital functions are performed by one vitamin or mineral, but most involve several micronutrients working as a team. This is the main reason for incorporating a variety of foods in the menu.

The food scientist needs to be aware not only of the nutritive value of these compounds but also the effects of processing on their presence in foods. Many of these nutrients are lost or damaged in processing. At this time, the law only requires the replacement of four vitamins and one mineral that are lost in processing: thiamin, riboflavin, niacin, folic acid, and iron.

The consumer needs to be aware that balance is an important key to understanding nutrition. Just adding vitamin pills to a poor diet will not necessarily prevent diet-related illnesses. Choosing foods that are highly processed can lead to imbalance and poor nutrition. Processed foods are an important part of today's diet, but they must be balanced with fresh produce and whole grain breads and cereals. Several steps can be taken at home to preserve the nutrients in food.

Check Your Understanding

1. List the three general functions of vitamins.
2. Name the two forms of vitamin A found in food and their sources.
3. How does the human body obtain vitamins D and K through nonfood sources?
4. Name the functions of the B vitamins.
5. Which vitamins function as antioxidants? What does an antioxidant do?

6. Explain the difference between major and trace minerals.
7. Identify the six vitamins and minerals that work as a team to build bone tissue.
8. List one substance that interferes with iron absorption and one that increases it.
9. Give two reasons for adding nutrients to processed foods and give an example of each.
10. List three factors that can affect vitamin and mineral content in processed foods.

Critical Thinking

1. A healthy man is concerned that the meals he has been eating on a business trip have not been meeting all his vitamin needs. Which of these nutrients should he consume as soon as possible after returning home?
2. Based on the information in this chapter, how would you respond to someone who says "Additives are harmful and should not be allowed in food"?
3. What are some possible ways for a vegetarian who avoids red and white meat to obtain enough iron in the diet?
4. If you don't like lemon with tea, what are three options you have to keep tea from interfering with iron absorption at a meal?
5. Explain why it is best to avoid rinsing pasta or rice after cooking.

Explore Further

1. **Technology.** Analyze one day's diet on a computer diet analysis program. List those nutrients that were below 50% of the recommended daily intake. For each, list three good food sources that you could eat.

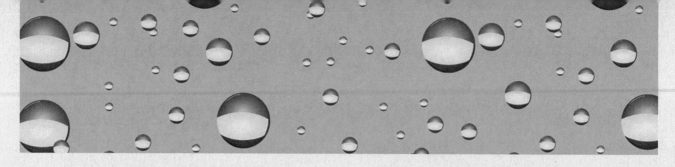

2. **Analytical Skills.** Propose a food vehicle, other than orange juice, to contribute sufficient calcium to the teen diet. Explain how your proposal would satisfy the criteria for an ideal fortified food.

3. **Math.** Calculate your sodium intake for one day. Examine the sources of sodium in your diet. List each source that has more than 200 mg per serving (read labels) and suggest a low salt substitute for each food.

4. **Food and Nutrition.** Plan one day's diet using MyPyramid. Compare the plan to what you ate yesterday. List the changes you need to make to meet MyPyramid's recommendations.

Experiment 13A
Minerals in Milk

Purpose

One way to measure the total mineral content of a food is to heat the food until only an ash remains. When a food is exposed to very high temperatures, the water evaporates and compounds break down into water and carbon dioxide. At high temperatures, these are both gases that escape into the air. The white ash that remains is minerals. In this experiment, you will determine the total mineral content of various milk products.

Equipment

crucible
tongs
electronic balance
10-mL graduated cylinder
glass rod

Supplies

10 mL assigned milk

Procedure

Part I

1. Heat the crucible on a range or over a Bunsen burner for about five minutes or until it glows red hot to burn off any unwanted residue.

2. Move the crucible to a heatproof surface with tongs and let it cool.

3. Mass the crucible on an electronic balance. Record the mass in a data table.

4. Pour 10 mL of assigned milk into the crucible and mass. Record the mass in the data table.

   Variation 1: whole milk

   Variation 2: 2% milk

   Variation 3: 1% milk

   Variation 4: fat free milk

   Variation 5: evaporated milk

   Variation 6: half-and-half

5. Place the crucible on a range or Bunsen burner and heat until most of the milk has simmered away. With a glass rod, pull any skin that forms to the sides of the crucible to keep steam pressure from building up.

6. Continue to heat until the milk burns.

7. Place the crucible on an oven rack in a self-cleaning oven.

8. Set the oven to the cleaning cycle and lock the door. The oven is designed to reach temperatures of 538°C (1000°F). This will burn off everything but minerals. The process takes two to three hours.

Part II

1. The next day, remove the crucible from the oven.

2. Mass the crucible and ash.

Calculations

1. Calculate the mass of the ash.

2. Calculate the percentage of milk that is minerals.

3. Approximately 28% of the mineral content of milk is calcium. Calculate the approximate mass of the calcium in your sample.

4. Calculate how many mg of calcium would be in 244 g (1 cup) of milk.

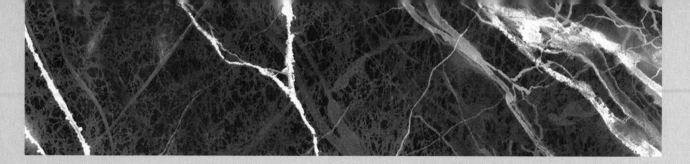

Questions

1. Why should you not simply remove the skin from the crucible as it forms?

2. How close was your calculation of calcium content to the figures given in nutrition analysis tables?

3. Does the mineral content differ from one type of milk to another?

Experiment 13B
Effects of Calcium on Coagulation

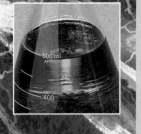

Purpose

Two chemical reactions occur that cause milk to coagulate and form cheese curds. First, the enzyme rennin reacts with the protein casein to form paracasein. Then, calcium ions combine with the paracasein to form calcium paracasein. This new compound forms an insoluble curd that contracts and squeezes out a clear liquid called whey. In this experiment, you will examine what happens if calcium is not present or is bound to other substances.

Equipment

wax pencil
4 test tubes
100-mL graduated cylinder
400-mL beaker
thermometer
thermometer holder
4 test-tube stoppers
test-tube tongs

Supplies

60 mL milk
20 mL chocolate milk
200 mL water
0.6 g rennin (¹/₂ rennet tablet)
0.1 g sodium citrate (< ¹/₈ teaspoon)
20 drops calcium chloride solution

Procedure

1. Use a wax pencil to label the test tubes 1 through 4. Fill test tubes 1 through 3 with 20 mL of milk each.

2. Fill test tube 4 with 20 mL of chocolate milk.

3. Pour 200 mL water into a 400-mL beaker.

4. Insert a thermometer into a thermometer holder and clip the holder to the side of the beaker. Place the beaker over medium heat until the temperature of the water reaches 37°C (99°F).

5. Place all four test tubes into the beaker.

6. Test tube 1 is the control.

7. Add 0.2 g rennin to test tube 2.

8. Add 0.2 g rennin and 0.1 g sodium citrate to test tube 3.

9. Add 0.2 g rennin to the chocolate milk in test tube 4.

10. Stopper the tubes and heat 5 minutes, being careful not to let the temperature of the water bath increase beyond 37°C (99°F).

11. Use test-tube tongs to remove the test tubes from the water bath. Examine the tubes. Carefully invert them. (Do not shake the tubes.) Record your observations.

12. Add 10 drops of calcium chloride solution to test tubes 3 and 4.

13. Return test tubes 3 and 4 to the water bath for 5 more minutes.

14. Record your observations.

Questions

1. How did the texture of the milk in the test tubes differ?

2. What happened to the calcium ions in test tubes 3 and 4 after the first heating in the water bath?

3. Explain what happened when the calcium chloride solution was added to test tubes 3 and 4.

4. What effect does cocoa have on the ability of milk to coagulate?

Experiment 13C
Determining Vitamin C Content

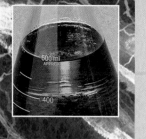

Purpose

When a substance gains electrons or loses hydrogen atoms, it is oxidized. The substance that loses electrons or gains hydrogen atoms is reduced. Such an oxidation-reduction reaction can be used to determine the presence of vitamin C (ascorbic acid). When ascorbic acid and the dye 2,6 dichloroindophenol are mixed, the ascorbic acid gives up two hydrogen atoms to the dye. When the dark blue dye is reduced or gains hydrogen atoms, it turns a light pink. When drops of 2,6 dichloroindophenol remain blue, there is no longer any vitamin C with which the dye can react. The more dye that is needed to react with all the vitamin C in a substance, the higher the vitamin C content of the substance is.

Equipment

5 100-mL beakers
100-mL graduated cylinder
3 Erlenmeyer flasks
titration stand with buret
strainer
thermometer

Supplies

50 mL minced bell pepper, cabbage, or tomato
50 mL distilled water
75 mL apple juice

0.1% solution of 2,6 dichloroindophenol
75 mL white grape juice

Procedure

1. Measure approximately 50 mL of minced bell pepper, cabbage, or tomato into a 100-mL beaker. Add 50 mL of distilled water and let the mixture stand for 15 minutes.

2. Measure 25 mL of apple juice into an Erlenmeyer flask.

3. Take an initial reading of the amount of 2,6 dichloroindophenol in the buret. Add the dye to the apple juice in the flask one drop at a time, swirling after each addition. If the solution changes from dark blue to colorless or a light pink, ascorbic acid is present. Add the dye until the dark blue color remains after swirling. Record the amount of dye dispensed from the buret (initial reading minus final reading).

4. Repeat steps 2 and 3 with the white grape juice.

5. Strain the liquid from the vegetable-water mixture into a clean 100-mL beaker.

6. Repeat steps 2 and 3 with 25 mL of the liquid strained from the vegetable-water mixture prepared in step 1.

7. Pour 50 mL of apple juice into a 100-mL beaker. Place the beaker over medum heat and simmer 5 minutes. (The juice should steam but not boil.)

8. Allow the apple juice to cool to 50°C or less.

9. Measure 25 mL of the heated apple juice into an Erlenmeyer flask and repeat step 3.

10. Repeat steps 7 through 9 twice, once with white grape juice and once with the remaining liquid strained from the vegetable-water mixture.

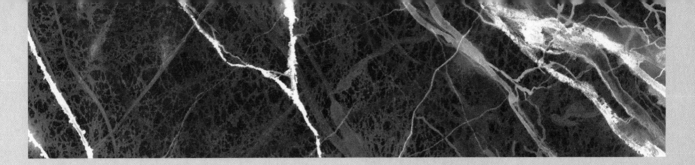

Questions

1. Rank the six solutions by vitamin C content from least to greatest.

2. What effect did heating have on the vitamin C content?

3. Why do you think the liquid strained from the vegetable-water mixture tested positive for vitamin C content? What does this indicate about the vitamin C content of the vegetables?

4. What recommendations would you make for preparing foods that are high in vitamin C?

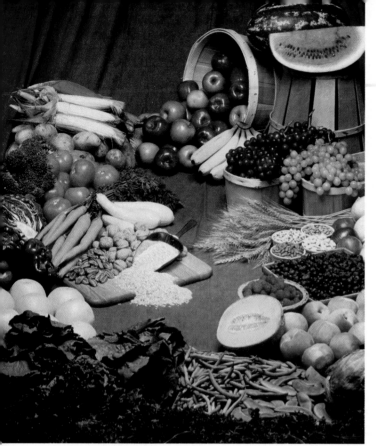

Agricultural Research Service, USDA

Fruits, vegetables, and grains provide a bounty of phytochemicals.

Chapter 14

Phytochemicals: The Other Food Components

Objectives

After studying this chapter,
you will be able to

list at least eight groups of phytochemicals and give a food source for each group.

identify possible links between phytochemicals and disease prevention.

describe ways in which food processing can affect the phytochemicals in foods.

plan menus that are rich in phytochemicals.

Key Terms

phytochemical
allyl sulfides
carcinogen
carotenoids
flavonoids
isoflavones
phytoestrogens
indoles
cruciferous vegetable
isothiocyanates
phenolic acids
phenols
polyphenols
saponins
terpenes
isomer
tannins
functional food
bioactive component

Much knowledge about vitamins and minerals was revealed through research in the second half of the twentieth century. This research led some people to believe they could make up for any nutritional deficiencies by taking vitamin pills. However, physicians soon learned that known nutrients were not sufficient for good health. Doctors found that patients who ate nutritious food recovered faster than patients who received calories and nutrients intravenously. This finding indicated food contains substances other than nutrients that affect health.

The more scientists study food, the more they discover. This chapter looks at recent research into the value of food components other than nutrients. Many of these components are called phytochemicals. You may also hear them called *phytonutrients*. However, these compounds are not recognized as nutrients because the body does not require them to function.

Phytochemicals

Phytochemicals are a group of compounds originally produced by plants. Many of these compounds are active in the human body. The name *phytochemical* is derived from the Greek word for plants—*phyto*. These compounds seem to help plants endure extreme weather; fight off disease; and, in some cases, resist pests. They are found naturally in vegetables, fruits, grains, herbs, and spices. Phytochemicals give these foods their colors and flavors.

For years, scientists have recognized that eating lots of fruits and vegetables seems to lower cancer risk. Part of the reason may be the phytochemicals present in nearly all fruits and vegetables. Orange juice is known to contain at least 59 phytochemicals. Forty phytochemicals have been identified in broccoli, and 50 have been identified in garlic and onions.

Like other food components, phytochemicals need to be consumed with balance and moderation. It is important to remember that no supplement can replace a good diet. There is no miracle pill that will enable you to eat anything you want. Failing to eat a nutritious diet increases the risks associated with nutrient deficiencies and excesses. See 14-1.

Until a few decades ago, phytochemicals had been largely ignored. Then in the 1960s, scientists began studying the properties of phytochemicals. Since that time, researchers have isolated thousands of these compounds. One problem facing researchers is that isolated phytochemicals may not provide the same

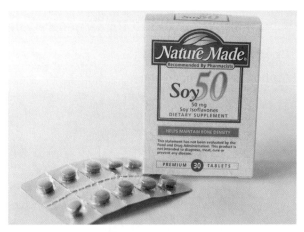

14-1 Although phytochemicals are available in pill form, most registered dietitians recommend getting these beneficial compounds from foods.

benefits as phytochemicals consumed with other compounds. Identifying the nutritional benefits of any one phytochemical will be a long, hard process.

Health Tip

Phytochemical pills are available in the vitamin sections of many stores. However, use caution before deciding to take pills to "boost your intake." You need to remember that research in phytochemicals is in its infancy. For many phytochemicals, scientists do not know what amounts are beneficial and what amounts are toxic. An example of the potential dangers is *taxol*. Taxol is found in the Pacific yew tree. It has been found to be effective in treating ovarian cancer. If it is taken incorrectly, however, it will cause death. Even in very low concentrations, taxol will cause such negative side effects as hair loss.

Phytochemical Families

Most of the work in phytochemical research has involved isolating and classifying the compounds and identifying their food sources. Phytochemicals are grouped by their chemical structures. See 14-2. Current research and reports in health, nutrition, and medical journals center around seven families of phytochemicals. Some of these families have subgroups that have been studied more extensively than others.

Chemistry Shorthand for Organic Compounds

Chemical Structure	Shorthand Symbol
Carbon and hydrogen chain 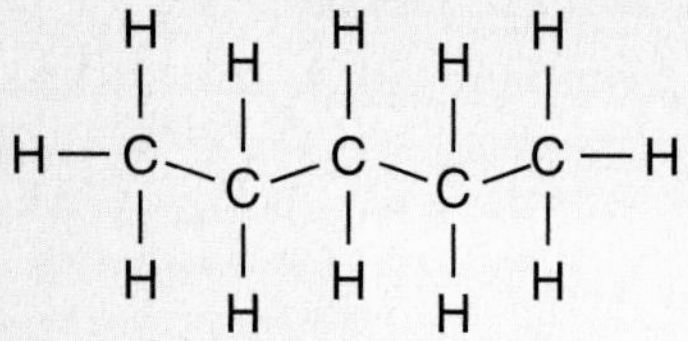	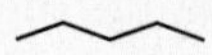
Double bond 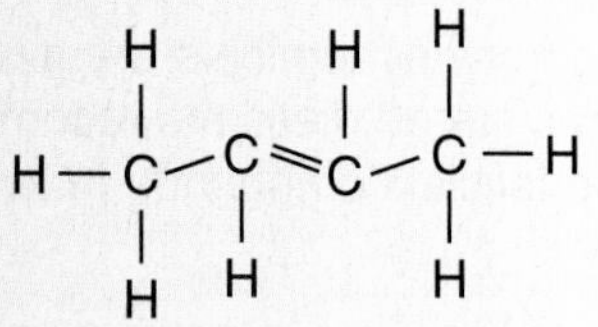	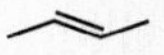
Carbon ring 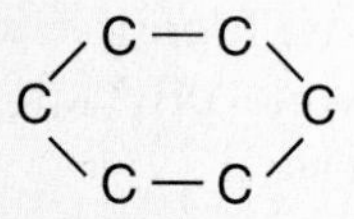	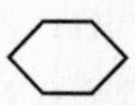
Benzene or aromatic ring with double bonds	or
	Because the location of the double bonds flutuates, the circle in the center of the hexagon is preferred

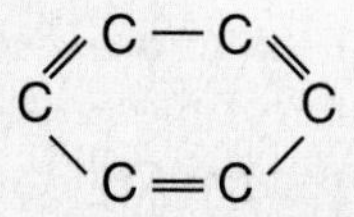

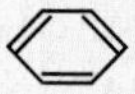

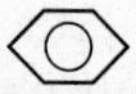

Each line represents a carbon-to-carbon bond. There is a carbon atom at each bend or line intersection and a carbon atom at each end. It is assumed that all remaining bonds (remember, carbon atoms bond four times) are to hydrogen atoms. Symbols of elements are only shown when the atom is not a carbon or hydrogen atom.

14-2 Complex organic molecules, such as phytochemicals, have large numbers of carbon and hydrogen atoms. To simplify the drawing of models of these molecules, scientists use the abbreviations shown above.

Allyl Sulfides

Allyl sulfides are a group of compounds that contain sulfur and increase enzyme reactions. There is evidence that these sulfur-containing compounds kill bacteria, fungi, and viruses. The enzyme reactions in which allyl sulfides are involved can help rid the body of cancer-causing substances. (Substances that are known to cause cancer are called *carcinogens.*)

Foods high in allyl sulfides that seem to help prevent cancer are onions, garlic, leeks, and chives. Allyl sulfides also seem to give garlic blood-thinning properties that are similar to those of aspirin. To receive the benefits of these phytochemicals, include foods that contain them in your daily diet. You can add garlic and onions to almost any casserole, soup, or vegetable combination. The milder or sweeter the onion, the lower the allyl sulfide levels. Chives make an attractive garnish to many potato dishes. Garlic is also available in pill form for those who do not like the flavor. See 14-3.

Cooking can change allyl sulfide compounds, which results in a change in the benefits they provide. To get a full range of benefits from sources of allyl sulfides, you should eat them in both raw and cooked forms. For example, raw garlic is high in the compound allicin, which has antibiotic and antifungal properties. When cooked, allicin changes into other allyl sulfides that act as anticoagulants.

Carotenoids

Carotenoids are a family of compounds known for their work as antioxidants. There are about 600 known carotenoids. Roughly 50 of these carotenoids can be used as precursors for vitamin A. Carotenoids are usually composed of a 40-carbon chain. Most have a ring shape at either end of the chain. See 14-4.

Carotenes

The carotenoids are divided into two subgroups based on their molecular structure. The first subgroup is the *carotenes*. These compounds include alpha-carotene, beta-carotene, beta-cryptoxanthin, and lycopene. Carotenes contain only carbon and hydrogen atoms. *Alpha-carotene* is found in pumpkins and carrots. *Beta-carotene* is found in dark green and yellow vegetables. Papayas, oranges, and tangerines are sources of *beta-cryptoxanthin*. Tomatoes, watermelon, guava, and red peppers are rich in *lycopene*.

The best known carotenoid is beta-carotene. This compound has been reported to have cancer-fighting properties. However, recent studies in Finland and China have led some people to think that beta-carotene does

Allyl Sulfides

Alliin reacts with the enzyme allinase to form allicin.

Allicin gives cut garlic its pungent odor.

Diallyl disulfide is the compound formed when garlic is heated in steam or boiling water.

14-3 The allyl group (CH_2=$CHCH_2$) bonds to sulfur to form allyl sulfides.

Carotenoids

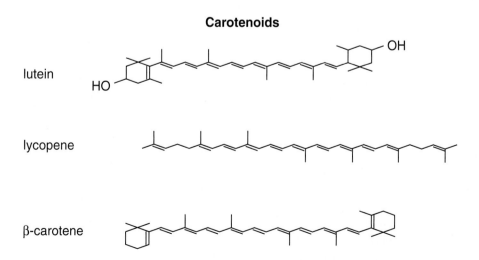

lutein

lycopene

β-carotene

14-4 These models represent just a few of the many carotenoids found in foods.

not work against cancer. The problem with these studies is that beta-carotene was isolated and given in pill form. Other research indicates the key to fighting cancer is green and yellow fruits and vegetables, not beta-carotene by itself.

There seems to be a link between the lycopene in tomatoes and a reduced risk of prostate cancer. One study found men who ate 10 servings of tomato-based foods a week were half as likely to develop prostate cancer. Consuming high levels of lycopene also seems to boost the physical and mental activity of older adults. Lycopene is not destroyed by heat. Therefore, tomato sauce is a richer source of this phytochemical than fresh tomato slices. This is because tomato sauce is concentrated.

Xanthophylls

The second subgroup of carotenoids is called *xanthophylls.* Xanthophylls contain a hydroxyl group and are yellow to orange in color. The xanthophylls that have received the most notice are *lutein* and *zeaxanthin.* These compounds help the eyes filter out harmful blue light. A study at Harvard Medical School found a link between lutein-rich spinach and a lower risk of cataracts. Other studies have focused on the effects of low levels of lutein and zeaxanthin. A link may exist between low levels of xanthophylls and some eye diseases that lead to blindness later in life. Some of the best sources of these phytochemicals are dark green leafy vegetables.

Reactions among phytochemicals or between phytochemicals and other compounds will vary from one food mixture to another. For instance, the color of carotenoids is related to the food systems in which they are found. Beta-carotene is orange. When it is combined with chlorophyll in spinach, however, the color that is visible is dark green.

The stability of carotenoids is also related to the food systems in which they are found. Carotenoids are fat soluble. Therefore, they are often found with lipids. Carotenoids in unsaturated lipids are more stable than those in saturated lipids. Lycopene is very stable within tomato tissue. However, it is unstable when purified and extracted. These examples show why food scientists cannot assume that a given phytochemical will be stable in any food mixture.

More research is needed to be certain of all the roles carotenoids play in nutrition and food preparation. However, studies currently point to several possible benefits. Carotenoids appear to

❖ act as antioxidants, changing potentially harmful free radicals into harmless compounds, such as water.

❖ reduce tissue damage that can lead to the formation of cancer cells.

❖ enhance the immune function.

❖ maintain healthy eye tissue and reduce the risk of age-related eye diseases, such as cataracts and night blindness.

Some experts suggest most people in the United States should double their current intake of carotenoids. You can increase your supply of these valuable phytochemicals by eating more deep orange and dark green fruits and vegetables. Large doses of carotenoids have been known to cause the skin to turn yellow. However, high levels of carotenoids have not been found to have any toxic effects. See 14-5.

Flavonoids

Flavonoids are a group of compounds responsible for many of the flavor characteristics of foods. They are also color pigments. Most are red or white in color. See 14-6.

Researchers have identified over 800 flavonoids. These compounds have been linked with a number of health benefits.

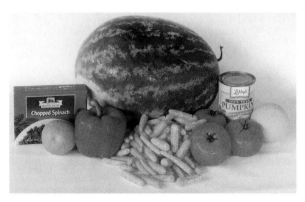

14-5 These colorful foods all serve as significant sources of various carotenoids.

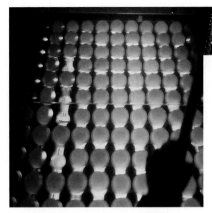

Technology Tidbit
A Designer Tomato

The red color in tomatoes comes from lycopene. Research shows this phytochemical plays a role in protection against various types of cancer. Research indicates that prostate cancer is one of those cancers affected by lycopene.

Researchers at the Royal Holland University of London have created a lycopene-rich tomato. They altered the genes so the tomato has twice the normal levels of lycopene. The new tomatoes taste the same as regular tomatoes. However, the higher lycopene levels create a redder color. Research teams are looking to see if the altered tomatoes provide the desired health benefits.

Watch for more "designer foods" in the future. Food scientists will continue to look for ways to create healthier versions of consumer favorites.

Flavonoids

catechin   quercetin

14-6 In addition to their potential health benefits, flavonoids give foods characteristic flavors and colors.

Scientists have recently found that many flavonoids may help fight cancer. One such flavonoid called HEMF is a powerful anticarcinogen found in soy sauce. Some flavonoids have anti-inflammatory properties. These phytochemicals may help guard against asthma attacks. Flavonoids isolated from grapes, fruits, nuts, teas, herbs, and spices have been found to relax artery walls. This reduces constriction of the arteries and lowers the risk of stroke. Dark chocolate, apples, and blueberries are good sources of flavinoids. *Quercetin* is a flavonoid that has been found to be antifungal, anti-inflammatory, antiviral, and antibacterial.

It also helps reduce the risk of heart disease. Good sources are yellow and red onions, red grape juice, apples, cranberries, broccoli, and tea.

Isoflavones

Isoflavones are a subgroup of flavonoids. They are found mainly in soy products. They have a hexagonal carbon ring structure like flavonoids. See 14-7.

Isoflavones seem to play a role in cancer prevention. Observing that people who ate soy products were at lower risk for many cancers led researchers to explore this role.

Isoflavones

HO—⬡⬡—O
       ‖
       O   —◯—OH

genistein

14-7 Many foods that are high in isoflavones are not part of a typical U.S. diet.

Researchers found that soy is the only significant source of two important isoflavones, *genistein* and *daidzein.*

Isoflavones are also called phytoestrogens. **Phytoestrogens** are plant hormones. They are similar in structure to the human hormone estrogen, but they are less potent. In the body, estrogen binds to sites called *receptors.* This binding can trigger the development of some cancers. Isoflavones appear to compete with estrogen for the receptors. When the weaker isoflavones bind to the receptors, cancer cell growth and division are blocked.

Eating soy products has also been linked with lowering the unpleasant symptoms of menopause. *Menopause* is the time in a woman's life when the menstrual cycle slows and stops. Menopause is a result of a decrease in the production of estrogen. Many women have uncomfortable hot flashes and night sweats during menopause. Researchers have observed that Asian women who have diets high in soy products have less severe menopausal symptoms. This indicates that isoflavones from soy help make up for the lack of estrogen in the body. Isoflavones seem to reduce bone losses that result from lower estrogen levels, too.

Studies link health benefits with 25 g or more soy protein and 50 mg isoflavones per day. Some health experts suggest consuming as little as 125 mL ($^1/_2$ cup) of tofu or one glass of soy milk a day can provide benefits. These amounts will provide an adequate supply of isoflavones. Tofu is relatively flavorless. It can be used in place of part of the cheese in many Italian foods like lasagna and stuffed manicotti. Soy milk, flour, or powder can be added to baked goods.

Besides soy products, isoflavones are present in chickpeas and licorice, 14-8. Other foods high in the isoflavone *genistein* are Chinese cabbage and bok choy. Isoflavones are also found in many processed foods. Food scientists have been adding soy protein to many processed foods because of its versatility and cost. It is relatively flavorless. It can be used in place of many animal-based proteins at a lower cost. The evidence of the healthfulness of isoflavones is another reason to expand the use of soy in processed foods.

Indoles

Indoles are a family of compounds found in large amounts in a plant group known as cruciferous vegetables. **Cruciferous vegetables** include broccoli, cabbage, kale, and cauliflower. This group of plants gets its name from the cross shape of the flower petals. Indoles are known to stimulate many enzymatic reactions. One such reaction seems to speed up the breakdown of the hormone estrogen. When estrogen is present in large amounts, the risk of breast cancer increases. By making estrogen less effective, indoles reduce the risk of breast cancer. See 14-9.

More of the indoles in cruciferous vegetables become available when the vegetables are cooked. The heat of cooking speeds the action of an enzyme that helps compounds in the vegetables turn into indoles. A lot of chewing will also speed this process. The mixing and grinding of the food with the digestive

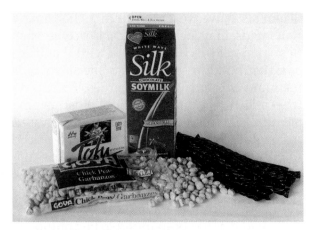

14-8 Incorporating these foods into your diet will help you increase your intake of isoflavones.

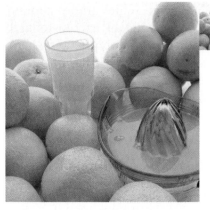

Nutrition News
Organics—Are They Worth the Cost?

The *Journal of Agricultural and Food Chemistry* reported in February 2003 that organically grown berries contain up to 58% more polyphenolics than commercial berries sprayed with herbicides and pesticides. In 1993 the *Journal of Applied Nutrition* had similar findings. A study of organic potatoes, apples, pears, and corn found this produce contained up to four times more trace minerals, 13 times more selenium, and 20 times more calcium and manganese than commercial produce. Organic produce also had less heavy metal content including 25% less lead and 40% less aluminum.

Indoles

sulforaphane   melatonin   serotonin

14-9 Broccoli, cabbage, and cauliflower are sources of compounds called indoles.

enzymes in saliva hasten the necessary chemical reactions.

Isothiocyanates

Isothiocyanates are a subgroup of indoles. They are also found in cruciferous vegetables. These compounds protect against cancer by affecting enzyme reactions. They are the source of the aromas in Brussels sprouts, cabbage, turnips, mustard greens, watercress, and radishes. See 14-10.

Phenolic Acids

Phenolic acids or **phenols** are weak organic acids that have a hydroxyl group attached to an *aromatic ring.* This ring of six carbons

Isothiocyanate

4-methylthio-3-t-butenyl

14-10 This phytochemical compound is found in radishes.

contains three carbon-to-carbon double bonds. These double bonds fluctuate or change from one side of the carbon to another.

Each of the six carbons has a bonding site facing out from the ring. A hydroxyl group is bonded to at least one of these six sites. See 14-11.

Ellagic acid is one type of phenolic acid. It has been found to reduce damage to the lungs caused by tobacco smoke and air pollution. It works on altering the carcinogens in these substances before they can damage genetic material in lung cells. Strawberries and raspberries are rich in ellagic acid. Citrus fruits, tomatoes, carrots, whole grains, and nuts are also good sources.

Polyphenols

Polyphenols are phenol compounds that have more than one carbon ring, 14-12. They have been identified as important compounds in fighting cancer and heart disease. People in Asia are at lower risk than people in Western countries for many kinds of cancer. Research has been conducted in the Far East to identify why. The research led scientists to focus on polyphenols found in tea. Although green tea seems to have higher levels, black teas common in the United States are also high in polyphenols.

The French eat a lot of butter and cream. However, they have a lower rate of heart disease than people in the United States. The reason for this may be the wine in the French diet. The polyphenols in red wine help reduce the risk of heart disease. These polyphenols are found in almost any red or purple grape product. The more color a grape product has, the more polyphenols it contains. White grapes and white grape juice have little or no polyphenols. (However, white grapes contain other helpful phytochemicals, such as ellagic acid.) To get the benefits of polyphenols, snack on fresh red grapes or drink a glass of purple grape juice. See 14-13.

Another food that contains helpful polyphenols may be the herb rosemary. This herb is commonly found in Italian chicken dishes. It may help prevent colon and breast cancers. Polyphenols are also found in sunflower seeds, barley, and apples.

Saponins

Saponins are molecules formed from a sugar reacting with an alcohol. See 14-14. Saponins appear to block the reproduction of DNA in cancerous cells. They do this by interfering with enzyme reactions.

The name *saponin* is derived from the Latin word for soap. This is because most saponins easily form a soapy foam and have a

Polyphenols

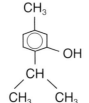

epigallocatechin-3-gallate (EGCG)

14-12 Polyphenols are being studied for their role in fighting cancer and heart disease.

Phenolic Acids

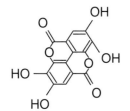

Ellagic acid is found in strawberries, tomatoes, whole grains, and nuts.

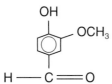

Vanillan is the main component in vanilla beans.

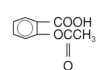

Thymol is in oil of peppermint.

Acetylsalicylic acid is the chemical name for aspirin.

14-11 Phenolic acids are found in aspirin as well as in a variety fof foods and flavorings.

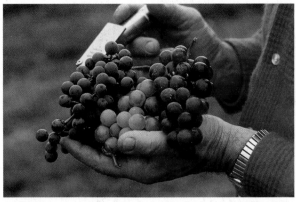

USDA

14-13 Because many phytochemicals are color compounds, foods with richer color will have more phytochemicals than light ones. For example, red and purple grapes are high in polyphenols. White grapes are not.

Saponins

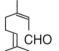

This is the chemical structure for a saponin in ginseng. R_1 and R_2 represent sugar chains.

14-14 Saponins are four-ring, steroidlike chemicals with a sugar side chain.

bitter taste. Saponins are found in spinach, potatoes, tomatoes, oats, beans, and legumes. They are also found in soybeans, sugar beets, peanuts, and asparagus.

Cooking Tip

Some saponins, such as those in raw lima beans, soybeans, and red kidney beans, form cyanide compounds when digested. These compounds are toxic. Thoroughly cooking and rinsing beans before eating helps remove the cyanide. When cyanide is eaten in small amounts, the body can quickly turn it into thiocyanate, which is not toxic.

Terpenes

Terpenes are a group of compounds responsible for the flavors of citrus fruits and many seasonings and herbs. Research indicates that terpenes block the development of tumors. They do this by reversing the growth of tumors and/or by changing tumors to a less malignant type. Terpenes appear to block the formation of cancer cells. One member of the terpene family has shown promise in treating pancreatic tumors in animals. This type of terpene is found in cherries. Another terpene, which is found in citrus peel, seems to block the development of breast tumors. See 14-15.

The best known terpene is *taxol*, which is being used to treat ovarian cancer. Taxol is not found in food. It is found in the Pacific yew tree and can now be reproduced in the laboratory.

Phytochemicals and Food Processing

As you read earlier, phytochemicals give many foods their colors and flavors. When developing food products, food scientists work to maintain these colors and flavors. Food scientists also want to preserve the phytochemicals in foods for their health benefits.

Maintaining the Colors of Foods

Phytochemicals are largely responsible for the colors in fruits and vegetables, 14-16. By maintaining the natural colors of food during processing, many of the phytochemical levels will also be maintained.

Terpenes

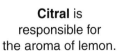

Citral is responsible for the aroma of lemon.

Limonene is the compound that gives limes their aroma.

14-15 Citrus fruits get their flavors from phytochemicals called terpenes.

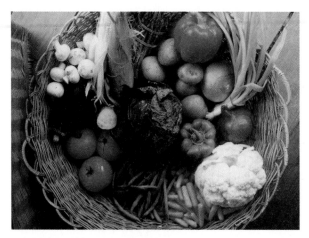

14-16 Fruits and vegetables get their rainbow of bright colors from phytochemicals.

The carotenoids are responsible for yellow, orange, and red pigments in fruits and vegetables. When carotenoids are present along with chlorophyll, the color that is visible is green. Carotenoids are insoluble in water. This allows them to remain stable in foods cooked by most methods. When carotenoid molecules are cooked in the presence of acid, they change shape. This causes the orange colors to become more yellow. However, the elements in the compound do not change. Two molecules with the same chemical formula but slightly different structures are called *isomers.* Research is needed to find out if all isomers of carotenoids have the same functions in the body. Carotenoids are sensitive to oxidation when dehydrated. The result is a loss of color and an inability to form vitamin A.

Lycopene is the carotenoid that gives tomatoes their red color. When isolated from plant tissues, it is changed by exposure to oxygen and light. However, studies have found that many home and commercial cooking processes make lycopene more absorbable. Lypocene reduces risk of cancers in reproductive tissue, enhances the immune system, and slows the aging process of eyes, skin, heart, and other body tissues.

Flavonoids are water soluble, and they often undergo changes during processing. The flavonoids in foods like red cabbage are red in acid and blue in base. Because acids evaporate as they are heated, the pH of foods containing acids rises during cooking. This is why red cabbage will change to a bluish color when cooked. The more alkaline the mixture is, the bluer the cabbage will be. Many red cabbage recipes call for apples or vinegar. The acid in these ingredients helps keep the cabbage red when it is cooked. Color changes obviously make some foods unappealing. However, more research is needed to determine whether the color changes also signal a change in nutritive value.

Flavonoid compounds will form salts of iron or tin when stored or cooked in these metals. These compounds are bluish red or violet in color. They give green vegetables such as asparagus an unattractive color when cooked in iron. The color change is a result of the metal reacting with a hydroxyl group (OH) on the carbon rings. Some food cans have a white coating inside. This coating helps reduce color changes by keeping flavonoids from reacting with the metal can.

The appearance of tea is affected by reactions between water and flavonoids in the tea. Tea brewed in alkaline water will have a dark brown color. This is caused by calcium and magnesium in the brewing water. These ions will form compounds with the flavonoids that cloud the tea as it cools. If lemon juice is added to the tea, the flavonoid-mineral compounds dissolve and stay suspended in the tea.

Another group of flavonoids is white to pale yellow. They become more yellow when the pH is 8 or higher. Apples and potatoes contain these flavonoids. These foods will retain a whiter color during cooking if the pH is 6 or lower.

> ### Storage Tip
> Reactions between flavonoids and some materials cause color changes in foods that are high in flavonoids. To prevent color changes, store foods high in flavonoids in glass, plastic, or stainless steel containers.

Maintaining the Flavors of Foods

The phytochemicals in foods affect the flavors of the foods. Food scientists need to be aware of how food processing can alter phytochemicals and the flavors they produce.

Allyl sulfides are unstable flavor compounds that are formed when plant tissues are disrupted. For instance, these compounds are released when onions and garlic are chopped. Cooking onions and garlic alters the allyl sulfides, resulting in milder flavors. Overcooking can cause allyl sulfides to break down, leading to a loss of flavor.

Isothiocyanates are other flavor compounds that are unstable in heat. The flavors of foods high in isothiocyanates become stronger after cooking. Examples of such foods include Brussels sprouts, cabbage, and turnips.

Polyphenols create an astringency in foods. In other words, they draw up the muscles of the mouth. Some people mistake astringency for bitterness. The astringency of polyphenols affects the flavor of tea, grape juice, and wines, 14-17. The British custom of adding milk to tea removes the astringency because the polyphenols bind to the milk proteins.

Tannins are a group of polyphenols that can cloud liquids. Tannins are involved in the enzymatic browning process. These polyphenols react with proteins and oxygen to form very large complexes of molecules. The heavier weight of these polyphenol and protein complexes causes them to eventually settle to the bottom of liquids.

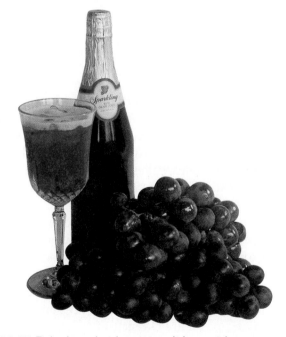

14-17 Polyphenols give grape juice astringency.

Tannins can cloud beer and processed apple juice and form an unpleasant sediment. Therefore, manufacturers often add a small amount of gelatin to these beverages. The hydroxyl group on the polyphenol forms a hydrogen bond with the peptide bonds in the gelatin protein. The polyphenol-gelatin complex is then filtered out of the liquid.

Food scientists still have much to learn about the effects of food processing on phytochemicals and the flavors they produce. This area of study is complicated by the fact that phytochemicals are a part of many ingredients in foods. The mixture of phytochemicals varies from plant to plant and from food to food. The mixture of compounds present will affect how the phytochemicals respond to pH and temperature changes.

Preserving Phytochemicals

Most phytochemicals will develop only in fruits and vegetables that ripen on the plant. These compounds form during the final stages of ripening or maturation. Fruits and vegetables are often harvested before they are fully ripe. This gives growers time to sort, pack, and ship produce to the point of sale. The produce is usually ripe by the time it is sold. However, the phytochemical content is lower than if the fruits and vegetables had ripened before picking.

Food scientists are trying to find ways to maximize the phytochemical content of produce. One technique they are using is rapid freezing of fruits and vegetables right after harvest. This technique requires production plants to be built near the point of harvest.

Food scientists are also working to develop new breeds of plants in which phytochemicals can develop before harvest. The first bioengineered food was the Flavr Savr tomato. This tomato was genetically altered to delay spoilage. These tomatoes can ripen on the vine. They will then keep for up to two weeks before spoiling. Flavr Savr tomatoes are no longer marketed because of high production and processing costs. Researchers are working to develop other fruits and vegetables with delayed spoiling characteristics. Other goals of bioengineering include nutritional enhancement and altered composition to aid processing without negatively affecting nutritional value.

Research is needed to determine the effects of processing on each of the identified phytochemicals. Food scientists also need information on the stability of these compounds when exposed to oxygen, acids, salts, and light. Data is currently limited. However, some studies have been conducted on soy products. These studies have shown the isoflavone genistein is lost when soy proteins are removed from the beans. By altering processing methods, genistein levels increase significantly. Studies also show that heating, freezing, and freeze-drying reduce isoflavones in soy products by 40% to 53%.

Manufacturers are working to come up with processing methods that will increase phytochemicals in foods. At the same time, manufacturers are trying to maintain or improve the appeal of these foods.

Potential Health Benefits of Phytochemicals

Research suggests that phytochemicals appear to help prevent disease. They seem to be able to stop a healthy cell from changing to a cancerous cell. Some phytochemicals act as antioxidants or enzyme activators. Others seem to protect the cell's genetic material. Some phytochemicals have antifungal, antiviral, and antibacterial properties. Foods high in phytochemicals seem to help the body fight off colds, influenza, and infections. Phytochemicals have been linked to lower rates of heart disease and reduced cholesterol levels. Phytochemicals may have many other health benefits that have not yet been discovered. See 14-18.

Increasing Phytochemicals in Your Diet

There are thousands of phytochemicals. Remembering their tongue-twister names is not as important as remembering the foods in which you can find them. You have read that some phytochemicals are destroyed by heat. However, some are created by cooking reactions, and others are unaffected. How can you be sure you are getting a full range of these valuable compounds? The best way is to eat a variety of foods. Does that advice sound familiar? Make sure the variety includes the following powerhouses of nutrition in both cooked and raw forms.

Broccoli tops the list of foods rich in phytochemicals. It also provides a variety of vitamins and minerals. There are few foods with the overall nutritional impact of broccoli. Close behind broccoli are the other cruciferous vegetables: cabbage, cauliflower, and kale.

Dark green vegetables are high in phytochemicals, vitamins, and minerals. The darker the green color is, the higher the nutritional value will be. Foods in this group include spinach, watercress, collard greens, and parsley.

Tea in any form is a good addition to the diet. A factor to remember is that polyphenols in tea will react with iron and calcium consumed at the same time. (For more information about this reaction, refer to the Recent Research box *Tea with Lemon Please!* in Chapter 13.) Herbal teas are not made from tea leaves. Therefore, they do not contain the polyphenols found in white, green, and black tea. However, many herbal teas, such as clove, cinnamon, and mint, contain other phytochemicals that may be of benefit.

Red and purple grapes, grape juice, and raisins that are not sun dried are good sources of polyphenols. Polyphenols help protect plants from damage caused by ultraviolet light. When fruits are sun dried, the ultraviolet light exposure uses up or chemically changes polyphenols.

Onions, garlic, leeks, and chives have a wide range of health benefits. Try to include them in your diet every day. Garlic has the highest levels of phytochemicals in this group.

Citrus fruits, including the "zest" or grated peel, are high in vitamin C and make excellent additions to the diet. Adding finely grated citrus peel to cookies, cakes, and muffins can create a deliciously fruity flavor while increasing phytochemical levels.

Tomatoes are packed with phytochemicals. They are versatile, economical, and available year round. Use fresh tomatoes on sandwiches or as garnishes. Try dried tomatoes in salads. Canned tomatoes are long-standing favorites in soups and casseroles. Tomato sauces on pizza and pasta are classic.

Phytochemicals in Your Diet

Phytochemical Family or Subgroup	Possible Health Benefits	Food Sources
Allyl sulfides	Increase enzymatic reactions that rid the body of carcinogens Thin blood Act as antibacterial, antifungal, and antiviral agents	Chives, garlic, leeks, onions
Carotenoids	Serve antioxidant functions Reduce tissue damage that leads to formation of cancer Help maintain healthy eye tissue	Broccoli, cabbage, carrots, guava, kale, oranges, papayas, pink grapefruit, pumpkins, spinach, tomatoes, tangerines, watermelon
Flavonoids	Provide anti-inflammatory properties Reduce risks of stroke and heart disease Act as antibacterial, antifungal, and antiviral agents	Apples, asparagus, broccoli, cranberries, grapes, herbs and spices, nuts, onions, red cabbage, soy sauce, teas
Isoflavones	Block estrogen, reducing risks of breast and ovarian cancers Reduce symptoms of menopause	Bok choy, chickpeas, Chinese cabbage, legumes, licorice, soybeans, soy milk, tofu
Indoles	Stimulate enzymes that reduce the effects of estrogen, possibly reducing the risk of breast cancer	Broccoli, Brussels sprouts, cabbage, cauliflower, kale, kohlrabi
Isothiocyanates	Stimulate the production of anti-cancer enzymes, helping the body ward off cancer	Broccoli, Brussels sprouts, cabbage, cauliflower, horseradish, kohlrabi, radishes, turnips, watercress
Phenolic acids	Protect cells' genetic material from carcinogens	Carrots, citrus fruits, nuts, raspberries, strawberries, tomatoes, whole grains
Polyphenols	Lower risks of many kinds of cancer Reduce risk of heart disease Lower LDL and cholesterol levels	Apples, grape juice, green and black tea, red and purple grapes, rosemary, sunflower seeds
Saponins	Interfere with DNA replication, preventing cancer cells from multiplying	Asparagus, beans, legumes, oats, peanuts, potatoes, soybeans, spinach, sugar beets, tomatoes
Terpenes	Block the growth of tumors, reverse tumor growth, and change tumors to a less malignant type	Cherries, citrus peel

14-18 Researchers are investigating a wide range of possible health benefits that phytochemicals may offer.

Many registered dietitians recommend you consume 5 to 10 servings of fruits and vegetables a day. These fruits and vegetables should include at least three colors. The kinds of phytochemicals consumed increase as food colors vary.

Dietitians suggest two servings of fruit for breakfast. For example, you might top a whole-wheat waffle with strawberries and drink a glass of orange juice with it. Eat one serving of fruit and two servings of vegetables at both lunch and dinner. Lunch might include lettuce, tomato, and onion on a sandwich eaten with carrot sticks and an apple. A fresh fruit salad, green beans, and a baked sweet potato would make great accompaniments to a dinner menu. You can include phytochemicals in your snack foods, too. Try frozen grapes instead of a flavored ice pop for a cool summer snack. A spicy salsa adds the benefits of tomatoes, onions, and green peppers to crunchy tortilla chips.

A closer look at a popular meal among teens will show how easily you can add phytochemicals to your diet. The next time you eat at your favorite pizza place, consider making the following phytochemical-rich choices:

❖ pizza with extra sauce and chopped vegetables instead of extra cheese and pepperoni, 14-19

❖ a side salad with extra tomato, broccoli, and bean sprouts instead of bread sticks

❖ ice tea with lemon instead of a soft drink

New Directions for Food Science

During the 1990s, food scientists developed hundreds of foods that were lowfat, fat free, and microwaveable. Many of these foods were developed because of consumer demands for healthier convenience foods. As research uncovers the value of phytochemicals, consumer demand for foods rich in these

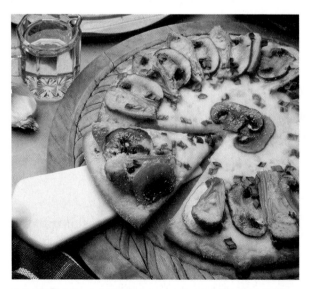

14-19 Extra vegetables on a pizza will add phytochemicals as well as flavor.

compounds is likely to grow. New challenges for food scientists will focus on preserving and enhancing phytochemicals in foods.

The idea of "designer foods" based on phytochemical content may be the nutrition trend of the next decade. Food scientists can already change the chemical composition of food through plant breeding techniques and food processing. In the future, they will continue to use their knowledge to design foods that help fight heart disease or cancer.

Food scientists are examining a new category of foods called functional foods. *Functional foods* are modified foods or food ingredients that may provide heath benefits beyond the traditional nutrients they contain. The concept of functional foods was first introduced in Japan. These foods contain bioactive components such as phytochemicals. *Bioactive components* are compounds that have physiological benefits. They improve normal body processes, reduce the risk of chronic disease, or block the development of cancer cells. Functional foods have one or more of the following characteristics:

❖ an ingredient that is known to create health hazards is removed from the food (cholesterol-free eggs)

❖ ingredients not normally found in the food are added or combined to provide known health benefits (calcium-enriched orange juice)

❖ the concentration of bioactive ingredients in the food is increased (lycopene-rich tomatoes)

Functional foods are consumed as a part of a normal diet. As research into phytochemicals continues, doctors may prescribe functional foods as part of a total health care program. The food prescribed will depend on the illness being treated.

The FDA currently has no official definition for the term *functional food*. Functional foods are not recognized as a legal category of food products in the United States. However, food-specific health claims can be put on product labels if the claims are FDA approved. Private companies must petition the FDA for the right to use health claims on labels. Each claim must be supported by scientific studies that document the health benefits the food provides. The first food to receive approval for a health claim label was oats. This claim was supported by 37 studies over 15 years that documented the effects of β-glucan fiber in oats on lowering cholesterol.

People need to know what compounds they should increase in their diets. Then they can determine how functional foods can play a role in health care by providing these compounds. How much is beneficial? How much is harmful? Are there any side effects from changing nature's balance? There is much for scientists to learn. There is also much for you to learn as a consumer. You will be able to make wiser choices if you keep up with the developments. Make a point of learning how scientific findings can affect your diet and food preparation methods.

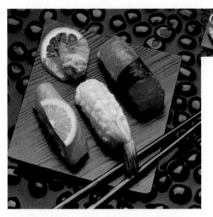

International Issue
Prescribing Food in Japan

Diseases such as heart disease, diabetes, and cancer are growing problems in Japan. This is due to a rapidly aging population and the Westernization of the diet. Part of Japan's plan to fight these growing health problems is food. Japan's Ministry of Heath and Welfare has created the concept of functional foods. The Ministry's goal is to encourage the development of food products that have specific health benefits. It is hoped that these foods will improve the health of the Japanese people.

In Japan, functional foods are based on the belief that food has three purposes

❖ to serve as a source of nutrition to maintain life

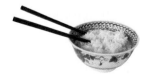

A low-allergen rice was one of the first functional foods to receive approval as a FOSHU food in Japan.

❖ to provide sensory appeal

❖ to prevent or cure disease or assist in recuperation from disease

In a broad sense, functional foods are foods that possess all three functions. Functional foods are more narrowly defined as products aimed at regulating body processes. A subgroup of functional foods was identified as "foods for specified health use," or FOSHU foods.

Japan is the first nation to promote the development of foods for specific health and disease-fighting functions. A formal approval process was set up to qualify a product as a FOSHU food. The first foods to receive this approval were a low-allergen rice and low-phosphorus milk. The approval process requires food scientists to submit evidence that shows a food meets a number of conditions. These conditions include

❖ the food is effective for the improvement of daily diet and for the preservation and promotion of health

❖ the medical and dietetic grounds on health preservation are evident in research

❖ appropriate servings are medically and dietetically defined

❖ the food is proven to be safe and different from a pharmaceutical pill form

Functional foods have a number of health benefits. These include disease prevention and recovery, body-rhythm regulation, and reduced effects of aging. New foods being formulated include

❖ carrots that supply three to five times the beta-carotene of regular carrots

❖ orange-flesh cucumbers that contain beta-carotene

❖ strawberries that contain more cancer-protective ellagic acid (a phenolic acid)

❖ orange juice that contains much higher levels of phytochemicals than normal

❖ snack foods that contain cholesterol-lowering phytochemicals

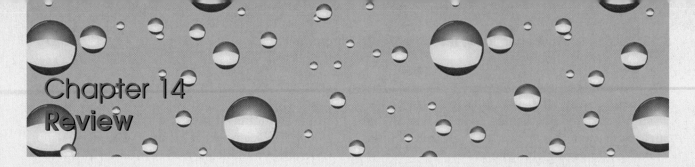

Chapter 14
Review

Summary

This chapter examined one of the newest areas of research related to nutrition and food science—phytochemicals. Phytochemicals are compounds found in plants that may help the body fight disease. Research is so new in this area that experts are only beginning to reach any definite conclusions. There is, however, enough evidence to indicate that researchers and consumers alike need to turn their attention to the study of these compounds.

Phytochemicals are mostly flavor and color compounds naturally found in foods that, in the past, have had no recognized nutritive value. They were considered to be neither harmful nor helpful. Many now appear to provide beneficial effects to human health, and some may even combat disease. Future research may lead to the development of foods designed to help fight specific diseases.

Recognizing the names of the families of phytochemicals will help you follow research developments as they are announced in the news. The families or categories of phytochemicals are: allyl sulfides, carotenoids, flavonoids, indoles, isoflavones, isothiocyanates, phenolic acids, polyphenols, saponins, and terpenes. The foods highest in many of these compounds include: soy products, broccoli, dark leafy green vegetables, tea, red and purple grapes, onions, garlic, leeks, chives, citrus fruits including the zest of the peel, and tomatoes.

Check Your Understanding

1. Explain why vitamin and mineral pills by themselves are not sufficient for good health.
2. List the three ways allyl sulfides may help the body fight disease.
3. Describe the difference in chemical structure between the carotenes and xanthophylls.
4. Name the carotenoid that seems to reduce the risk of prostate cancer and its most common source.
5. For what are flavonoids responsible?
6. Which type of cuisine is highest in isoflavones? Why?
7. List the two ways to increase the availability of indoles.
8. What do tea and grape juice have in common?
9. Identify three sources of terpenes and the cancers they attack.
10. Why is it important to maintain the flavor and color of plant foods?
11. Describe two ways researchers are working to preserve or increase phytochemical levels in foods.
12. What is the purpose of functonal foods in the diet?

Critical Thinking

1. Explain the problems with trying to lose weight by eating and drinking only vitamin- and mineral-fortified beverages.
2. Describe the diet you would recommend to a family member who was diagnosed with cancer.
3. Why is hard water more likely to result in cloudy ice tea than soft or distilled water?
4. Based on information in the chapter, what is a good response to this comment: "Nothing good will come from tampering with the genes of fruits and vegetables."
5. What are the potential problems with taking large amounts of phytochemical supplements?

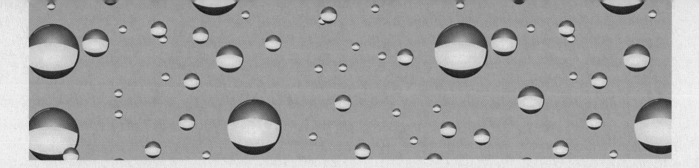

Explore Further

1. **Food and Nutrition.** Plan a diet for one day that contains at least one good source of each of the ten families of phytochemicals. Label each. Does this diet meet the guidelines of MyPyramid? What changes, if any, are needed?

2. **Technology.** Use the Internet to find two research studies related to the same phytochemical. Summarize the conclusions of the studies and report your findings to the class.

3. **Analytical Skills.** Describe a new functional food that would appeal to teens. What "function" would the new product address? Design a package label or advertising campaign for this new food.

4. **Communication.** Write an article for your school newspaper that explains what phytochemicals are and why teens need more of them.

5. **Research.** Examine the research reports that have studied the health value of chocolate. Report on the phytochemicals found in chocolate and the compounds that may negatively impact health.

Experiment 14A
Effect of pH Changes on Chlorophyll

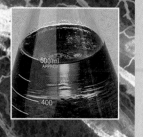

Purpose

In this experiment, you will examine the effect of acids and bases on chlorophyll, which is a color pigment found in green vegetables. A change in the color of a food usually indicates a change in the color compounds present. Under certain conditions, chlorophyll will become pheophytin, which has an olive green color.

Equipment

chef's knife

cutting board

wax pencil

4 250-mL beakers

metric measuring spoons

electronic balance

pH paper or meter

beaker tongs

4 serving spoons

fork for each lab group member

Supplies

100 g fresh spinach

400 mL distilled water

3 g (½ teaspoon) salt

1 g baking soda

5 mL (1 teaspoon) vinegar

aluminum foil

4 disposable cups for each lab group member

Procedure

1. Wash, chop, and divide 100 g of spinach into four equal portions.

2. Use a wax pencil to label four 250-mL beakers *A, B, C,* and *D.* Prepare the following solutions:

   Beaker A: 100 mL distilled water

   Beaker B: 100 mL distilled water plus 3 g salt

   Beaker C: 100 mL distilled water plus 1 g baking soda

   Beaker D: 100 mL distilled water plus 5 mL (1 teaspoon) vinegar

3. Measure the pH of the solution in each beaker. Record the results in a data table.

4. Bring the solutions in the beakers to a boil. (The beakers can be placed in a circle on the same burner.)

5. Add a portion of the spinach to each beaker.

6. Lay a square of foil on top of each beaker and simmer for 10 minutes.

7. Use beaker tongs to remove the beakers from the heat.

8. Record observations regarding the color and texture of the spinach in each beaker.

9. Measure the pH of each solution. Record the results in the data table.

10. For each lab group member, label the outside of a set of four disposable cups with the letters *A, B, C,* and *D.*

11. Use a clean spoon to place a small amount of each spinach variation in the appropriately labeled cups. Taste the spinach samples.

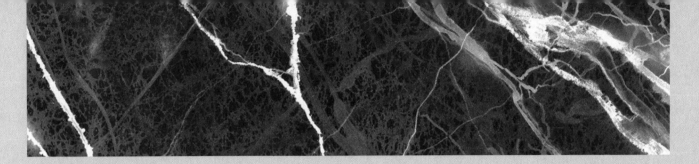

Questions

1. How did the color, texture, and flavor of the vegetables compare?

2. Is chlorophyll water soluble? How do you know?

3. What are the effects of acids, bases, and salts on chlorophyll?

4. How can you apply this information to food preparation?

Experiment 14B
Effect of pH Changes on Flavonoids

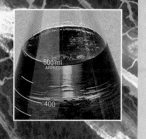

Purpose

Anthoxanthin and anthocyanin are flavonoid pigments. The pH of a food mixture will affect the colors of these pigments. In this experiment, you will determine what color changes occur in acidic, basic, and neutral solutions.

Equipment

chef's knife

cutting board

wax pencil

3 250-mL beakers

electronic balance

metric measuring spoons

pH paper or meter

beaker tongs

glass rod

Supplies

300 mL distilled water

salt

1 g baking soda

5 mL (1 teaspoon) white vinegar

250 mL assigned fruit or vegetable

aluminum foil

Procedure

1. Wash your assigned fruit or vegetable and chop, if necessary. Describe the color of the food prior to cooking.

   Variation 1: cauliflower

   Variation 2: potato

   Variation 3: blackberries

   Variation 4: blueberries

2. Use a wax pencil to label three 250-mL beakers *A*, *B*, and *C*. Prepare the following solutions in the beakers:

   Beaker A: 100 mL distilled water

   Beaker B: 100 mL distilled water plus 1 g baking soda

   Beaker C: 100 mL distilled water plus 5 mL (1 teaspoon) vinegar

3. Measure and record the pH of each solution.

4. Bring the solutions in the beakers to a boil. Add one-third of the assigned fruit or vegetable to each beaker.

5. Cover each beaker with aluminum foil and simmer for 5 minutes.

6. Use beaker tongs to remove the beakers from the heat and measure the pH. Conduct a sensory evaluation. Record your observations of the color, texture, and flavor of the food.

7. Combine Beakers B and C. Stir briefly. Note any color changes.

Data

Record your data and observations on a class data chart on an overhead projector.

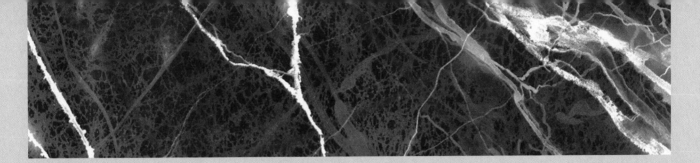

Questions

1. What changes occurred to fruits and vegetables cooked in distilled water?

2. What changes occurred to fruits and vegetables cooked in the basic solutions?

3. What changes occurred to fruits and vegetables cooked in the acid solutions?

4. Are the flavonoids in these fruits and vegetables water soluble? How do you know?

5. Are the color changes reversible?

6. What application does this have to food preparation?

Experiment 14C
Effect of Blanching on Chlorophyll

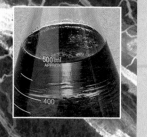

Purpose

Fresh spinach contains several phytochemical pigments that give the vegetable its deep green color. They include chlorophyll A, chlorophyll B, carotenes, and xanthophylls. The enzyme chlorophyllase is also present. During mild heating, bright green pigments known as chlorophyllides are formed. When more severe heating occurs, the chlorophyllase breaks the chlorophyllides down into pheophytins. The pigments in spinach can be separated using a simple process called paper chromatography.

Equipment

metric ruler
coin
hair dryer
pencil
250-mL beaker
rubber band

Supplies

filter paper
fresh spinach leaf
blanched spinach leaf
tape
ethanol (95%)
plastic wrap
paper towel

Procedure

1. Cut a strip of filter paper 8 cm long and 3 cm wide.

2. Lay the strip so one of the 3-cm sides is at the bottom. Draw a pencil line across the strip 1 cm from the bottom. This is the spotting line. Draw a second pencil line across the strip 6 cm above the first line. This is the solvent front line.

3. Below the bottom line on the left half of the strip, write F for fresh. Below the line on the right half of the strip, write B for blanched. (See illustration below.)

4. Place a fresh spinach leaf on the spotting line above the F. Gently press down with the edge of a coin until a heavy green pigment spot, about 0.5 cm in diameter, is visible.

5. Repeat step 4 with a blanched spinach leaf on the spotting line above the B.

6. Dry the strip with a hair dryer.

7. Tape the top edge of the strip to the middle of a pencil.

8. Lay the pencil across the top of a 250-mL beaker so the bottom of the paper strip touches the bottom of the beaker.

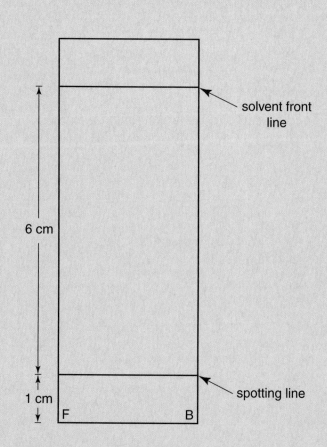

solvent front line

6 cm

1 cm

F   B

spotting line

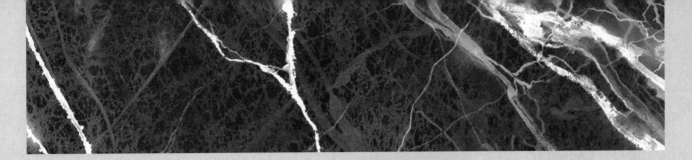

9. Carefully add enough ethanol to the beaker to submerge the end of the paper strip. Do not cover the spotting line or the pigment spots with the ethanol. The pigment spots should be just above the line of ethanol.

10. Cover the top of the beaker tightly with plastic wrap to keep the ethanol from evaporating. Hold the wrap in place with a rubber band.

11. Allow the strip to remain in the ethanol until the ethanol reaches the solvent front line. (This will take about 12 to 15 minutes.)

12. Remove the strip from the beaker and lay it on a paper towel. Blot the strip dry.

13. With a pencil, circle each spot of color that appears above the spotting line. Construct a drawing of your strip or attach your strip to your data table.

14. Record the distance from the spotting line to the solvent front line in a data table. Measure the distance from the spotting line to each spot of color you circled in step 13. Record the distances and color of each spot in the data table.

Calculations

Calculate the retardation factor (R_f) for each color spot. You will calculate the R_f value by dividing the distance the color spot traveled by the distance the solvent (ethanol) traveled. The R_f value is a number between 0 and 1. If conditions are constant, the R_f value for any given pigment is also constant. Compare your calculations to the R_f values for the pigments in spinach given below.

chlorophyll B = 0.17

chlorophyll A = 0.37

carotenes = 0.63

xanthophylls = 0.87

Questions

1. Based on your calculations, which pigments were visible in the fresh spinach? Which pigments were visible in the blanched spinach?

2. What differences did you observe between the fresh and blanched spinach?

3. What is the effect of heating on color pigments?

4. How can this be applied to food preparation and phytochemicals?

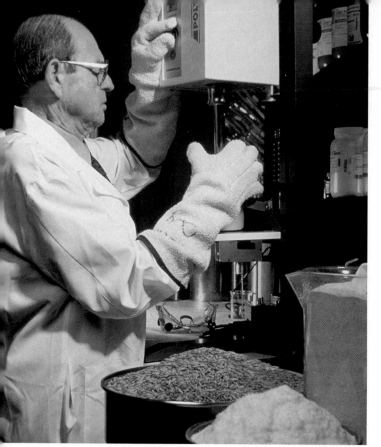

This chemist is working with a starch-based product he developed that can take the place of fat in some foods.

Objectives

After studying this chapter,
you will be able to

list the four main functions of food analogs.

distinguish between nutritive and nonnutritive sweeteners.

compare the performance of fat replacers to the performance of fat.

describe advantages and disadvantages of potassium chloride as a salt substitute.

Chapter 15

Food Analogs: Substitute Ingredients

Key Terms

saccharin	polyols
aspartame	bulking agent
acesulfame K	Simplesse
sucralose	olestra

Imagine everyone in a family being able to eat ice cream made to order for his or her health needs. Grandmother might select a lowfat, sugar-free variety because of her diabetes. Mom might order the same kind to help her lose weight. Dad might choose a salt free, fat free product because of his high blood pressure. The son who cannot tolerate milk might pick ice cream that is milk free and still high in calcium. The daughter who wants to store energy for sports competition could choose ice cream made with a complex-carbohydrate fat replacer. All these frozen dessert products would be tasty and satisfying. They would resemble ice cream in texture, color, and taste. However, they would not contain the same ingredients as traditional ice cream. See 15-1.

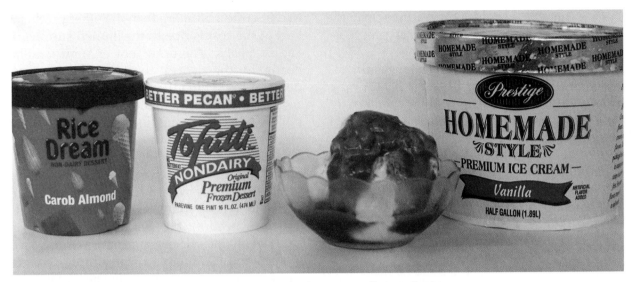

15-1 Rice and soy can be used to create nondairy ice-cream-like products.

You may have heard the expression "A rose by any other name is just as sweet!" All sugars are sweeteners, but not all sweeteners are sugar. Bacon-flavored bits on your salad may not be bacon. Grocery stores are filled with imitation flavored drinks, fat free ice cream, and sugar-free candy. How does the nutritional value of these food substitutes compare to the "real thing"? Food scientists have the ability to create foods that have the qualities consumers want without some of the negatives.

Functions of Food Analogs

Food analogs make up an area of research that grew significantly in the last half of the twentieth century. As you learned in Chapter 1, *food analogs* are natural or manufactured substances. They are used in place of traditional food products or ingredients. Food analogs are designed to serve one or more of the following functions:

❖ save money

❖ change the nutritive value of foods

❖ improve the performance of foods or compounds

❖ take the place of foods or food ingredients that are restricted for health reasons

In some cases, food analogs are created to reduce food costs for consumers. For example,

soybeans are cheaper to produce than beef. Soybeans can be treated with an alkali bath. A sticky liquid of protein is formed that can be forced through small holes into an acid bath. The new soy product is a texturized protein that lacks color or flavor. This product can be given a consistency that resembles chicken or beef. With the addition of flavorings and colorings, this texturized soy can become an analog for bacon bits. Different flavorings and colorings allow it to be used as a beef analog to stretch hamburger dishes.

Some soybean analogs also change the nutritive value of foods. Unlike hamburger, texturized soy protein is fat and cholesterol free. Studies found that people who regularly consume soy protein have lower blood cholesterol levels than people who consume animal proteins. Soy products contain some beneficial phytochemicals, too.

Nondairy whipped topping is a food analog whose performance is in many ways an improvement over the original food. Whipped topping has a longer shelf life, a less-greasy mouth feel, greater foam stability, and fewer Calories than whipped cream. Many people are so accustomed to whipped topping that they prefer it to whipped cream.

Another example of a food analog that improves the performance of a food is instant pudding. Traditionally, pudding had to be cooked for the starch to be able to thicken and gel. Instant puddings are made with a starch analog that gels at cold temperatures instead of hot ones. The result is a shorter preparation time.

Many food analogs are the result of research to make a substitute for health reasons. Artificial sweeteners allow people to sweeten foods without using sugar. These analogs taste sweet, but their chemical structures cause them to be digested in a manner different from sugar. This is especially helpful for people who have diabetes. Many people with high blood pressure use salt substitutes. These products make foods seem salty without increasing blood pressure the way sodium chloride can.

The Pros and Cons of Food Analogs

Foods are very complex and need to be understood. Some people believe food analogs are a drawback to the current food supply. These consumers may prefer "natural" foods that are free from "chemicals." These consumers may not realize that all foods are made up entirely of chemical elements. Analogs are just made from different chemical components than traditional foods.

Some people think food analogs offer great advantages in shaping the food supply. These people may assume analogs will eventually allow them to eat anything they want without restricting their intake. Many analogs offer the benefits of lowfat, reduced Calorie options to traditional foods. However, analogs will never be able to take the place of all traditional foods in your diet. You know your body needs a variety of foods. No single food provides all the nutrients you need. Even scientists with a deep knowledge of how food delivers nutrition do not know how to meet all the body's needs. Anytime food scientists create an analog, they study it carefully to look for any potentially harmful side effects.

Analogs keep the prices of many food products reasonable. The supply of many "natural" foods is too small to economically meet current demand. Vanilla ice cream illustrates this point. Compare a brand containing natural vanilla beans with a brand containing artificial vanilla flavoring. The two flavorings have equivalent nutritional values. However, the product flavored with vanilla beans is likely

to cost quite a bit more than the other product. Part of the cost is due to the limited supply of vanilla beans. There are not enough vanilla beans in the world to meet the present demand for vanilla flavorings. See 15-2.

The true place of analogs in the food supply lies between the views of those who oppose analogs and those who favor them. You do not have to choose between an economical, abundant food supply and a healthful one. To make wise decisions, you need to understand how your body uses food analogs. You also need to be aware of the nutritive value of analogs. They can easily become part of a healthful eating plan. You simply need to check their nutrition labels, just as you would for any food product.

This chapter cannot cover all the possibilities. However, it will look at the most popular food analogs on the market that are used as substitute ingredients. It will also review some current research that is in the news. By looking closely at a few analogs, you will learn how to determine whether these products should be part of your balanced diet. You will learn what questions to ask. This will help you

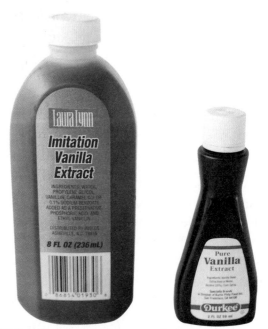

15-2 Imitation vanilla extract helps meet the demand for vanilla flavorings, and it costs consumers about one-tenth as much as pure vanilla extract.

decide whether a product is right for you and your family.

The three types of food analogs in widest use today are sugar substitutes, fat substitutes, and salt substitutes. The use of these products has been boosted by health problems linked to traditional sugars, fats, and salt. These problems include obesity, heart disease, diabetes, and cancer. Consumers want the flavors and textures traditional sugars, fats, and salt give food products without the health risks. Food scientists all over the world have been working to fill this tall order through food analogs.

Sugar Substitutes

Most people's favorite taste is sweet. This may have something to do with the fact that the brain can use only glucose as fuel. An excess of Calories from sugar can lead to weight gain. For diabetics, too much sugar in the diet can cause fainting, coma, and even death. Finding a sugar substitute has health benefits for many people.

Consumer demand for lower-Calorie foods that taste like high-Calorie favorites has led to the development of several sugar substitutes. These popular food analogs change the nutritive value of food. They add sweetness to the taste of a food without adding many Calories. Several types of sugar substitutes are presently approved for use in the United States. The number of Americans consuming sugar-free foods or beverages has risen from 68 million in 1984 to 180 million in 2004.

Nonnutritive Sweeteners

Nonnutritive sweeteners are also called artificial sweeteners. They are nonnutritive or artificial because they provide virtually no energy. They add a sweet flavor to foods without adding sugar or Calories. Current research indicates that artificial sweeteners pose no health risks when used appropriately. The American Dietetic Association advises they be used in moderation as part of a nutritious diet. See 15-3.

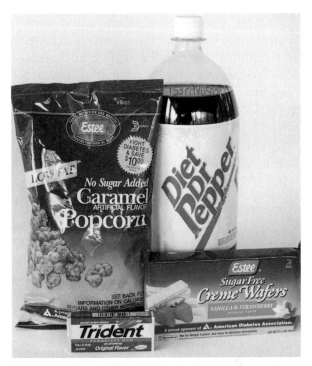

15-3 A wide variety of sugar-free foods is available for consumers seeking to limit sugar and/or calorie intake.

Saccharin

Saccharin is an artificial sweetener that is stable in a wide range of foods under extreme processing conditions. Discovered in 1879, it was the only artificial sweetener available for the first half of the twentieth century. An advantage of saccharin is that it is economical to produce. Its sweetening power is at least 2,000 times that of sugar.

Two main drawbacks have caused saccharin to become less popular than other artificial sweeteners. The first is that saccharin has a bitter aftertaste at higher concentrations. Many people do not care for the flavor of saccharin unless it is combined with other nonnutritive sweeteners. The second drawback of saccharin involves evidence that saccharin caused bladder tumors in rats. This evidence led the Food and Drug Administration (FDA) to ban saccharin as a food additive in 1977. Strong public opinion against the ban and the lack of an acceptable alternative led Congress to allow its use. However, Congress did require warning labels on all food products that contain any saccharin.

Twenty years of research have shown there is not a connection between saccharin consumption and bladder cancer in humans. In 2000 saccharin was removed from the National Toxicology Program's list of carcinogens. Consumers can be assured the "pink packets" are safe for human consumption. Saccharin is found in artificially sweetened foods and beverages. It is also used as a table-top sweetener.

Aspartame

Aspartame is a dipeptide made from the amino acids aspartic acid and phenylalanine. Aspartame is the most popular of the artificial sweeteners. This is due mostly to aspartame's flavor, which is almost identical to sugar. Aspartame first received limited approval from the FDA in 1981. In 1983, aspartame was approved for use in carbonated drinks. It is now used extensively in drinks and drink mixes, puddings, gelatins, chewing gum, frozen desserts, and presweetened cereals. Aspartame is about 200 times sweeter than sugar.

Aspartame in its original form is not heat stable. At 30°C (86°F), aspartame breaks down into compounds that are not sweet. This is why soft drinks containing aspartame should not be stored at warm temperatures. Aspartame can be successfully added to hot drinks because it can withstand the short time exposure to heat.

In 1993, the FDA approved a special aspartame formulation for use in heated products. This happened after researchers developed a method of protecting aspartame from breaking down during the heating process. Commercial baked goods made with specially treated aspartame are safe. However, baked goods prepared with aspartame at home will not have the desired sweetness.

During digestion, aspartame breaks down into methyl alcohol. The body quickly converts this substance into formaldehyde and then into carbon dioxide. Methyl alcohol and formaldehyde are naturally present in many foods. However, they are restricted as additives in food because they are toxic compounds. Because of this, aspartame had to undergo extensive testing. Researchers needed to determine the levels at which these com-

pounds would cause no harm. The FDA has set the maximum safe level for aspartame at 50 mg per kilogram of body weight per day. A 60-kilogram (132-pound) person would have to consume 15 aspartame-sweetened drinks in one day to reach this level.

A second caution regarding aspartame use is related to the phenylalanine from which it is made. A genetic disorder called phenylketonuria (PKU) causes some people to be unable to digest this amino acid. High levels of phenylalanine will build up in body tissue causing damage. Anyone with PKU should not use aspartame.

Concern about aspartame arose in the mid 1980s after several preschoolers were rushed to emergency rooms with seizures. This occurred on a hot day, and the children had refused to eat because of the heat. They had consumed nothing other than eight to nine glasses of aspartame-sweetened drinks. The problem turned out to be one of balance. Having eaten no nourishing food or beverages, their bodies were not equipped to withstand the heat stress. Had the children drank water instead, their reactions to the stressful condition would probably have been similar. Most people should have no problems with aspartame if they eat a nutritious diet.

Acesulfame Potassium

Acesulfame potassium, or *acesulfame K*, is an organic salt used as an artificial sweetener. The FDA approved it in 1988. It is almost as sweet as aspartame and has the advantage of being very stable at high temperatures. It has an initially sweet taste with a slight aftertaste. It is 130 times sweeter than sugar. It has been approved for use in chewing gum, drinks, instant tea, instant coffee, gelatins, and puddings. It can be used alone or in a mixture of aspartame and saccharin. People with PKU can use it without any known side effects. Because it is heat stable, it can be used in baked goods and hot beverages.

Stevioside

Stevioside is a natural extract from the leaves of a plant (*Stevia rebaudiana Bertoni*). On a sweetness scale of sucrose equals one, stevioside equals 300. It is stable at high temperatures and in acids. Some stevioside extracts have a menthol-like aftertaste.

Sucralose

A more recent addition to the lineup of approved nonnutritive sweeteners is *sucralose.* The FDA approved sucralose in the Fall of 1995 for use beginning in 1998. This sugar substitute is made by adding chlorine atoms to sugar. It is a disaccharide made in a five-step process that replaces three hydroxyl groups with chlorine. Sucralose is 4 to 800 times sweeter than sugar and cannot be digested. It is very stable in processing, soluble in water, and easily added to foods using traditional processing methods.

Neotame

On July 5, 2002, after extensive study, the FDA approved Neotame as a nonnutritive sweetener. Neotame is made of amino acids L-aspartic acid and L-phenylalanine combined with a methyl ester group and a neohexyl group. It is 7,000 to 13,000 times sweeter than sugar, stable in high heat, and has been approved for baking applications. It also works as a flavor enhancer when used in low levels.

> ### Cooking Tip
> One packet of artificial sweetener equals 10 mL (2 teaspoons) sugar. It takes 24 packets to equal the sweetening power of 1 cup of sugar. In baked goods, replace up to half the sugar with an artificial sweetener to reduce Calories. Remember, some sugar is needed to tenderize the product, develop texture, and brown the surface.

Nutritive Sweeteners

Polyols, also known as sweet alcohols, are a group of low-calorie sweeteners. They provide 1.5 to 3.0 Calories per gram as compared to 4.0 for sugar. They are found naturally in apples, berries, and plums. Because polyols are digested slowly, some reach the colon where they are broken down and used by bacteria. This causes a reduction of available Calories.

The polyols commonly used include sorbitol, mannitol, xylitol, maltitol, maltitol syrup, lactitol, erythritol, isomalt, and hydrogenated starch hydrolysates. Polyols that are produced by hydrolysis of corn, wheat, or potato starch followed by hydrogenation at high temperatures are called *hydrogenated*

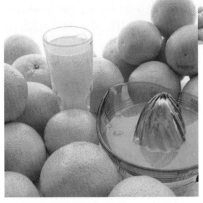

Nutrition News
Do Artificial Sweeteners Help People Lose Weight?

Consumption of diet carbonated soft drinks rose from 4.3 gallons per person in 1977 to 11.7 gallons in 1997. Use of artificial sweeteners in coffee, tea, fruit drinks, and desserts also grew. During that period, obesity in the United States increased among all age groups.

Studies have shown that artificial sweetners do no cause an increase in appetite. However, many health experts fear that sugar substitutes may be giving people a false sense of security. They believe many people may be eating larger servings and snacking more frequently

because of the Calories saved from artificial sweeteners.

You need to keep the proper perspective when using sugar substitutes. These products do not enable you to eat all you want whenever you want. You still need to use moderation, balance, and variety when making food choices.

starch hydrolysates (HSH). HSH were first developed in Sweden in the 1960's. They are 40% to 90 % as sweet as sugar with maltitol and xylitol being the sweetest. They are used extensively in sugar-free candies because they do not crystallize, they blend well with other flavors, and work well in mixtures of artificial sweeteners.

HSH that contain 50% or more of a single polyol are listed as syrups. For example, if an ingredient label contains maltitol syrup, it has HSH that is 50% or higher maltitol content. HSH are ingredients that are generally recognized as safe and can be used without limits. They are found primarily in baked goods, ice cream, candy, and chocolates. They have allowed manufacturers to create a wider variety of sugar-free, low-calorie choices for people with diabetes.

Polyols help control moisture content, improve texture, reduce browning, and extend shelf life. They do not promote tooth decay. Consuming large amounts of some polyols such as sorbitol can have a laxative effect.

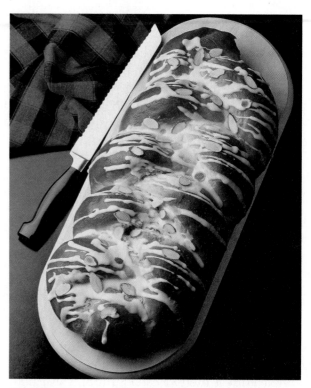

15-4 Besides providing sweetness to baked products, sugar helps tenderize the dough and promotes a brown crust.

New Developments in Sweeteners

Food scientists are working to develop some new sugar substitutes. One sweetener they are looking into is a supersweet protein found in a vine plant with reddish, grapelike fruit. This protein is called *brazzein*. It consists of 52 amino acids and is 2,000 times sweeter than sugar. Brazzein is heat stable at 98°C (208°F) for at least two hours. It is also stable in a wide range of acidic and alkaline solutions. Electrical recordings of taste bud responses on animals show brazzein has a pure sweet taste with no aftertaste.

Bulking Agents

The use of artificial sweeteners is more complex than simply comparing the sweetness to sugar. Sugar has other functions in foods. For instance, in baked goods it helps provide body, color, volume, and texture, 15-4. Researchers are challenged to find an approved substance that will provide the bulk and texture of sugar without adding Calories. So far, they have found no single ingredient that will replace all the qualities of sugar.

In most cases, artificial sweeteners are combined with a bulking agent. A *bulking agent* is a substance added to foods to enhance texture or thicken the consistency. Polydextrose has been found to be a safe bulking agent that mimics the mouth feel of sugar in food mixtures. Polydextrose has 1 Calorie per gram, which is one-fourth the Calories of sugar. The Calorie content of polydextrose is why many artificially sweetened foods are labeled as "Reduced Calorie" instead of "Calorie Free." See 15-5. Small amounts of other bulking agents, such as alginates, gum acacia, pectin, and xanthan, are often used in diet soft drinks.

Fat Substitutes

The average U.S. diet provides a larger percentage of Calories from fat than recommended. Many consumers want all the pleasure and none of the guilt associated with eating fat. Fat carries flavor and improves the mouth feel of many foods. However, few people want the risks that go with a high-fat diet. Fat is linked

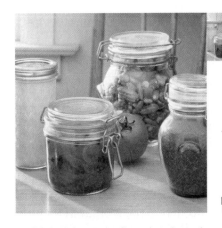

Historical Highlight
Margarine—A Modified Fat

Margarine was first developed in 1869 by the French chemist Mege-Mouries. Napoleon III had offered a prize to the person who could develop a tasty, nutritious, economical alternative to butter. The first margarine was made mainly from beef fat. It was sold commercially as Oleo. This name came from the large amount of oleic acid used in the early margarines. Today, most margarines and vegetable oil spreads are made from corn or soybean oils.

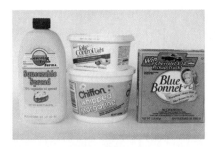

Margarines and vegetable oil spreads are available in stick, tub, and liquid forms to meet a variety of consumer needs.

Margarines did not gain popularity in the United States until the 1940s. Three factors caused margarine to become more widely accepted. One factor was the rationing of butter during World War II. This caused many homemakers to turn to margarine to fill the gap.

A second factor that increased acceptance of margarine was adding color. The first margarines were white. Customers had a hard time accepting a butter substitute that did not look like butter. This led manufacturers of margarines to add beta-carotene to their products. This precursor to vitamin A remains suspended in fat and produces a yellow color similar to butter.

A third factor to increase margarine's popularity came in the 1960s. People in the United States became more aware of the link between heart disease and saturated fat in the diet. Butter is high in saturated fat. Margarines made from

hydrogenated vegetable oils are much lower in saturated fat. Therefore, many people switched from butter to margarine in the belief that margarine was more heart healthy.

However, the hydrogenation process that turns liquid vegetable oils into solid margarine produces trans-fats. Research indicates the body cannot properly digest trans-fats. It appears they are no healthier than saturated fat. Therefore, although margarine may be less costly than butter, it is not likely to be any healthier for the heart.

New recommendations are to reduce use of both butter and margarine. Also, remember the softer a margarine or spread is, the less trans-fat it will contain. Liquid vegetable oil spreads are lower in trans-fat than soft products in tubs. Margarines and spreads in tubs are lower in trans-fat than stick varieties.

to weight gain. It has been associated with three of the leading causes of death: heart attack, stroke, and cancer. Evidence also indicates that fat consumption is related to the ability to prevent and control diabetes. These health concerns have made the development of fat substitutes the subject of intense research for many food scientists.

Like sugar, fat has many functions in food

products. Researchers must do more than find a flavor substitute. Food scientists are looking for ways to keep the positive qualities of fat while reducing or eliminating negative ones. Fat helps stabilize mixtures; carry flavor compounds; and add smooth, creamy textures. Fat also tenderizes doughs, controls ice crystal formation in frozen foods, and forms foams such as whipped cream. Food scientists have used starches, proteins, and chemically altered fats to develop fat replacers that perform some of these functions.

Starch-Based Fat Replacers

Manufacturers use a variety of modified starches and gums to replace fats in foods. These starch-based products mimic the mouth feel of fat, but they are lower in Calories than fat. The most commonly used starch-based fat replacers are vegetable gums, dextrins, maltodextrins, polydextrose, and pectin. One example is carrageenan, which comes from red algae. When mixed with

water, carrageenan helps lowfat hamburgers retain juices. Another example of a starch-based fat replacer is the cellulose gel used in many low-Calorie salad dressings. Although these substitutes help create the feel of fat, they cannot imitate fat's flavor. The advantage of these fat replacers is they are safe ingredients commonly used in foods.

In 1993, the United States Department of Agriculture (USDA) developed the starch-based fat replacer Oatrim. This product is derived from oat flour and, like oats, is high in soluble fiber. It may be called "hydrolyzed oat flour" on ingredient labels. It is being used in several lower-Calorie products, such as cheeses and ground beef. Food scientists have found Oatrim easy to use in baking, 15-6. It has only one Calorie per gram as compared to fat's nine Calories per gram. There is some evidence that Oatrim can help improve control of blood sugar and cholesterol levels.

The kinds of foods in which starch-based fat replacers will work are limited. For instance, many nutritionists recommend using applesauce and pureed prunes instead of fat in homemade muffins, cakes, and fruit breads. These fruit products work because they are high in pectin. Although pectin works well in an applesauce spice cake, it cannot

---

Food Label Nutrient Claims

Calorie free. Less than 5 calories per serving.

Fat free. Less than 0.5 grams of fat per serving.

Free. An amount that is nutritionally trivial.

Less. The described nutrient is reduced by at least 25%.

Light. Calories are at least one-third less than the comparable product.

Low. Allows frequent consumption of that type food without exceeding dietary guidelines.

Low calorie. Less than 40 calories per serving or 100 grams of food.

Low fat. 3 grams of fat or less per serving or 100 grams of food.

Low in saturated fat. 1 gram or less of saturated fat per serving and not more than 15% of the calories from saturated fat.

Low sodium. Less than 140 milligrams per 100 grams of food.

More fiber. At least 2.5 grams more per serving than the reference food.

Reduced. Can be used for calories, cholesterol, fat, sodium, or sugar if the food contains 25% less than the comparison food.

Reduced fat. No more than 25% of the fat of the comparable food.

Salt or sodium free. Less than 5 milligrams of sodium per serving.

Sugar free. Less than 0.5 grams per serving.

15-5 Nutrient claims made on food product labels must meet the above definitions.

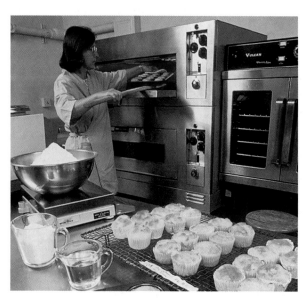

Agricultural Research Service, USDA

15-6 Fat free baked goods made with Oatrim are prepared in ARS test kitchens to evaluate their quality.

make an acceptable biscuit or pie crust. Biscuits and pie crust are flaky because solid fat is cut into the flour. The gluten structure is separated into tender layers of dough as the fat melts when the product is heated. Starch-based fat replacers cannot mimic the flaky, tender quality solid fats give to these baked goods.

Protein-Based Fat Replacers

A fat substitute made from protein is known by the trade name *Simplesse.* Simplesse is made by a process called microparticulation. Milk and egg proteins are heated and blended in such a way that tiny round particles are formed. The heating causes the proteins to denature. They can then rebond with one another in a random coil with a ball shape. When suspended in water, these particles swell and have the mouth feel of fat.

Taste tests have found that particle size affects the way people identify food textures. People perceive particles smaller than 0.1 micrometer as watery. People perceive particles larger than 5 micrometers as powdery. Simplesse microparticles range in size from 0.1 to 3 micrometers. The size and shape of these microparticles cause them to roll over the tongue. This creates a feel of smoothness and creaminess.

In 1989, the FDA approved Simplesse for use in frozen desserts, mayonnaise, and salad dressings. Simplesse is also approved for use in yogurt, dips, butter, puddings, cheese, and some baked goods. The body digests and absorbs Simplesse, which provides a little more than one Calorie per gram. Although this is fewer than the nine Calories per gram provided by fat, it is not Calorie free. Products made with Simplesse can be used in most recipes prepared with heat. The biggest drawback of Simplesse is that it gels when heated, making it unsuitable for frying.

Two other lesser known protein-based fat replacers are LITA and Trailblazer. LITA is made from corn gluten. Trailblazer, like Simplesse, is made from egg whites and milk proteins.

A problem with starch- and protein-based fat replacers is related to flavor. Most flavor compounds are fat-soluble and are gradually released when eaten. Researchers working with fat replacers point out that starch- and protein-based fat replacers release flavor compounds all at once. The result is too much flavor and then none. See 15-7.

Fat and sugar both play key roles in how foods taste, feel, and look. It is difficult to remove both fat and sugar and still have an acceptable product. In fact, many manufacturers increase sugar in products made with fat replacers to make up for the lack of flavor. Therefore, although fat grams are reduced, total Calories may not be.

Manufactured Fats

Some of the fat substitutes food scientists are developing are neither starch-based nor protein-based. These products can be described as manufactured fats. The FDA approved the first of these products, olestra, in January 1996. *Olestra* is a sucrose polyester. It looks like fat, feels like fat, and performs like fat.

You learned in Chapter 9 that fats have one to three fatty acids attached to a glycerol molecule. You also learned that a fatty acid joins to glycerol where there is a hydroxyl group. Olestra was made by attaching six to eight fatty acids at the site of hydroxyl groups

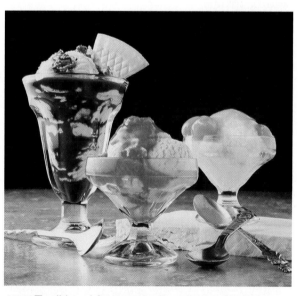

15-7 Traditional fats gradually release the flavors of foods. Food scientists have had trouble mimicking this quality with fat replacers.

on a sucrose molecule. The characteristic of a fat is determined by the fatty acids attached to the molecule. Therefore, olestra can be either solid or liquid. If a solid fat is needed, fatty acids with high melting points, such as palmitic and stearic acids, are used. If a liquid fat is needed, then fatty acids like oleic and linoleic are used.

The body has no enzyme to break down this manufactured fat. Therefore, olestra provides no Calories. It passes through the body undigested.

Olestra may sound like an ideal product. However, the FDA requires warning labels on all products that contain olestra, 15-8. One reason for this is that olestra may cause diarrhea when consumed in large amounts. A second reason for the warning labels has to do with the way olestra absorbs or bonds with fat-soluble vitamins. As olestra passes through the body undigested, so do all the fat-soluble vitamins bonded to it. Food scientists have gotten around this problem by saturating olestra with the fat-soluble vitamins. This keeps the olestra from picking up any other fat-soluble vitamins that are consumed from other foods. Olestra also tends to carry carotenoids out of the body, but the FDA found no evidence that this could be harmful. Some drugs are fat-soluble, too. Olestra can interfere with the body's ability to absorb fat-soluble drugs.

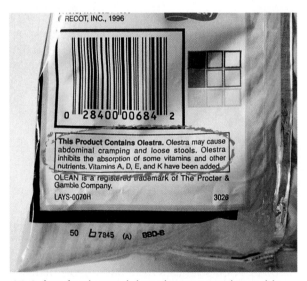

15-8 Any food containing olestra must have this warning on the label.

SALATRIM, available since 1994, is another fatlike compound developed by food scientists. The name SALATRIM is an acronym for short- and long-chain acid triglyceride molecules. Like Simplesse, SALATRIM will not stand up in frying. It has five Calories per gram instead of the nine in most fats. It is derived from soybean oil and other natural fat sources. SALATRIM is made of three fatty acids attached to a glycerol molecule. The Calorie reduction is a result of the fatty acids used. One of the fatty acids used is stearic acid, which the body has difficulty absorbing. Short-chain fatty acids, which are lower in Calories, are also used. Many cannot tell the difference in chocolate products made with SALATRIM versus high-fat chocolate. It is digested and metabolized normally. The average expected daily intake is 10 grams or less. People may experience abdominal discomfort, nausea, bloating, and headaches when they consume 40 grams or more per day.

Salt Substitutes

The third major source of flavor behind sugar and fat in most diets is salt. As you know, salt is a major source of sodium in the diet. The average U.S. diet supplies many times more sodium than needed. To meet current health recommendations, many people are trying to use less salt. Studies have repeatedly linked sodium and high blood pressure, which is a risk factor for heart disease. Therefore, health experts especially urge people with high blood pressure to reduce their intake of salt and sodium, 15-9. This has prompted researchers to look for salt substitutes that provide the desired taste without the negative consequences.

Potassium Chloride

Potassium and sodium are members of the same family of elements in the periodic table. These elements are both soft metals that combine with chlorine to form salts. Table salt is sodium chloride. Potassium chloride can be used in place of table salt to flavor foods without adding sodium to the diet.

Potassium chloride has an advantage for heart patients who are placed on no-salt diets. These patients often need extra potassium due

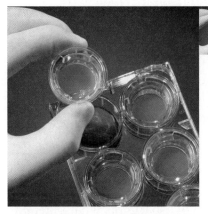

Recent Research
Can You Tell the Difference?

Taste tests were held at Rutgers University to assess the way people perceive the fat content in foods. The participants tasted five versions of six common foods. Only the amount of fat in each food was altered.

It was discovered that people could notice the fat content difference in some foods and not others.

Participants could not tell the difference in scrambled eggs and chicken spread. Participants could tell the difference in crunchy snacks, mashed potatoes, and milk-based foods such as pudding. The conclusion was that food scientists can make relatively large changes in fat content in some foods without people

noticing. New fat replacers or processing techniques may be needed before such foods as lowfat crunchy snacks can be marketed successfully. Consumers can begin reducing fat consumption in foods where fat content has minimal changes on flavor and texture, such as egg products.

to losses caused by heart medications. A disadvantage of potassium chloride is its flavor. It has a slightly bitter aftertaste.

Other Salt Substitutes

Adding other seasonings to food is an alternative to using salt. There are endless combinations of herbs and spices that can flavor your food without adding sodium. Herb and spice blends are not analogs of salts because they do not have a saltlike flavor.

Do not assume all seasoning mixes can act as sodium-free salt substitutes. The names and descriptions on the fronts of food packages often give no clues about the products' salt contents. For instance, you may not think of a coating mix for meat, fish, and poultry as a source of sodium. However, some coating mixes have as much as 660 mg of sodium per serving. That is over one-fourth of the Daily Value listed as a recommendation on food

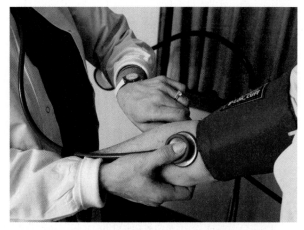

15-9 For some people, reducing sodium intake can reduce blood pressure.

product labels. Always read the Nutrition Facts panel and ingredient list for the sodium content.

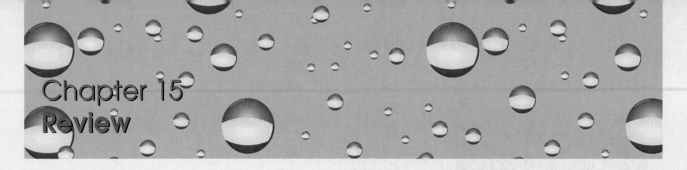

Chapter 15
Review

Summary

Food analogs are nontraditional replacements for traditional food ingredients. The most common food analogs are those developed to replace the main flavor agents in foods: sugars, fats, and salts. Because food analogs become a part of the diet, it is important to know how they react in cooking, storage, and digestion.

As with all other foods, food analogs must be eaten in moderation, variety, and balance for a healthful diet. No food component allows you to safely eat all you want of any food without creating imbalances. Although analogs have many positive characteristics, they also have some drawbacks. Becoming aware of these factors will help you when choosing food products containing analogs.

Check Your Understanding

1. What are the functions of food analogs?
2. List three examples of food analogs.
3. List one of the nonnutritive sweeteners and explain pros and cons related to its use.
4. Why should diabetics monitor their use of sweet alcohols?
5. Explain why bulking agents are added to foods made with artificial sweeteners.
6. List two starch-based fat replacers and a food in which each is used.
7. Why is Simplesse not used in fried foods?
8. How does olestra differ chemically from fat molecules?
9. Describe two problems with eating large amounts of olestra.
10. Name two alternatives to salt for flavoring food.

Critical Thinking

1. Which artificial sweetener is the best choice for making caramel candies? Why?
2. If you make a batch of muffins with the regular form of aspartame, what potential problem will likely result?
3. How would you respond to this common question: Why are fat free foods so expensive when all they do to make them is cut out the fat?
4. If a food scientist wanted to develop a new fat free, sugar free pancake mix, which analogs would definitely be avoided?
5. Explain how researchers have solved most of the problem olestra poses for nutrients such as beta-carotene in the body.

Explore Further

1. **Analytical Skills.** Construct models of each of the three main sugar replacers.
2. **Communication.** Debate the advantages and disadvantages of using food analogs.
3. **Science.** Conduct a taste test of real ice cream next to fat free and sugar free substitutes. Be sure the test compares the same flavors. Can teenagers tell the difference? Report your findings in class and/or the school newspaper.
4. **Math.** Create bar graphs comparing the fat, sugar, and calorie totals of the various ice creams used in Experiment 15B.
5. **Analytical Skills.** Develop a homemade low fat and sugar-reduced or sugar free baked product. Conduct taste evaluations to compare the new product to the original recipe. How does flavor and texture differ? Is the new product enjoyable?

Experiment 15A
Artificial Sweeteners

Purpose

In this experiment, you will evaluate hot and cold beverages sweetened with various artificial sweeteners. Some artificial sweeteners are not Calorie free. However, they still reduce the total Calories in foods because less of the artificial sweeteners are needed to sweeten to the same level as sugar.

Equipment

wax pencil

5 250-mL beakers

100-mL graduated cylinder

metric measuring spoons

5 glass rods

2-quart saucepan with lid

Supplies

12 3-ounce paper cups per lab group member

2 packets aspartame

2 packets acesulfame K

2 packets saccharin

2 packets sucralose

20 mL (4 teaspoons) sugar

500 mL (2 cups) chilled unsweetened fruit drink

500 mL (2 cups) water

1 tea bag

Procedure

1. Use a wax pencil to label a set of five 3-ounce paper cups for each lab group member with the first three letters in the name of each of the following sweeteners: *asp*artame, *ace*sulfame K, *sac*charin, *suc*ralose, and *sug*ar.

2. Label five 250-mL beakers with the same letters.

3. Pour 100 mL of prepared unsweetened fruit drink into each beaker.

4. Add one packet of aspartame to the beaker labeled *asp.* Add one packet of acesulfame K to the beaker labeled *ace.* Add one packet of saccharin to the beaker labeled *sac.* Add one packet of sucralose to the beaker labeled *suc.* Add 10 mL (2 teaspoons) of sugar to the beaker labeled *sug.*

5. Use a clean glass rod to stir each mixture thoroughly.

6. Divide each beaker of drink into your lab group's labeled paper cups. Wash the beakers.

7. Prepare a sixth cup filled with water for each group member.

8. Describe the flavor of each sample in a data table. Take a sip of water between each sample.

9. Heat 500 mL (2 cups) of water to the boiling point in a 2-quart saucepan. Remove the pan from the heat.

10. Steep one tea bag in the hot water for 4 minutes. Cover the pan while the tea is steeping.

11. Repeat steps 1 through 8 with the hot tea.

12. Record calories and ingredients from the package labels of each sweetener in a data table.

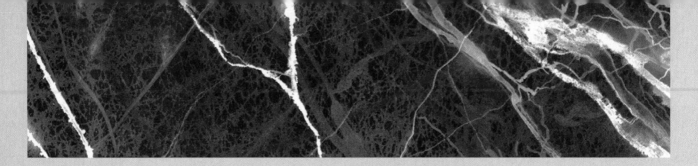

Calculations

The FDA has established an acceptable daily intake (ADI) for aspartame. Aspartame is quickly absorbed. Seizures have occurred in individuals who have exceeded their ADI. This is especially true when no food is eaten. The ADI is based on a person's body weight. The acceptable intake per day is no more than 50 mg of aspartame per kilogram of body weight (50 mg/kg). Calculate your ADI.

weight in pounds ÷ 2.2 kg/lb
= weight in kilograms

weight in kilograms × 50 mg/kg
= ADI for aspartame in mg

Using the chart below, calculate approximately how much aspartame you consume per day.

Food	Average Aspartame Content
Equal packet	35 mg
Diet soft drink (12-ounce serving)	170 mg
Diet drinks prepared from mix (12-ounce serving):	
Crystal Light	180 mg
Koolaid	260 mg
Tang	200 mg
Iced tea mix	110 mg
Sugar free gelatin	75 mg
Sugar free pudding	90 mg
Sugar free cereals (1 cup serving)	50 mg
Sugar free hot cocoa	100 mg

Questions

1. Which artificial sweetener(s) had an aftertaste?

2. Which artificial sweetener(s) tasted like sugar?

3. Which, if any, of the artificial sweeteners did not work well in hot beverages?

4. How much aspartame do you usually consume? How does this amount compare to your ADI?

5. How can you apply what you have learned to food preparation?

Experiment 15B
Lowfat Ice Cream

Purpose

During this lab, you will evaluate the role fat plays in the texture and flavor of ice cream. You will compare batches of ice cream made with cream, milk, and fat free half-and-half. The fat free half-and-half contains carageenan gum to mimic the texture of fat. Each lab group will make one batch of each variation.

Equipment

wax pencil

100-mL graduated cylinder

metric measuring spoons

thermometer

3 terry cloth towels

electronic balance

1 spoon per lab group member

Supplies

125 mL (½ cup) half-and-half

75 mL (⅓ cup) whipping cream

175 mL (¾ cup) whole milk

175 mL (¾ cup) fat free half-and-half

90 mL (6 tablespoons) sugar

9 mL (2¼ teaspoons) vanilla

90 mL (6 tablespoons) pasteurized egg substitute

3 1-gallon resealable plastic bags

3 dashes salt

3 1-quart resealable plastic bags

690 g ice

270 g rock salt

3 disposable paper cups per lab group member

Procedure

1. Use a wax pencil to label three 1-quart resealable plastic bags as follows: *control, Variation 1,* and *Variation 2.* Pour the appropriate liquid(s) into each bag.

    Control: 125 mL (½ cup) half-and-half and 75 mL (⅓ cup) whipping cream

    Variation 1: 175 mL (¾ cup) milk

    Variation 2: 175 mL (¾ cup) fat free half-and-half

2. Add 30 mL (2 tablespoons) sugar, 3 mL (¾ teaspoon) vanilla, 30 mL (2 tablespoons) pasteurized egg substitute, and a dash of salt to each bag.

3. Record the temperature of the mixture in each bag. Squeeze out the excess air and seal all three bags.

4. Mass 230 g of ice to place in each of three 1-gallon resealable plastic bags.

5. Mass 90 g of rock salt to add to the ice in each gallon bag. Place one of the 1-quart bags into each gallon bag and seal.

6. Wrap the gallon bags with terry cloth towels and gently knead the bags until the mixtures become firm. Record the time required for each mixture.

7. Label a set of three disposable cups for each lab group member as follows: *C* (for control), *1* (for Variation 1), and *2* (for Variation 2).

8. Remove the 1-quart bags from the gallon bags. Clean the outside of the 1-quart bags before tasting each variation to avoid contaminating the ice cream mixture with salt.

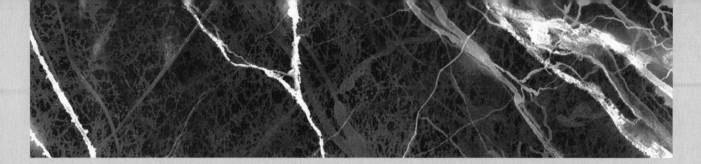

9. Divide the variations among the appropriately labeled cups. Conduct a sensory evaluation of all three variations. Describe the appearance, flavor, and consistency of the ice cream.

Questions

1. What difference did the amount of fat make to the ice cream flavor?

2. What difference did the kind of fat make to the ice cream texture?

3. Which variation gave the best quality ice cream product?

4. How can you apply this lab to other food situations?

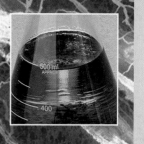

Experiment 15C
Fat Replacers in Muffins

Safety

❖ Follow sanitation procedures for food preparation.

❖ Wash hands before handling food products.

❖ Clean all utensils after use.

❖ Use hot pads to protect hands and counters.

Purpose

"Low fat" labels are common in today's grocery stores. Many consumers are striving to lower their fat intake because of fat's association with heart disease and obesity. Although commercial fat replacers are not available to the home cook, there are some options that can reduce fat. In this experiment, you will evaluate three types of starch-based fat replacers available to consumers. The first type is commercial pectin, which is a complex carbohydrate that can mimic fat to some degree in baked goods. Pectin is available in liquid and powdered form for making jams and jellies. The second type is fruit purees. Fruits such as apples and prunes are high in pectin. They can be pureed and used in place of fat in many recipes. The third type of starch-based fat replacer you will evaluate is instant pudding mix with modified starch.

Equipment

electronic balance

large mixing bowl

100-mL graduated cylinder

small mixing bowl

wooden spoon

muffin tin

serrated knife

Supplies

250 g all-purpose flour

65 g sugar

5 g salt

7 g baking powder

1 egg

250 mL (1 cup) lowfat milk (omit in variation 5)

assigned fat or fat replacer

12 paper baking cups

Procedure

1. Preheat the oven to 425°F.

2. Combine flour, sugar, salt, and baking powder in a large mixing bowl.

3. Combine the egg and milk in a small mixing bowl. (Omit milk in Variation 5.) Add your assigned fat or fat replacer.

   Control: 50 mL (¼ cup) vegetable oil

   Variation 1: 50 mL (¼ cup) pureed prunes

   Variation 2: 50 mL (¼ cup) applesauce

   Variation 3: 30 mL (2 tablespoons) liquid pectin and 15 mL (1 tablespoon) water

   Variation 4: 25 mL water and 30 mL (2 tablespoons) powdered pectin

   Variation 5: Combine 500 mL (2 cups) fat free milk and 1 package vanilla instant pudding to make 500 mL (2 cups) prepared pudding.

4. Make a well in the center of the dry ingredients.

5. Add the liquids all at once.

6. Use a wooden spoon to stir the liquids into the dry ingredients just until all the flour is moistened. *Do not beat! The batter will be lumpy.*

7. Spoon the batter into 12 paper-lined muffin cups. Fill each muffin cup two-thirds full.

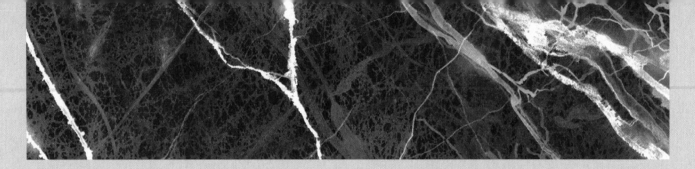

8. Bake 18 to 20 minutes. Muffins will be lightly browned and will spring back when gently pressed.

9. Remove muffins from muffin tin. Allow muffins to cool for 2 to 3 minutes. With a serrated knife, cut the muffins in half from top to bottom.

10. Evaluate each variation for cell size, color, and shape before taste testing.

Questions

1. Which variation produced the tallest muffins? Which variation produced the shortest?

2. Which variation produced the best flavor?

3. How did the textures of the variations compare?

4. Which fat substitutes would you recommend? For what types of foods would you recommend these substitutes? Explain your answers.

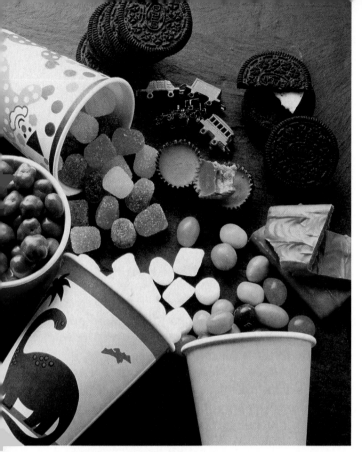

These treats owe their desired characteristics largely to such additives as flavorings, colorings, emulsifiers, and preservatives.

Chapter 16

Additives: Producing Desired Characteristics in Foods

Objectives

After studying this chapter,
you will be able to

differentiate between intentional and incidental food additives.

state the role of the Food and Drug Administration in regulating additives.

describe four main functions of additives.

weigh the advantages and disadvantages of additives in the food supply.

Key Terms

ingredient

food additive

intentional food additive

incidental food additive

margin of safety

GRAS list

controlled-use substance

Delaney Clause

preservative

antimicrobial agent

sulfite

ester

anticaking agent

humectant

maturing and bleaching agent

pH control agent

Supermarkets are filled with foods that have been formulated in some way. Each product has an ingredient list that tells you what has been combined to make that food. Food scientists define *ingredients* as substances that are generally recognized as safe and are component parts of food products. However, some of the compounds in food product ingredient lists may not fit this definition. This chapter looks at these compounds, which are added to foods in their development and manufacture.

What Is a Food Additive?

The average person in the United States eats over five pounds of food additives each year. A *food additive* is a substance added to a food to cause a desired positive change in the product's characteristics. Additives may or may not have nutritional value. They can be put into a food at any point from the farm to the kitchen table, 16-1. USDA and FDA regulations control the use of food additives. Legal guidelines for using food additives are established after extensive testing and research to confirm their safety.

Intentional and Incidental Additives

One way to group additives is based on how they get into a food product. *Intentional food additives* are added on purpose. They are used to give foods specific characteristics or resistance to spoilage. For example, vitamin D is purposely added to milk at the dairy processing plant. *Incidental food additives* get into foods unintentionally. If milk is packed in a wax-coated carton, some of the wax will get into the milk. The wax fragments are an example of an incidental food additive. Incidental additives may enter a food during production, processing, storage, or packaging. Food scientists must look at all aspects of food preparation and handling. They must monitor any substance that could enter the food supply.

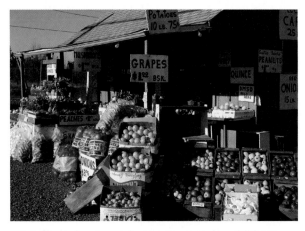

16-1 Even fresh produce can contain additives.

Both intentional and incidental food additives are regulated to protect the consumer from health hazards.

Regulating Additive Use

Because additives do not naturally occur in food, some consumers are concerned about the safety of additives. These consumers may worry about "chemicals" being added to the food supply. At this point in your study of food science, you know that all food components have a chemical structure. It should also be clear to you that few chemicals in food are all good or all bad. Most compounds in foods can be helpful or harmful. For example, glucose is used as a sweetener in some food products. This chemical compound is helpful as a source of energy for the body. However, too much glucose can be harmful by causing obesity.

The United States has a very strict, detailed set of regulations regarding food additives. No country in the world keeps a closer watch on the safety of its food supply. Foods are constantly monitored, tested, and reevaluated. Food regulations and guidelines change to keep up with new scientific knowledge.

The Food and Drug Administration

The average consumer cannot monitor the safety of his or her food without help. The United States Congress recognized the need to monitor the food supply for safety. In 1938, the Federal Food, Drug, and Cosmetic Act was passed. It gave the Food and Drug Administration (FDA) authority over food and food ingredients. This act also defined requirements for the truthful labeling of ingredients. It is the basis of modern food law in the United States. (Refer to Chapter 1 for more information on this topic.)

The FDA is a branch of the Department of Health and Human Services. The FDA is responsible for regulating all foods except red meat, poultry, and eggs. These foods are monitored by the United States Department of Agriculture (USDA). The FDA supervises the use of additives in the food supply. They also set the guidelines by which manufacturers can use additives.

Additive Guidelines

Congress passed the Food Additives Amendment on September 6, 1958. This amendment states that no additive can be used in foods unless the FDA is convinced it is safe. Evidence used to persuade the FDA must be based on thorough scientific study.

The manufacturer who develops an additive is required to provide proof of safety. To receive approval to use a new additive, a manufacturer must go through a series of steps. See 16-2.

Additives are considered a hazard if they can produce injury under certain uses. The FDA establishes *margins of safety* for each additive. This is the zone between the concentration in which an additive is normally used and the level at which a hazard exists. The margin of safety for table salt is 1/5. That means the average consumption of salt is one-fifth as much as the level that can produce injury. Most additives that involve any risk have a margin of safety of 1/100. A person would have to eat 100 servings of that food in a short period to be at risk.

By law, the FDA can approve only new additives that are found to be safe. Health and safety are not the only requirements additives must meet. The law also requires that

❖ An intentional additive must perform a useful function.

❖ An additive cannot be used to deceive the consumer or cover up faulty manufacturing practices.

❖ An additive cannot cause a substantial loss of nutritive value in a food.

❖ An additive cannot be used in place of good manufacturing practices.

❖ A method must exist for analyzing the presence of the additive in food.

The FDA can reject an additive if any of the requirements cannot be met.

The GRAS List

The careful testing of additives takes time. Requiring this testing of all additives already in use in 1958 would have brought most U.S. food production to a stop. Most commonly used foods would have had to be removed from the market until proven safe.

Food additives that had long been used with no known health hazards were exempted from immediate testing. There were over 600 of these additives placed on a *"generally recognized as safe"* list. The name of this list was abbreviated to the *GRAS list.* Additives on the GRAS list would still have to be tested eventually. However, food manufacturers could legally continue using these additives until testing proved them to be hazardous. See 16-3.

In 1969, President Nixon ordered that GRAS substances be reexamined. By the 1980s, 415 GRAS ingredients had been examined. Any additive shown to be a potential hazard was removed or reclassified. For instance, many of the original GRAS list food colors were removed from the list or restricted in use.

After being reexamined, ingredients on the GRAS list were divided into five classifications. The majority of ingredients were given a Class 1 status. They are considered safe at present and anticipated levels of use. Class 2 substances are safe at current usages. However, further study is advised to see if an increase in use could be hazardous. This list includes alginates, zinc salts, and vitamins A and D. Manufacturers were permitted to continue restricted use of Class 3 substances.

Food Additive Approval

❖ test the effectiveness of the additive (does it do what the manufacturer claims?)

❖ measure the amount of additive present in the final food product

❖ feed the additive in large doses to animals under controlled conditions to prove it is safe

❖ present all test results to the FDA for review

❖ submit to an FDA hearing at which the public is invited to offer testimony

❖ yield to the FDA's written regulations stating how much and in what foods the additive may be used

16-2 Manufacturers of food additives must take a number of steps to receive FDA approval for a new additive.

GRAS List Additives

ferrous gluconate

propylene glycol

citral

calcium silicate

glutamic acid

tocopherols

sodium phosphate

16-3 Do not allow long names on food product ingredient lists to concern you. The additives named above are all on the GRAS list, which means they are generally recognized as safe.

Further research is needed to answer questions about these substances. This class includes caffeine, BHA, and BHT. Class 4 includes items for which the FDA should establish safer guidelines. This list includes salt and four modified starches. Class 5 ingredients are recommended to be removed from the GRAS list. More data needs to be collected regarding the safety of these ingredients.

The FDA continually examines scientific studies for evidence that an approved additive might be harmful. The GRAS list is under constant revision as a result of new research.

More than 3,000 additives are approved for use in foods. Most of these are *controlled-use substances,* which do not appear on the GRAS list. These substances must be used within set guidelines. The guidelines vary according to the type of food to which the substance is added. Additive use is defined in *parts per million (ppm),* usually by weight. The same additive may be allowed in one food at 100 ppm and in another food at 25 ppm. This means that for every 100 (25) molecules of the additive, there must be 1 million molecules of other types.

Unlike controlled-use substances, GRAS additives do not have set ratios for use in foods. GRAS additives may be added at levels consistent with good manufacturing practices.

For instance, oregano is an herb on the GRAS list that has no known harmful effects. Manufacturers can add any amount of oregano to a food product needed to produce the desired taste. On the other hand, oxytetracycline is an antibiotic used in poultry feed. It is a controlled-use substance. Farmers and poultry packers must not allow this substance to exceed 0.0007% of the edible tissue of poultry.

The Delaney Clause

The Food Additives Amendment of 1958 and the Color Additive Amendment of 1960 contain a restrictive clause. This clause is named for its sponsor, Representative James Delaney from New York. The *Delaney Clause* bars the approval of any food additive found to cause cancer in humans or animals.

This clause sounds simple enough, but there are a few problems. The first is that an additive may cause cancer in animals under conditions not related to use in food. The second problem is the advance of technology. Additives once detectable at levels of only parts per thousand can now be detected in parts per billion.

An FDA official points out that with current technology, all foods could be found to contain at least one carcinogen. Scientists now realize that it is impossible to keep all

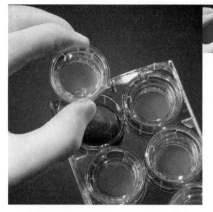

Recent Research
Caffeine: The Good, the Bad, and the Ugly

What is caffeine? Caffeine, which was placed on the GRAS list in 1958, is a mild stimulant. It is a flavoring agent with a slightly bitter taste. It occurs naturally in over 60 plants, including tea leaves and coffee and cacao beans.

What are the recommended consumption levels per day? Up to 300 mg of caffeine per day is considered a moderate dose. This equals the amount of caffeine in 2 to 3 cups of coffee or 7 to 10 cans of cola.

What are the physical effects of caffeine? Caffeine has undergone more testing than most compounds on the GRAS list. The National Research Council reports there is no established link between normal caffeine consumption and an increased health risk. However, moderate consumption has been shown to increase

❖ respiration rate
❖ heart rate
❖ blood pressure
❖ secretion of stress hormones
❖ production of stomach acid

❖ water loss through urination
❖ release of fatty acids

Caffeine also causes some people to experience stomach upset, nervousness, sleeplessness, irritability, headaches, and diarrhea. In addition, caffeine appears to reduce delicate muscular coordination. Caffeine does not speed the elimination of alcohol from the blood. However, recent research has found that caffeine reduces drowsiness and increases awareness of tasks at hand.

The effects of caffeine vary depending on how much is consumed. Doses of up to 750 mg per day may produce nausea, tense muscles, and irregular heartbeat. More than 750 mg daily can produce symptoms similar to anxiety attacks. These symptoms may include delirium, ringing in the ears, and light flashes.

The weight of an individual and the tolerance he or she has developed also influence the effects of caffeine. Therefore, a serving of food or beverage containing caffeine will have a greater effect on a child than on an adult.

Caffeine's effects begin 15 to 45 minutes after consumption. The effects reach maximum levels in 30 to 60 minutes. For most people, it takes 5 to 7 hours for the body to remove all the caffeine from the bloodstream.

How much do you consume? The amount of caffeine in tea and coffee varies. The variety, brewing method, and brewing time can all affect caffeine levels.

Is caffeine addictive? Caffeine is not addictive in the same sense as drugs like morphine and cocaine. However, people who consume large amounts of caffeine often feel discomfort after suddenly stopping caffeine use. Withdrawal symptoms usually last for two to three days. These symptoms may include headache, shakes, and irritability. Babies born to heavy caffeine users may also display withdrawal symptoms. These symptoms appear right after birth and can include an irregular heartbeat. It is recommended that caffeine users reduce consumption gradually to avoid these symptoms.

Food or Beverage	Serving Size	Caffeine Content
Coffee, brewed	8 oz	65–120 mg
Tea	8 oz	20–90 mg
Cocoa	6 oz	2–25 mg
Cola	12 oz	30–46 mg
Chocolate	1 oz	1–35 mg

carcinogens out of food. Today, the FDA views an additive "safe" if the risk of cancer is one in a million or less. New guidelines allow the use of these substances if they are required or cannot be avoided. Then regulations are to be established to limit quantities to such an extent as necessary for the protection of public health.

International Regulation

A growing number of food items sold in the United States are produced overseas. Regulations on additives vary from one country to another. The rise in use of imported foods has created a greater need for international standards. See 16-4.

The United Nations has set up two organizations that deal with international food supplies. The Food and Agricultural Organization (FAO) was formed in 1944 to reduce hunger and improve nutrition worldwide. The World Health Organization (WHO) was founded in 1948 to help improve the general health of all people. A large part of their budget is spent on nutrition issues.

The FAO and the WHO worked together to form a commission to set international food standards. The standards set by the commission are not binding. A nation's food standards may or may not match those set by the commission. More work is needed to ensure cooperation among nations on the use of additives in foods.

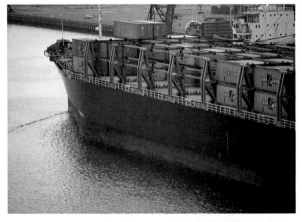

16-4 A growing number of imported food products on U.S. grocery shelves reinforces the need for international regulation of food additives.

Functions of Additives

All additives are in food for a reason. Additives are allowed in foods when their benefits outweigh their risks. The functions of additives in food are to

❖ maintain product quality and/or prolong shelf life

❖ enhance flavors and/or colors

❖ control product consistency

❖ improve or maintain nutritive value

This section will examine the more common additives for each function. It will also discuss foods in which additives are used and how additives work.

Preserve Product Quality

One of the main functions of food additives is to maintain freshness. *Preservatives* are substances added to food to prevent or slow spoilage and maintain natural colors and flavors. Food can spoil in two main ways. It can become contaminated with bacteria, mold, or fungus. Food can also become rancid due to fats reacting with oxygen. Food scientists select preservatives that are functional, nontoxic, flavorless, and economical.

Antimicrobial Agents

Spoilage that results in foodborne illness is dangerous. A key factor in providing a safe food supply is keeping harmful microbes out of food. *Antimicrobial agents* are preservatives that prevent growth of microbes in food. The type of antimicrobial agent used depends on the food and how that food is most likely to spoil.

The oldest and most frequently used antimicrobial agents are salt and sugar, 16-5. At high concentrations, salt and sugar preserve foods by dehydrating microbes. They draw water from the food and from any microbe that is present. Microbes cannot grow without water. Salt is used in foods like beef jerky, salted fish, and country ham. Sugar serves the same purpose in jams and jellies. Canned and frozen fruits often have sugar added, too.

Salt and sugar are considered food ingredients rather than food additives. They are food components that have multiple functions

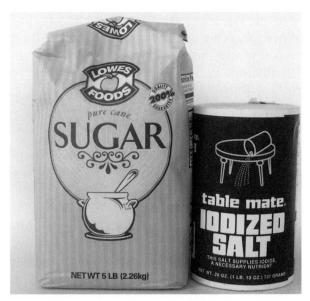

16-5 Salt and sugar have been used for centuries as additives that help preserve foods.

in foods. For example, although salt and sugar are used in many processed foods, their main role is usually flavor, not preservation. As a result, foods with salt and sugar may also contain other preservatives.

Nitrites

One group of antimicrobial agents is *nitrites*. The most common of these substances is sodium nitrite ($NaNO_3$). Nitrites are used in many foods to prevent the growth of the bacteria that causes botulism. These foods include bologna, hot dogs, smoked fish, sausage, salami, bacon, and ham. Nitrites help preserve color and flavor as well as protecting against microbes.

Nitrites are controversial because they can react with some amino acids during digestion to form nitrosamines. Some nitrosamines are known to cause cancer. Therefore, use of nitrites in food is illegal according to the Delaney Clause. The problem is that a ban on nitrites would put people at a greater risk for botulism. Special legislation allows a gradual phase out of nitrites as safe alternatives become available.

Acids

Many acids are used as antimicrobial agents. They include acetic, ascorbic, citric, lactic, and propionic acids. They prevent

microbe growth by lowering the pH of food products. Calcium propionate ($C_6H_{12}CaO_5$) is added to bread products to prevent mold growth.

Sorbic acid and benzoic acid are examples of two preservatives being used together. Sorbic acid ($C_6H_8O_2$) is widely used to slow or stop the growth of mold and yeasts. It is effective below pH 6.5. Benzoic acid ($C_6H_6O_2$), which is commonly used in soft drinks, is most effective on yeast and bacteria. It works best in an acid environment of pH 2.5 to 4.0. Together, these acids protect foods with a pH range of up to 6.5 from all three groups of microbes. Sorbic acid is easily digested, and benzoic acid is easily eliminated from the body. Both have been found to have no side effects or hazards when used as recommended.

Antioxidants

The second way food spoils is a result of exposure to oxygen. Oxidation can cause changes in color, texture, flavor, and nutritional value. These changes are usually not health hazards, but they are often undesirable. For example, few people want to eat mushy, brown apples.

Antioxidants are preservatives that protect food from changes caused by exposure to oxygen. Antioxidants interfere with the formation of free radicals. A *free radical* is an atom or group of atoms that contains one or more unpaired electrons. Free radicals are unstable. This makes them highly reactive. They can cause fats to become rancid and trigger enzymatic browning. They can also cause carcinogens to form. Antioxidants work by donating hydrogen atoms to free radicals to create stable compounds.

Antioxidants are added to foods in four main ways. The first method is to add them directly to the fats or oils. Water-soluble antioxidants are first combined with glycerol-water emulsions. Foods can also be sprayed with or dipped in a solution containing antioxidants. Lastly, foods can be packaged in wraps that contain antioxidants.

GRAS List Antioxidants

Three natural antioxidants appear on the GRAS list. Two of these are vitamin C (ascorbic acid, $C_6H_8O_6$) and vitamin E (tocopherols,

$C_{26}H_{44}O_2$). The presence of either of these vitamins in a food containing nitrites can interfere with the production of nitrosamines. Some cured meats have ascorbic acid added to maintain color as well as to prevent nitrosamines from forming. Vitamin E occurs naturally in most plants, and it helps keep many vegetable oils stable. See 16-6.

Citric acid is the third natural antioxidant on the GRAS list. Citric acid works to prevent oxidation in lipids by holding metal ions in solution. It is also added to many other foods to react with metal ions. Metal ions can start oxidation in food mixtures.

Vitamin E can be regenerated by ascorbic and citric acids. When vitamin E reacts with free radicals, new stable compounds are formed. Vitamin E then becomes unavailable. When ascorbic or citric acid is present, it removes and inactivates the free radical from the vitamin E. The vitamin E is then free to react with another free radical.

Controlled-Use Antioxidants

Hundreds of antioxidants have been evaluated for use in food. Only four synthetic antioxidants are used extensively in food. They are BHA, BHT, propyl gallate, and TBHQ.

BHA (butylated hydroxyanisole, $C_{11}H_{18}O_2$) is a waxy white solid. It is used in ice creams, candy, chewing gum, dry dessert mixes, and gelatin desserts. It is also used in instant potatoes, breakfast cereals, lard, shortening, unsmoked sausages, baked goods, and snack foods.

BHT (butylated hydroxytoluene, $C_{15}H_{24}O$) is an inexpensive synthetic antioxidant. It is a white crystalline solid that works well in conjunction with BHA. BHT is used in chewing gum, instant potatoes, breakfast cereals, animal fats, and shortenings. Both BHA and BHT are effective in animal fats. They are not as effective in vegetable oils.

Large doses of BHA and BHT were found to inhibit the growth of cancer in animals. However, approved levels of use in foods are below the level needed to receive much protection from cancer.

Propyl gallate ($C_{10}H_{12}O_5$) is a white crystalline solid synthetic antioxidant. It has some water solubility. It is used in cereals, snack foods, and pastries. It helps stabilize vegetable oils but decomposes at its melting point of 148°C (298°F).

TBHQ (tertiery-butylhydroquinone, $C_{10}H_{12}O_4$) is a synthetic antioxidant that is a white to tan powder. It works well in vegetable oils. After extensive testing, TBHQ was approved as an additive in 1972. It works best in frying applications and to some extent in baking.

Sulfites

A controversial group of antioxidants is the sulfites. *Sulfites* are salts containing sulfur. The sulfites include sulfur dioxide, sodium sulfite, sodium and potassium bisulfite, and sodium and potassium metabisulfite.

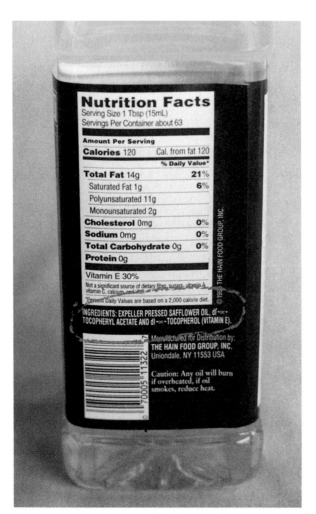

16-6 This safflower oil, like many vegetable oils, contains added tocopherols (vitamin E) to help preserve the quality of the product.

Sulfites are added to frozen and dried fruits and vegetables to help prevent browning. At one time, they were also used to keep raw fruits and vegetables looking fresh on salad bars. In 1986, the FDA banned the use of sulfites on fresh fruits and vegetables. This ban occurred after some people developed dangerous allergic reactions to sulfites.

Sulfites must be declared on the ingredient list of any product containing them in amounts of 10 ppm or higher. Sulfites may not be used as a preservative in any food that is a recognized source of the vitamin thiamin. This is because sulfites destroy thiamin. Any food containing sulfites will not help meet the daily requirements for thiamin.

Enhance Sensory Characteristics

A second main function of additives is to make foods more appealing. Four kinds of additives are used to enhance the sensory characteristics of food. Additives in this group are coloring and flavoring agents, flavor enhancers, and sweeteners.

Coloring Agents

Colors make foods more appetizing. They also help identify products. Consumers expect chocolate candy to be brown and grape candy to be purple. See 16-7.

Two main types of coloring agents are used in foods: natural and synthetic. Natural colors are extracted from plant, animal, and mineral sources. Beta-carotene, a plant extract, gives foods a buttery yellow color. Spices, such as turmeric, saffron, and paprika, are also plant sources of color. Squid ink, a fluid used by the squid for defense, is used to dye gourmet pastas black. Ferrous gluconate is a coloring agent that comes from a mineral source. It is used to color black olives. See 16-8.

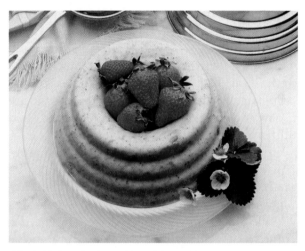

16-7 Pink coloring gives this dessert mold eye appeal and helps you identify the flavor as strawberry.

Natural Coloring Agents

Additive	Color
Annatto	Yellow-red
Beet powder	Red
Beta carotene	Yellow
Caramel	Brown
Carrot oil	Orange
Cochineal extract	Red
Grape skin	Purple-red (beverages only)
Paprika	Red-orange
Riboflavin	Yellow
Saffron	Orange
Toasted cottonseed flour	Brown shades
Turmeric	Yellow

16-8 These coloring agents have no restrictions on their use.

Synthetic food coloring agents are used more widely than natural colors. This is because synthetic dyes provide the most stable colors. They are easier to produce, more economical, and do not add unwanted flavors. They also blend nicely and can be used in small quantities due to their strong coloring ability.

Most synthetic colors were originally made from aniline, which was derived from coal. They were called *coal-tar dyes.* Many of the coal tar dyes are no longer used because they were found to be carcinogenic. Of the approximately 200 coloring agents on the GRAS list in 1960, there are only about 30 remaining.

Today, synthetic colors are made from petroleum. They are tested and retested before being approved. In fact, coloring agents are the most screened and tested category of food additives.

Each approved coloring agent has a specific chemical formula. Each substance can be analyzed to check its composition. The manufacture of coloring agents involves complex chemical reactions. This causes each batch of color to be a little different. Therefore, every batch of synthetic color made must be tested and certified as to its content. If the composition does not meet narrow guidelines, the whole batch is rejected.

Synthetic dyes are identified by use, shade, and number. Abbreviations indicate the uses for which a dye has been approved. Dyes approved for use in food are labeled with an *F. A D* shows that a dye can be used in drugs, and *C* means it can be used in cosmetics. Therefore, FD & C Red No. 40 is a red coloring agent approved for use in food, drugs, and cosmetics.

Some coloring agents cause allergic reactions among a small percentage of people. Therefore, all FDA certified colors are now required to be listed by name on product labels.

Flavoring Agents

Flavoring agents are the largest group of food additives. Added flavors are often used to replace natural flavors lost during processing.

Flavoring agents include natural and synthetic flavors. Natural flavoring agents are often overlooked as additives. They are not limited in use and do not have to be listed by name on ingredient labels. Their presence in a food is represented by the words *natural flavorings* or *spices.* Examples of natural flavorings are cinnamon, dill, ginger, basil, poppy seed, and thyme. These natural flavorings come from dried leaves, bark, roots, buds, flowers, fruits, and seeds.

There are close to 2,000 synthetic flavoring agents and flavor enhancers. One reason for the widespread use of synthetic flavors is consumer demand. Synthetic flavors are cheaper and more abundant than natural flavors. For example, there are not enough strawberries or vanilla beans to meet the demand for these flavors. Many of the synthetic flavors are organic compounds called esters. *Esters* are produced by combining an organic acid and an alcohol. For example, salicylic acid plus methanol produces an ester with wintergreen flavor. See 16-9.

The way a product is labeled indicates the type of flavoring agents it contains. A product labeled "strawberry yogurt" means the yogurt is flavored with strawberries. "Strawberry-flavored yogurt" means that at least some of the flavor comes from synthetic flavoring agents. "Imitation strawberry yogurt" has only synthetic flavors added.

Food scientists develop synthetic flavors by studying the complex chemicals that are responsible for the natural flavors of food. The scientists then combine synthetic flavor chemicals in ratios that are as close as possible to the natural flavors. Synthetic flavors often differ from natural flavors due to lack of complexity. It is hard to identify all the flavor chemicals that affect a food's flavor. For instance, chocolate is viewed as one of the most complex flavors. It is believed to consist of over 500 flavoring chemicals. Synthetic flavors rarely contain all the chemicals involved in a natural flavor.

Flavor Enhancers

Flavor enhancers improve an individual's ability to taste the natural flavors in a food. The most widely used flavor enhancer is salt. When salt is used to give a product a salty taste, it is a flavoring agent. When salt is used in small amounts, however, it can enhance flavors without creating a salty taste. For

Artificial Flavoring Esters

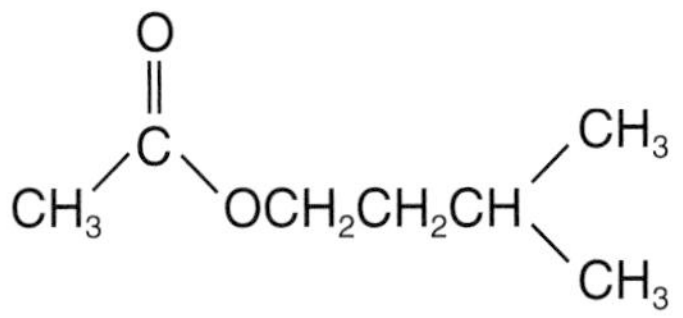

isoamyl acetate
Banana

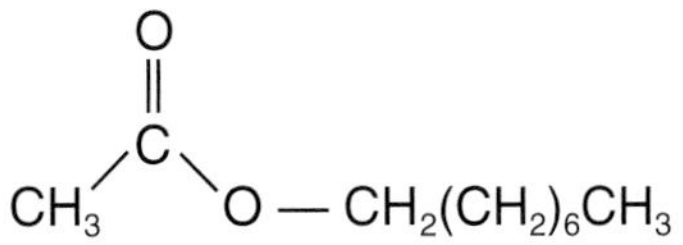

octyl acetate
Orange

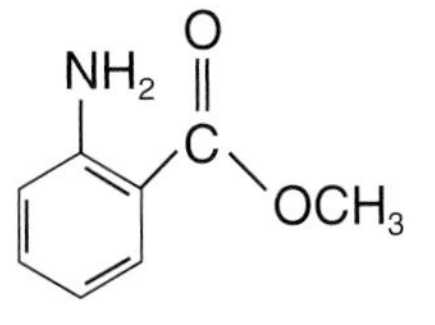

methyl anthranilate
Grape

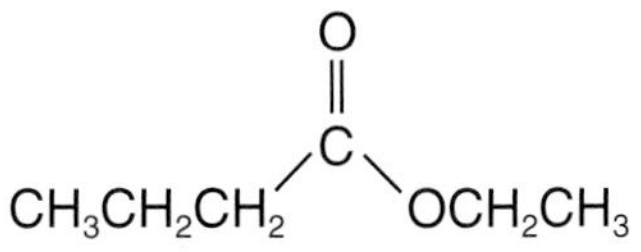

ethyl butyrate
Pineapple

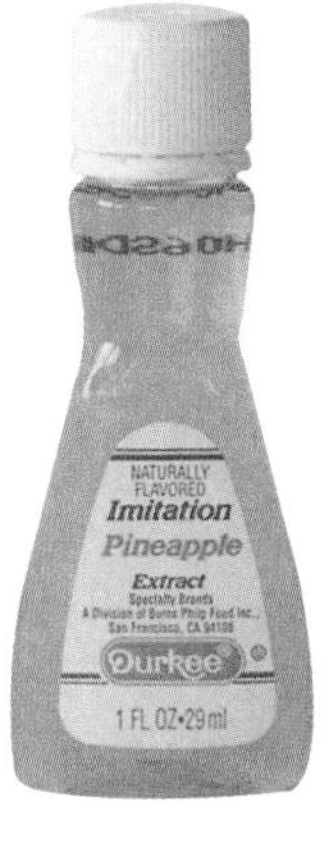

16-9 These are just a few of the hundreds of artificial flavoring compounds that have been developed for use in foods.

instance, studies found that salt gave soup a better balance of flavor. It changed people's perception of the sweetness, bitterness, and mouth feel of the soup. Salt also enhances the flavor of chocolate.

Health Tip

One flavor enhancer that has received much publicity is MSG, monosodium glutamate ($C_5H_8NO_4^-$, Na^+). This is because a number of people have reacted to Chinese food flavored with MSG. Those who react complain of burning sensations, chest and facial flushing, and severe headaches. Studies have had mixed results in attempting to confirm reactions to MSG, but research is continuing. If you have experienced any of these symptoms, you may want to consider ordering your Chinese food without MSG.

Sweeteners

Sweeteners are used to make the tastes of many food products more appealing to consumers. Natural sugars are widely used to sweeten processed foods. Besides sweetening, sugars alter textures and aid in browning.

Sweeteners are classed as nutritive or nonnutritive. Nutritive sweeteners provide calories to the diet. They include sucrose,

glucose, and fructose. They also include the sugar alcohols, such as mannitol and sorbitol. Nonnutritive sweeteners do not supply calories. These sweeteners include saccharin and aspartame.

Control Product Consistency

A third main function of food additives is to control the consistency of foods. Seven groups of additives perform this function by creating various desired effects during food processing. These additives affect the texture and appearance of foods. Interactions of these compounds within a food may also affect the flavor of the product. This group of additives has had the least controversy.

Anticaking Agents

Anticaking agents absorb moisture. They are used to keep powdered and crystalline ingredients from caking or forming lumps. Products such as table salt, baking powder, and confectioner's sugar contain small amounts of anticaking agents. Calcium silicate ($CaSiO_3$), silicon dioxide (SiO_2), and dicalcium phosphate ($CaHPO_4$) are among the agents to keep foods free-flowing.

Emulsifiers

Oil and water do not mix unless there is an emulsifier around. Emulsifiers help distribute tiny particles of one liquid in another. They keep salad dressings mixed and help maintain ice cream's creamy texture. Emulsifiers also disperse flavors in candies, pickles, and beverages. See 16-10.

The most widely used emulsifiers are extracted from natural food sources. Lecithin is an emulsifier found in milk, soybeans, and egg yolks. It is used in chocolates, baked goods, margarine, ice creams, mayonnaise, and salad dressings. Mono- and diglycerides are emulsifiers extracted from vegetables or animal fat. They help stabilize margarine and keep peanut butter from separating. In addition, these fatty acids work as lubricants and binders. For example, they help make bread products soft. (You will read more about emulsifiers in Chapter 22.)

Humectants

Humectants are additives used to help products retain moisture. They are used mainly in flaked coconut, marshmallows, soft candies, chewing gum, and confections. Besides moisture retention, these additives can help control crystal growth and regulate water activity. They also affect texture and carry flavor compounds.

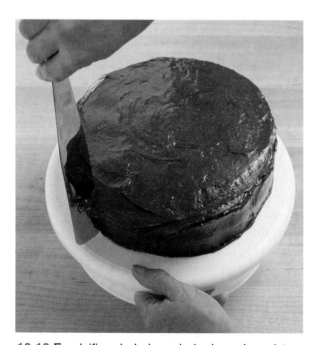

16-10 Emulsifiers help keep baked goods moist and frostings creamy.

The most common humectants are propylene glycol ($C_3H_8O_2$), glycerol or glycerin ($C_3H_8O_3$), sorbitol ($C_6H_{14}O_6$), and mannitol ($C_6H_{14}O_6$). These are sweet alcohols. Propylene glycol is one of the few humectants not found naturally in foods. Glycerol is a by-product of fermentation. Sorbitol is found in small amounts in some fruits. Mannitol is made from seaweed.

Leavening Agents

Leavening agents are added to foods to increase volume and alter texture. They make baked goods light and airy.

Two main types of leavening agents are added to foods. The first type is yeast. Fresh, moist yeast cells are grown, harvested, and compressed into blocks, which are sold in grocery stores as "compressed yeast." Yeast may also be dried and vacuum-packed to stop its growth until needed. This type of yeast is sold in grocery stores as "active dry yeast." Many products containing yeast also contain ammonium sulfate [$(NH_4)_2SO_4$] to help promote the yeast's growth. (You will read about how yeasts function in Chapter 17.)

Chemical leavening agents are the second main type of leavening agents added to foods. Chemical leavening agents include baking soda and baking powder. These additives cause an acid-base reaction that results in the formation of a salt, carbon dioxide (CO_2), and water. Baking soda is sodium bicarbonate ($NaHCO_3$). Baking soda combined with one or more dry acids is the basis for baking powders. (Refer to Chapter 6 for a description of how these compounds work.)

Maturing and Bleaching Agents

If flour is used without aging, the result is an inferior baked product. This is because the gluten characteristics needed to form an elastic dough are poorly developed in freshly ground flour. The result is a sticky dough that is hard to handle. Freshly ground flour also has a pale yellow tint.

Storing flour for several months allows time for the carotenoids in flour to oxidize. This aging process causes the flour to whiten. Aging flour makes dough less sticky and improves the quality of baked products.

In the early 1900s, scientists discovered chemicals that would speed the aging process and whiten flour. These chemicals are called *maturing and bleaching agents.* Some of these agents mature, others bleach, and some do both. These compounds eliminate the need for time-consuming storage of flour, which is costly. See 16-11.

Some maturing and bleaching agents are added to flour during the milling process. They improve the flour and then break down, leaving little chemical residue on the flour.

Maturing and Bleaching Agents

Name	Chemical Formula	Function
Benzoyl peroxide	$[(C_6H_5CO)_2\,O_2]$	Bleach
Chlorine gas	Cl_2	Bleach and mature
Chlorine dioxide	ClO_2	
Nitrosyl chloride	$NOCl$	
Nitrogen dioxide	NO_2	
Potassium bromate	$KBrO_3$	Condition dough and mature
Potassium iodate	KIO_3	
Ammonium phosphate	$(NH_4)_3\,PO_4$	Facilitate yeast growth by providing nutrients and controlling pH levels
Calcium phosphate	$CaHPO_4$	
Cellulose	Polysaccharides	Improve water holding ability of dough
Locust bean gum		
Methylcellulose		
Carboxymethylcellulose	Polysaccharides	Decrease fat absorbed by dough during frying
Carrageenan	Polysaccharides	Soften texture of sweet baked goods

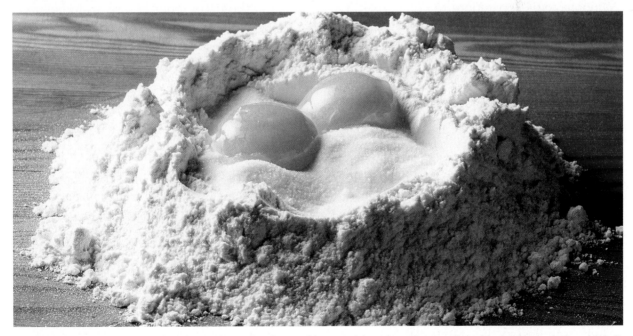

16-11 Maturing and bleaching agents make flour whiter and improve the quality of baked goods in which it is used.

Other maturing and bleaching agents are added during the dough mixing process in commercial baking. These compounds work as dough conditioners.

pH Control Agents

Changing the acidity or alkalinity of a food mixture can affect its safety, flavor, and texture. An additive that alters or stabilizes the pH of a mixture is a *pH control agent.* Acids, bases, buffers, and salts can all work as pH control agents.

Acids

Making the pH of foods more acidic can serve a number of functions. As you read earlier, acids are added to some foods as preservatives. For instance, vinegar (acetic acid) is added to pickles to keep them from spoiling.

Acids can give foods a tart flavor. This is why citric acid is added to some lemon-lime soft drinks.

Another important function of acids in mixtures is to alter texture. Acids in the pectin gels of jams and jellies enable the pectins to form a three-dimensional network. This network traps water and forms the gel. Acids also affect the texture of some candies. Acids help hydrolyze sugar and reduce crystal growth. This is necessary for fudges to have a smooth creamy texture.

Some acids serve more than one role in a food product. For instance, phosphoric acid (H_3PO_4) is used in colas, root beers, and other nonfruit soft drinks. It enhances flavor and, along with CO_2, protects against microbial growth.

Bases

Besides controlling pH, bases can enhance the color and flavor of some foods. An example is chocolate. After cocoa beans are picked, they are allowed to dry and ferment. Bases are added to neutralize the acids produced during fermentation. The addition of the base also deepens the color and produces a milder flavor.

Like acids, bases can affect the texture of food products. For instance, bases are necessary for the thickening of instant pudding mixes. Bases are used to modify or alter starch granules so the starch can thicken at low temperatures.

Strong bases are used to peel various fruits and vegetables. Peaches and apricots are often dipped in a 3% sodium hydroxide solution at 60°C to 82°C (140°F to 180°F) before peeling. This basic solution softens the fruit skin, making it easier to remove. This results in less waste.

Buffers

Buffers are added to food mixtures to stabilize the mixtures at a desired pH. Sodium salts, citrates, and phosphates are widely used buffers. Examples of naturally occurring buffers are proteins, lactic acid, organic acids, and phosphate salts. Organic acids and phosphate salts act as buffering systems in many plants. They can be extracted for use as food additives. See 16-12.

Stabilizers and Thickeners

Other additives used to help control the consistency of food products are stabilizers and thickeners. These compounds can improve the appearance and mouth feel of a food.

Stabilizers keep chocolate from settling out of chocolate milk. They keep flavors from evaporating in cake, pudding, and gelatin mixes. Stabilizers also prevent ice crystals from forming in ice cream.

Thickeners increase the viscosity of mixtures. In some cases, they help form gels. Ideally, these compounds are water-soluble.

Common Sources of Buffering Agents

Organic Acids in Natural Buffering Systems	Plant Sources
Citric acid	Lemons, tomatoes, rhubarb
Malic acid	Apples, tomatoes, lettuce
Oxalic acid	Rhubarb, lettuce
Tartaric acid	Grapes, pineapples

16-12 Some plants rely on natural buffering agents to maintain the pH level needed for normal growth and reproduction. These agents can be extracted from the plant sources for use in foods.

They are often used in icings, frozen desserts, chocolate milk, and gelled candies such as gummy bears.

Most of the stabilizers and thickeners are natural carbohydrates. Gelatin comes from the bones and hooves of animals as well as the breakdown of collagen in meaty tissues. Pectin comes from apples and citrus peel. Other commonly used compounds are alginates, carageenan, and propylene glycol ($C_3H_6O_2$).

Vegetable gums from plants such as tropical trees and seaweed are also used as stabilizers and thickeners. These gums have a much greater thickening power than starches from wheat and corn. Two of these, tragacanth gum and gum arabic, may cause allergic reactions in susceptible people.

Improve or Maintain Nutritive Value

The fourth key function of food additives is to improve or maintain the nutritional quality of food products. Most nutrient additives are vitamins or minerals. Initially, nutrients were added to widely eaten foods to reduce or eliminate illnesses due to nutrient deficiencies. Iodine was the first nutrient added to food. It was added to salt to prevent goiter. Another example of a nutrient additive is vitamin D in milk. Iron and B vitamins are added to refined grain products.

A new trend in the food industry is fortifying foods with nutrients to improve health benefits. An example is calcium-fortified orange juice. It is promoted as a healthy way to increase calcium intake, especially for people who do not drink milk.

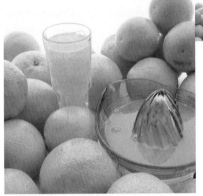

Nutrition News
Cholesterol-Lowering Spreads

The Functional Food: Benecol and Take Control are vegetable oil spreads with added ingredients that lower cholesterol.

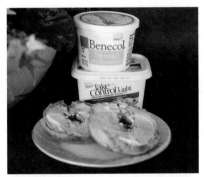

These vegetable oil spreads contain additives to help lower the cholesterol levels of people who consume the products.

The Active Ingredient: Benecol contains pinewood stanol esters. Take Control contains sterol esters extracted from soybeans. After looking at the research, the FDA has declared these two esters as "generally recognized as safe."

The Research: Research has found that 2 grams per day of the esters in Take Control lowered cholesterol levels by 8%. A one-year study showed that 3 grams per day of the active ingredient in Benecol lowered LDL by 14%. People in the study had an average cholesterol level of 235. Three pats of Take Control or Benecol per day provide the amounts of active ingredients shown to be effective.

The Caution: Research has found that Benecol lowers blood beta-carotene levels by as much as 20%. In the study, this was still in the normal range for beta-carotene. Further research is needed to determine if more than three pats of spread a day would pose a health threat.

The Recommendation: Using Benecol or Take Control appears to be a safe way to lower cholesterol without drugs. It is important to limit intake to within the tested levels. People using these products should also include fruit and vegetable sources of beta-carotene in their diets.

The problem with nutrient additives is they can lead to false thinking. Some people may believe fortified foods will provide all the nutrients needed for good health. Remember that no single food, regardless of how many nutrients are added to it, can meet all nutrient needs. Eating a variety of foods is the only sure way to get all the needed nutrients.

Balancing Benefits and Risks

Additives have made possible an abundant and varied food supply. The financial impact of additives is enormous. Additives, technological advancements, and rapid transportation systems have made it possible to have thousands of food choices every day. Think about how many jobs exist because of the production of these foods. Also think about how much money flows into the U.S. economy from food purchases. People in the United States spend over $400 billion a year in supermarkets. They spend over $210 billion a year eating away from home.

How would your life differ if you could not use packaged, shelf stable, frozen, and quick-fix foods? The amount of time you spent obtaining and preparing food each day would probably increase quite a bit. Most convenience products are only possible due to the use of additives. See 16-13.

Although food additives offer many benefits, their use also creates concern for some consumers. Some concern comes from the removal of additives from the GRAS list. Consumers may wonder what other compounds added to foods will later be found to be harmful. Consumers might also worry about additives that have caused allergic reactions among some people. The FDA gives consumers the chance to express their concerns when hearings are held to approve or review additives.

In general, the more processing a food undergoes, the more additives it is likely to contain. However, because additives cost money, manufacturers only add what is needed to accomplish the desired result. In addition, the FDA operates an Adverse Reaction Monitoring System (ARMS) to monitor the safety of additives. A computerized database tracks complaints regarding additives and dietary supplements. ARMS is used to help decide if reported adverse reactions represent a real public health hazard.

It is impossible to test all possible combinations of additives in a diet. Therefore, limiting your use of processed foods can help you reduce any risk additives might pose. The following guidelines can help you reduce possible risks linked with food additives:

❖ Wash all produce before eating to remove additives such as soil and pesticide residues.

❖ Choose fresh fruits and vegetables for snacks instead of processed snack foods like fruit rolls and potato chips.

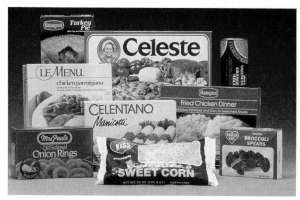

USDA

Benefits of Food Additives

❖ greater variety of low-cost foods available year-round

❖ reduced risk of foodborne illness

❖ less waste due to spoilage

❖ less time required for food preparation tasks

❖ greater variety of processed, convenience foods

16-13 Additives have allowed food scientists to develop many convenience foods that help consumers save time when preparing meals.

❖ Learn to prepare foods from scratch to limit your use of highly processed convenience foods.

❖ Read food product labels to be aware of the additives you consume.

❖ Read current newspapers and magazines to keep informed about new findings related to food additives.

Remember that FDA margins of safety vary from one additive to another. With some additives, harmful levels may be reached when a diet is imbalanced. This can happen when one food is consumed to the exclusion of others. The responsibility for keeping your food safe does not lie only with the FDA or food manufacturers. The responsibility also lies with you.

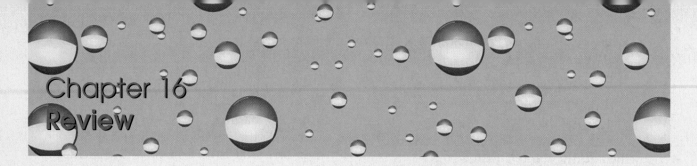

Summary

An additive is any substance added to a food to cause a change in the food's characteristics. Additives may be intentional or incidental. All sources of additives are monitored to protect consumers. A series of laws have been passed to provide guidelines for monitoring additives. These laws include detailed instructions on the approval and use of additives in foods, drugs, and cosmetics. The GRAS list includes all additives that are generally recognized as safe. Additives on the GRAS list are usable by food manufacturers. The Delaney Clause bars the approval of any additive found to cause cancer in humans or animals.

The functions of additives can be divided into four main categories: preserving product quality, enhancing sensory characteristics, controlling product consistency, and improving or maintaining nutritive value. Many additives are found naturally in foods, but synthetic additives are also used. In many cases, synthetic additives are more economical to produce and more consistent in their results.

Additives have made a wide variety of foods possible. In addition, they have helped provide a safer food supply. However, food additives also cause consumers some concern. The FDA monitors the safety of the food supply in general, but consumers must also take responsibility for monitoring what they eat.

Check Your Understanding

1. Describe the difference between intentional and incidental additives. Give an example of each.
2. What law is the basis of modern food regulations? Who oversees this law?
3. List three of the requirements an additive must meet before it can be approved for use in the United States.
4. Why was the GRAS list created?
5. List two problems related to the Delaney Clause.
6. Name two organizations that work to establish international food standards.
7. Name the two categories of preservatives and their functions in foods.
8. Explain how salt and sugar preserve foods.
9. List two natural and two synthetic antioxidants used in foods.
10. List the four types of additives that enhance sensory characteristics of foods and give an example of each.
11. List and describe the types of additives that control product consistency.
12. What are three guidelines for reducing possible risks linked with food additives?

Critical Thinking

1. If two loaves of wheat bread—one with preservatives and one without—were wrapped in unlabeled packages, how could you tell them apart?
2. Explain how you would know which of the following imaginary coloring agents could be used with food:
   ❖ F Yellow No. 8
   ❖ D Yellow No. 111
   ❖ C Yellow No. 40
   ❖ FD&C Yellow No. 23
3. Explain the likely effect of substituting pineapple juice for half the milk listed on the label of instant vanilla pudding.
4. When a food containing vitamin B_1 is preserved with a sulfite, what can be concluded?

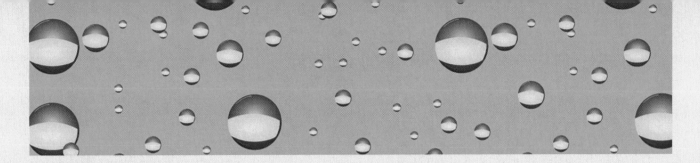

Explore Further

1. **Analytical Skills.** Examine the labels on two of your favorite snack foods that contain 10 or more ingredients. Identify the functions of each additive in the food.

2. **Math.** Survey the foods eaten by your class in the last 24 hours. Calculate the percentage of items that contained food additives versus those that did not. Illustrate the results in a pie chart.

3. **Technology.** Examine the total amounts of salt and sugar you eat during a weekend. Read food labels to find out how much of these ingredients your meals contain and measure the extra amounts you add. Total your intake of each for the two days. On the Internet, find a recent research brief addressing each. What conclusions can you draw from examining your diet and recent research? Report to the class.

4. **Analytical Skills.** Construct a model of the ester that creates the wintergreen flavor.

5. **Writing.** Write an article for your school newspaper explaining the use of additives in the food supply.

Experiment 16A
Pectin as a Texturizer

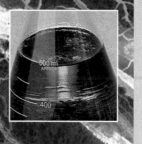

Purpose

One of the functions of some food additives is to add texture or stability to food products. Many stabilizers and thickeners are found in nature, including pectins, gums, mono- and diglycerides, and lecithin. In this experiment, you will examine the role of pectin in developing the gummy texture in a category of popular fruit-flavored candies. These candies also rely on artificial flavoring and coloring agents to provide distinctive flavors and the corresponding colors.

Equipment

2 saucepans, 1½- to 2-quart

2 large spoons

9-inch square pan

container with a lid

Supplies

1 49-g package commercial pectin

60 mL (¼ cup) water

2 mL (½ teaspoon) baking soda

250 mL (1 cup) sugar

250 mL (1 cup) corn syrup

2 to 5 mL (½ to 1 teaspoon) imitation flavoring or extract of your choice

food coloring of your choice

butter

125 mL (½ cup) confectioners' sugar

waxed paper

Procedure

1. Combine one package of commercial pectin with 60 mL (¼ cup) of water in one saucepan.

2. Add 2 mL (½ teaspoon) of baking soda to the pectin and water. The mixture will foam.

3. Combine 250 mL (1 cup) of sugar and 250 mL (1 cup) of corn syrup in a second saucepan.

4. Cook both mixtures over high heat at the same time. Have one lab group member stir each of the mixtures.

5. Cook and stir until the corn syrup mixture boils rapidly while stirring and the foam breaks down in the pectin mixture (approximately 4 to 5 minutes).

6. Pour the pectin mixture into the corn syrup mixture. Cook 1 more minute.

7. Remove the mixture from the heat and add 2 to 5 mL (½ to 1 teaspoon) of an imitation flavoring or extract and a corresponding food coloring. For example, you might add grape flavoring and purple food coloring.

8. Pour the mixture into a buttered 9-inch square pan. Let it stand until cool and firm.

9. Turn the candy out of the pan onto waxed paper dusted with confectioners' sugar.

10. Dust the top of the candy with more confectioners' sugar. Cut the candy into 1-inch cubes.

11. Place the candy on waxed paper inside a sealed container and allow it to sit overnight.

12. Evaluate the texture and flavor of the candy the next day in class.

Questions

1. How does the texture of the candy you made compare to commercial gummy candies?

2. What ingredients are used to create the gummy texture in commercial candies?

374

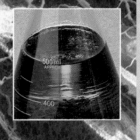

Purpose

American cheese slices are an example of process cheese. Process cheese is made by shredding aged cheeses and melting them with emulsifiers. The emulsifiers keep the fat from separating from the solids, giving the process cheese a smoother melting quality. This quality is preferred when using cheese in such foods as cheeseburgers and macaroni and cheese. In this experiment, you will compare process cheese prepared with various amounts of the emulsifier sodium phosphate (Na_2HPO_4).

Equipment

electronic balance

grater

double boiler

thermometer

large spoon

muffin pan

knife

cookie sheet

Supplies

100 g Cheddar cheese

sodium phosphate (Na_2HPO_4)

foil baking cup

wax pencil

Procedure

1. Grate and mass 100 g of cheese. Place it in the top of a double boiler.

2. Mass the assigned amount of Na_2HPO_4 and add it to the cheese in the double boiler.

   Control: no Na_2HPO_4 is added

   Variation 1: 0.5 g Na_2HPO_4

   Variation 2: 1.0 g Na_2HPO_4

   Variation 3: 2.0 g Na_2HPO_4

   Variation 4: 4.0 g Na_2HPO_4

3. Heat the cheese mixture to 66°C (150°F). Do not stir with the thermometer. Stir gently with a large spoon.

4. Pour the cheese mixture into a foil-lined muffin cup. Set aside to cool until firm.

5. Preheat the oven to 350°F.

6. When the cheese is set, remove the foil baking cup and slice the cheese in half. Observe and record any differences in appearance of the interiors of the five samples.

7. Lay half of each cheese variation, cut side down, on a cookie sheet or piece of foil on a cookie sheet. Label each variation with a wax pencil. Place the cookie sheet in the preheated oven. Open the oven and examine the cheese every 60 seconds. Record differences in melting characteristics of the samples.

Calculations

Calculate how many moles of Na_2HPO_4 were used in each variation.

Questions

1. Which cheese sample melted fastest? Which cheese sample melted slowest?

2. Which cheese sample(s) had curd showing?

3. Which level of Na_2HPO_4 would you recommend for making process cheese with the best melting qualities?

Experiment 16C
Preservatives in Cured Meat

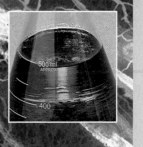

Purpose

One of the oldest methods of preserving meat is to cure it in salt. After curing, the meat would appear gray unless the salt was contaminated with sodium nitrate. Today, sodium nitrate and nitrites are deliberately added to develop the characteristic red color associated with hot dogs, bologna, and ham. In this experiment, you will observe the differences in the color of fresh and cooked meat with and without sodium nitrite added.

Equipment

electronic balance
wax pencil
2 150-mL beakers
2 rubber scrapers
large saucepan

Supplies

200 g fresh hamburger
1-quart resealable plastic bag
0.02 g sodium nitrite
plastic wrap
375 mL (1½ cups) water

Procedure

Day 1

1. Mass 200 g fresh hamburger and divide it into two equal parts.

2. Put one half of the hamburger into a 1-quart resealable plastic bag and sprinkle the meat with 0.02 g sodium nitrite. Seal the bag and knead it for 3 minutes to mix the nitrite into the hamburger.

3. Use a wax pencil to label two 150-mL beakers as follows: *with* and *without.*

4. Transfer the hamburger from the plastic bag into the beaker labeled *with.*

5. Put the other half of the hamburger from step 1 in the beaker labeled *without.*

6. Use a clean rubber scraper to tightly pack the hamburger in each beaker to remove as much air as possible.

7. Describe the odor of each sample in a data table and then tightly cover the beakers with plastic wrap.

8. Examine each sample and record the surface and interior colors in a data table.

9. Refrigerate the beakers overnight.

Day 2

1. Examine both samples for odor and surface and interior colors. Record your observations in the data table.

2. In a large saucepan, heat 375 mL (1½ cups) water to boiling.

3. Place the beakers in the boiling water bath and heat for 15 to 20 minutes or insert a thermometer into the center of the meat and cook to 68°C (155°F).

4. Examine both samples for odor and surface and interior colors. Record your observations.

Calculations

1. The legal limit of nitrite (NO_2) for meat is 156 ppm. How many milligrams of nitrite

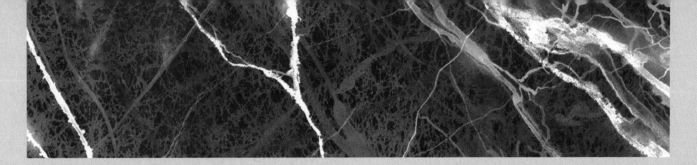

are allowed in one kilogram of meat? (Hint: Start by calculating how many milligrams are in a kilogram.)

2. Calculate the mass of 1 mole of nitrite (NO_2) and 1 mole of sodium nitrite ($NaNO_2$).

3. Use the answers from calculation 2 to figure what percentage of $NaNO_2$ is made up of NO_2.

$$\frac{\text{mass of 1 mole of } NO_2}{\text{mass of 1 mole of } NaNO_2} = \text{percentage of } NaNO_2 \text{ made up } NO_2$$

4. What is the maximum amount of $NaNO_2$ that can be added to 1 kg of meat? (Hint: Divide the answer from calculation 1 by the percentage from calculation 3.)

Questions

1. Which of the samples most closely resembles the odor of ham or sausage?

2. What effect does cooking have on the samples?

In the last two units, you have examined the chemical composition of the food supply. You have read about carbohydrates, lipids, proteins, vitamins, minerals, phytochemicals, and food analogs. You have studied their structures, reactions in food mixtures, and nutritional value.

You may have learned in science classes that biology is the study of living organisms. Some organisms are too small to be seen by the human eye. They are called *microbes.* Food microbiology is the study of microbes that are found in foods. In this unit, you will study many of the positive and negative effects microbes have on the food you eat. These effects include

❖ producing new food products

❖ causing spoilage

❖ contaminating food and causing foodborne illness

In Chapter 17, you will look at the benefits of microbes in the food supply. You will examine how foods are changed into new products through the planned addition of microbes. In Chapter 18, you will study the unwanted contamination of food by microbes. Analyzing how foods spoil will help you take steps to reduce or eliminate undesirable and unhealthful changes caused by microbes.

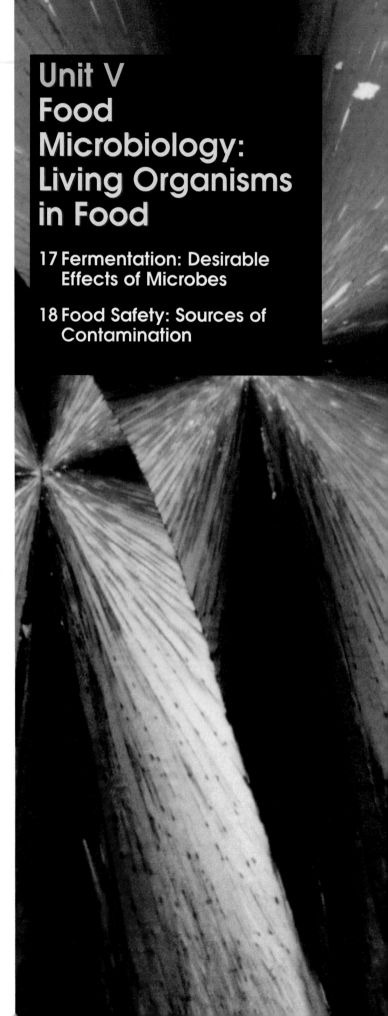

Unit V
Food Microbiology: Living Organisms in Food

17 Fermentation: Desirable Effects of Microbes

18 Food Safety: Sources of Contamination

A substance as common as bread takes on a unique appearance when viewed through an optical microscope. Bread is a product of fermentation, which results from the activity of microorganisms in food.

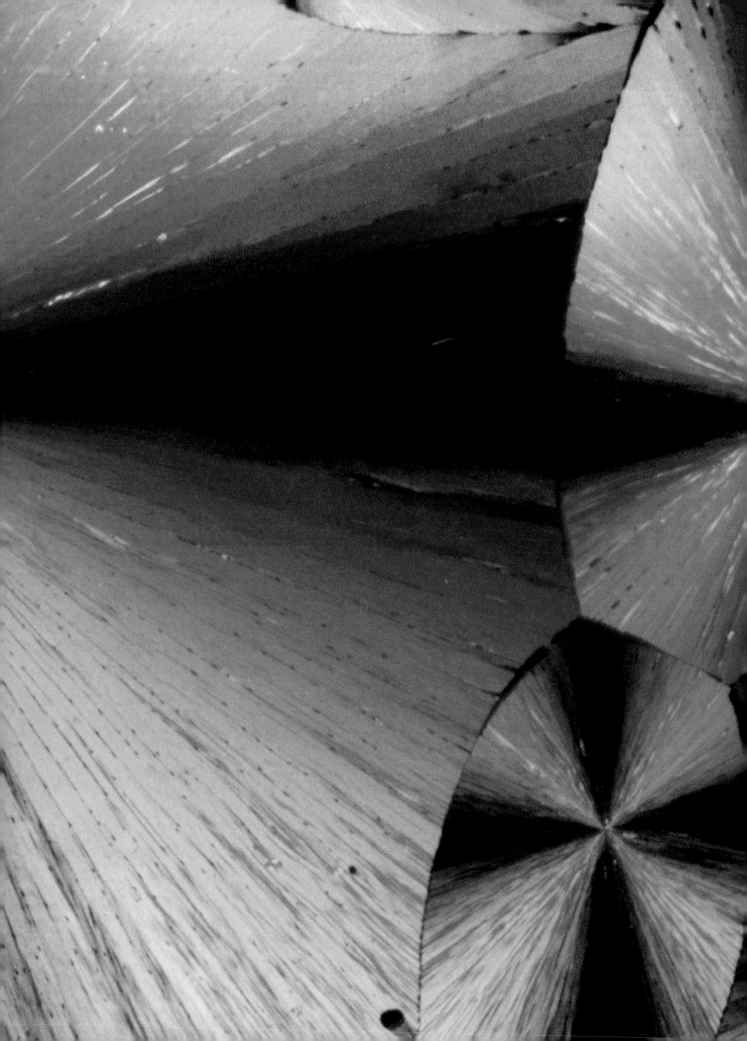

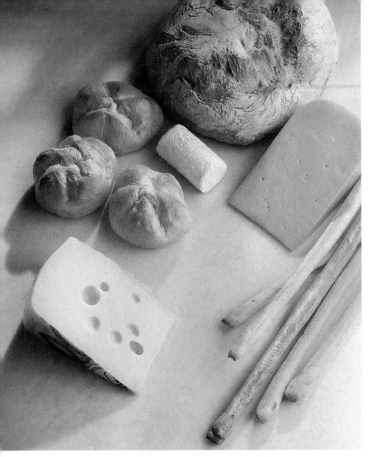

Cheese and bread are just two of the many food products that are produced by fermentation.

Chapter 17

Fermentation: Desirable Effects of Microbes

Objectives

After studying this chapter,
you will be able to

describe the types of microbes that impact the food supply.

list factors that impact the growth of single-celled organisms.

differentiate among yeast, bacterial, and mold fermentation.

identify food products that are a result of fermentation.

Key Terms

microbiology	mycelium
microorganism	spore
microbe	mold
Monera	yeast
Fungi	pure culture
bacteria	starter
micrometer	proteolytic
cytoplasm	lipolytic
bacilli	halophilic
cocci	genus
spirilla	species
Gram's stain	pasteurization
aerobic	fermentation
anaerobic	by-product
facultative	brine
fungus	curd
hyphae	

Microbiology is the study of living organisms too small to be seen by the unaided human eye. Living organisms that are only visible through a microscope are called *microorganisms* or *microbes.* Microbes are all around you. They are in the soil under your feet and on the desk in front of you. They are in the air you breathe, the water you drink, and the food you eat. They multiply rapidly, transfer from one surface to another easily, and blow around in the wind.

You may be unaware that microbes are unavoidable. Perhaps you would rather not think about the fact that microbes live on and in you. However, you can think of many microbes as friends and allies. There are thousands of different microorganisms. Several hundred of these are associated in one way or another with the production of food products. Without microbes, many foods you enjoy would not be possible. Foods produced with the help of microbes include chocolate, coffee, tea, cheese, soy sauce, pickles, sauerkraut, and yeast breads.

This chapter will look at the main kinds of microbes. You will study how they multiply and how they change food into new products. You will also read about how the nutritional value of foods is affected by microbes.

The Types of Single-Celled Organisms

Three categories of microbes can have positive uses in foods. They are bacteria, yeasts, and molds. These microbes have some similarities. Individually, they cannot be seen by the human eye. They reproduce very rapidly when given the right environment. They also depend on outside sources of food to grow and multiply.

Research in the twentieth century changed scientific understanding of microscopic organisms. This led to disagreement on how to classify microbes. Most of the microbes that affect the food supply belong to one of two kingdoms of organisms. Most biologists classify bacteria as members of the *Monera* kingdom. Yeasts and molds are members of the *Fungi* kingdom.

Bacteria

Bacteria are extremely small single-celled organisms that multiply through cell division. The head of a pin can hold thousands of bacteria. These microbes must be magnified 1,000 times with a microscope to make them visible. Bacteria are usually one to three micrometers (μm) in length. A *micrometer* is one-thousandth (0.001) of a millimeter. Suppose you were to lay bacteria that are 1 μm in length end to end. It would take 1,000 of them to equal 1 millimeter. It would take one million of these bacteria to equal 1 meter.

Bacteria cells have rigid walls and no nucleus. The cells are filled with a gelatinous liquid called *cytoplasm.* The processes of metabolism and reproduction take place within this liquid. Bacteria are classified according to their shape, their cell wall structure, and their oxygen needs.

Bacteria have three basic shapes: rod, spherical, and spiral. Rod-shaped bacteria are called *bacilli.* Spherical bacteria are called *cocci.* Spiral bacteria are called *spirilla.* See 17-1.

Bacteria have two basic types of cell wall structures. The two types of cell walls are identified by their ability to be stained by a crystal violet dye. One of the first steps in identifying a type of bacteria is a staining process called *Gram's stain.* Hans Christian Gram developed Gram's stain in 1884. He developed the process because bacteria cells are nearly colorless. This makes them difficult to see, even with a microscope. Gram-positive cell walls will turn blue-violet during the staining process. Gram-negative cells will turn red. See 17-2.

Doctors need to be able to tell the two types of bacteria cell wall structures apart. This allows doctors to decide what medicine to prescribe for a bacterial infection. Many antibiotics will kill either gram-negative or gram-positive bacteria but not both. Plant cell walls and animal cell membranes are not made of the same material as bacteria cell walls. This is why antibiotics can kill bacteria without damaging body tissue.

The oxygen needs of bacteria are important to food scientists who work with food-related bacteria. Some bacteria need oxygen to

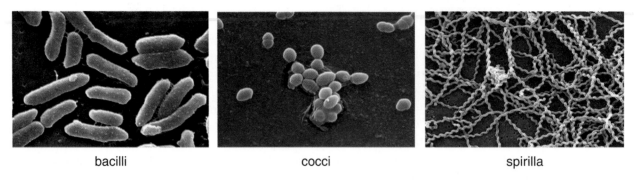

bacilli   cocci   spirilla

17-1 The three basic shapes of bacteria are bacilli (rods), cocci (spheres), and spirilla (spirals).

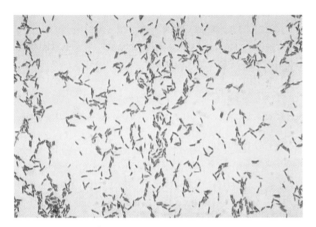

Gram-positive bacteria

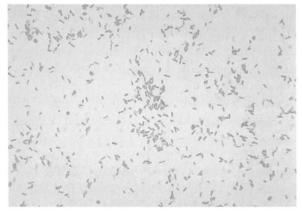

Gram-negative bacteria

17-2 The blue-violet color of the bacteria on the top indicates they are Gram-positive. The red bacteria on the bottom are Gram-negative.

multiply. Others will multiply only in an oxygen-free environment. Bacteria that must have oxygen to function are called *aerobic.* Bacteria that function best in an oxygen-free environment are called *anaerobic.* Bacteria that can function in either environment are called *facultative.*

You can get an idea of how aerobic and anaerobic bacteria work from the example of cabbage. Cabbage spoils when aerobic bacteria are present and given time to multiply. Aerobic bacteria must have oxygen present for respiration to occur. In simple terms, *respiration* is the transfer of electrons to release energy for cellular function. In aerobes, oxygen is the electron receptor. In contrast, the enzymes in anaerobes will not function in the presence of oxygen. They use carbon dioxide or sulfur- or nitrogen-based compounds as electron receptors. If cabbage is submerged in water, where oxygen levels are low, anaerobic bacteria will begin to multiply. Sauerkraut is made by submerging cabbage in salt water. In this environment, the aerobes cannot spoil the cabbage because oxygen is unavailable. However, the anaerobes can grow, and they are responsible for developing the characteristic flavor and texture of sauerkraut.

Bacteria's rate of growth depends on their environment. When temperature, air, pH, and food supply are right, bacteria can reproduce in as little as 20 minutes. Bacteria reproduce by increasing their cell size. The cytoplasm material divides equally in half, and the cells split into two daughter cells. Every time the cells divide, the number of cells doubles.

Fungi

A *fungus* is a plant that lacks chlorophyll. It also lacks definite roots, stems, and leaves. Unlike bacteria, fungi are not always single-celled, and their cells contain a nucleus. Fungi include mildews, molds, mushrooms, rusts, smuts, and yeasts. They are widely distributed in nature and play a major role in helping organic matter decay. They break down the complex macromolecules of organic matter into usable nutrients, which they absorb.

Fungi are classified by their structure and reproduction methods. The basic structure of most fungi is made of filaments or tubes called *hyphae.* Hyphae are elongated cells or chains of cells that absorb nutrients from the environment. As the hyphae lengthen, they intertwine and form a branched network called a *mycelium.* Part of the mycelium grows down into an energy source to absorb nutrients. The other part remains in the air above the energy source and reproduces through spores.

Spores could be called the seeds of fungi. Spores usually develop in a sac- or balloonlike structure. This structure explodes when full, sending spores out into the surrounding air. Spores are microscopic, resistant to harsh environments, and easily carried to other surfaces. See 17-3.

Mycelia tend to grow in a circular pattern. This pattern is created as the hyphae extend outward from a spore or a single cell. When a mycelium becomes large enough, it is visible without magnification.

Of the various types of fungi, molds and yeasts play key roles in food processing. Most yeast and mold cells are three to five times larger than the cells of bacteria. Molds and yeasts vary in length, width, and structure.

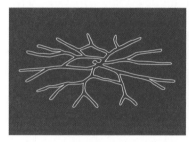 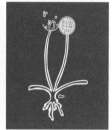

mycelium   spores

17-3 Fungi absorb nutrients through their mycelium structure and reproduce through spores.

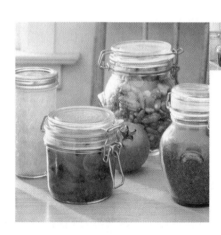

Historical Highlight
Food Poisoning in Salem, MA?

In Salem, Massachusetts, in 1692, over 100 people were accused of witchcraft. Twelve were found guilty and hanged. The teenage girls who made the accusations suffered from a number of symptoms. These symptoms were similar to those of people who take hallucinogenic drugs like LSD.

A fungus that grows on rye when the weather is especially cool and wet is called *Claviceps*

purpurea. (Its common name is ergot.) One of the by-products of this fungus is LSD, a powerful hallucinogen. The fungus can cause a foodborne illness known as *convulsive ergotism.* The symptoms range from mild to severe and can even cause death, especially among the young. The disease causes prickling feeling to severe pain in the joints. There may also be blindness, deafness, hallucinations,

fits, and laughing and crying spells.

Outbreaks of ergotism occur throughout the world when rye crops are weakened by cold and damp weather. Historical records indicate these conditions existed in New England from 1690 to 1692. This is one of many possible explanations proposed for the events in Salem.

Molds

Molds are fungi that form a mycelium structure with a fuzzy appearance. Visible molds have a wide range of colors. These colors include yellow, rust, red, green, and black. Many molds give off an antibiotic that kills bacteria likely to be growing in the same area.

Like other fungi, molds reproduce through spores. During their reproductive stage, some molds produce a visible spore case. This spore case is called a *basidiocarp.* The basidiocarp has a stem, a cap, and gills. The gills, which contain the spores, are located under the cap. The stem lifts the cap and gills into the air so the wind can disperse the spores. Mushrooms, toadstools, and puffballs are examples of basidiocarps produced by molds, 17-4.

Yeasts

Yeasts are fungi with a single-celled structure. They reproduce by budding. This means they form buds that swell and separate into a duplicate cell or form a chain of cells. Reactions involving yeast result in the production of alcohol.

A unique feature of some fungi, including some yeasts, is the ability to form both mycelium and single-celled structures. When a spore from one of these fungi lands on soil or plants, it produces a mycelium structure. When these fungi are found in people or animals, they reproduce by budding. See 17-5.

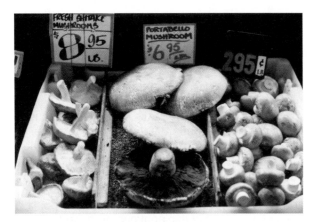

17-4 Mushrooms are the visible spore-carrying structure of the basidiomycetes group of fungi. The stem holds the mushroom above the ground so the breeze can catch and disperse the spores that form along the gills under the cap.

Common Characteristics of Microbes

Both bacteria and fungi grow very rapidly and can be good sources of edible protein. Microbial sources of protein are used in animal feed. Research is underway to develop microbial proteins that are safe for human consumption. Microbes enhance or add to the nutritional value of foods. An example is yeast bread. When yeast dough is held at room temperature for one hour, it will double in volume. The increase in volume is caused by carbon dioxide, which is released as the yeast feed, grow, and multiply. Yeast cells in baked bread add small amounts of protein, vitamins, and minerals. Baking kills the yeast but does not destroy the nutritive value of the yeast.

Bacteria and fungi can also enter a dormant, or inactive, state. This last characteristic allows these microbes to protect themselves. When temperature, pH, moisture level, or the surrounding air becomes harsh, the cells will dehydrate themselves. The dehydrated cells can remain dormant for long periods. As soon as the environment matches a cell's growth needs, the cell will rehydrate and begin to reproduce again.

The ability of microbes to go into a dormant state helps manufacturers mass-produce them. Manufacturers isolate the desired microbe and create ideal conditions for it to grow. The result is a *pure culture,* which is a large volume of one type of microbe that has purposely been grown in a nutrient medium. After mass-producing a desired microbe, manufacturers create an environment that encourages the microbes to dehydrate themselves. Manufacturers can ship cultures or

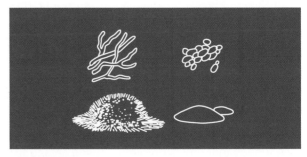

17-5 Yeasts form fuzzy mycelium structures when they grow in plants and soil. In animal sources, yeasts have smooth cells and reproduce by budding.

dehydrated microbes to food processing plants. At processing plants, large volumes of microbes are used in the development of foods such as cheeses, pickles, and beverages. When a pure culture is mixed with a food source, a starter is made. A *starter* is a substance containing microorganisms that is added to food to bring about desired flavor, texture, and/or color changes. Once starters are mixed, the microbes come out of the dormant state. Then they can begin to reproduce and change a food product.

Microbial Enzymes

Changes in food products are usually a result of enzymes produced by the microbes in the food. Microbes use large organic molecules as a food source. However, most organic molecules are too large to be transported through a microbe's cell wall. To access the energy in these compounds, microbes excrete digestive enzymes. These enzymes break down the large molecules. Then the microbes can absorb the resulting fragments and use them as fuel.

Another way to classify microbes is by the type of organic molecules they use as food sources. The classifications are based on the types of enzymes produced by the microbes. Most microbes rely on sugars and starches for their energy source. These microbes produce a variety of carbohydrases. See 17-6.

A few microbes rely on protein as their food source. Microbes that make enzymes to digest protein are called *proteolytic.* Proteolytic microbes change proteins to amino acids. Some uses of proteolytic bacteria in food production are tenderizing meat and clotting milk. Proteolytic bacteria also help remove the outside pulp and develop the chocolate flavor of cacao beans.

Lipolytic microbes produce enzymes that digest fats. Some uses include flavor production in cheese and removing egg yolk from egg white. A nonfood use of lipolytic bacteria is to help clean up industrial oil spills. The bacteria digest the oil and change it into a form that is easily removed from the environment.

A few microbes thrive in salty environments. They are found in nature in salt deposits that result from the evaporation of seawater. Microbes that require high salt concentrations to function are called *halophilic.*

Uses for Sugar- and Starch-Digesting Microbes

Enzymes Produced	Microbial Sources	Uses
Amylases	Aspergillus Rhizopus Bacillus	Convert starch to sugar for baking, brewing, and syrup production
Cellulases	Aspergillus	Change cellulose to fermentable products Clarify fruit juices
Sucrases	Saccharomyces Streptomyces Aspergillus Penicillium	Convert maltose to glucose in brewing Convert glucose to fructose in corn syrup Convert glucose to gluconic acid in liquid eggs
Invertases	S. cerevisiae Candida utilis	Convert sucrose to glucose and fructose Prevent crystallization in soft-centered candies Aid in production of artificial honey
Pectinases	Aspergillus Rhizopus	Clarify wine and fruit juice Release juice from fruit for increased yields Remove pectin for the production of concentrated fruit juices

17-6 Microbes that produce carbohydrate-digesting enzymes are used for a variety of food processing functions.

Such microbes are used in Asia to make several fish- and soybean-based products, including Chinese cheese and bean cake.

Bacteria have varying tolerances for salt. The addition of salt to cabbage helps slow the growth of spoilage bacteria, which have a low tolerance to salt. The bacteria that develop the characteristic flavor and texture of sauerkraut tolerate higher levels of salt.

Scientific Names for Microbes

Microbes are classified by two Latin names. The first is the name of their genus. A *genus* is a group of living organisms that have similar characteristics. You could say that the genus is a family name like your last name. The name of the genus is always capitalized.

The second Latin name used to classify microbes is the name of the species. *Species* is the basic category of the classification of living organisms. It identifies the type of microbe within the family and is never capitalized.

An example of a microbe name is *Lactobacillus acidophilus.* This is the name of a bacterium used in the processing of fruits, vegetables, meats, and dairy products. *Lacto-* refers to milk. It is the same root used in the term *lactose,* which is milk sugar. The *-bacillus* ending on the first name indicates the bacteria cells have a rod shape. The endings *-bacter, -monas,* and *-ella* also indicate rod-shaped bacteria. The *-coccus* ending is used if the genus of bacteria has a spherical shape. (None of the spiral-shaped bacteria are used in food production.) The species name *acidophilus* indicates the bacteria give off an acid. Therefore, the name *Lactobacillus acidophilus* tells you this bacterium probably lives in or feeds on milk. From the name, you can also tell the bacterium has a rod shape and produces an acid.

Scientists often abbreviate these long Latin names when referring to particular microbes. Scientists typically use only the initial of the genus name. For example, *Lactobacillus acidophilus* is shortened to *L. acidophilus.* In this book, the first time a bacterium is discussed, the full name will be written. After that, the name will be abbreviated.

Factors Affecting Microbe Growth

A number of factors are known to affect the growth of microbes. These are food supply, water availability, pH, and temperature. However, the specific conditions that best support growth differ for each type of microbe. Each microbe has a preferred range within each factor. Therefore, there is no one set of guidelines that can be followed for every bacterium, mold, and yeast.

Food Supply

Microbes are composed of complex molecules made from carbon, oxygen, nitrogen, and hydrogen. Therefore, microbes need a food supply that provides these four chemical building blocks. Most microbes use organic compounds (carbohydrates, lipids, or proteins) as a main source for these chemicals.

Some microbes need protein for their food supply. Other microbes need lipids, and others need starches. Some microbes can feed off several types of macromolecules. The food supply needed by a microbe depends on the enzyme systems the organism can make. If a bacterium can only produce proteolytic enzymes, then it will only be able to digest proteins. A proteolytic bacterium could be surrounded by sugar and never reproduce. This is not because there is no source of energy. It is because the energy is in a form the bacterium cannot use.

Microbes need small amounts of minerals to enhance enzyme activity. Microbes need vitamins, too. Many vitamins act as coenzymes. Therefore, a microbe's need for vitamins varies according to the enzyme reactions the microbe performs. The microbe must absorb directly from its food supply any vitamin it cannot produce.

Water

Like all living organisms, microbes need water to function. Some microbes are able to remain alive in a dried condition. These microbes survive but cannot grow or reproduce

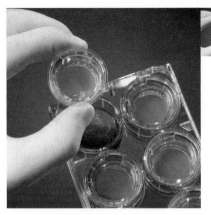

Recent Research
Bacteria Turns Pollution into Protein

Microbiologists have found a group of bacteria called *carboxydobacteria*. These bacteria use carbon monoxide from automobile exhaust as their energy source. They reproduce rapidly in an environment of 50% air and 50% exhaust. The bacteria cells contain 65% crude protein. There are about 350 million cars in the world. Experts estimate these bacteria could produce 500,000 tons of protein per year from all the exhaust.

In the future, scientists could develop a method for producing this protein from carboxydobacteria. Then they can mass-produce carboxydobacteria to turn poisonous car exhaust into nutritious protein. Food scientists may have a new source of protein to use in producing tasty foods.

without water. On the other hand, microbes cannot grow in pure water. This is because pure water does not provide many of the nutrients microbes need. Each microorganism has a range of water content that it prefers. Generally, bacteria need more water than yeasts, and yeasts need more water than molds for growth.

Food scientists measure water needs in terms of water activity, a_w. (See Chapter 7.) Pure water has an a_w of 1.0. A saturated salt solution has an a_w of 0.75. See 17-7.

Determining water needs of microbes can be difficult. This is because factors such as temperature and pH also impact whether a microbe will grow. Freezing temperatures make water unavailable to microbes. High water temperatures can kill microbes. For example, yeast dies when the water used in bread dough is too hot. The pH level also affects which type of microbe can grow at a given a_w level. For example, the a_w of most fruits is around 0.97. Bacteria should multiply rapidly in such an environment. However, the reason bacteria do not spoil many fruits has to do with the fruits' acidic pH. The low pH kills bacteria. This allows molds that usually prefer a lower a_w to grow.

Preferred a_w Ranges for Microbes	
Microbe	**Preferred a_w**
Bacteria	0.83–0.96
most spoilage bacteria	0.90–0.91
Most yeasts	0.87–0.94
Most molds	0.70–0.80

17-7 Like all living things, microbes need a certain amount of water to grow and reproduce.

A safe a_w for most food storage is considered to be 0.70 or lower. There are three main ways to lower water activity level. These are removing water, adding solutes to the solution, and freezing. Removing water from the environment causes microbes to dehydrate. Adding solutes, such as sugar or salt, creates an imbalance that pulls water out of the microbe cells. Freezing locks water molecules into a crystalline structure and limits access to the water.

pH

Each type of microbe has a different preferred pH range. Many fruits have a pH of less than 4. Most bacteria are killed if the pH is below 4.6. Molds, on the other hand, can survive with a pH as low as 1.5. This explains why molds are more likely than bacteria to spoil fruits. However, as molds grow on fruit, they release substances that can cause the pH of the fruit to rise. The pH of the fruit can become high enough for bacteria to begin to grow. This is especially true of bacteria that give off lactic or acetic acid. These bacteria will usually tolerate a lower pH than proteolytic bacteria, which produce ammonia. See 17-8.

Temperature

The last factor that affects microbe growth is temperature. You have already studied how freezing can slow enzyme activity and cell reproduction. Extreme cold generally does not kill microbes. It slows them down or causes them to enter a dormant or resting state. On the other hand, heating can kill microbes. The temperatures that support microbe growth are between the freezing and boiling points of water. The temperature at which microorganisms die is usually 5°C to 12°C (9°F to 22°F) above the temperature at which maximum growth occurs.

Food processors often use high temperatures to kill harmful microbes. Processors must think about how heating foods will affect quality and production costs as well as microbes. For example, *pasteurization* is a process in which a liquid is heated until pathogens and some spoilage bacteria have been destroyed. This process is used to help prevent disease that can be caused by harmful bacteria. It also helps lengthen the shelf life of milk. However, it can affect the flavor of milk. At a low pasteurization temperature of 63°C (145°F), it takes 30 minutes to kill the bacteria. This affects milk flavor to a more noticeable degree. Using a high pasteurization temperature of 72°C (161°F) for 15 seconds reduces the damage to the milk flavor. See 17-9.

Food scientists can successfully grow cultures of microbes for use in food processing. A culture can be a specific microbe or a mixture of select microbes. To produce the desired culture, scientists must create the right growing conditions. They need to know the microbe's preferred food supply, water activity level, pH, and temperature. Trained technicians are needed to keep track of these factors at each step in the growth process.

Ideal conditions for growing microbes are created in large vats or tanks. Producers mix the necessary food supply with a small amount of the desired microbe. The vats holding the food-microbe mix are kept within the

pH Ranges for Microbe Growth

Microbe	Minimum	Preferred	Maximum
Bacteria (most)	2.9–6.0	6.5–7.5	8.0–10.0
Yeasts	1.5–3.5	4.0–6.5	8.0–8.5
Molds	1.5–3.5	4.0–6.8	8.5–10.5

17-8 The pH level of a food product affects what types of microbes can live in the product.

Pasteurization Times and Temperatures

Process	Temperature	Time
Vat processing	67.2°C (153.0°F)	30 min.
High temperature-short time pasteurization	71.7°C (161.1°F)	15 sec.
Ultrapasteurization	138.0°C (280.4°F)	2 sec.

17-9 By increasing pasteurization temperatures, food processors can reduce the amount of time a product must be exposed to heat.

preferred temperature and pH levels to maximize microbe growth. The cultures are then shipped to manufacturers for use in various food products.

Fermentation

Food manufacturers often add microbes to foods to bring about fermentation. *Fermentation* is an enzymatically controlled change in a food product brought on by the action of microorganisms. Some desired changes in food products occur as microbes release digestive enzymes. These enzymes break down components in the food product. Other changes are caused by the release of by-products. A *by-product* is a substance that is produced in addition to the main product of a reaction. The primary product of a microbial reaction is energy. In producing energy, microbes also produce by-products such as carbon dioxide, acetic and lactic acids, and ethanol. Such by-products can change the color, texture, flavor, aroma, and pH of a food.

Fermentation is an anaerobic process. It relies on microorganisms that use organic compounds for their food supply. These microbes release enzymes to break down proteins, carbohydrates, and lipids that are nearby. After the enzymes break down these large molecules, the microbes absorb the smaller molecules through their cell walls. The microbes use these nutrients for growth and energy. Fermentation is the part of the process in which the nutrients are converted to energy.

Glucose is the energy source for most living organisms. It is converted into two *pyruvate* molecules. The next step is where fermentation occurs. Pyruvate is broken down into either an acid or alcohol and carbon dioxide. Many organisms can also break protein and lipids down into pyruvate for energy. Energy is released as by-products are formed from pyruvate.

Fermentation varies in terms of the by-products that are created. Microbes are grouped as to the by-products they give off as a result of fermentation. You will study the fermentation process, the types of by-products, and foods produced by yeasts, bacteria, and molds.

Yeast Fermentation

Foods fermented by yeast have been used since the dawn of recorded history. Babylonians used yeast to make beer as early as 6000 B.C. Egyptian tomb reliefs show the apparent commercial production of leavened bread, wine, and beer around 2400 B.C.

All yeast breads, alcoholic beverages, and vinegar require yeast in the production process. The most commonly used yeast is *Saccharomyces cerevisiae*. *S. cerevisiae* grows best in a warm, moist environment where sugars and/or starches are available. See 17-10. It is the main yeast in brewer's yeast and is also used for breads.

Saccharomyces means sugar fungus. The *S. cerevisiae* family of yeasts relies on sugar as its main energy source. It can also feed on honey (high in fructose), molasses, or corn syrup. However, high levels of sugar in bread dough will slow yeast growth. This is because high sugar levels lower the a_w. When the a_w drops too low, microbes cannot reproduce.

Although some types of yeast can hydrolyze starch, *S. cerevisiae* cannot. Some breads, such as Italian and French breads, do not contain an added sweetener. Therefore, these breads rely on added enzymes or amylases naturally found in the flour to break down the starch.

Some breads are prepared with quick-rising yeast. This is a commercially produced hybrid product made from two yeast strains.

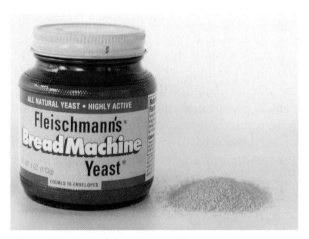

17-10 Yeast used for breads (*Saccharomyces cerevisiae)* is dehydrated and then packaged in cakes, packets, or jars.

The result is a yeast that releases both amylases and sucrases. This speeds the production of carbon dioxide as a by-product.

Before the commercial production of yeast, starters were the main source of yeast for baking. A yeast starter is a mixture of equal parts of flour and water that has natural yeast growing in it. Natural yeast is present in the air in small amounts. This yeast would settle onto the flour and water mixture. The yeast would use the mixture as a food source to grow and multiply. Bakers learned that adding the mixture to bread dough created a light, airy product when baked. The bakers discovered how to add some of the starter to the bread and save some for later. The saved portion would have equal amounts of flour and water added. It would be stirred and covered daily until the yeast had multiplied and it was time to bake bread again.

Cooking Tip

You can make a yeast starter by combining 250 mL (1 cup) water, 250 mL (1 cup) flour, and 1 package of yeast. The container used to store the starter should be no more than half full. This allows room for the starter to expand as the yeast feeds on the flour.

Bread

Yeast fermentation changes heavy, dense yeast dough into light, porous bread. Yeast is affected by several important steps in the bread-making process. The first step is mixing. Most yeast bread recipes call for warming liquids, which activates the yeast. Mixing the flour, liquid, and other ingredients distributes the yeast evenly throughout the dough. The dough is kneaded, or worked with the hands, to develop gluten. Gluten is an elastic protein substance formed when flour is combined with liquid and manipulated.

The second step in the bread-making process that affects yeast is proofing. *Proofing* means allowing the dough to sit in a warm environment. During the proofing time, the yeast releases enzymes so it can feed, grow, and multiply. These enzymes break down sugars in the dough, releasing alcohol (ethanol) and carbon dioxide as by-products. The carbon dioxide becomes trapped in small pockets throughout the dense dough. The pressure of the increasing volume of this trapped gas causes the gluten to stretch. This is what makes the dough rise.

Baking is the final step in bread making that affects yeast. During baking, the alcohol produced during proofing quickly evaporates and the yeast cells are killed. The remains of the yeast stay in the dough, providing some flavor and nutritional value. The yeast bread will continue to rise in the oven until a crust forms and the protein structure is set. This is because the carbon dioxide expands as it is heated. The result is a moist, light product.

If guidelines are not followed when making bread, the product may be unsatisfactory. For instance, yeast is killed by relatively low temperatures. The ideal temperature for yeast fermentation is 30°C to 35°C (86°F to 95°F). If the *S. cerevisiae* is hotter than 40°C (104°F), it will begin to die. If the yeast is killed before the dough is proofed, the bread will be heavy and flat. Bread recipes recommend heating the liquids to 41°C to 46°C (105°F to 115°F). This is because the addition of yeast cools the mixture to the ideal fermentation temperature range.

Two things happen if the dough is proofed too long. Keep in mind that the longer the dough sets, the more by-products are produced. When too much carbon dioxide is produced, the dough will be stretched too far. This will cause it either to collapse or develop a coarse, dry texture during baking. When too much alcohol is produced, the bread will have an undesirable flavor.

All bread products have the following ingredients in common: flour, yeast, salt, and water. Additional ingredients that are often used in yeast breads are eggs, milk, sugar, honey, molasses, spices, and seeds. These ingredients change the flavor, nutritive value, and/or texture of the finished bread.

Wine

Wine is the fermented juice of plant products. Honey, dandelions, and various fruits are used to produce wine. However, classical wines are made from fermented grape juice.

The quality of wine depends partly on which microbes are present. Therefore, many wine makers treat the crushed grapes to kill all wild yeasts, bacteria, and fungi that may be present. Sulfur dioxide (SO_2) or potassium metabisulfite is added to inhibit the growth of unwanted organisms. These sulfites also stabilize the wine color. The crushed grapes then have commercially produced yeasts (*S. cerevisiae* and *S. ellipsoideus*) added.

The yeast feeds on sugars naturally found in the fruit juice, releasing alcohol and carbon dioxide as by-products. The fermentation requires anaerobic conditions for one to four weeks. The fermenting juices are held in small oak barrels or large stainless steel tanks, 17-11. The fermentation process is complete when bubbling from carbon dioxide production stops. The wine is then put in barrels or vats for aging. Chemical interactions within the new wine slowly develop the characteristic flavors.

The original sweetness of wine is determined by the degree of fermentation and sugar content of the fruit. In sweeter wines, the fermentation process is stopped before the yeast breaks down all the sugar. These wines have an alcohol content of 8% to 9%. Less sweet, or dry, wines are allowed to ferment until the yeast has broken down all the sugar.

These wines contain 12% to 14% alcohol. However, the sweetness and alcohol content of finished wines is sometimes adjusted by the addition of unfermented juice, sugar, and/or alcohol.

During wine production, the carbon dioxide produced as a by-product may be allowed to escape. It may also be collected, compressed, and sold for commercial uses. Sparkling wines, such as champagne, are made by retaining some of the carbon dioxide as a gas solute.

Other Alcoholic Beverages

In processes similar to wine making, yeast is used in the fermentation of other alcoholic beverages. The flavors and names of these beverages are determined by the food source used to feed the yeast. Beers are usually made from fermented, *malted* (germinated) barley. Sake is a Japanese beverage made from fermented rice.

After the fermenting process, whiskey is made by distilling the fermented mixture to concentrate the flavor and alcohol content. Irish whiskey is made from a variety of grains. Scotch whiskey is made mainly from barley.

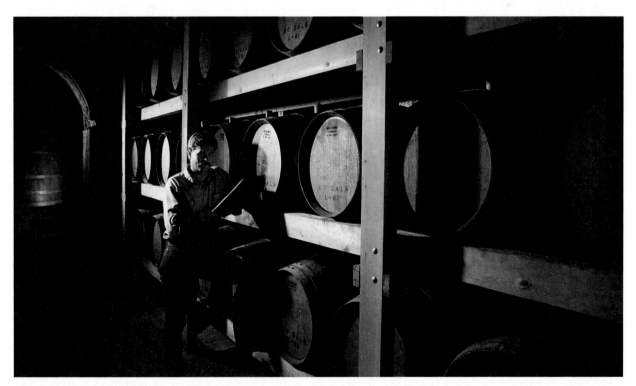

17-11 Oak barrels are used to give a characteristic flavor to wine as it ferments.

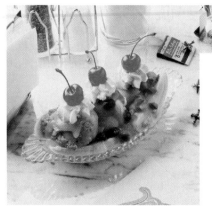

Item of Interest
The Color Is in the Skin

The amount of contact grape juice has with the grape skins determines the color and flavor of wine. If the skins are removed one to two days after fermentation begins, the wine will be a rosé wine. This is a wine with a pink color. If the skins stay in the fermentation tanks for 5 to 10 days, the wine will be red. White grapes produce white wine.

However, red grapes can also be turned into white wine. This requires the skins to be removed before adding the yeast. Notice the next time you eat a red grape that only the skin has color.

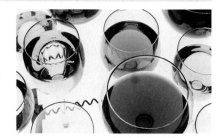

Wine gets its color from the skins of the grapes used to make it.

Bourbon is a whiskey that originated in Kentucky. It is made from corn.

Fermented ingredients are distilled to make a number of other alcoholic beverages. Rum is made from sugar cane or molasses. Brandy is distilled wine or fermented fruit juice. Liqueurs and cordials usually have a brandy base with sugar and flavorings added. Popular liqueurs are *crème de menthe*, which is flavored with mint and *curaçao*, which is made from bitter oranges.

Bacterial Fermentation

Foods are fermented by microbes other than yeast. A number of types of bacteria are used to ferment food products. There are three main classes of bacterial fermentation. These are lactic acid, proteolytic, and acetic acid fermentation. Some foods require two separate fermenting agents.

Bacterial fermentation often causes texture changes and a unique sour flavor in foods. For instance, the thick texture and sour flavor of yogurt result when bacteria ferment milk. The sour taste is caused by acids that are released

as by-products. The acids also act as preserving agents.

Lactic Acid Fermentation

Many of the foods produced through bacterial fermentation are fermented by bacteria whose major by-product is lactic acid. Some lactic acid bacteria also produce other by-products. These include acetic acid, formic acid, and carbon dioxide. Lactic acid bacteria are found in the genera (plural of genus) of *Streptococcus, Pediococcus, Leuconostoc,* and *Lactobacillus.* Lactic acid bacteria are used to ferment vegetables, meats, and dairy products. See 17-12.

Sauerkraut

Sauerkraut means acid cabbage. Sauerkraut is the result of lactic acid fermentation of cabbage submerged in a vat of brine. **Brine** is a mixture of salt and water. In this case, a 2% to 3% salt solution is used. The salt helps discourage the growth of unwanted bacteria and fungi by controlling water activity level. The salt also pulls water with dissolved

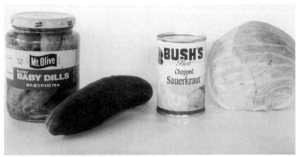

17-12 Lactic acid fermentation changes cucumbers into pickles and cabbage into sauerkraut.

sugar and nutrients to the surface of the cabbage. This provides the water and food source needed for the bacteria to grow. If there is too little salt, the sauerkraut will be soft with a poor flavor. If there is too much salt, the lactic acid bacteria are slowed. The sauerkraut will be darkened, and yeast may begin to grow.

Three types of lactic acid bacteria that prefer the slightly salty environment work in succession over a three-week period. The bacteria feed on the sugar present in the cabbage. The cabbage is shredded to expose more surface area on which the bacteria can feed. The bacteria release mainly carbon dioxide and lactic acid into the brine. The result is a creamy white, shredded product with a soft but firm texture.

Air must be kept from the fermentation process to control the growth of yeasts and molds. The cabbage is weighted down below the surface of the brine. Sheets of plastic are laid over the vat to keep out dirt and air. This creates the necessary salty, anaerobic environment needed to make sauerkraut.

Pickles

Cucumbers can be turned into pickles by three basic methods. They may be heated in a spiced vinegar solution. They can be refrigerated in an acid brine. However, the oldest method is by fermentation with lactic acid bacteria. These processes are used to pickle foods other than cucumbers. Such foods include watermelon rinds, beets, cauliflower, okra, and onions.

When cucumbers are pickled, they are packed in a salt brine for the same reasons as cabbage. It is important that all carbohydrates used during the pickling process be fermentable. This is because bacteria, molds, and yeasts are found on cucumbers. If extra salt is not added during fermentation and simple carbohydrates remain, yeasts can begin to multiply. The yeast can feed off the lactic acid produced by the bacteria. This raises the pH and allows spoilage bacteria to contaminate the pickles.

Commercial pickling starts by washing the cucumbers in a chlorine solution. This removes unwanted yeasts and molds. If these microorganisms are not removed, they can cause softening and bloating. (Bloating is the formation of a large air pocket in the center of the pickle.)

After the cucumbers are washed, they are placed in brine and a pure culture of *Lactobacillus* is added. The bacteria feed on natural sugars from the cucumbers and release lactic acid into the brine. This lowers the pH and gives pickles their crisp texture and sour taste.

Some picklers choose to make pickles by a natural process. For this process, cucumbers are placed in a brine of the same salt concentration used in the commercial process. Then salt is gradually added to the brine during the fermentation period. The salt level is more than doubled by the end of the process. The additional salt is not needed in the commercial process. This is because the chlorine washing process has already removed the undesirable microbes the salt is used to control.

The commercial process has two advantages. First, it requires less salt, which is important for low-salt diets. Second, it helps picklers meet Environmental Protection Agency (EPA) standards regarding the dumping of brine into streams.

Olives

Olives are fermented by the same types of lactic acid bacteria as cucumbers. However, fermenting olives calls for an added preparation step that is not required in making pickles. Olives are washed in a lye solution to remove bitter flavor compounds. The lye can remove needed microbes, and rinsing removes nutrients as well as the lye. To overcome these problems, lactic acid is added to neutralize any lye remaining after the olives are rinsed. This reduces the amount of washing needed.

Sugar is added, and lactic acid bacteria start the fermentation process.

Fermenting olives also requires a higher salt concentration than making pickles. The salt solution in which olives are fermented needs to be kept between 5% and 15%. This range is ideal for lactic acid bacteria to grow and multiply but is too salty for most spoilage bacteria. As the olives ferment, sugar is pulled out of the olives and salt is pulled into them. This lowers the salt concentration of the brine. Salt must be added anytime the brine drops below the 5% level. Fermentation of olives can take two weeks to several months.

Green or Spanish olives are picked when they have reached full size but before they have ripened. They are then cured and often pitted and stuffed, most commonly with pimento. Black or ripe olives are picked at a riper stage. They have a deep green color when picked. The lye curing process and oxygenation turns them black. Olives that are tree ripened have a dark brown to black color. Most tree-ripened olives are pressed for their oil.

Meats

Meats are fermented with lactic acid bacteria to make semidry and dry sausages. The fermentation process increases the acid level. This tenderizes the meat and adds a tart flavor. Fermentation, along with smoking and drying, lowers the a_w level to prevent spoilage.

Fermented sausages are made by mixing chopped meat with sugar, spices, and salt. The sugar provides food for the lactic acid bacteria. The spices and salt add desired flavor. Sodium nitrate, sodium nitrite, or a combination of these is mixed into the meat. These additives prevent the growth of spoilage bacteria. Lactic acid bacteria are added to ensure proper color and flavor of the sausage.

Cultured Dairy Products

Cultured dairy products include sour cream, yogurt, and buttermilk, 17-13. These products are made with the help of lactic acid bacteria. The strains of bacteria used vary depending on the desired end product. Several kinds of *Streptococci* are used because they are the fastest lactic acid producers. They enable the milk base to acidify quickly. This reduces preparation time and the risk of

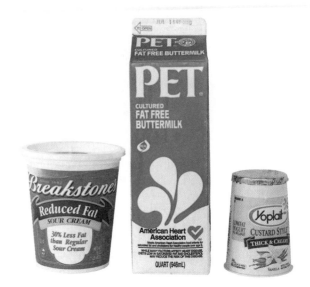

17-13 Cultured dairy products are fermented with bacteria that feed on lactose.

contamination. *Leuconostoc* and *Lactobacilli* strains are added to produce the desired flavors.

Fresh milk contains microorganisms that would cause it to spoil. Therefore, milk being used for cultured dairy products is pasteurized. Pasteurization ensures that unwanted microbes are destroyed. This helps produce a consistent, high-quality product.

After pasteurization, starter cultures of bacteria are added to the milk. The bacteria feed off the lactose in the milk. They release carbon dioxide, lactic acid, and a number of flavor compounds. The acid denatures the proteins and causes them to coagulate. The degree of coagulation is determined by the combination of bacteria. Temperature, pH, fermentation time, and added enzymes also affect the texture of the product.

Most cultured dairy products are made by similar processes. The products are heated, cooled, mixed with a culture, and fermented. The fermentation process is stopped by cooling. The products are then ready for packaging.

Cultured dairy products are often suggested for people with lactose intolerance. This is because the bacteria use the lactose as their energy supply. The result is low-lactose products that are easier to digest.

People with lactose intolerance can also use lactose-free milk products. These products are made by adding *L. acidophilus.* The

L. acidophilus releases an enzyme that breaks lactose down into glucose and galactose. The products that result are sweeter than milk because glucose tastes sweeter than lactose. People with lactose intolerance can add commercially produced lactase drops or tablets to dairy products, too.

> ### Health Tip
> **Antibiotics will often destroy helpful microbes in the intestines as well as disease-causing bacteria. Eating yogurt that contains "active cultures" can help replenish intestinal microbes after the use of antibiotics.**

Cheeses

Like making cultured dairy products, making cheese starts with pasteurizing the milk. The proteolytic enzyme rennin and a culture of lactic acid bacteria are then added to help form the curds. *Curds* are clumps of coagulated protein. In this case, the protein is casein. The lactic acid bacteria lower the pH so the proteolytic enzymes in rennin will coagulate the casein more effectively.

The curds are cut into small cubes. The mixture is then heated to 38°C to 40°C (100°F to 104°F) for about 45 minutes. The cutting and cooking process helps the whey separate from the curds. *Whey* is a liquid high in soluble whey proteins. The whey is drained off and collected to be used as an additive in processed foods such as baked goods, mixes, and margarine. The curds are then salted to add flavor and reduce the risk of spoilage.

At this point, the cheese making process varies according to the type of cheese being made. Curds being used to make cottage cheese are mixed with cream that has had cultured skim milk added. Curds for aged cheeses, such as Cheddar, Edam, Swiss, brick, and blue, are put in presses. The presses squeeze out excess moisture.

Most cheeses need a ripening period. Bacteria remaining in the curds will ripen some cheeses. For other cheeses, microorganisms such as mold are added to the salted curds to do the ripening. During ripening, the cheeses are wrapped or covered with wax and placed in curing rooms. The curing rooms have controlled humidity and temperature levels. These conditions are designed to match the growth needs of the microorganisms doing the ripening.

Specific types of fermenting bacteria and/or molds are used to give each type of cheese its characteristic flavor. Propionic acid bacteria are added to Swiss cheese. These bacteria develop the carbon dioxide that forms the characteristic eyes, or holes, in Swiss cheese, 17-14. Molds are used to make cheeses such as Limburger and blue cheeses. Limburger uses a mold at the beginning of the ripening process. This mold lowers the acidity so proteolytic bacteria can develop the cheese's characteristic flavor, texture, and aroma. Blue cheeses, such as Roquefort, have a blue-green mold added. This mold needs oxygen to grow. Therefore, the surfaces of blue cheeses are pierced with needles to allow oxygen to reach the mold within the cheese.

The *sharpness* of cheese refers to the strength of its flavor and aroma. Sharpness is caused by acids and a variety of aroma compounds. These compounds are formed as bacteria and enzymes in cheese continue to ferment lactose and other organic compounds during a curing process. Therefore, the sharpness of cheese depends on the length of time the cheese is cured. For instance, mild Cheddar cheese is cured for four months. Sharp Cheddar is cured for about a year. Extra sharp Cheddar is cured for up to two years. Tasting samples of mild, sharp, and extra sharp Cheddar cheese will illustrate

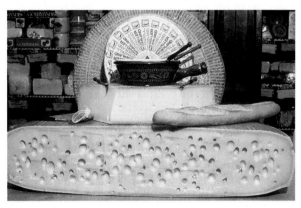

USDA

17-14 The holes in Swiss cheese are a result of propionic acid fermentation.

these flavor differences. You will also note texture differences. Cheeses that are cured longer tend to have firmer textures, are more crumbly, and melt into sauces more readily.

Mold Fermentation

Some fermented foods are produced by the action of molds. Molds create a wide range of by-products. These by-products include antibiotics, flavor compounds, and enzymes.

Soy Sauce

Soy sauce, an important flavoring ingredient in Asian cooking, is a fermented mix of soybeans and wheat. The fermenting agent is a mixture of cooked rice and several strains of mold from the *Aspergillus* family. When added to the soy-wheat mixture, the molds produce enzymes. These enzymes hydrolyze the proteins and carbohydrates in the soybeans and wheat. Once mold covers the soy-wheat mixture, a brine is added. The brine stops the growth of unwanted microbes. Lactic acid bacteria can then multiply, causing the pH of the mixture to drop. Toward the end of the fermentation period, yeasts are added. They ferment the sugars remaining from the hydrolysis of the carbohydrates. The fermented mixture is filtered, pasteurized, and bottled.

Tempeh

Another soy product produced through mold fermentation is tempeh. *Tempeh* is an Asian soybean cake. The soybeans are cooked, mashed, and formed into cakes. The cakes are inoculated with *Rhizopus* molds. The cakes are then wrapped in banana leaves and fermented for one to two days.

Two-Step Fermentation

Many fermented foods are made with two or more fermentation steps. Each step may require a different kind of microbes. Some two-step fermentation processes involve lactic acid bacteria plus other microbes. Acetic acid fermentation is an example of a two-step process. It requires yeast as well as bacteria.

Lactic Acid Plus Other Microbes

Two-step fermentation often involves lactic acid bacteria in one step and other microbes in a second step. The aged cheeses you read about earlier are examples of this type of fermentation. Lactic acid fermentation is used to make the cheese. Then other microbes are used to develop the characteristic flavors and textures.

Sourdough bread is another example of a food product made with a two-step fermentation process involving lactic acid bacteria. The first step of the process requires lactic acid bacteria to ferment the yeast starter. This step is what gives sourdough bread its characteristic sour flavor. See 17-15. The second step of the process is the same yeast fermentation used to make other yeast breads.

The strain of bacteria used in sourdough starter is *Lactobacillus sanfrancisco*. This bacterium is *indigenous*, or native, to the San Francisco bay area. During the Alaskan gold rush, many prospectors would keep jars of yeast starter in their parkas. This would keep the starter warm. The prospectors would use part of the starter to make bread, biscuits, or pancakes. Then the prospectors would add more flour and water to feed the base starter for the next day. Many of these prospectors would sail from San Francisco or return to the bay area for the winter. The bacteria would get into their starter when they were in San Francisco.

Acetic Acid Fermentation

The first step of acetic acid fermentation is yeast fermentation. Yeasts are added to a food product under anaerobic conditions. The yeasts use sugars in the food product for their

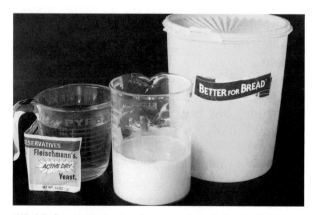

17-15 A yeast starter for sourdough is a mixture of equal amounts of flour and warm water with a package of yeast.

food supply. The yeasts release alcohol as a by-product as they break down the sugars. After the yeast fermentation is complete, the second step of acetic acid fermentation can begin.

For the second step, *Acetobacter* bacteria are added to the food product. These bacteria are aerobic. They use the alcohol produced by the yeast as their food supply. They release acetic acid as a by-product as they break down the alcohol. The chemical changes caused by *Acetobacter* are shown by the following chemical formula:

$$C_2H_5OH + O_2 \xrightarrow[\text{bacteria}]{\text{acetic acid}} CH_3COOH + H_2O$$

$\quad$ alcohol $\quad$ oxygen $\qquad\qquad$ acetic acid $\quad$ water

Vinegar is one of the foods produced as a result of acetic acid fermentation. Acetic acid is what gives vinegar its sour taste. Acetic acid bacteria will produce different types of vinegar depending on the food on which it feeds. When acetic acid bacteria are present in red wine, red wine vinegar is produced. A mixture of water and wheat will produce white vinegar. Apple juice with acetic acid bacteria will yield apple cider vinegar. The FDA requires that vinegar contain at least 4 mL of acetic acid per 100 mL of water. This means vinegar is a 4% solution.

Other foods that require acetic acid fermentation are cacao beans and candied citron. This two-step process helps turn cacao beans into chocolate. Candied citron is a fermented product of citron lemons used in baked goods such as fruitcake.

Benefits of Fermentation

Fermenting food products has a couple of key advantages. First, microbes help preserve some foods. Milk will keep for about a week in the refrigerator. Cheese can keep for

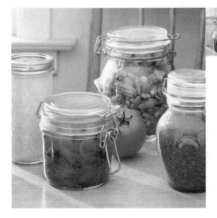

Historical Highlight
Louis Pasteur: One of the World's Greatest Scientists

During his lifetime, Louis Pasteur (1822-1895) made major contributions to science, medicine, and the food industry. His science contributions began with his work in chemistry with the structure of crystals. He then turned to studying microbes. He was the first to prove the theory of *spontaneous generation* was false. This theory stated that living things (microbes) could come from nonliving material, such as dirt.

Pasteur made several contributions in the areas of human and animal medicine. He helped prove that microorganisms are the source of infectious disease. He worked to prevent the death of silkworms. He also focused on the development of immunity to disease through vaccination. He developed vaccines to protect sheep from anthrax and chickens from cholera. He also developed the vaccine for rabies.

Pasteur made an impact on the food industry in his day. In 1857, he wrote in his journals that alcoholic fermentation was caused by yeast. He noted that lactic acid fermentation was caused by round organisms (now known as lactic acid bacteria). In 1861, he identified rod-shaped organisms as the source of butyric acid fermentation. He also noted these bacteria were anaerobic. In 1864, Pasteur began researching the cause of bitter flavors in wine. He found that microbes were the cause. He developed the pasteurization process to protect wine from these microbes. He applied this method to the preservation of milk and beer as well as wine.

months when properly stored. Cucumbers will spoil in a week or so in the refrigerator. Pickles will keep in unopened jars on the shelf for a year or more.

A second benefit of fermentation is variety. Fermented products have added a wider range of food options to diets around the world.

Nutritional Changes in Fermented Products

The nutritional value of fermented foods often differs from the value of their unfermented counterparts. The types of microbes added and the energy sources they consume affect the nutrient content. For instance, cheeses are higher in fat than milk. This is

because portions of the casein molecules that form the curds are attracted to fat. When the water-soluble whey is drained off, the fat concentration is increased. Calcium is also concentrated in cheese. One ounce of Cheddar or Monterey Jack cheese contains as much calcium as six ounces of milk. The iron in one cup of raw cabbage is 0.4 mg. One cup of sauerkraut contains 3.47 mg of iron.

Other ingredients added during processing also affect the nutritional quality of fermented foods. For instance, all pickles have more sodium than cucumbers. This is because of the salty brine used during fermentation. Soybeans contain 1 mg of sodium per cup. "Light" soy sauce contains as much as 530 mg of sodium per tablespoon. See 17-16.

What Microbes Do to Food Value

Food	Serving Size	Cal	Protein (g)	Carb (g)	Fat (g)	Sodium (mg)	Calcium (mg)	Iron (mg)	Vit A (RE)	Vit C (mg)
Cucumbers	15 slices	11	<1	3	<1	3	11	0.22	3	3
Pickle, dill	**1 med**	**12**	**<1**	**3**	**<1**	**833**	**6**	**0.34**	**21**	**1**
Grape juice	4 oz	78	<1	19	<1	4	11	0.31	1	<1
Red wine	**3.5 oz**	**74***	**<1**	**2**	**0**	**6**	**8**	**0.22**	**0**	**0**
Vinegar	**4 oz**	**8**	**0**	**4**	**0**	**60**	**4**	**0.36**	**0**	**0**
Soybeans	1/4 c.	75	7	4	<1	<1	43	2.21	<1	1
Soy sauce	**1/4 c.**	**36**	**4**	**8**	**<1**	**4116**	**12**	**1.44**	**0**	**0**
Miso	**1/4 c.**	**142**	**8**	**20**	**4**	**2516**	**46**	**1.89**	**6**	**0**
Cabbage	1 c.	16	1	4	<1	12	32	0.4	9	33
Sauerkraut	**1 c.**	**44**	**2**	**10**	**<1**	**1561**	**72**	**3.47**	**4**	**35**
Milk	1 c.	150	8	11	8	120	291	0.12	76	2
Yogurt	**1 c.**	**138**	**8**	**11**	**7**	**104**	**275**	**0.11**	**68**	**1**
Cottage Cheese	**1 c.**	**215**	**26**	**6**	**9**	**850**	**126**	**0.30**	**101**	**<1**
Cheddar Cheese	**1 c.**	**455**	**28**	**1**	**37**	**701**	**815**	**0.77**	**342**	**0**

*Alcohol provides 7 calories per gram.

17-16 The nutritional profile of a fermented food differs from its unfermented equivalent due to added ingredients and microbial activity.

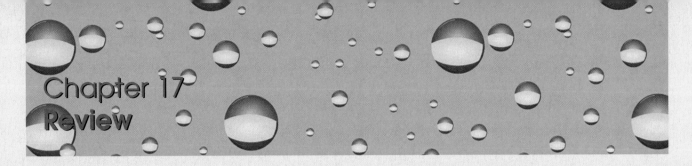

Chapter 17 Review

Summary

Microbes are used to produce a wide variety of foods. Three categories of microbes that have positive uses in foods are bacteria, yeasts, and molds. All three are organisms that grow and reproduce in foods. They change food by breaking down molecules in the food and creating waste called by-products.

Several factors affect the ability of microbes to grow and multiply. These factors include food supply, water, oxygen, pH, and temperature. Food scientists can recreate ideal conditions to successfully grow cultures of microbes. The microbes can then be mass-produced and sent to food processing plants.

Microbes change foods through fermentation. In fermentation, nutrients are converted to energy in an anaerobic process. Foods can be fermented by yeasts, bacteria, molds, or a combination of microbes working together. The final food product is affected by the initial food, the microbes, and fermenting or curing time. Fermentation requires careful monitoring to ensure a quality product.

Microbes play a major role in producing the foods you enjoy every day. However, you should also be aware of nutritional changes caused by fermentation. For instance, fat and sodium may be increased in the fermentation process.

Check Your Understanding

1. On what three characteristics are bacteria classified?
2. Describe the three shapes of bacteria and give the name for each.
3. What two types of fungi play key roles in food processing?
4. Why is it important to food producers that microbes can become dormant?
5. What is the function of microbial enzymes?
6. How do scientists determine what name a microbe should have?
7. Identify three ways to lower water activity level for food storage.
8. Explain how food products are changed by the process of fermentation.
9. How does quick rising yeast speed the production of bread?
10. Why is salt important in lactic acid fermentation?
11. What causes cultured dairy products to coagulate?
12. What microbe is used in the production of soy sauce?
13. Describe the two fermentation steps required to make vinegar.
14. Name two benefits of fermented foods.

Critical Thinking

1. Explain what has likely happened to a homemade loaf of yeast bread with a mis-shaped top crust and several large air pockets.
2. What type of microorganism is likely to first attack fresh pineapple chunks left in the refrigerator too long?
3. In what ways would you expect Swiss cheese to differ from aged Swiss?
4. Which grows faster in pure water—bacteria or yeast?

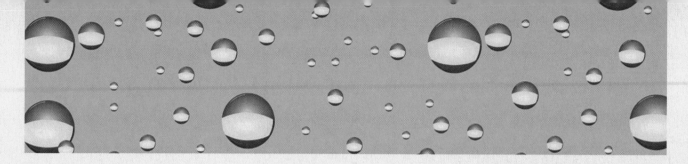

Explore Further

1. **Foods and Nutrition.** Make a salad dressing recipe with white, apple cider, and red wine vinegars. Prepare evaluation sheets to examine flavor and color differences. Serve dressing samples on iceberg lettuce to class members. Report the evaluation results to the class.

2. **Communication.** Via the Internet or by letter, contact a manufacturer of a fermented food product and request materials describing the production process. Share the information received with the class.

3. **Reading.** Research the history of an industry whose product(s) rely on fermentation. Report to the class the major scientific and technological developments that made the industry possible.

4. **Foods and Nutrition.** Study the process for making pickles, sauerkraut, or cheese. Develop a procedure for producing the fermented product and make one batch. Compare its flavor, texture, and color to that of a purchased product.

5. **Math.** Research the nutritional differences in four fermented foods and their original food sources. Create bar graphs to compare and contrast the nutritional differences. Report your findings to the class.

Experiment 17A
Factors Affecting Yeast Growth

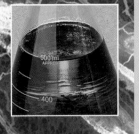

Purpose

Yeast provides the leavening for many bread products. With moisture, a food supply, and warm temperatures, yeast cells will grow and multiply. Yeast cells digest food and release two by-products: carbon dioxide and alcohol. The carbon dioxide is trapped in bread dough, creating a light, airy texture. The alcohol evaporates. In this experiment, you will determine whether salt and sugar enhance or inhibit the production of carbon dioxide by the yeast.

Equipment

wax pencil

4 16-ounce soft drink bottles or 4 250-mL Erlenmeyer flasks

100-mL graduated cylinder

metric measuring spoons

Supplies

400 mL warm tap water

4 packages yeast (11 mL or 2 ¼ teaspoons each)

15 mL flour

15 mL sugar

15 mL salt

4 balloons

Procedure

1. With a wax pencil, label four soft drink bottles or Erlenmeyer flasks as follows: *control, flour, sugar,* and *salt.*

2. Pour 100 mL of warm tap water into each container.

3. Add 1 package of yeast to each container.

4. Add 15 mL of flour, sugar, or salt to the appropriate containers.

5. Cover the top of each container with the mouth of a balloon.

6. Record you observations at 5 minute intervals for 20 minutes.

Questions

1. Which container had the greatest carbon dioxide production? How do you know?

2. Which container had the least carbon dioxide production?

3. What predictions can you make about rising times for yeast breads that contain sugar? What predictions can you make about rising times for yeast breads that contain high levels of salt? What predictions can you make about rising times for yeast breads that are sugar free?

Experiment 17B
Making Sourdough Starter

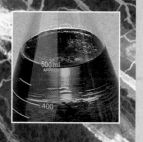

Purpose

Your ancestors did not have active dry yeast available at the local grocery store. Starters were the source of yeast. A starter is a flour and water mixture that contains yeast. When bread was made, part of the starter was set aside. The reserved starter would be "fed" to help the yeast multiply for the next day. Starters have been known to be kept alive and in use for hundreds of years. Over time, these starters would become contaminated with various types of bacteria. The bacteria would produce acidic by-products. These acids, combined with the alcohol released by the yeast, would give the breads a sour flavor. In this experiment, you will make a starter and observe changes as it ferments.

Equipment

1000-mL beaker

250-mL dry measure

large spoon or whisk

inoculating loop

microscope slide

clean linen towel

microscope

Supplies

250 mL (1 cup) tap water

250 mL (1 cup) flour

1 package active dry yeast (11 mL or 2 1/4 teaspoons)

Procedure

Day 1

1. Measure 250 mL (1 cup) of tap water in a 1000-mL beaker.

2. Add 250 mL (1 cup) of flour and 1 package of active dry yeast to the water in the beaker.

3. Use a large spoon or whisk to stir the mixture until smooth. Record observations of the starter's appearance and odor in a data table.

4. Use the inoculating loop to smear a small thin sample of the yeast onto the center of a microscope slide.

5. Cover the beaker with a clean linen towel and set aside until tomorrow.

6. Examine the slide with a microscope. Sketch what you see. Try to identify the flour and yeast cells. Look for yeast cells that are budding, or forming new cells.

7. If possible, stop by the classroom later in the day. Record observations regarding the starter's appearance and odor. Stir the starter and re-cover.

Day 2

1. Record your observations of the starter's appearance and odor in the data table.

2. Prepare another slide smear of the starter and examine under the microscope. Sketch what you see.

Questions

1. How did the appearance and odor of the starter change over a 24-hour period?

2. Were you able to distinguish the yeast cells from the flour cells?

3. Which slide had more budding yeast cells?

4. Why are starters that have been used for years safe to use in bread products?

5. How do starters become contaminated with bacteria?

Experiment 17B Extension
Comparing Traditional Pancakes to Sourdough Pancakes

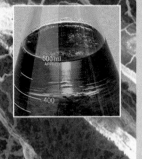

Purpose

Any change in ingredients can alter the flavor, texture, and appearance of a food product. In this experiment, you will conduct a sensory evaluation of sourdough pancakes and pancakes made with chemical leavening agents. Each lab group will prepare only one type of pancake. Then you will share pancakes with a group preparing the other variation. The sourdough starter made in experiment 17B will be used to make the sourdough pancakes. Note that both types of pancakes are made with equal amounts of flour and liquid. The proportions given result in thinner, almost crepelike pancakes that cook quickly. To make thicker, cakelike pancakes, increase the flour by 50 mL (¼ cup) in each recipe. Decide as a class on the thickness of the batter to use to avoid an extra variable.

Equipment

metric dry measuring cups
metric measuring spoons
large mixing bowl
whisk
medium mixing bowl
500-mL (2-cup) liquid measuring cup
6- to 10-inch nonstick skillet or griddle
pancake turner

Supplies
Traditional Pancakes

250 mL (1 cup) flour

10 mL (2 teaspoons) baking powder

2 mL (½ teaspoon) salt

15 mL (1 tablespoon) sugar

1 egg

30 mL (2 tablespoons) vegetable oil

250 mL (1 cup) milk

Sourdough Pancakes

1 batch sourdough starter

15 mL (1 tablespoon) sugar

2 mL (½ teaspoon) salt

1 mL (¼ teaspoon) baking powder

30 mL (2 tablespoons) vegetable oil

1 egg

1 mL (¼ teaspoon) baking soda dissolved in 5 mL (1 teaspoon) water

Procedure
Traditional Pancakes

1. Combine 250 mL (1 cup) flour, 10 mL (2 teaspoons) baking powder, 2 mL (½ teaspoon) salt, and 15 mL (1 tablespoon) sugar in a large mixing bowl.

2. Beat egg in a medium mixing bowl.

3. Add 30 mL (2 tablespoons) vegetable oil and 250 mL (1 cup) milk to the beaten egg.

4. Add the liquid ingredients to the dry ingredients all at once.

5. Stir until blended.

6. Pour approximately 50-mL (¼-cup) portions of batter onto a preheated skillet or griddle. (The skillet or griddle has reached an appropriate temperature when water drops dance and sizzle as they hit the hot surface.)

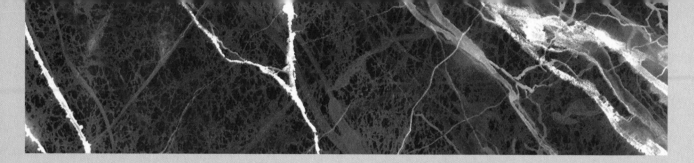

7. Cook pancakes until the top surfaces are bubbly and set around the edges.

8. Flip and cook until browned. (The pancakes will rise in the center and then flatten down slightly when finished cooking.) Do not push down on the pancakes with the pancake turner after flipping!

Sourdough Pancakes

1. Reserve 125 mL (½ cup) starter. Place the remaining starter in a large mixing bowl and add 15 mL (1 tablespoon) sugar, 2 mL (½ teaspoon) salt, 1 mL (¼ teaspoon) baking powder, and 30 mL (2 tablespoons) vegetable oil. Stir until combined.

2. Beat in an egg.

3. Gently fold in 1 mL (¼ teaspoon) baking soda dissolved in 5 mL (1 teaspoon) water.

4. Cook pancakes following steps 6 to 8 under the procedure for traditional pancakes.

5. Add 250 mL (1 cup) of flour and 250 mL (1 cup) of water to the 125 mL (½ cup) reserved starter. Place the starter in a covered plastic container and refrigerate for up to one week before using or "refeeding." (The container should have at least twice the volume of the starter)

Tasting

1. Each member of two lab groups should receive one of each type of pancake.

2. Conduct a sensory evaluation of each type of pancake. Evaluate color, appearance, and flavor. Record your observations in a data table.

Questions

1. How did the flavor of the two types of pancakes differ? Which type did you prefer?

2. How did the texture of the two types of pancakes differ? Which type did you prefer?

3. Which method of mixing pancakes is faster (disregard the time required to make the starter)?

4. For what types of products could a sourdough starter be used?

5. What types of changes would be needed in a standard recipe if it was to be made with sourdough?

Experiment 17C
Lactic Acid Bacteria and Yogurt

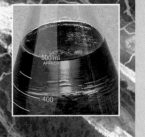

Purpose

To successfully make yogurt, several conditions must exist. Undesirable bacteria must be killed by heating the milk. Heating also denatures proteins and aids in forming the thick texture of yogurt. The milk must have living lactic acid bacteria added to it. Then the mixture is *incubated,* or held at warm temperatures until the yogurt is formed. In this experiment, you will use an active yogurt culture as a starter to *inoculate,* or add bacteria to the milk.

Equipment

1000-mL graduated cylinder

1000-mL beaker or 1-quart saucepan

thermometer

15-mL measuring spoon

glass rod or spoon

wax pencil

2 250-mL beakers

incubator

Supplies

400 mL (1²/₃ cups) milk

30 mL (2 tablespoons) unflavored yogurt with active cultures

30 mL (2 tablespoons) nonfat dry milk
   plastic wrap

Procedure

1. Measure 400 mL (1²/₃ cups) milk into a 1000-mL beaker or a 1-quart saucepan.

2. Heat the milk to 82°C (180°F) and hold it at that temperature for 15 minutes.

3. Cool the milk to 43°C (109°F).

4. Add 30 mL (2 tablespoons) of unflavored yogurt with active cultures to the cooled milk and stir until blended.

5. Use a wax pencil to label two 250-mL beakers with your group number. Label one of the beakers *milk added.*

6. Divide the yogurt mixture evenly into the two beakers.

7. Add 30 mL (2 tablespoons) nonfat dry milk to the beaker labeled *milk added.*

8. Cover both beakers with plastic wrap and place them in an incubator set at 40°C to 43°C (104°F to 109°F).

9. Leave the beakers in the incubator for at least 2 hours, or until the gel has set. (The yogurt may be kept in the incubator overnight if necessary.)

10. Remove the beakers from the incubator and place them in a refrigerator to chill thoroughly.

11. Compare the appearance, flavor, and texture of both yogurt samples. Record your observations in a data table.

Questions

1. Which yogurt sample has the firmer texture?

2. Was there a difference in flavor between the two samples?

3. What changes in nutrition will result from adding nonfat dry milk to yogurt?

4. What are the similarities between making yogurt with lactic acid bacteria and making sourdough with a yeast starter?

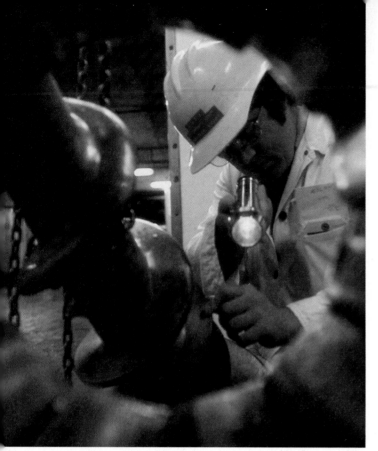

USDA

Making regular sanitation checks of food processing equipment is a critical step in preventing contamination.

Chapter 18

Food Safety: Sources of Contamination

Objectives

After studying this chapter, you will be able to

identify three main types of food contaminants.

differentiate among the types of foodborne illnesses.

name pathogens that cause foodborne illnesses.

describe the two main ways pathogens enter the food supply.

use food handling procedures that will help prevent the growth of illness-causing microbes.

list the seven steps in developing a HACCP system.

Key Terms

contamination
biodegradable
food spoilage
foodborne illness
pathogen
toxin
food intoxication
food infection
salmonellosis

parasite
host
trichinosis
virus
capsid
hepatitis
cross-contamination
HACCP (Hazard Analysis and Critical Control Point)

A toddler is hospitalized as a result of drinking contaminated apple juice. A preschooler dies because he eats a hamburger that is not thoroughly cooked. A cruise ship comes back to port early because many passengers have become ill with the same symptoms. A school cafeteria is unable to operate because half the staff is out with symptoms of vomiting, diarrhea, and fever. In each case, the illness or death was traced to something in the food supply.

Types of Food Contamination

The United States has the safest food supply in the world. Even with this record, some people get sick from eating food. Some experts estimate up to half of all cold and flu cases in this country may really be foodborne illnesses. People's lives depend on a reliable, safe food supply that is free from harmful contamination. *Contamination* is the state of being impure or unfit for use due to the introduction of unwholesome or undesirable elements. Food can be contaminated by insects, rodents, chemicals, microbes, or other foreign particles.

The addition of microbes is not necessarily bad. As you read in the last chapter, adding microbes to foods can result in many new food products. You could say that baked apples are contaminated if juice from a peach pie drips in from the rack above. Fortunately, the baked apples are still safe to eat unless you are allergic to peaches. However, the baked apples are no longer pure. They have been contaminated by, inoculated with, or mixed with peach juice. This has made them impure but not unfit or harmful.

In this chapter, you will study how and when harmful contamination occurs. You will find out what steps you can take to help prevent it. You will also read about the differences among contamination, spoilage, and foodborne illness.

Contamination occurs when something not normally found in the food is added. Contamination implies the addition is not intended or planned. The substance added may or may not cause problems. Three main sources of contamination are from physical, chemical, and microbial sources.

Physical Contaminants

Physical contaminants are substances that become part of a food mixture. They may not change or damage the food itself. However, their presence can create health hazards for the consumer. For instance, metal filings or broken pieces of glass have occasionally gotten into foods. These materials would not spoil food, but they could cause injury if swallowed. Other examples of physical contaminants

include packaging material, insects, and rodent droppings.

Insect and rodent contamination present two major problems. The first is the large volume of food that insects or rodents can eat and/or destroy. It is estimated that as much as 10% of the U.S. grain crop is destroyed annually by insects. The second concern is the microbes that may enter the food because of the insects or rodents. For example, flies pick up microbes on their hairy feet. When flies walk on food, microbes can transfer from the flies' feet to the food. Insects and rodents also damage the surfaces of foods such as fruits and vegetables. This creates openings that allow microbes to enter and multiply within the foods.

Insects and rodents can contaminate the food supply at any stage of growth or production. For example, some insects lay eggs in wheat while it is growing in fields, 18-1. These eggs are not visible, and their presence in small amounts is not harmful to human health. Keeping all insect eggs out of the wheat supply would be extremely expensive. On the other hand, cockroaches are likely to enter the wheat supply during the processing

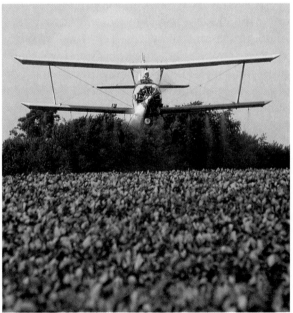

USDA

18-1 Aerial spraying of fields with pesticides protects crops from insect and some microbial types of damage.

stage. Their presence is less acceptable and can be affordably controlled by the food manufacturer.

The FDA examines food products for insect parts. FDA inspectors want to identify the types of insects present. To do this, the inspectors must be able to recognize insects from fragments, such as antennae. Inspectors also need to know about the habits of insects and the processes used to produce foods. This helps the inspectors determine the amount of contamination and the point at which the contamination occurred.

Chemical Contaminants

Keeping insects and other pests under control can lead to chemical contamination. *Insecticides* are chemicals used to improve crop yields by reducing losses due to insects. *Herbicides* are used for the same reasons to control weeds. Both types of substances are *pesticides*. If pesticide residues remain on food, they enter the food supply. The United States Department of Agriculture (USDA) monitors all pesticides. Any substance used on crops must undergo thorough testing to see how effective it is. Foods are examined for residues. Tests are conducted to determine whether residues pose a health hazard.

A second way chemical contaminants can enter the food supply is in water. Water is used in the processing of nearly every food product. Water is an excellent solvent. Therefore, many poisonous substances will dissolve in and pollute water supplies. The term *toxic* is used for substances that are harmful in low concentrations. Mercury, cadmium, lead, chloroform, benzene, and polychlorinatedbiphenyls (PCBs) are among the toxic substances that may get into water supplies.

Whether a substance is considered toxic or nutritious is often a matter of volume. Everyone needs very small amounts of zinc for good health. However, in high levels, zinc can lead to death. Too much of a good thing may not be a good thing!

City and industrial water supplies are often checked for toxic substances. However, there are no requirements for checking most private well water sources. Homeowners are advised to test well water routinely to protect their families from pollution.

Sources of Toxic Substances

Two main sources of toxins in water supplies are pesticides and industrial waste. The use of some pesticides has been banned because they are not *biodegradable.* This means that, in time, biological systems will break them down into chemical parts that nature can safely recycle. When pesticides do not break down, rain washes them into streams and rivers. They travel on to lakes and oceans. In time, they can build up to toxic levels in the flesh of fish.

Pollutants from industry can enter the water supply in a number of ways. Exhausts emitted into the air can be carried to the earth by rain. Wastes may be dumped directly into bodies of water. Groundwater can filter through buried dump sites and carry pollutants into the water supply. Frequent testing of factory waste products and water sources is needed to ensure the safety of the public.

One of the substances often dumped in industrial waste is mercury. In the mid 1970s, the FDA warned consumers to stop eating swordfish. The FDA was concerned about the high levels of mercury found in the flesh of the fish. Today, the tuna industry checks mercury levels as the tuna is packed. Standards are updated as research reveals new information regarding toxins and their hazards.

Another case of a surprising pollution source occurred in 1998 in Crescent, Oregon. The city water supply was contaminated when leaks formed in old, buried petroleum tanks. The tanks were from a bankrupt service station. Their removal was only 1 of 702 approved underground tank cleanups for Oregon in 1998. Building new subdivisions over old gas stations, landfills, or industrial sites increases the chance of pollutants reaching underground water tables. This, in turn, increases the risk of contaminants getting into the food supply.

Lead

The level of lead in the U.S. food supply was 90% lower in 1992 than in 1980. This reduction was due to tighter FDA regulations, changes in gasoline, and voluntary changes from the food canning industry. A major source of lead was leaded gas, which created exhaust that settled on crops and in water.

Another source of lead was the lead solder used to seal the seams on tin cans. The Can Manufacturers Institute announced that, as of November 1991, lead was no longer being used to solder cans. Lead solder was responsible for as much as 45% of the lead found in food before this time.

Consumers need to be aware of the other ways lead can leach into water. The main sources are glazed ceramic dishes (including china), lead crystal glassware and decanters, and silver-plated hollowware, 18-2. The FDA recommends that you avoid storing acidic beverages or foods in any of these containers. Heat and low pH increase the rate at which lead leaches into water. This is why cups used to serve hot, acidic coffee must meet the toughest standards for dinnerware.

Health Tip

To avoid risk of lead contamination, look for labels ensuring that ceramic cookware and dishes are lead free. When serving hot beverages, make sure you are using lead-free cups.

Microbial Contaminants

Physical and chemical contaminants do not change the food itself. They are potential hazards when consumed with the food. When undesired changes occur in the food itself, the food is considered to be spoiled.

Most of the time, a food is described as spoiled when its appearance, texture, flavor, or odor has changed. You would say a tomato is spoiled if it has black fuzzy patches on it. You probably would not choose to eat a mushy apple over a crisp one. You would not be likely to drink your milk at lunch if it has a bad odor. You probably would not eat many potato chips if they have a rank flavor. Each of these is an example of food spoilage. *Food spoilage* is a change in a food that makes it unfit or undesirable for consumption. Food spoilage occurs when a contaminant or naturally occurring enzymes cause the food to deteriorate or change in undesirable ways. You read about food spoilage as the result of enzymatic changes in Chapter 12.

This chapter will look mainly at microorganisms that cause food spoilage. You know that bacteria, fungi, and mold can cause desirable changes in food. They can also cause undesirable changes. Often enzymes and microorganisms work together to spoil food. Softening caused by enzymes can make it easier for molds and bacteria to enter and feed on a food product. See 18-3.

Signs of Spoilage

❖ discoloration

❖ off odor

❖ fuzzy growth on the surface

❖ slimy feel on the surface

❖ foaming or gas bubbles in the product

❖ bulging or corroded can

❖ cloudy appearance

❖ off flavor

❖ mushy texture

❖ soft spots or breaks in the skin on fruits and vegetables

If you suspect a food is spoiled, DO NOT TASTE IT.

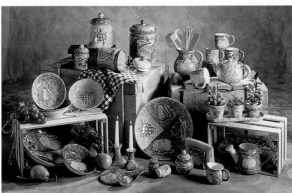

Tabletops Unlimited

18-2 Glazes used on commercially made ceramic dinnerware are regulated for lead safety. However, you may want to use handmade and hand-painted items for decorative purposes only unless they are labeled *lead free.*

18-3 This list describes noticeable changes in food or food packaging that indicate food spoilage has occurred. However, note that some foods in early stages of spoilage may not exhibit any of these signs.

Many changes in food caused by spoilage make the food unpleasant to eat. This does not necessarily mean the food is unsafe. However, microorganisms often bring about unpleasant changes in food that can also cause illness. A sickness caused by eating contaminated food is called *foodborne illness.*

Types of Foodborne Illness

Many people who think they have "stomach flu" are really sensing the symptoms of a foodborne illness. These symptoms often include diarrhea, stomach cramps, and vomiting. There are approximately 76 million cases of foodborne illness each year.

An outbreak of foodborne illness is easier to detect when two or more people have the same symptoms. However, some people are more sensitive than others to foodborne pathogens. Therefore, two people can consume the same contaminated food, but they may not both become sick.

Most cases of foodborne illness are a result of pathogens in food. *Pathogens* are microorganisms that can cause illness in humans. The pathogens that cause foodborne illness do not necessarily cause undesirable changes in food. Many times, pathogens cause a food to be unsafe to eat before there are any visible signs of spoilage. Pathogens can cause illness in one of two ways: intoxication or infection.

Food Intoxication

Some microbes can give off a by-product that causes illness. Substances released by microbes that are harmful to humans are called *toxins.* In this case, it is not the microbe that makes people sick but the toxin it produces. A foodborne illness caused by a toxin released by microbes is called a *food intoxication.*

It is important to remember that killing the microbes may not be enough to prevent cases of food intoxication. If the toxin is still present and has not been damaged or altered, the person will still become ill. The severity of the illness will depend on the amount of toxins present in the food eaten. It will also depend on how susceptible the person is to illness.

A number of microbes cause food intoxication. The following sections discuss those that cause some of the most common illnesses.

Clostridium Perfringens

The bacterium *Clostridium perfringens* causes one of the most frequent and, fortunately, mildest forms of food intoxication. This gram-positive microbe is anaerobic, but it survives in an oxygen environment. Its spores are very heat resistant, and small numbers often remain in cooked foods, 18-4. These organisms can multiply to toxic levels during cooling and storage of prepared foods. *C. perfringens* is widespread in nature. It is found in soil, water, air, sewage, and on many food products.

Foodborne illness caused by *C. perfringens* is often traced to eating protein-based foods. This is because of changes these foods cause in the pH of the stomach. The low pH of stomach acid will normally kill *C. perfringens*. However, consumption of protein foods raises the stomach pH. This rise in pH allows the more acid-resistant spores to survive and enter the intestines, where conditions allow rapid growth. The toxin is a protein that is part of the spore coat. It causes fluids to move into the intestines. Enzymes released by *C. perfringens* damage the cells of the lining of the small intestine.

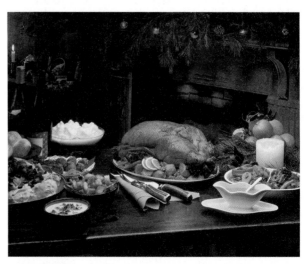

18-4 To prevent *C. pefringens* from multiplying, it is important to keep meats, gravies, and stuffings hot (above 60°C, 140°F) during serving.

Onset of the illness can occur anywhere from 2 to 29 hours after eating contaminated food. Symptoms include diarrhea, which is a result of the toxin pulling water into the intestines. The by-products of the pathogen include acids and large amounts of gas, which cause bloating and cramps. The symptoms last for 12 to 24 hours. A person with this illness can usually return to normal activities the next day. Because recovery rarely requires medical help, many cases go unreported. Death rarely occurs unless a person is already weakened by other illnesses.

Outbreaks of *C. perfringens* usually occur where large volumes of food are prepared at one time. Examples include catering services, hospitals, nursing homes, and school and workplace cafeterias. Protein-based foods involved in outbreaks have often been prepared a day or two in advance and then chilled. Large amounts of food are slow to chill and allow for rapid growth of the bacteria.

Controlling *C. perfringens* can be accomplished in three ways. First, food handlers must limit contamination. Preventing contamination is very difficult, but following sanitation procedures helps limit microbe populations. It takes a large number of *C. perfringens* cells to cause illness. The body is usually able to handle small amounts at a time.

The second method for controlling this illness is to prevent growth. Refrigeration temperatures slow the growth of *C. perfringens*, and most of the cells are killed when frozen. Maximum growth occurs at 50°C to 52°C (122°F to 125°F). Therefore, keep heated foods well above these temperatures. Place leftovers in shallow containers. Place the containers in a bath of water and ice so food will quickly drop below 50°C (122°F). Then place the leftovers in the refrigerator for storage.

The third way to control *C. perfringens* is to destroy the organism. Cooking easily kills active cells. Over 99% of the cells were killed in beef cubes held at 53.3°C (127.9°F). However, some spores are so heat resistant that food would be destroyed before the spores were. Therefore, it is safest to assume that spores have survived the cooking process. Gravies and sauces that may be contaminated need to be reheated by boiling for

10 to 15 minutes. Always throw away food that has not been properly heated or cooled.

Staphylococcus Aureus

Staphylococcus aureus is a gram-positive bacterium that occurs singly, in pairs, and in clusters. These bacteria can survive in aerobic or anaerobic conditions. They do not compete well with other bacteria. This means when other bacteria are present, *S. aureus* will not grow rapidly. Most strains of *S. aureus* will grow in salt solutions that kill or stop other bacteria. This is why *S. aureus* is a common cause of foodborne illness traced to cured meats. Pasteurization and reheating will kill *S. aureus*. However, the toxin it produces is more heat stable and can still cause illness after the microbe has been destroyed. Therefore, it is necessary to prevent contamination with and growth of the microbe to avoid illness.

S. aureus is found on healthy humans and most warm-blooded animals. It is found in pimples, boils, and open wounds. It is also on the skin and mucous membranes, such as the lining of the nose. The bacteria are easily transferred to the hands by touching infected surfaces, such as blemishes, the nose, or soiled tissue.

Growth of *S. aureus* occurs most rapidly at temperatures of 33°C to 38°C (91°F to 100°F). It takes about 3 hours at room temperature after contamination has occurred to produce enough toxin to cause illness. The illness usually begins within 30 minutes to 8 hours after eating the contaminated food. The symptoms can include nausea, diarrhea, vomiting, and abdominal cramps. The illness is rarely fatal and lasts only one to two days. The severity of the illness will depend on the amount of food consumed and the individual's resistance to the toxin.

Foods most likely to be contaminated with *S. aureus* include red meats, especially ham. Poultry; potato, macaroni, and tuna salads; and custard- or cream-filled bakery products may also be involved in *S. aureus* contamination. In most cases, the food is contaminated after it is cooked. See 18-5.

Humans are the main source of *S. aureus*. Therefore, monitoring the health, hygiene, and work habits of food handlers is the best

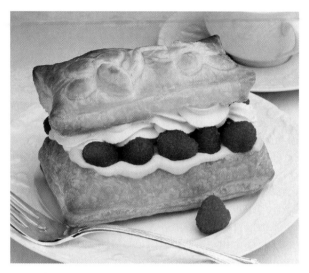

18-5 Some cases of illness caused by *S. aureus* have been traced to cream-filled pastries.

prevention method. Anyone who has excessive acne, infected cuts, or symptoms of the common cold should not handle food. Food handlers should frequently wash their hands and avoid touching their faces while working with food. Cleaning and sanitizing equipment is also important. *S. aureus* can be transferred from humans to work surfaces and then to any food that touches those surfaces.

Controlling *S. aureus* means rapidly cooling susceptible foods or serving them quickly. Any susceptible food should be placed in containers that are no more than three inches deep for rapid cooling. Foods should reach a temperature of 4°C (40°F) within four hours. Foods that may be contaminated with *S. aureus* should not be eaten. This is because, although reheating will kill the bacteria, it does not destroy the toxin that causes illness.

Clostridium Botulinum

Unfortunately, the third most common source of food intoxication can be extremely dangerous. *C. botulinum* is a gram-positive, rod-shaped, anaerobic bacterium. It is commonly found in all soil types and in the sediments of marshes and lakes. Fish have been found to be carriers. The bacteria can live in fish intestines but do not multiply there. Because of their presence in soil, *C. botulinum* are commonly found on the surface of vegetables.

C. botulinum produce a toxin called *botulin,* which passes through the intestinal wall and

enters the bloodstream. It then travels to nerve cells. The presence of the toxin at nerve fiber junctions will prevent nerve impulses from being transmitted. This results in paralysis of the muscles.

Foodborne illness caused by *C. botulinum* is called *botulism.* Symptoms can appear anywhere from 12 to 24 hours after eating a contaminated food. The first signs of botulism are blurred vision; progressive weakness; and red, sore mouth, tongue, and throat. The patient may also experience diarrhea followed by constipation and abdominal pain. Paralysis begins in the throat and progresses to the chest, arms, and legs. The patient needs prompt medical attention to avoid death due to suffocation. The sooner treatment begins, the better the chance of survival.

Infants up to 12 months of age are more susceptible to botulism than people in other age groups. Honey can be a source of *C. botulinum* spores and should never be fed to infants. Spinach, which can promote the growth of botulism, is another high-risk food for infants. Some studies indicate 5% of infants who reportedly died of sudden infant death syndrome (SIDS) were infected with botulin.

Most cases of botulism are caused by home-canned foods that were improperly processed, 18-6. Other likely sources of botulism are improperly processed peppers, soup, asparagus, mushrooms, spinach, and ripe olives.

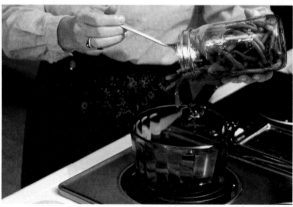

USDA

18-6 Green beans canned at home need to be processed in a pressure canner to avoid risk of *Clostridium botulinum.*

C. botulinum need a pH of 4.6 or greater and an oxygen-free environment to multiply. The bacteria grow best between the temperatures of 25°C and 37°C (77°F and 99°F).

Prevention of botulism begins with washing vegetables to remove soil and as many *C. botulinum* organisms as possible. Fish should be carefully gutted and thoroughly washed. Growth of *C. botulinum* can be prevented by freezing food.

Care needs to be taken when processing and preparing home-canned foods. This is especially true of low-acid foods, such as corn and green beans. The spores of *C. botulinum* can survive temperatures in excess of 100°C (212°F) for several hours. Therefore, low-acid foods need to be processed at a temperature of 121°C (250°F) to destroy the spores. (The toxins are destroyed at lower temperatures than the spores.) It is recommended that low-acid canned foods be heated to boiling (100°C, 212°F) after opening. Before these foods are eaten, they should be simmered for 10 to 15 minutes to guarantee the toxin has been destroyed. Home-canned low-acid vegetables should never be eaten cold.

Cured and processed meats would be ruined at temperatures high enough to destroy *C. botulinum* spores. Therefore, chemicals must be used to destroy botulism in meat products. Cases of botulism have been traced to chicken liver pâté, luncheon meats, ham, sausage, lobster, and smoked and salted fish. Sodium nitrite can be added to these foods to fix the color and prevent growth of *C. botulinum*.

Escherichia Coli

Escherichia coli are gram-negative, rod-shaped bacteria that live in the colons of mammals. They are transported to the food supply by sewage-contaminated water or infected food handlers.

There are four strains of *E. coli* that are known to cause foodborne illness. One strain causes illness when present in large numbers in the small intestine. A second strain seems to produce a toxin while in the small intestine. A third strain invades the mucous lining of the intestines. A fourth strain causes bleeding in the colon and kidney failure. This last strain is

the deadliest, especially among small children and older adults. It can cause illness with as few as 10 cells in the food supply.

The time from exposure to onset varies from less than 1 day to 13 days. Most patients begin to exhibit symptoms between 18 and 44 hours after eating the contaminated food. The illness usually lasts from 3 to 4 days. The main symptom is diarrhea, but nausea, fever, cramps, weakness, aches, and vomiting may also occur. Treatment centers on replacing fluids and electrolytes.

Outbreaks of *E. coli* have occurred as a result of consuming soft cheeses, hamburgers, salads, and apple juice. Any food exposed to raw fecal matter is at risk of being contaminated. Ground meats are at risk because the grinding process can mix any *E. coli* present throughout the meat. Any patty not cooked until done would then have *E. coli* present in the center of the meat. See 18-7.

Steps for preventing contamination can be taken by communities as well as by individuals. Communities chlorinate water supplies to eliminate harmful bacteria. Anyone handling food must thoroughly wash his or her hands after using the bathroom. People who

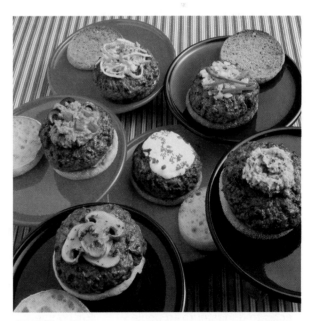

18-7 Hamburgers and other ground meat products need to be cooked to an internal temperature of 71°C (160°F). This will kill any *E. coli* that may be present.

cook ground meat must be sure to cook it thoroughly. These efforts will help reduce the risks of an *E. coli* outbreak.

Food Infection

The second major cause of foodborne illness is the microbes themselves. Microbes release digestive enzymes that begin to damage body tissue and cause illness. This type of foodborne illness is called *food infection.* A food infection cannot occur if the microbes are killed.

Food infections may be caused by bacteria, parasites, and viruses. A large number of living organisms is usually required to cause illness. Symptoms are related to damage caused by the organisms feeding on their hosts.

Listeria Monocytogenes

Listeriosis is a foodborne infection caused by *Listeria monocytogenes.* This is a rod-shaped, gram-positive bacterium. It is found in soil, water, and many species of animals. Food sources include soft cheeses, uncooked meats, unwashed vegetables, and unpasteurized milk.

L. monocytogenes is harder to kill than many other foodborne pathogens. It can grow

and multiply at refrigerator temperatures. It is aerobic, but it grows best at reduced oxygen levels combined with increased carbon dioxide. It can grow in 10% salt solutions and at a pH of 9.

Symptoms of listeriosis include fever, headache, nausea, diarrhea, and vomiting. Listeriosis can also cause infections in pregnant women, which can result in miscarriage or stillbirth. Nearly 25% of serious cases result in death.

Those at greatest risk are pregnant women, newborns, and people with weakened immune systems, including many older adults. General guidelines for reducing the risk of listeriosis include thoroughly cooking raw meat and poultry and carefully washing raw vegetables. In addition, people in high-risk groups should avoid eating soft cheeses, such as feta, Brie, and blue-veined cheeses. Those at risk should also heat all precooked foods and processed meats, such as deli meats and hot dogs, until they steam. See 18-8.

Salmonellae

Salmonella is a genus of rod-shaped, gram-negative, anaerobic bacteria. These microbes cause an illness called *salmonellosis.* The bacteria attach to the lining of the intestines and

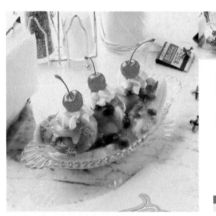

Item of Interest
Outbreaks of E. coli

In October 1996, an outbreak of *E. coli* infection occurred in the western United States. Thirteen cases of *E. coli* infection were traced to unpasteurized apple juice packaged by Odwalla Apple Juice. The company recalled all drinks that contained apple juice.

In July 1997, an outbreak of *E. coli* infection occurred in Colorado. The Colorado Department of Health and Environment traced this outbreak to frozen hamburger patties from Hudson Foods Company. The source was believed to be meat

grindings. Apparently leftover meat grindings from one day's processing had been saved and used the next day. The FDA conducted further investigation. This led the FDA to order a recall of 25 million pounds of hamburger produced by a Hudson Foods plant.

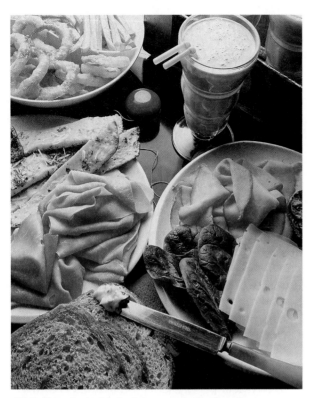

18-8 People in high-risk groups for foodborne illness should heat cold cuts until they are steaming hot to reduce possible exposure to *L. monocytogenes.*

release digestive enzymes. These enzymes damage the tissue of the intestinal lining. It takes a large number of salmonellae to cause symptoms. However, a small number of bacteria can attach to the intestines and reproduce until illness results. Body fluids are pulled into the intestines, which causes diarrhea. Other symptoms include cramps, fever, nausea, vomiting, chills, and headache. Treatment includes giving fluids to prevent dehydration. Use of antibiotics has no noticeable benefit and leads to strains of salmonella that are resistant to antibiotics.

Less than 1% of all reported cases of salmonellosis end in death. This makes salmonellosis far less dangerous than botulism. However, there are so many cases of salmonellosis that far more people die from it than from botulism. Young children, older adults, and people with other illnesses are at the greatest risk.

The time between eating a contaminated food and the onset of salmonellosis is generally 6 to 48 hours. Symptoms in adults usually last only 2 to 3 days. However, symptoms may last longer in children.

The Centers for Disease Control estimate that eggs are involved in about 75% of all salmonellosis outbreaks. Other foods most likely to be contaminated with salmonellae are poultry, beef, dairy products, and pork. Poultry and livestock producers are working to reduce the number of salmonellae that occur in animals before and during slaughter.

Poultry and poultry products are major sources of salmonellae for two main reasons. The first is that salmonellae live in poultry without causing the birds to become sick. The second is the broad use of antibiotics in poultry feed to increase poultry production. Many of the strains of salmonellae that commonly cause illness are resistant to antibiotics. Salmonellae also multiply quickly when other microbes have been killed or reduced in number by antibiotics.

Care needs to be taken to prevent salmonellae contamination during food preparation. Salmonellae are often spread from one food to another by food handlers. These bacteria can survive on people's hands for hours before being transmitted to foods where they will thrive and multiply. Therefore, food handlers should keep work surfaces and hands clean.

To prevent salmonellae growth, cold foods need to be kept cold, and hot foods need to be kept hot. Salmonellae grow very quickly between 10°C and 50°C (50°F and 122°F). When heating and chilling, foods need to be moved through this temperature range as quickly as possible. Foods that are cooked just before eating will usually be free of salmonellae.

Care must be taken to cook ground meat and poultry until they are thoroughly done. When meat is ground, the salmonellae can be mixed all through the meat. If hamburgers are still pink in the middle, salmonellae could still be alive in the center of the patty. Poultry should always be cooked until the juices run clear. See 18-9.

Raw or improperly cooked eggs are a potential hazard. Many uncooked recipes for homemade ice cream, Caesar salad, hollandaise sauce, and mayonnaise call for raw eggs.

Pasteurized eggs should be used in place of raw eggs in these dishes. Pasteurized eggs have been heated to kill bacteria such as salmonellae. Shell eggs should be cooked until the yolk is thickened and the white is firm. Scrambled eggs should be cooked until they are no longer runny. See 18-10.

Parasitic Infections

Most of the pathogens that cause foodborne illness are bacteria. However, some illnesses are caused by parasites. *Parasites* are organisms that live in and feed on a host. A *host* is an animal or plant from which a parasite receives nutrients. Some parasites that cause foodborne illness are commonly found in contaminated water supplies. Raw fish can be sources of these parasites. Fresh fruits and vegetables cleaned with contaminated water can be sources, too. Hogs, cattle, and wild animals are common hosts of other illness-causing parasites.

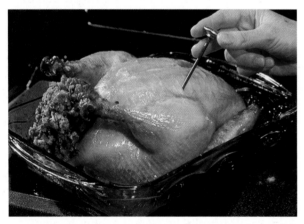

USDA

18-9 Checking poultry with a food thermometer ensures the internal temperature is high enough to kill any salmonellae that may be present.

Trichinella Spiralis

Trichinella spiralis is probably the best-known parasite that causes foodborne illness. This parasite is a microscopic roundworm. It occurs in hogs and wild animals, such as bears, boars, and rabbits. Humans can also serve as hosts of *T. spiralis*. This parasite can enter a host as adult worms or larvae through infected food. *Larvae* are immature parasites that are often surrounded and protected by a *cyst*, or pocket. Within the host, digestion breaks down the cysts, releasing the larvae into the host's small intestines. The larvae feed and grow into adult roundworms. The adult worms attach themselves to the intestinal walls, where they produce new larvae. The new larvae penetrate the intestinal walls and travel in the bloodstream to muscle tissue. Once imbedded in the muscle, the larvae form protective cysts. *T. spiralis* can survive for years in the muscle tissue of the host.

An infection caused by *T. spiralis* is known as **trichinosis.** During the first phase of the illness, the symptoms include nausea, abdominal pain, and diarrhea. Once the larvae enter the muscle tissue, symptoms will include muscle pain and fever.

Prevention is the best protection against trichinosis. *T. spiralis* larvae are destroyed when meats are adequately cooked. Curing, smoking, and fermenting processes will also destroy the larvae. Pork used to be the most widely eaten source of this parasite. Inspection and production procedures have effectively eliminated *T. spiralis* from commercial pork, 18-11. The USDA has recommended processing procedures that should destroy any *T. spiralis* in cured pork products. The main source of *T. spiralis* in the United States today is game meats. Like pork, fresh game, such as bear, boar, and rabbit, should always

Recommended Cooking Times for Eggs	
Sunny side up	7 minutes, uncovered 4 minutes, covered
Over easy	3 minutes on one side then 2 minutes on the other side
Poached	5 minutes in boiling water

18-10 Salmonellae are destroyed when egg dishes reach an internal temperature of 71°C (160°F).

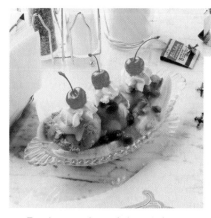

Item of Interest
Salmonellae—Who's the Culprit?

Poultry and poultry products have been identified as major sources of salmonellae contamination. Statistics from the Centers for Disease Control also show outbreaks in which beef and veal are the sources. (An *outbreak* is when two or more people are known to become ill from eating the same food.) The reason for this is that chicken is usually eaten well done. However, many people eat beef and veal rare.

In outbreaks in which the food source was identified, 80% were caused by undercooked or raw eggs. In August 1990, the FDA released recommendations for the use of eggs in all commercial food settings. These recommendations include using pasteurized eggs in place of shell eggs whenever possible.

be cooked to an internal temperature of 71°C (160°F). Freezing will kill the larvae if the meat is held at -15°C (5°F) for at least 30 days.

Viral Infections

Viruses are a third type of pathogen that can cause foodborne illnesses. A *virus* is a microscopic disease-causing agent made up of genetic material surrounded by a protein coating. The protein coating is called a *capsid.* Viruses do not multiply in food, but some viruses can be transmitted in food.

A virus must attach to a host cell. Genetic material from the virus is injected into the host cell. The genetic material can attach to the host cell's genes. This causes the host cell to make more virus particles. Eventually the large number of virus particles causes the host cell to rupture and die. The virus particles are then freed to find new host cells and repeat the process. The nature of viral infections is related to which cells the virus can attach to and destroy.

Health experts do not know how many virus particles a person must ingest for illness to occur. This is because viruses are difficult to detect in food. Experts do know that viruses must survive stomach acids and digestive enzymes for any illness to develop. Studies have found that viruses remain stable and

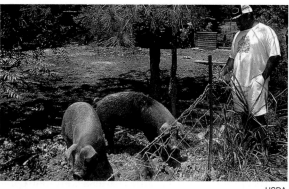

USDA

18-11 Hogs are inspected to ensure they are free of *Trichinella spiralis.*

able to contaminate food in a wide range of situations. For instance, poliovirus was found on fruit and vegetable crops fertilized with contaminated sewage sludge. This virus was able to survive on the fruits and vegetables up to 36 days. Viruses can also survive

❖ on glass, stainless steel, and tile for up to eight weeks at room temperature

❖ on low-moisture foods for over two weeks at room temperature and more than two months when refrigerated

❖ in ground meat for 8 to 14 days at 4°C (39°F)

Viruses are usually transmitted through the *fecal-oral route.* This refers to the consumption of any food or beverage that has come in contact with feces. A viral infection can be transmitted from contaminated feces to food in two main ways. The first is failing to wash hands after going to the bathroom and then handling food. The second is using sewage-contaminated water or fertilizer on food crops.

Four main types of viruses have been found to cause foodborne illness. These include Rotavirus, Norwalk virus, and hepatitis. Threat of the fourth type, poliovirus, has largely been eliminated in the United States by vaccinations.

Rotavirus

Rotavirus occurs most often in young children. By age five, most children have been infected with this virus and developed immunity. Flulike symptoms, including vomiting, diarrhea, and low-grade fever, will last for 2 to 10 days. This viral infection is most common during winter months. Good hygiene practices are the best prevention. Any food handled by an infected person and then eaten without further cooking is a potential risk.

Norwalk Virus

Norwalk virus is named for the first documented outbreak, which occurred in 1968 among school children in Norwalk, Ohio. This virus causes a mild flulike illness that lasts one to two days. It occurs among all age groups and during any time of the year. Outbreaks have been traced to green salads, raw oysters, cake frosting, and chicken sandwiches. Humans are the only carriers. Prevention involves good personal hygiene. It is also important that people with any flu or cold symptoms avoid handling or preparing food.

Hepatitis

Hepatitis is a viral infection that attacks the liver cells. Hepatitis A, or *infectious hepatitis,* is the strain of hepatitis that can be transmitted through contaminated food. Flulike symptoms will last for one to three days. Three to four weeks later, symptoms of liver infection develop. Cases are usually mild.

More severe infections can lead to liver failure and death.

Hepatitis A is destroyed when food is cooked. Foods at risk are uncooked salad ingredients, raw shellfish, and any food requiring handling after cooking. People who buy shellfish should make sure the seafood has come from clean waters that are free from raw sewage. Shellfish should not be eaten raw. Clams dropped in boiling water until they opened seemed to be the cause of one hepatitis outbreak. This indicates that limited heating is not sufficient to destroy the virus. See 18-12.

Most outbreaks of hepatitis have been traced to infected food handlers. Infected food handlers can transmit hepatitis for 7 to 10 days before they develop any symptoms. Therefore, food handlers need to monitor their health and wash their hands frequently to help prevent the spread of hepatitis. They should also wear disposable gloves when handling foods just prior to serving. Anyone who has been exposed or is at risk of exposure can be given a vaccine called *immune serum globulin.*

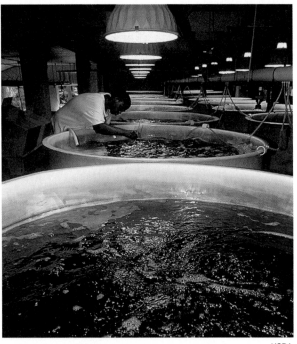

USDA

18-12 Commercially raised clams are tested for microbial contamination as an important part of the inspection process.

How Pathogens Enter the Food Supply

Why is there a problem with pathogens in the food chain? One reason is the development of new, hardier strains of microbes. The speed with which bacteria reproduce enables new strains to develop quickly. A genetic change in a bacterium takes less than 24 hours to appear in thousands of new bacteria. By contrast, a genetic change in a human takes around twenty years to appear in a few children.

New strains of microbes develop due to minor genetic differences in a small percentage of microbes. For instance, when antibiotics are given to chicken, most of the bacteria present are killed. However, a small percentage of the bacteria has some minor difference. This makes them harder to kill and allows them to survive. These bacteria will reproduce. The result will be a new strain of bacteria that is resistant to the antibiotic. New strains of microbes that withstand higher temperatures, lower pH ranges, or different air mixes develop in the same way.

It is important to understand how microbes can get into the food supply. There are two main ways food can become contaminated with pathogens. Pathogens can be transmitted by animals and through improper handling procedures.

Transmission by Animals

You may have noticed that many of the foods linked to food infections and food intoxications are from animal sources. Animals are hosts or carriers for many microbes. Protein-based foods from animal sources also provide an environment in which microbes can grow and multiply.

Warm-Blooded Animal Carriers

All warm-blooded animals have microbes living in and on them. Animals can transfer these microbes to food products. One way this can happen is by allowing food products to come in contact with animal feces.

An example of this is found in apple juice contaminated with *E. coli* bacteria. One way this juice might have been contaminated is by deer. *E. coli* live in the colons of humans and other mammals, including deer. If *E. coli* enter the stomach and small intestines, they can cause illness. In the colon, however, these bacteria help break down waste products. *E. coli* can be passed out of the body in feces.

Deer will feed on apples that grow on the lower branches of apple trees. Deer also excrete in apple orchards while eating. Apples that fall from the trees may come in contact with deer feces. These fallen apples are likely to be bruised and will quickly spoil. They can, however, be pressed to make apple juice. The apples need to be thoroughly washed or the juice needs to be pasteurized. Otherwise, the apple juice can become contaminated with *E. coli* from the deer feces.

Another way microbes from animals can end up in foods happens when the animals are used as meat sources. During slaughter and packaging, microbes on the surfaces of an animal are often transferred to the cuts of meat. If the meat is not properly handled and prepared, it can become a source of foodborne illness. See 18-13.

Raw Fish

Various parasites live in fish and shellfish. If the fish is eaten raw, these parasites can enter the digestive tract, causing illness and death. Popular raw fish dishes that are at risk of causing illness include sushi, oysters, clams, and mussels. The FDA has recommended a procedure for fish that will be consumed raw. The

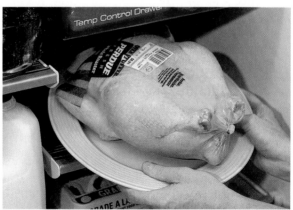

USDA

18-13 Store raw meats and poultry on trays in the refrigerator to avoid contaminating other foods with dripping juices.

fish should be quick-frozen to -35°C (-31°F) for 15 hours. The fish can also be held in a commercial freezer at -20°C (-4°F) for 24 hours. The fish may then be thawed and eaten.

Meat and Dairy Products

Meats, milk, and eggs are often associated with foodborne illness. There are three key reasons for this. First, these foods all provide a medium in which microbes can thrive. Second, these are popular foods that are widely consumed in the U.S. diet. Third, many people are uninformed about how to handle these foods to prevent illness. For example, some people believe raw eggs are a healthful ingredient in a protein shake. These people are unaware that salmonellae can get into an egg before the shell is formed. They do not realize that drinking a shake containing raw egg puts them at risk for salmonellosis.

Avoiding food from animal sources is not a wise way to prevent foodborne illness. These foods are important sources of nutrients in the diet. Learning how to properly handle these foods is a more appropriate prevention strategy.

Improper Handling Procedures

Once food is contaminated, improper handling can allow the microbes to multiply and cause illness when eaten. Improper handling procedures can be divided into three groups.

❖ time and temperature abuse
❖ poor personal hygiene
❖ cross-contamination

Time and Temperature Abuse

The number one cause of foodborne illness is the failure to properly cool food. Most pathogens multiply rapidly between 4°C and 60°C (40°F and 140°F). This temperature range is referred to as the *temperature danger zone*. Foods at risk for pathogens should be kept cold or hot during storage, transportation, preparation, holding, and service. All refrigeration units must be below 4°C (40°F) and heating units must be at or above 60°C (140°F). As a rule, the total time a perishable food is in the danger zone should not exceed two hours. This time includes mixing time at room temperature, standing time before or after cooking, and holding time during meal service.

Poor Personal Hygiene

The food industry works hard to provide a safe food supply that is as free from contaminants as possible. The FDA, EPA, and USDA inspect and monitor the food supply. They strive to protect consumers from contaminants during the growth, production, and processing of food. However, food handlers and customers are one of the major causes of unsafe food. Sources of human contamination include hands, breath, hair, wounds, unshielded coughs and sneezes, and perspiration.

Cross-Contamination

Cross-contamination occurs in food when a contaminated substance comes in contact with another food. Any surface that comes in contact with food will cause cross-contamination if microbes are present. For example, suppose you use a cutting board for deboning and slicing a raw chicken breast for a stir-fry. Salmonellae are on the surface of the chicken. The salmonellae get on the cutting board. You give the board a quick rinse with warm water. You then use the board to slice raw vegetables for a salad. The salmonellae will be transferred from the cutting board to the salad ingredients. Although salmonellae on the chicken will be killed during cooking, the salad is not cooked prior to eating. See 18-14. Cross-contamination can also occur when plant foods are harvested and come in contact with the soil around them.

Uninformed or Careless Consumers

All three major causes of foodborne illness are related to uninformed and careless consumers and food handlers. It does not matter whether food is contaminated by improper heating, poor personal hygiene, or cross-contamination. The result is illness for anyone who eats the contaminated food. It is important to remember that pathogens can make people ill long before the food will show signs of spoilage.

Any food, if improperly handled, can cause foodborne illness. The leading cause of food-related illnesses is consumers and food handlers who are ignorant or careless. A

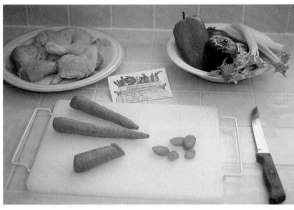

18-14 To prevent cross-contamination, be sure to thoroughly wash cutting boards, knives, and hands after preparing poultry before handling fresh vegetables.

salad. Those who ate the salad were too sick to report to work the next day. This type of problem can easily occur at picnics, community dinners, church potlucks, restaurants, and family gatherings.

> ## Storage Tips
> Observe the following precautions to reduce the risk of foodborne illness:
>
> ❖ **When in doubt, throw it out!**
>
> ❖ **Use older foods first. (Remember this tip by the acronym *FIFO*, which stands for first in, first out.)**
>
> ❖ **Reheat leftovers only once. Discard any uneaten reheated food.**
>
> ❖ **Use refrigerated leftovers within three to four days.**

certain hunter is an example of a consumer who was ignorant of the dangers associated with eating some foods. This hunter decided to feed bear meat to friends at a cookout. The hunter mixed the bear meat with ground beef to conceal the taste. He did not tell anyone that part of the meat came from bear. Those who chose to have their burgers cooked to the well-done stage were fine. Those who chose to have their burgers cooked to the rare or medium stage became ill. In this case, the hunter did not know that bear meat is often contaminated with parasites. The guests were uninformed as to what they were eating.

The school cafeteria workers mentioned at the beginning of the chapter are an example of careless food handlers. The health department traced the illness to a potato salad made by a cafeteria worker trained in food safety. The worker had made the potato salad for a potluck luncheon held to honor retiring cafeteria workers. The worker left the potato salad on her kitchen table while she dressed for the potluck. Then she left the salad in her hot car when she made some stops on the way to the luncheon. (The temperature in a closed car on a hot, sunny day can quickly exceed 38°C, 100°F.) At the potluck, the potato salad was placed on the serving table almost an hour before everyone was served. By the time the salad was eaten, it had been at or above room temperature for over two hours. Half of the county cafeteria workers ate some of the

Food Industry Sanitation Procedures

Monitoring the safety of the food supply involves two key aspects. The first is a voluntary effort by the food industry to set and follow standards that will help prevent contamination. The second part of the monitoring process is government regulation.

Developing a HACCP System

The food industry works with government agencies to set up guidelines that will prevent contamination or growth of microbes in foods. The food safety system used most often by U.S. food producers is called *HACCP (Hazard Analysis and Critical Control Point)*. A HACCP system looks at every point in the food production process where contamination can occur. This system views a hazard as anything that could cause harm. Hazards include microbes, toxins, chemicals, and foreign objects in food. A critical control point is any point in a food operation where hazards can be removed, prevented, or minimized.

Meat and fish producers became required to phase in HACCP systems between 1998 and 2000, 18-15. The FDA published rules mandating HACCP for fruit juice producers in January 2001. For producers of other food products, HACCP is voluntary. However,

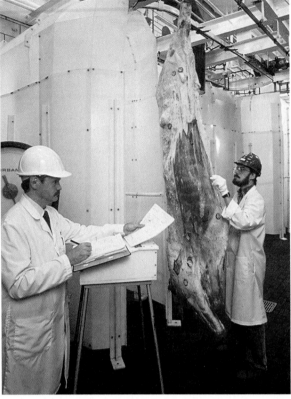

USDA

18-15 Meat producers are required to use a HACCP system to help ensure the safety of meat products.

many food producers choose to use a HACCP system because it reduces the producer's risk of liability. HACCP also increases profits by working to prevent outbreaks of foodborne illness.

The HACCP concept was originated by NASA and Natick Laboratories in the 1960s. Pillsbury worked with NASA and Natick Laboratories to develop the HACCP system in 1971. The system was designed to be flexible enough to adapt to any aspect of the food industry. It can help prevent contamination at any stage from growing crops to serving the food.

Developing a HACCP system involves seven main steps. The first step is to determine potential hazards. Is the company working with high-risk foods, such as meat, poultry, seafood, or egg and dairy dishes? How does food move through the system? Where and how is it stored or packaged? When does it come in contact with humans, chemicals, and machinery?

The second step is to develop a flowchart for each procedure in the company, plant, or restaurant. Each point in the process where hazards can occur is identified.

The third step is to set standards that are needed at each control point. Standards must be specific and measurable. This step also involves determining procedures for maintaining the standards. Examples include monitoring temperatures of heating and cooling units, identifying cooking times, and defining cleaning procedures. Employees must be trained to follow procedure directions exactly.

Step four is to monitor the critical control points. Regularly checking equipment for accuracy and keeping thorough records of procedures are part of this process.

The fifth step is to correct any problems as soon as they are discovered. For example, chili is to be held at 60°C (140°F) until it is served. A supervisor performs a temperature check and discovers the chili is at 57°C (135°F). The supervisor then checks the records to see how long the chili has been on the holding unit. If the chili has been held for longer than two hours, it is discarded. If the holding time is less than two hours, the chili is immediately reheated to 74°C (165°F) for 15 seconds.

Step six is keeping records. Procedures are to be clearly written and posted. Time and temperature logs are dated and kept for each batch of food prepared or processed. These records provide legal verification of procedures used.

The last step is to have the HACCP system verified once it is in place. This is usually done by an official inspector from the FDA, USDA, or local health department.

HACCP in the Meat Industry

Beef Products, Inc. is one of the world's leading producers of boneless lean beef. Their HACCP system is a 24-hour process. A sample of finished product is pulled from the line every 10 seconds. A sample is pulled from each box on every pallet. Samples are combined from enough beef packages to fill a pallet. This composite sample is analyzed for fat, water activity, and protein levels. Each box on each pallet is bar coded with the date and pallet information. Every two hours, a portion of all samples drawn are sent to an independent lab for microbial testing. Each 2-hour sample is tested for total plate count, *E coli*, coliform, *Salmonella, Listeria, Staphylococcus,* and *E coli* 0157:H7. In addition, a daily composite sample is sent to an independent outside lab for central nervous tissue testing. All packaged products are moved immediately after packaging to a 15-level cold storage unit that holds up to 28 million pounds of meat.

Once the meat is packaged, a fully automated system moves the packages through temperature-controlled areas. The pallet packing area is held at 27°F, the holding freezer is 0°F to -5°F, and the loading dock is kept at 40°F. In addition, none of the meat is released for shipping until all the microbial profiles have been completed and the meat is found to be safe. No matter how thorough such a HACCP system is, the final safety of any food product depends on the retailer and the consumer continuing to handle, store, and prepare all foods appropriately.

Government Regulation of the Food Industry

The FDA and USDA are two of the federal agencies that monitor the safety of the food supply. They are mainly responsible for food produced and shipped across state lines. These agencies set standards that often represent the minimum needed for safety. For example, the standard for chilling a food after cooking may be to reach 0°C (32° F) within one hour. It is fine if the chilling time is less than one hour. However, it cannot exceed one hour.

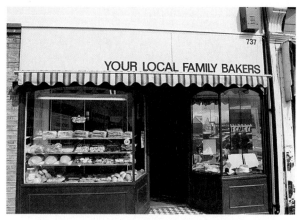

18-16 Businesses that make and sell food products must undergo periodic health inspections.

Local and state health departments monitor foods produced and sold within states. Local health departments also regulate food-service operations. Local regulation agencies use guidelines established by federal and state agencies.

Before any food business can open, it must get a permit and be inspected. This is to make sure safety and sanitation regulations are being followed. Once a business is operating, the FDA recommends that inspections be carried out at least twice a year. Fewer inspections are needed when efficient HACCP systems are in place. Violations of regulations can result in warnings, fines, and/or closure of the business. See 18-16.

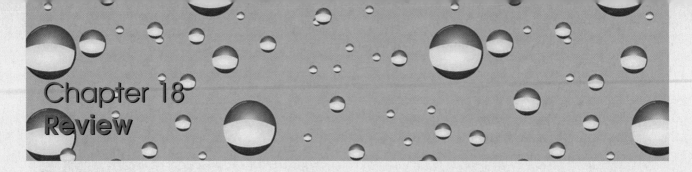

Summary

Food becomes spoiled when contamination causes undesirable changes. Spoiled food is unpleasant but not necessarily harmful to your health. Spoiled food has an unpleasant taste, texture, odor, and/or appearance. Spoilage is usually a result of enzymes and microbes naturally found in the food.

Illness can result when foods become contaminated with harmful substances. Some food illness is caused by the toxins released by microbial action as a by-product. Both the bacteria and the toxins produced must be destroyed to prevent illness. Other cases of food illness are caused by the microbes themselves. To protect your family and yourself from food contamination, it is helpful to understand the pathogens that cause illness. You need to know what they require to survive, grow, and multiply. Each microbe has a preferred food source, temperature, and pH range. This information is your best weapon for fighting food contamination.

Pathogens have been found to enter the food supply in several ways. The first source is through animal carriers. The second source is improper handling procedures. Uninformed and careless consumers are a major source of pathogens in food.

Government agencies and the food industry work together to monitor and maintain a safe food supply. HACCP is an efficient food safety system that reduces the risk of foodborne illness and the need for frequent inspections. A safe food supply requires the cooperation and education of everyone involved in the handling of food.

Check Your Understanding

1. List the primary sources of contamination and give two examples of each.
2. Describe two ways that insects and rodents can damage or contaminate food.
3. Explain the difference between contamination, spoilage, and foodborne illness.
4. Compare and contrast the two ways that pathogens can cause illness.
5. List four common microbes that cause food intoxication and a common food source for each.
6. Why are poultry and eggs the main sources of salmonellosis?
7. Name a parasite that can cause foodborne illness and its most common food source.
8. List three viral infections that can contaminate food
9. What are the three reasons that meat and dairy products are often sources of foodborne illness.
10. Name three basic ways that food is handled improperly. For each, name a safety guideline to follow to reduce risk of foodborne illness.
11. List the seven steps of the HACCP process.
12. Who is responsible for monitoring the safety of the food supply?

Critical Thinking

1. After enjoying a buffet at a family reunion, many guests report having diarrhea, stomach cramps, and bleeding in the colon 24 hours later. Which microbe is the likely cause?
2. Why are county fair entries of low-acid canned goods simmered for 15 minutes before judges sample them to select the winners?
3. After eating Brie that has been kept well chilled, an older adult experiences diarrhea, vomiting, and fever. What microbe is the likely cause?
4. Why is it best to sweeten an infant's hot breakfast cereal with sugar rather than honey?

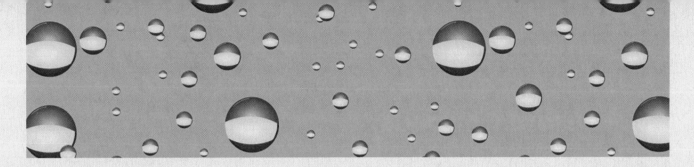

Explore Further

1. **Math.** Research the number of cases of foodborne illness last year reported by the Center for Disease Control. Calculate the percentage of foodborne illness caused by intoxication versus infection.

2. **Technology.** Use the computer to create an attractive, attention-getting poster or handout on food safety procedures for the school's Family and Consumer Sciences food labs.

3. **Writing.** Write an article for the school newspaper on how to safely handle and store foods to prevent foodborne illness.

4. **Application.** Use the HACCP process to develop a procedure for monitoring the safety of the laboratory during and after conducting this chapter's experiments. How will you ensure that bacteria samples do not contaminate surfaces that will be used for food production by other classes.

5. **Analytical Skills.** Read a recent article on the use of antibiotics in our society. Report how antibiotics are made, why they become ineffective, and what you recommend regarding the food industry's use of antibiotics in the future.

Experiment 18A
Mold Growth in Foods

Safety

❖ **Do not taste any of the samples.**

❖ **Clean all surfaces with a sanitizing solution at the end of the experiment.**

Purpose

Molds are found nearly everywhere. Molds are hardier than bacteria and yeast. They grow over a wider range of pH and temperature and at higher salt concentrations. Although molds spoil food, most are not a health hazard. In 1961, a *mycotoxin* (a toxin generated by some molds) named aflatoxin was discovered. Aflatoxin damages the liver and is a known liver carcinogen. These toxins are extremely lethal and frequently heat stable. Cooking mold-contaminated food will not destroy the toxins. In this experiment, you will examine how molds grow on foods. This will help you determine the safety hazards of unidentified molds.

Equipment

paring knife
microscope slides
microscope

Supplies

1 slice apple
½ slice preservative-free bread
1 slice cheese
3 closed containers or resealable plastic bags

Procedure

1. Cut a piece as thin as possible off slices of apple, bread, and cheese.

2. Place each sample on a microscope slide.

3. Observe each sample under a microscope. Record your observations and draw a sketch of what you see in a data table.

4. Place the rest of the half slice of bread in a container or resealable plastic bag so there are 3 to 5 cm of airspace above the bread. Seal the container and label it with your lab group name or number.

5. Place the apple slice in a second container and the cheese slice in a third container, just like the bread. Label both containers with your lab group name or number.

6. Place all three containers on a table or window sill as directed by your teacher.

7. Each day, examine the food samples for visible mold growth.

8. When mold is visible, use a knife to remove a small piece of the *aerial* (above the food) mold from the bread. Place it on a slide.

9. Observe the mold under a microscope. Record your observations and draw a sketch in the data table.

10. Repeat steps 8 and 9 for the apple and cheese.

11. Scrape the visible mold from the surface of each food.

12. Cut a thin, cross-sectional sample of each food.

13. Place each sample on a slide and observe it under a microscope. Look for signs of *submerged* (under the surface) mold growth in the food. Record your observations and draw a sketch in the data table.

14. Discard all food samples and clean all surfaces with a sanitizing solution.

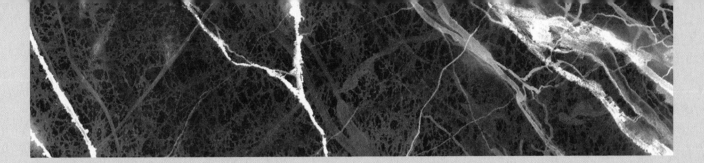

Questions

1. What texture changes occurred on moldy samples?

2. What, if any, differences were there in the appearance of the molds on each of the three samples?

3. How deeply does mold appear to grow into each of the three foods?

4. How can mold growth be prevented or delayed?

Experiment 18B
Growing Bacterial Cultures

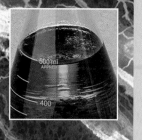

Purpose

Bacteria is present everywhere. It is not visible unless it has grown into a large colony known as a *culture*. Cultures can be isolated and studied by microbiologists. Bacteria is placed in petri dishes on a substance called agar. Agar cools into a gel and contains nutrients that aid the growth of bacteria. In this experiment, you will collect bacteria samples and incubate them to grow cultures.

Equipment

wax pencil

incubator

Supplies

1 disposable petri dish with agar per student

clear cellophane tape

Procedure

Day 1

1. Use a wax pencil to write your name on the outside of the lid of your petri dish. Draw two intersecting lines on the bottom of the dish to divide the dish into four quarters.

2. Tear off a short piece of cellophane tape. It should be long enough to fold in half with the sticky side out.

3. Gently press the sticky side of the folded tape against the surface to be tested. Immediately lift the lid of the petri dish and gently press the folded tape against the agar in one section of the petri dish. Quickly re-cover the petri dish and label the quarter on the bottom of the dish to indicate the surface tested.

4. Repeat steps 2 and 3 to test one other surface, as assigned by your teacher.

5. Lift the lid of the petri dish and gently place your thumb on a third quarter of the agar. Light pressure will reveal a thumbprint. Too much pressure will crack the agar. Label this quarter *unwashed*.

6. Wash your hands and then place a thumbprint in the last quarter of the petri dish. Label this quarter *washed*.

7. Tape the lid onto the petri dish. Turn the dish upside down and place it in an incubator as instructed by your teacher.

8. Your teacher will incubate the petri dishes at 37°C for 24 to 48 hours.

Day 2

1. Record descriptions of the bacteria colonies on your petri dish.

2. Examine the samples prepared by your teacher and record descriptions. One is the control that did not have the lid removed. The second was left open to the air for 15 minutes while samples were collected.

3. Examine the samples prepared by your classmates.

Questions

1. What procedure did you use to wash your hands?

2. How did the culture from your thumbprint compare to the cultures of your classmates' thumbprints?

3. What, if any, difference did the hand-washing procedure used make in bacterial growth?

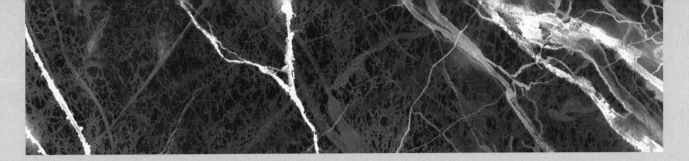

4. Did you find any sterile surfaces (surfaces that were free of bacteria)?

5. How easy is it to transfer bacteria from one place to another?

6. What differences did you observe between the control and the petri dish that was left open for 15 minutes? How could a culture start to grow on the dish that was left open?

Experiment 18C
The Gram's Stain Test for Bacteria

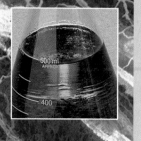

Safety

❖ Do not taste any of the samples.

❖ Clean all surfaces with a sanitizing solution at the end of the experiment.

❖ Dispose of all bacterial cultures according to teacher directions.

Purpose

Bacteria are small and hard to see, even if magnified 1,000 times. To examine bacteria, scientists spread a mixture of bacteria and distilled water on a slide to prepare a smear. The slide is air dried before being passed over an open flame several times to *heat fix* the bacteria to the slide. Failing to dry the slide before heating will cause the heated water to distort the shape of the cells. Heating the slide also denatures enzymes in the cells, which prevents deterioration of the cells. Once bacteria are heat fixed to a slide, they can be stained so they are easier to see. Stains also help identify the types of bacteria. Gram's staining is usually the first step in identifying bacteria. In this experiment, you will prepare slide samples from the bacteria you collected in Experiment 18B. After staining, you will determine whether the bacteria is gram-positive or gram-negative. You will also identify the shape of the bacteria cells.

Equipment

wax pencil

inoculating loop

gas flame source (Bunsen burner, gas stove)

1 clothespin per student

beaker or bowl

eyedropper

2 wash bottles

oil immersion microscope

Supplies

1 new microscope slide per student

distilled water

petri dish with bacteria cultures from Experiment 18B

1 to 2 drops crystal violet

Gram's iodine

ethyl alcohol

safranin

microscope tissue paper

2 drops immersion oil

Procedure
Preparing a Smear

1. Handle a new microscope slide by the edges. With a wax pencil, make a dime-sized circle in the center of the slide.

2. Sterilize your inoculating loop by holding it over a gas flame source until the loop is red hot.

3. Using the inoculating loop, place 1 or 2 loopfuls of distilled water in the center of the circle.

4. Sterilize your loop again. Allow the loop to cool so any bacteria you pick up with it will not be destroyed. Cooling takes about 30 seconds.

5. Use the sterilized loop to scrape a small amount of one of the bacteria cultures grown in Experiment 18B from the petri dish. Mix the culture with the water on the slide.

6. Spread the bacteria evenly within the ring.

7. Allow the smear to air dry. This will take about 2 to 4 minutes. Do not blow on the slide, as this will cause cell positions to shift.

8. After the slide is completely dry, use a clothespin to hold the slide as you pass it over the gas flame two or three times.

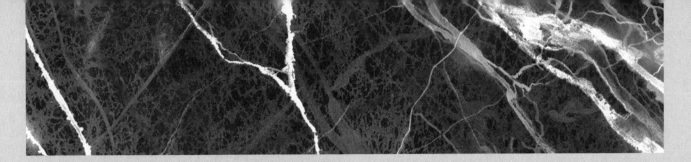

Gram's Staining

1. Hold the slide over a beaker, bowl, or sink.
2. Use an eyedropper to cover the smear with 1 or 2 drops of crystal violet. Wait 30 seconds.
3. Wash the slide with distilled water from a wash bottle. Do not squirt the water directly on the smear but on the slide above it.
4. Cover the smear with 1 or 2 drops of Gram's iodine. Wait 30 seconds.
5. Wash the slide with ethyl alcohol from a wash bottle until the alcohol runs clear.
6. Cover the smear with 1 or 2 drops of safranin. Wait 30 seconds.
7. Wash the slide with water from a wash bottle. Blot dry with microscope tissue paper.
8. Place the slide on the stage of an oil immersion microscope. Focus the microscope on the lowest setting.
9. Increase the magnification and fine-tune the focus.
10. Turn the lenses so 2 drops of immersion oil can be placed in the center of the circle on the slide.
11. Turn the 1000x immersion oil lens into place. Fine-tune the focus.
12. Sketch the bacteria and record observations. Identify the shape and gram type of bacteria seen.
13. If time allows, move to other stations to examine bacteria smears prepared by classmates.
14. Dispose of petri dishes with bacteria cultures and slides according to teacher directions. Wash all surfaces used with a sanitizing solution.

Questions

1. What types of bacteria were found?
2. Why is it important to wash the slide after each staining step?
3. Why do many doctors' offices swab patients' throats and conduct Gram's stain tests on the bacteria collected?
4. What can food preparation workers do to help reduce contamination of food by bacteria?

Foods begin to deteriorate as soon as they are harvested, slaughtered, or manufactured. As you have studied in previous chapters, a number of factors can also cause foods to spoil. Enzymes, microbes, oxygen, light, insects, and rodents can all contribute to food spoilage. To have a variety of foods available year round, deterioration and spoilage must be slowed or stopped.

Foods can spoil in many ways. Therefore, many methods have been developed to help protect food from spoilage. Chapter 16 discussed chemicals that can be added to foods to help slow or stop spoilage. Chapter 18 revealed the role of microbial fermentation in extending the shelf life of food. However, chemicals are not enough to prevent all forms of spoilage, and not all foods can be fermented.

The following chapters will look at other processing and packaging methods used to preserve today's food supply. Chapter 19 examines thermal preservation, which is the use of heat or cold to slow deterioration. Chapter 20 studies controlling water activity through dehydration and concentration. The last chapter in this unit explores current trends in food preservation.

Spoilage will quickly destroy food quality. However, preservation methods can also change the flavor, texture, and nutritional value of foods. These changes, along with the costs of preservation, must be weighed against the increase in shelf life. Food scientists face the task of finding a balance between preventing spoilage and maintaining quality.

Unit VI
Food Preservation and Packaging

19 **Thermal Preservation: Hot and Cold Processing**

20 **Dehydration and Concentration: Controlling Water Activity**

21 **Current Trends in Food Preservation: Irradiation, Packaging, and Biotechnology**

This photomicrograph provides an unusual look at polypropylene, which is a common food packaging material.

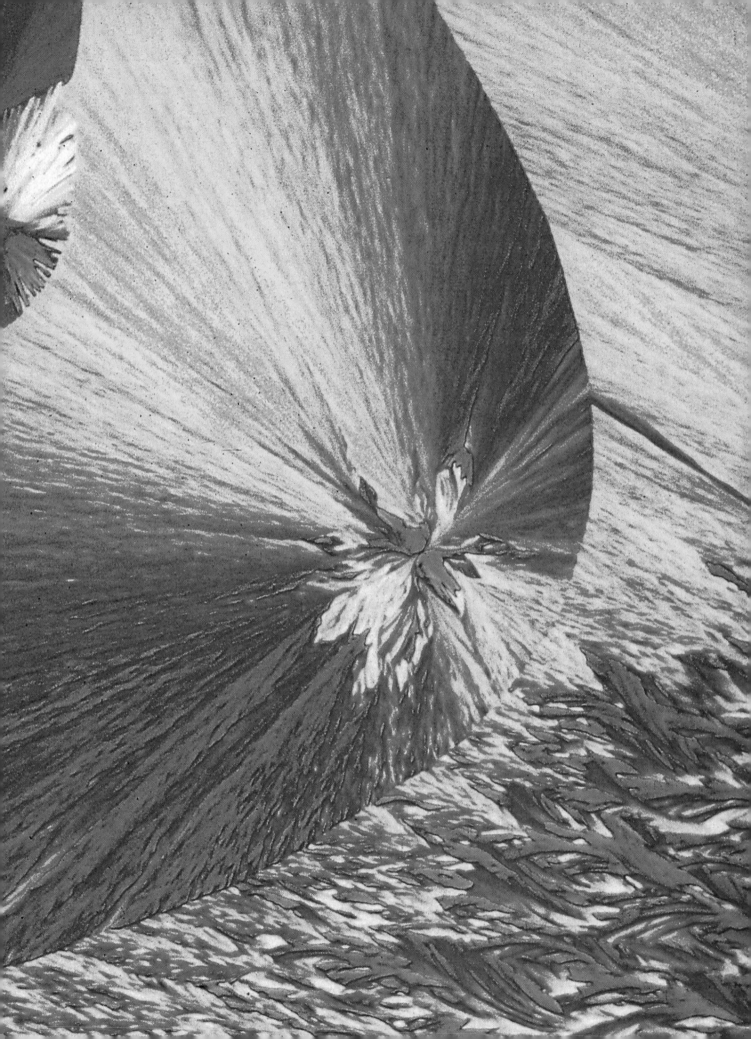

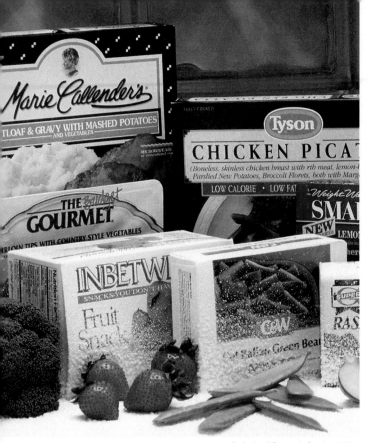

Agricultural Research Service, USDA

The freezing process has created a lot of new food options for consumers.

Chapter 19

Thermal Preservation: Hot and Cold Processing

Objectives

After studying this chapter,
you will be able to

identify the four degrees of heat preservation.

explain factors a food producer must consider before choosing a heat-preservation method.

describe commercial heat-processing methods.

determine which processing method should be used for various foods canned at home.

list variables that must be controlled to maintain the quality of refrigerated foods.

contrast the various methods used for commercial freezing.

Key Terms

shelf life
cold point
thermal death curve
retort
headspace
hydrostatic cooker
   and cooler
aseptic
cold pack method

hot pack method
water-bath processing
pressure processing
humidity
respiration
sharp freezing
blast freezer
refrigerant
cryogenic liquid

Thermal preservation involves changing the temperature or heat energy of a food. Most foods can be preserved by adding or removing heat energy. Heat processing transfers heat energy into a food. This destroys enzymes and bacteria that cause spoilage. Canned foods and bottled drinks are examples of foods that have had heat added. Cold processing pulls heat energy from foods. This slows molecular movement, which slows deterioration from enzymes and bacteria. Refrigeration and freezing are cold processing methods that remove heat energy.

Heat Processing

A goal of any food preservation method is to increase the shelf life of the food. *Shelf life* is the time a food can be stored and still be safe to eat. Cooking food is a form of preservation. This is because heat can denature enzymes and destroy microorganisms—two major factors that lead to food spoilage and contamination. However, heating food will not extend the shelf life very much unless the food is also packaged to prevent recontamination.

Degrees of Preservation

There are varying degrees of preservation as a result of heating. For example, raw milk will keep in the refrigerator for only a few days. Pasteurized milk will keep in the refrigerator for one to three weeks. Milk that has been heated to ultra-high temperatures will keep without refrigeration up to six months in a sealed package.

The food industry uses four levels of heat preservation. These are blanching, pasteurization, commercial sterilization, and sterilization.

Blanching

Blanching involves suspending food in boiling water or steam for a short period. This process denatures naturally occurring enzymes. Blanching is most often used to prepare fruits and vegetables for freezing.

Pasteurization

Pasteurization is a low-heat treatment used to preserve foods. It is designed to destroy pathogenic microorganisms and stop enzyme activity. The processing time and temperature depend on the types of enzymes and microbes commonly found in the food. Foods that are pasteurized to stop or slow enzyme activity include beer, wine, and fruit juices. Milk, oysters, and eggs are products that are pasteurized to kill harmful microbes.

Pasteurization has allowed restaurants, schools, and nursing homes to safely serve dishes that call for raw eggs. Pasteurized eggs are heated just enough to destroy any salmonellae that might be present. The eggs are still fluid. They provide a safe substitute for raw eggs in such dishes as chiffon pies, Caesar salad dressing, and eggnog. See 19-1.

Commercial Sterilization

Commercial sterilization is the level of heat preservation used for canned foods in sealed containers, including foods canned at home. All microbes that can cause illness, produce toxins, or result in spoilage are destroyed during commercial sterilization. Food may still contain small numbers of resistant bacterial spores. However, the spores cannot multiply in the canned environment. Most canned and bottled foods will keep for up to two years. Longer storage periods usually result in flavor and texture changes but not growth of microorganisms.

Sterilization

Sterilization refers to the complete destruction of all microorganisms. The temperature and length of exposure required to kill microbes varies from one microbe to another. To make sure all microbes are destroyed, all parts of a food must reach a temperature of 121°C (250°F) for 15 minutes. The heat must be *wet heat*, which means the food is in the presence of water or water vapor. This type of heat is also called *moist heat*. Wet heat is more deadly to microorganisms than dry heat at the same temperature.

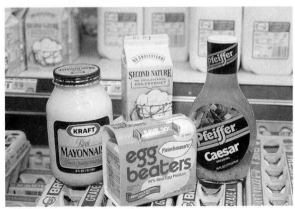

USDA

19-1 Food products like these are possible because of pasteurized eggs.

This is because water is a better conductor of heat than air. Water also penetrates microbes faster, moving heat energy to the inside of the cells.

The time required to sterilize a food depends on the amount of food. It could take several hours for every particle of food to reach the desired temperature. In many cases, complete sterilization would destroy other qualities of the food, making it inedible. As a result, sterilization is limited to foods that are in pureed or liquid form.

Variables Affecting Method

Heat processing does more than destroy microorganisms and denature enzymes. It also causes changes in texture, color, and nutritive value. The type of heat processing used must provide enough heat to preserve a food product. At the same time, the processing method must maintain as many of the food's original qualities as possible.

A number of factors identify a specific heat-preservation process. These include the kinds of foods, sizes of food particles, and desired end product. The types of processing equipment and containers are factors, too. Due to the many combinations of factors that exist, there are over 100,000 distinct heat-preservation processes. Each has been registered with and is monitored by the Food and Drug Administration (FDA).

A food producer must look at several factors before choosing a heat-preservation method. These include heat transfer in the food and cooking time versus temperature. Other factors are the components of the food product and pH.

Heat Transfer

In canning, heat is transferred through conduction and convection. (See Chapter 5, "Energy: Matter in Motion.") The method of heat transfer depends on the food.

Conduction is used when the food does not move in the can. Some foods that rely on conduction for heat transfer are corned beef hash, pumpkin pie filling, and tomato paste. Heat in these foods must be transferred by molecular collisions from the outside into the can. The more viscous the food is, the more

limited the molecular movement and the slower the heat transfer will be. The size and shape of the can become important considerations in conduction. This is because food on the outside edges of larger cans can overcook before the center has received sufficient heat.

Convection in canned foods occurs when the heating sets up currents in a liquid. Liquids near the bottom and sides of a can or bottle are heated through conduction. This causes the liquid to become less dense and rise to the top. These currents set up a stirring motion that speeds the transfer of heat energy throughout the container. Canned chicken broth and juices are examples of foods that reach the desired temperature quickly due to convection. See 19-2.

In some canned foods, such as fruit cocktail, heat is transferred through conduction and convection. These food mixtures have a liquid that heats quickly through convection. They also have chunks of food that rely on conduction to transfer heat to the center of each chunk. The timing and temperature for processing these foods are based on the largest, densest chunk of food. Manufacturers must estimate how long it would take heat to travel through this chunk if it were in the center of the can.

Processing times are based on how long it takes an entire can of food to reach the necessary temperature. The last point in a can or mass of food to reach the desired temperature

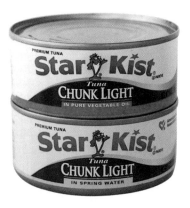

19-2 Tuna is packed in oil or spring water. Because oil is a poor heat conductor, it takes longer to process tuna in oil than tuna in water.

is called the *cold point.* In conduction, the cold point is the center of the container. When convection is involved, the cold point will be below the center point of the can. This is because the coldest portion of the liquid is also the densest. This portion will sink toward the bottom of the container. Processing times can be determined by running a test batch of the food. Temperature probes are inserted into the cans to measure progress.

Time Versus Temperature

Canning involves balancing the effects of heat on pathogens against the effects of heat on food products. A thermal death curve is used to determine the cooking time and temperature needed to kill a specific microorganism. A *thermal death curve* is a line plotted on a graph. It shows how long it takes to destroy a microorganism at a given temperature. The lower the temperature is, the longer the cooking time needs to be.

Table 19-3 shows the thermal death curve for *C. botulinum.* According to the chart, green beans could be cooked to 127°C (261°F) for 0.78 minutes. They could also be cooked to 100°C (212°F)for 330 minutes. The first temperature is fast and causes minimal damage to the beans. However, home canning equipment cannot achieve this temperature. On the other hand, boiling beans at 100°C (212°F) for

330 minutes would result in mushy beans with a brownish-green color. Few people would care to eat green beans that had such an unappealing texture and appearance. People who can green beans at home use a pressure canner. When used at a specified pressure, pressure canners can reach a sterilizing temperature for a length of time between these extremes.

Food Components

The food itself will affect the heat-processing method that should be used. Potential microorganisms, ingredients, particle size, and food density must all be considered.

The type of microbe with which a food is likely to be contaminated helps determine the choice of processing methods. This is because different microbes are destroyed by different temperatures. Foods like green beans may be contaminated with *C. botulinum.* They require higher processing temperatures than eggs, which are at risk for salmonellae.

Some ingredients can protect microorganisms from heat, making it necessary to increase processing time and/or temperature. Some food components can interfere with wet heat penetrating the food. Food components that have protective qualities are sugar, starch, protein, fats, and oils.

In addition to protective effects, some ingredients will slow the conduction process. Fat is a poor conductor of heat as compared to water. This is one reason tuna in vegetable oil will take longer to process than tuna in water.

The particle size and the density of a food product can also affect the choice of processing methods. The larger the particles in a food product are, the more the product must rely on conduction. Similarly, dense products must rely on conduction more than products with a thin consistency. For example, fruit in a heavy sugar syrup must be processed longer than fruit in light syrup.

If a liquid is thickened with starch, it can change from a convection heating system to a conduction heating system. The gravy in beef stew would be an example of a starch-thickened liquid that acts as a conduction heating system. Modified food starches have been developed that do not thicken until late in the heating process. Some modified starches do

Thermal Death Curve for
C. Botulinum

| Temperature | | Processing Time |
°C	°F	(minutes)
127	261	0.78
124	255	1.45
121	250	2.78
118	244	5.27
116	241	10.00
110	230	36.00
104	219	150.00
100	212	330.00

19-3 This chart shows the minimum processing times and temperatures that will kill *C. botulinum* in low-acid foods (pH 4.6 or higher).

not thicken until the food product begins to cool. This allows mixtures to be processed more quickly. Damage to the food is reduced while the desired thickness of the finished product is maintained, 19-4.

pH of the Food

A key factor that affects the choice of heat-processing methods is the pH of a food. The reason this factor is so critical is simple. The microbes that contaminate high-acid (low pH) foods can make you sick. *Clostridium botulinum*, which contaminates low-acid (high pH) foods, can kill you!

Most microbes can be destroyed by the temperature of boiling water. However, *C. botulinum* requires higher temperatures to be destroyed. Therefore, high-acid foods can be heat processed at 100°C (212°F). However, low-acid foods must be processed by methods that can bring the food to higher temperatures.

Remember that pH is a measure of acidity or alkalinity. A pH of 7 is neutral. A pH higher than 7 is alkaline, and a pH lower than 7 is acidic. The dividing line between high-acid and low-acid foods is a pH of 4.6. High-acid foods have a pH between 2.0 and 4.6, and low-acid foods have a pH of 4.6 or higher. Low-acid food will allow *C. botulinum* to survive and multiply.

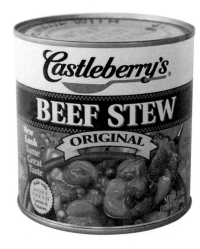

19-4 Thickened canned foods, like this stew, use modified food starches that do not thicken until late in the canning process. This shortens processing times.

Commercial Heat Processing

The commercial food processor must think about three main points when choosing a heat-processing method. The first point is safety. The method selected must destroy harmful microbes. The food processor's second consideration is food quality. The processor will decide which treatment will destroy microorganisms while maintaining the highest food quality possible. A third point is the cost of the production method. A cost study must look at packaging material, equipment costs, energy use, shelf life, and shipping costs.

The heat-processing methods available can be divided into two broad categories. The first category is heating food after it has been packaged. This is the method used in all home canning processes. The second category is heating food prior to packaging. This category involves sterile conditions and equipment that cannot be obtained in the home kitchen.

Heating Food After Packaging

Most heat-processing methods that heat food after packaging use one of two basic systems. These are an enclosed canning system and a conveyor belt system.

Retort

The huge pressure canners that are used by commercial food processors are called **retorts.** All retorts have a large, sealed chamber with special locks and valves to hold the filled cans. Internal pressure and temperature can be monitored throughout the heating process.

The simplest commercial canner is a *still retort*. It works on the same principle as a home pressure canner. The cans of food remain still during processing. This makes it possible for food to burn or stick to the can walls. For this reason, still retorts are limited to temperatures of 121°C (250°F) or lower. Still retorts are economical to produce but require long cooking times to bring the cold point to sterilizing temperatures. See 19-5.

Agitating retorts gently shake the cans during processing. This reduces the processing time for liquid and semiliquid foods. Not only does a shorter cooking time save energy, it

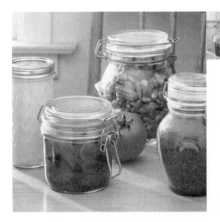

Historical Highlight
History of Canning

Canning is a common method of food preservation that combines heat and vacuum-sealed packaging to extend shelf life. The canning process was developed in 1795 by a French chef named Nicholas Appert.

Napoleon wanted a food source his troops could use on long marches. He offered 12,000 francs to anyone who could find a suitable way to preserve the food. After receiving his prize money, Appert further developed

the process. He then established the first commercial canning factory. However, it was not until Louis Pasteur's work with microorganisms 50 years later that anyone could explain why canning worked.

---

also means improved food quality. Agitating retorts can use temperatures higher than 121°C (250°F) to further reduce cooking times. This is because food is less likely to stick to the can walls. Agitating retorts require more headspace in the can to allow for the motion of the shaking food. *Headspace* is the space left in a container after adding food. This space allows for the expansion of the food during heating.

Hydrostatic Cooker and Cooler

A *hydrostatic cooker and cooler* is a modified U-shaped tube filled with water and steam. It is usually an agitating-type cooker that has processing times and temperatures similar to an agitating retort. The cooker has a conveyor belt to continuously transport filled cans, bottles, and jars from one end to the other. As the food containers move on the conveyor belt through the tube, temperature and pressure are gradually increased then reduced. This prevents sudden changes that could cause glass containers to burst.

As food containers enter the first leg of the U, they move into hot water. The water gradually increases the temperature in the containers. The lower section of the U is enlarged and raised so it fills with steam from the hot water.

This is the sterilizing zone where temperature and pressure can be controlled as in a retort canner. The last leg of the U holds cool water to gradually reduce the temperature in the containers. See 19-6.

Heating Food Before Packaging

Foods that are easily damaged by heat need processing times to be as short as possible. Many heat-sensitive foods are processed by methods that involve heating the food before packaging. These methods help minimize processing times.

Batch Pasteurization

The oldest method of heating prior to packaging is batch pasteurization. This method works best with liquids like milk. The liquid is heated in a large vat with mild stirring. Once the processing is complete, the liquid is pumped over a cooling plate and packaged and sealed. In batch pasteurization, milk is heated to 63°C (145°F) and held for 30 minutes. This method is still used in many smaller dairies.

Cooking time and temperature depend on the pathogens that may be present in a food. Dairy products need 63°C (145°F) to destroy *Mycobacterium tuberculosis.* Salmonellae in

Retort Processing Sequence

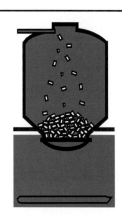

1. Loading. The retort is filled with water to cushion the cans and prevent damage. Then cans are loaded into the retort.

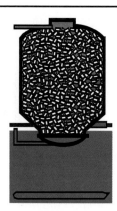

2. Start-up. Steam replaces the water in the fully loaded retort.

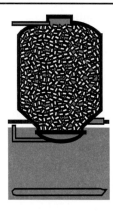

3. Processing. The cans are processed for the required time at the proper pressure and temperature.

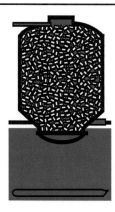

4. Cooling. The retort is filled with water to cool the cans.

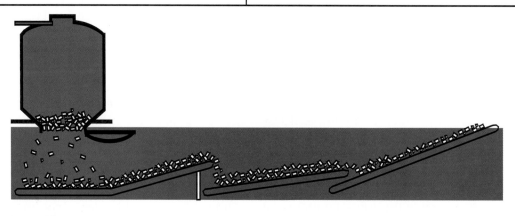

5. Discharge. The cans are discharged into a water-filled canal for final cooling before proceeding to labeling.

■ water   ■ steam

Malo, Inc.

19-5 Using the same principles as home canning equipment, commercial retorts process hundreds of cans of food at one time.

Hydrostatic Cooker and Cooler

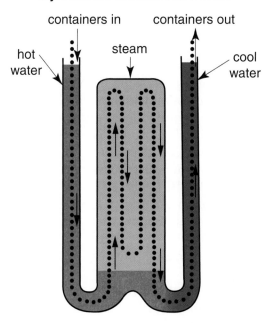

19-6 Food containers move through a hydrostatic cooker and cooler on a conveyor belt. Temperature and pressure are gradually increased and decreased in the U-shaped tube to process the food.

eggs is destroyed at 60°C (140°F). Mold spores in grape juice are killed at temperatures of 75°C to 85°C (167°F to 185°F).

High Temperature-Short Time Pasteurization

High temperature-short time (HTST) pasteurization rapidly heats and cools liquids. This system pumps the liquids through lengths of tube wrapped around a heat exchanger. The lengths and diameters of the tubes allow every food particle to reach the sterilizing temperature for the necessary time. The temperature is monitored and the fluid reheated if necessary. HTST pasteurized milk is heated to 72°C (161°F) for 15 seconds. After heating, the liquid moves through cooling tubes and is immediately packaged and sealed.

Aseptic Canning

Aseptic means free of pathogens. Aseptic canning involves preserving food to the commercial sterilization or sterilization level. The food is then placed in sterilized containers in a sterile environment. Aseptic canning requires large, self-contained processing machinery. The machinery must be carefully laid out and monitored. It completes all steps from the time the food enters the system until sealed packages exit at the other end. Aseptic canning is sometimes referred to as ultrahigh-temperature (UHT) sterilization. It can use temperatures as high as 150°C (302°F) for as little as 1 to 2 seconds.

Aseptic canning can be used for containers ranging from individual packets up to tank cars, 19-7. For instance, aseptic canning can be used to process tomato paste in 55-gallon drums. This provides a low-cost way to supply tomato paste to a company that makes pizza sauce.

Aseptic canning can be designed to use a wide variety of packaging materials. Packaging material that is heat sensitive can be sterilized with sprays of hydrogen peroxide, heated air, or ultraviolet light. This allows the use of lightweight plastics, paper, or thin foil. For instance, large plastic bags in cardboard boxes are used to hold aseptically packaged liquid eggs.

Home Canning Methods

Home canning can be a good way to store home-grown fruits and vegetables. It can also help people take advantage of low, seasonal food prices.

Aseptic Packaging

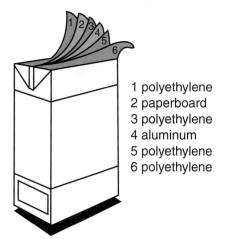

1 polyethylene
2 paperboard
3 polyethylene
4 aluminum
5 polyethylene
6 polyethylene

19-7 One of the most familiar aseptic containers is the drink box, which is made of multiple layers of packaging material.

Effective home canning involves choosing the right packing and processing method for each food to be preserved. First, the appropriate packing method is selected. Then the food is processed with the correct method for its pH. Keeping foods safe means using the right equipment and following guidelines exactly when canning foods at home. See 19-8.

Packing the Food

Food can be packed in canning jars before or after heating. In the *cold pack method,* food is prepared and packed in sterilized containers without preheating the food. Boiling water or syrup is poured over the food in the container. The container is then sealed and processed. The cold pack method is recommended for foods that are easily damaged. Peaches and berries that tend to fall apart during cooking are foods that might be packed this way. Foods prepared by the cold pack method will be firmer and hold their shapes better. However, a longer processing time is usually required than for hot-packed foods.

In the *hot pack method,* foods are heated in syrup, juice, or water prior to packing in containers. This method is used for foods, such as tomato sauce, that would be diluted if boiling water was added. The hot pack method softens foods like green beans. This allows the food to pack more closely, reducing the number of containers needed to store the food.

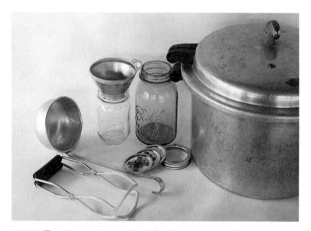

19-8 Equipment needed for home canning includes a pressure canner, jar lifter, ladle, large funnel, canning jars, caps, and rings.

Methods of Processing

After the food is packed, it must be processed. The major factor in determining which processing method to use is the pH of the food.

Water-bath processing involves submerging the sealed containers in boiling water. This method is recommended only for high-acid foods, with a pH below 4.6. The length of time a food is processed depends on the food and the size of container used. The cold point must reach at least 88°C (190°F). This is the temperature needed to destroy pathogens found in high-acid foods. Foods that can be safely processed using the water-bath method include most fruits, pickles, and acidified tomatoes.

Pressure processing is heating containers of food under pressure. This is the method that must be used when processing low-acid foods. Pressure processing is done in a pressure canner. This type of canner has a lid that locks into place. It also has a steam gauge or vent that allows the atmospheric pressure to be raised. The containers of food are set in about 1 inch of boiling water, and the lid is locked in place. Steam is allowed to build up in the canner as air is vented, causing the pressure to rise. The boiling point of the food depends on the kind of liquid in which it is packed. The boiling point also depends on the temperature and the atmospheric pressure. The pressure in the canner must become high enough to raise the boiling point to 121°C (250°F). This is the temperature required to destroy *C. botulinum* spores. Foods that must be pressure processed include corn, green beans, carrots, and meats. See 19-9.

Cold Processing

Most food spoilage is the result of chemical reactions that involve microbes or enzymes. The speed of chemical reactions is directly related to the temperature. For every 10°C (18°F) increase in temperature, chemical reaction rates are roughly doubled. Cold processing methods preserve food by slowing the chemical reaction rate in the food. Chilling does not kill most microbes or denature enzymes. It merely slows the deterioration of

pH of Foods

High-Acid Foods	pH	Low-Acid Foods	pH
Dill pickles	3.2–3.5	Meats	5.1–7.0
Jams and jellies	3.1–3.5	Melons	5.2–7.1
Most fruits	3.0–4.6	Most vegetables	4.9–7.5
Tomatoes	4.2–4.9	Poultry	5.7–6.8
Vinegars	2.0–3.5	Seafood	4.8–7.3

19-9 Although foods fall within a range of pH levels, they can be generally classified as high-acid (2.0 to 4.6) or low-acid (4.6 or higher). The pH of soups, stews, and other combination dishes depends on their ingredients, but they are usually treated as low-acid foods.

the food, thereby extending the shelf life. When chilled foods are brought back to room temperature, the rate of the spoilage process will increase.

Refrigeration

Refrigeration is the gentlest method of food storage. It causes few changes in taste or texture. Although refrigeration will not stop spoilage, it slows spoilage enough to avoid waste and stretch the use of many foods. For example, cooked poultry held at room temperature should be discarded after two hours. However, cooked poultry that has been properly refrigerated can be safely eaten for up to two days.

Ideally, refrigeration begins right after produce is harvested or an animal is slaughtered. Enzymatic deterioration can begin in some fruits and vegetables as soon as they are picked. For this reason, many processors begin refrigeration in the fields with portable coolers. Sweet corn changes 25% of its sugar content into starch within 24 hours if the temperature is 20°C (68°F). At 0°C (32°F), only 20% of the sugar is lost after 4 days. (Newer varieties of hybrid sweet corn bred for the lasting quality of sugar content will keep much longer.) Meat must be cooled from 38°C (104°F) to 2°C (36°F) within 24 hours of slaughter to maintain its quality. The more rapidly a manufacturer can chill a food, the better the quality and nutritive value will be maintained. This is true whether the food is to be eaten fresh or preserved by canning, freezing, or drying.

Variables to Control

There are variables that must be controlled with refrigeration. Just as each food responds differently to heat processing, each food has unique requirements for refrigeration. These variables are temperature, air circulation, humidity, and gas atmospheres.

Temperature

The temperature that is best for each food is different. Lettuce and tomatoes for a tossed salad keep best at 0°C to 1°C (32°F to 34°F). The cucumbers and bell peppers for the same salad prefer temperatures of 3°C to 5°C (37°F to 41°F). The variety of a food or changes in growing conditions can affect storage needs. For example, a Red Delicious apple stores best at 0°C (32°F). However, a McIntosh apple prefers 2°C to 5°C (36°F to 41°F). See 19-10.

Refrigerators must be designed to maintain temperatures below 4°C (40°F). A properly designed refrigeration unit will maintain the desired temperature within ±1°C (2°F). The temperature in home refrigerators varies from one section to another. Because cold air sinks, the lower sections are colder than the top. Many refrigerators have the meat drawer at the bottom of the refrigerator where the air is coldest. Fruit and vegetable drawers should be higher to prevent freezing.

Preferred Refrigeration Temperatures for Perishable Foods

	Storage Temperature		
Food	**°C**	**°F**	**Storage Life***
Fruits			
Apples	-1–0	30–32	varies by variety
Berries			7 days
Cherries			10–14 days
Dried fruits			9–12 months
Grapes			3–8 weeks
Cranberries	2–4	36–40	1–3 months
Grapefruit	0–10	32–50	4–8 weeks
Oranges	0–1	32–34	8–12 weeks
Papayas	7	45	2–3 weeks
Pineapple	4–7	40–45	3–4 weeks
Vegetables			
Asparagus	0–4	32–40	3–4 weeks
Cabbage			3–4 months
Carrots			4–5 months
Celery			2–4 months
Corn			4–8 days
Onions			8 months
Spinach			10–14 days
Broccoli	4–7	40–45	7–10 days
Cauliflower			2–3 weeks
Green beans			8–10 days
Green peas			1–2 weeks
Peppers			8–10 days
Cucumbers	7–10	45–50	10–14 days
Eggplant			10 days
Sweet potatoes			4–6 months
Squash, acorn			4–5 weeks
Dairy			
Butter	0–2	32–36	2 months
Cheese	2	35	varies by type
Eggs			
Shell	-2– -1	29–31	8–9 months
Meat			
Beef, fresh	0–1	32–34	1–6 weeks
Hams	0–1	32–34	7–12 days
Poultry	0	32	1 week

*Storage life is in commercial refrigeration systems where optimum temperature, humidity, and air circulation can be maintained.

19-10 Each food has a preferred temperature range for maximum keeping quality in a refrigerator.

Air Circulation and Humidity

Air circulation must be maintained to help move heat away from food stored in a refrigerator. If foods are stored close together, areas in the center of foods will not be able to cool quickly. This will allow food spoilage to begin.

The air circulating within the refrigerator must be at the right humidity level to maintain maximum food freshness. *Humidity* is the measure of water vapor in the air. This measure is compared to how much water vapor the air can hold at a given temperature. If the air is too dry, it will cause moisture in food to evaporate. The moisture will then condense onto the cooling coils or colder wall spaces. This causes foods like fresh fruits and vegetables to dry out and become limp. Moisture on the cooling coils will reduce the efficiency of the refrigerator. If the air in a refrigerator is too moist, molds can begin to grow.

Each food has a preferred humidity level. Crisp vegetables need high humidity levels of 90% to 95%. On the other hand, cheeses, margarine, and nuts prefer a humidity of 70%. In some foods, the preferred humidity range is very narrow. Conventionally aged beef hangs in cold storage lockers for several weeks at 2°C (36°F). If the humidity falls below 90%, the beef becomes dry. If the humidity rises above 90%, mold will grow on the surface.

The best way to control humidity levels is with proper packaging. Eggs are coated with a thin layer of mineral oil to help prevent moisture and carbon dioxide from escaping. To avoid removing this protective coating, eggs should never be washed until just before they are used. Eggs will also keep fresh longer if stored in the cardboard or foam carton in which they were sold. Cheeses are packaged in plastic films or wax prior to ripening in cold warehouses. This maintains the proper humidity next to the cheese. Many vegetables, including cucumbers, turnips, and rutabagas, are covered with a thin layer of wax to keep moisture from evaporating.

Gas Atmospheres

Animal and plant tissues absorb and give off gas. For instance, fruits and vegetables consume oxygen and give off carbon dioxide. This process is called *respiration.*

Many enzymatic reactions involved in food deterioration require oxygen. For example, fish lose fluid and red meats turn brown when exposed to oxygen. Although respiration is slowed when food is cooled, it is not stopped. If respiration is allowed to continue in cold storage, the food's shelf life is reduced.

Changing the gas content of the air in a refrigeration unit can halt respiration and extend a food's shelf life. Most of the oxygen in a refrigeration unit can be replaced with carbon dioxide. When this is done, the lack of oxygen prevents the chemical reactions that cause foods to spoil. This is why fresh apples that are locked in a gas-tight, cold-storage warehouse will keep for over six months. Red Delicious apples that ripen in late September are now available year round. See 19-11.

Food Changes During Refrigeration

Food products can change in a number of ways during refrigeration. Some of these

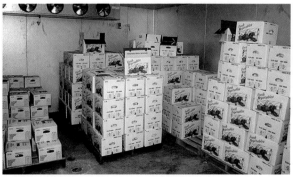

USDA

19-11 The atmosphere in cold storage rooms is adjusted to keep perishable foods fresh for extended periods.

changes are caused by the cool temperatures. For instance, bananas will turn black when they are chilled. This is because low temperatures slow enzymatic activity that helps the skins retain their yellow color. Other changes during refrigeration are due to the humidity level or the closed environment of a refrigerator. Bread will stale faster if stored in a refrigerator than if stored at room temperature. Many foods can absorb flavors and odors from other foods stored in the same refrigerator.

These changes make refrigeration a poor choice for some food products. As an example, potatoes keep best at temperatures above 4°C (40°F). With proper packaging, however, refrigeration is a good way to maintain the safety, quality, and nutritive value of most foods. For instance, carefully covering butter and wrapping cut onions will prevent odor exchange. This will keep the butter from tasting and smelling like onion.

Role of Refrigeration in Food Processing

The main function of refrigeration is preservation. However, food processors also rely on reducing the temperatures of some foods to aid in processing. Chilling is necessary for proper aging of cheese, beef, and wines. Citrus juice will have better flavor if the fruit is refrigerated prior to processing. Freshly baked bread needs to be cooled to room temperature to minimize damage to the loaf structure during slicing. Soft drinks will hold more CO_2 if the water is chilled before carbonation.

Freezing

Freezing has made possible a wide array of convenience foods. Many time-consuming preparation steps have been shifted from the chef or homemaker to the food processor. For example, you avoid spending time to mix, bake, and frost when you buy a frozen cake. You do not have to schedule time to wash, batter, and fry chicken that is ready to heat and eat.

A number of factors have led to an increase in the types of frozen foods sold in stores. These factors have, in turn, had an effect on the way people in the United States eat. Increased labor costs and a shortage of skilled chefs have prompted the development

of restaurant-quality frozen foods for home use. People no longer have to leave home to enjoy some of their favorite restaurant foods. The increase in two-career and single-parent households has spurred the frozen food industry to bring out more single-serving products. The ease of simply reheating frozen products has resulted in fewer families preparing foods from scratch. It has also allowed many family members with busy schedules to eat different foods at different times. Children may prepare a frozen pizza for an early supper following after-school activities. Parents may opt for frozen entrees later in the evening after getting home from work.

The main advantage to freezing is the increased shelf life. The fresh poultry that keeps up to 2 days in refrigeration will safely keep for 8 months at -7°C (20°F). It will keep for 15 months at -12°C (10°F) and 27 months at -18°C (0°F). These storage times and temperatures are for commercial freezers. Home freezers are opened and shut frequently. This causes temperature fluctuations that can speed deterioration. Therefore, for maximum quality, frozen poultry parts stored in a home freezer should be used within 9 months. Frozen whole birds should be used within 12 months.

It is important to follow storage charts regarding the shelf life of frozen food, 19-12. Although a pork roast will keep for a year in a deep freezer, bacon will keep only two months. In general, larger cuts of meat keep longer than small ones.

Factors That Affect Rate of Freezing

Food processors must examine several factors before determining the best method for freezing food. These factors are food components, package size, temperature, and airflow.

Different food components freeze at different rates and temperatures. Water conducts heat away from food faster than fat, and fat conducts heat faster than air. Meat surrounded by a thick layer of fat will freeze more slowly than meat with the fat layer removed. Frozen ice pops, which are flavored water, will freeze faster than ice cream bars, which are high in fat.

The thicker a package of food is, the longer it will take to freeze in the center. A roast that is four inches thick will take longer to freeze than a one-inch steak.

The colder the temperature is, the faster a food will freeze. All the principles of heat transfer discussed in heat processing apply to the freezing process. The difference is that heat is being removed from the food rather than added to it.

When airflow is increased, freezing will occur at a faster rate. This is because the air helps move heat energy away from the food.

Freezing Methods

In home freezers, food is frozen by exposure to still cold air. Commercial food processors use three basic methods to freeze foods. These are contact with cold air, indirect contact with a cooling medium, and immersion into a cooling medium.

Still Air Contact

Contact with still cold air is the oldest and cheapest method of freezing food. It is also the slowest. Food is placed in an insulated room with a temperature of -23°C to -30°C (-9°F to -22°F). Home chest freezers are closer to -18°C (0°F). The freezing time depends on the food, the package size, and the space left between packages. It may take hours or days.

The still air method is referred to as *sharp freezing.* By circulating the air in the freezing area, processing time can be shortened. Freezers that use airflow to speed freezing are called *blast freezers.* Blast freezers can be as

Shelf Life of Frozen Foods

Food	Recommended Storage Time
Beef	6–12 months
Bread	2–3 months
Fish	3–4 months
Fruits and vegetables	9–12 months
Ground meat	3 months
Ice cream	2 months
Lamb	6–9 months
Pork	3–6 months
Poultry	6–8 months
Processed meats (ham, hot dogs)	2 months

19-12 For best quality, use frozen foods within recommended storage times.

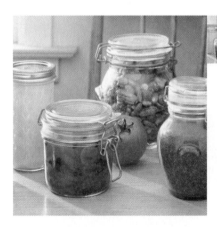

Historical Highlight
A Brief History of Frozen Food

Chilling food is an old method of preservation. Years ago, people in cold northern climates hung animal carcasses in sheds. The meat stayed frozen until it was cut off and taken inside to cook and eat. People also lowered containers of milk onto shelves inside hand-dug wells. This kept the milk cool during hot summer weather.

In the 1920s, Clarence Birdseye began research into quick freezing methods. He also studied freezing equipment, frozen food products, and packaging. One result of his research was the founding of the first frozen food packaging and distribution business. The invention of refrigerated vehicles and warehouses allowed the frozen food industry to grow. As refrigerators and freezers became common in many homes, the use of frozen foods became widespread.

simple as adding fans to circulate air in a cold room. They can be as complex as wind tunnels. This type of blast freezer uses conveyor belts to move foods through the freezing area at carefully timed speeds. The addition of airflow can reduce freezing times from hours to minutes.

There are several benefits to decreasing the processing time. These benefits include saving labor and energy costs for the food processor. Another major benefit is the rapid slowdown of microbe growth and enzyme activity that leads to spoilage. The less time it takes to completely freeze a food, the less the food can deteriorate. In addition, smaller ice crystals are formed, resulting in less cell damage than that caused by large crystals formed during slower freezing. Shorter freezing times also decrease the chances of contamination. See 19-13.

Indirect Contact

Indirect contact freezing requires the use of a refrigerant. A *refrigerant* is a fluid that can be used to remove heat energy from its environment. Refrigerants are liquids in subzero temperatures. Most refrigerants are also toxic.

In indirect contact freezing, a refrigerant flows through or around one surface of tubes or plates. Food is then placed in contact with the opposite surface of the tubes or plates. This is why the method is called *indirect* contact. The food never directly touches the refrigerant, only the metal surface the refrigerant has cooled.

Solid and packaged foods are frozen by contact with metal plates that are continuously chilled. Liquid foods, such as ice cream, are moved through tubes until the liquid forms a partially frozen slush. The slush is then packaged and frozen in blast freezers or by immersion.

Customized Blast Freezer

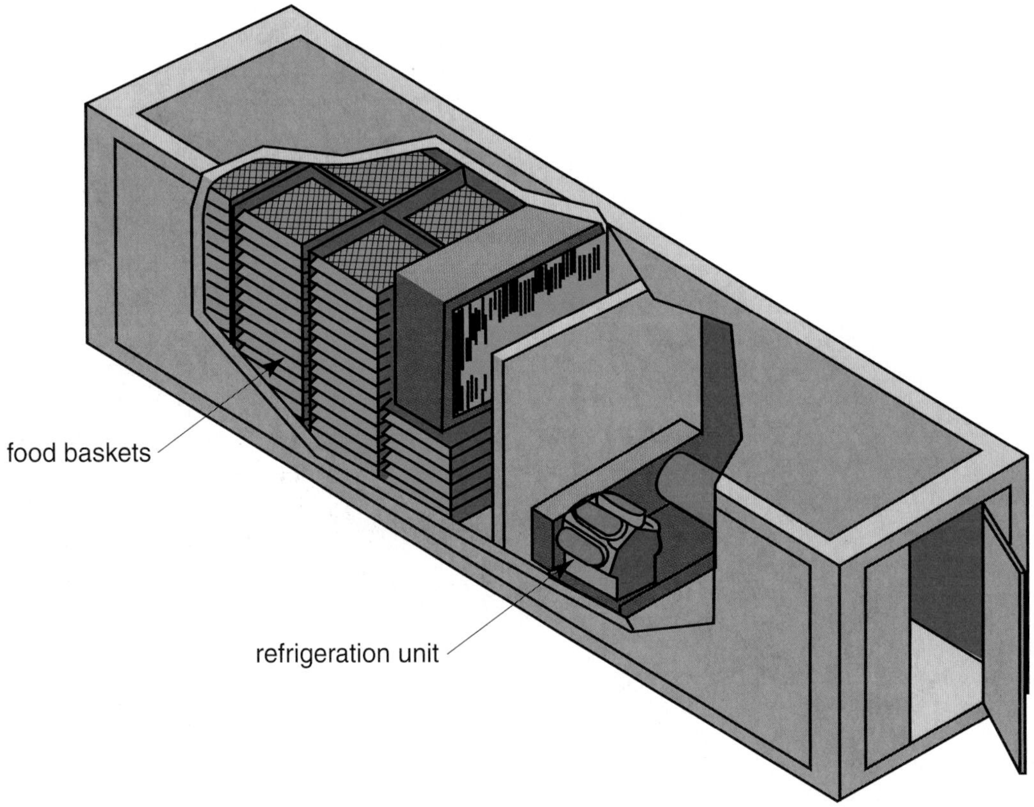

food baskets

refrigeration unit

19-13 Blast freezers contained in semitrailers can be moved near the point of harvest. They freeze thousands of pounds of food within a few hours.

Immersion

Immersion freezing surrounds foods with liquids chilled to temperatures below the freezing point of water. Because foods are immersed in the liquid, the liquid must be nontoxic and odor- and contaminant-free. There are two categories of liquids currently in use for immersion freezing. These are low-freezing point liquids and cryogenic liquids.

Low-freezing point liquids are sugar, salt, and glycerol solutions whose freezing points are lower than -18°C (0°F). For example, a 21% saltwater solution is used on commercial fishing vessels to freeze fish while still at sea. Fruits that can be sweetened can be frozen in mixtures of sugar and water or glycerol and water.

Cryogenic liquids are liquefied gases that have very low boiling points. The most common cryogenic liquid used in food processing is liquid nitrogen. Liquid nitrogen has a boiling point of -196°C (-321°F). Liquid carbon dioxide is also used in immersion freezing. It has a sublimation point of -79°C (-110°F).

Foods or food packages are sprayed with the liquefied gases, which quickly evaporate. The evaporation rapidly cools the food. Many food items can drop from 0°C (32°F) to -45°C (-49°F) in as little as one minute.

Immersion freezing has a number of advantages. One advantage is the even freezing of irregularly shaped foods, such as shrimp. A second advantage is that the speed of freezing reduces damage to foods because smaller ice crystals are formed. A third advantage is that oxygen is kept from the food by the cryogenic liquid. This minimizes oxidation damage.

The major disadvantage of immersion freezing is the high cost of the equipment and the cryogenic liquids. However, some foods, such as mushrooms, cannot be successfully frozen any other way. For these foods, the cost becomes a less important consideration.

Changes During Freezing

It is important to remember that all foods do not freeze equally well. Examples of foods that freeze well are meats, fish, poultry, blueberries, cranberries, raspberries, broccoli, corn, and peas. However, some foods, such as lettuce, green onions, and radishes, are destroyed by the freezing process.

Frozen foods often undergo textural changes. See 19-14. Frozen foods have been chilled to the point that liquid portions of the food reach a solid state. Before most frozen foods can be used, these solid portions must be thawed back into a liquid state. The phase changes of freezing and thawing create a greater possibility of damage to frozen foods than to refrigerated foods.

Most changes to frozen foods are due to the formation of ice crystals as the water in food freezes. Think about what happens to an unopened soft drink can left in the freezer. Water expands as it freezes. The pressure caused as water expands and forms ice can cause the metal can to burst. Water in food has the same ability to cause damage during the freezing process. The pressure caused as water within food cells expands can force cell walls to rupture.

Concentration Effects

Water and minerals are found in and around the cells that make up food. As free water around cells freezes, solute concentrations of salt, sugar, and other substances outside the cells increase. Water is pulled outside the cells in an attempt to balance the solute concentrations inside and outside the cells.

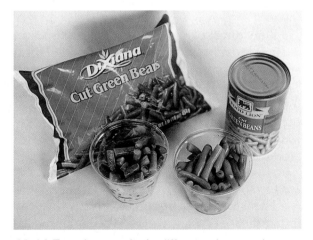

19-14 Freezing results in different changes in food quality than those caused by canning. The frozen green beans on the left have a brighter color and a crisper texture even after cooking.

The water pulled out of the cells then freezes. Not all the water pulled from cells during freezing will go back into the cells. This is partly because the freezing process damages cell tissue. The result is soggy textures in foods like lettuce.

As the concentration of solutes outside cells increases, the freezing point drops. This will slow the freezing process because it will take more time to reach the lower freezing point. A slowed freezing process can have several effects on food products. One effect is the formation of larger ice crystals. Stirring during freezing helps keep ice crystals small. Frozen sweets like ice cream can develop a gritty texture due to sugar crystals. As water freezes, lactose concentration in the unfrozen portions increases. This can cause large lactose crystals to form. A second effect of a slowed freezing process is a loss of volume in ice cream. This is because air has time to work its way out of the ice cream mixture. Another effect of slow freezing is that concentrated solutes such as salt can cause proteins to denature. This is why milk has a curdled texture if it is frozen and then thawed.

Another problem with the lower freezing point is that total freezing may not occur in the center of a food. Therefore, some microorganism growth and enzymatic activity can continue. This is a main cause of deterioration of quality in frozen foods. To ensure that freezing has occurred throughout the food, the freezer temperature must be -18°C (0°F) or lower.

Blanching prior to freezing is used to reduce microbe contamination and denature enzymes in some foods, such as vegetables. The result is higher quality vegetables with a longer shelf life. Blanching must be carefully timed to avoid overcooking the food. Once the food is blanched, it must be rapidly chilled to stop the cooking process.

Ice Crystal Damage

The slower the freezing process is, the larger the ice crystals will be. The larger the ice crystals are, the more likely they are to rupture

cell walls of plant and animal tissue. Large crystals are also more likely to break foams and gels. The jagged ice crystals will rupture the fragile bubbles in a foam, allowing air to escape. This affects the texture of whipped toppings, ice creams, and frozen puddings and custards.

Syneresis

Syneresis is leakage of water from a gel. In puddings and meats, water is squeezed from between protein and starch molecules during the freezing process. This causes these macromolecules to realign more tightly. Hydrogen bonds will form between the macromolecules. This can toughen and dry the food.

Freezer Burn

Freezer burn is damage caused by ice sublimating or evaporating out of a frozen food product, 19-15. As free water freezes, it can evaporate into open spaces in packaging or through holes in damaged packages. The evaporated water can recondense as frost either on the food, the packaging, or the walls of the freezer. Food cannot regain this loss of moisture and therefore becomes tough and dry. Freezer burn can be limited by using airtight packaging. Freezing foods quickly and avoiding thawing and refreezing will also reduce the likelihood of freezer burn.

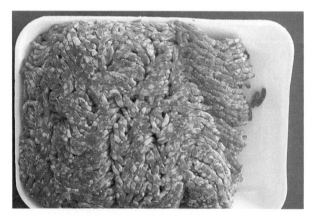

19-15 The top left corner of the hamburger in this tray is a slightly darker shade due to early stages of freezer burn.

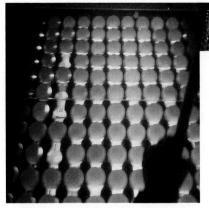

Technology Tidbit
Magnetic Resonance Imaging

Magnetic Resonance Imaging (MRI) has found wide use in the medical field. It enables doctors to capture computer images of the inside of a patient without surgery or damaging X rays. MRI works by measuring the difference in the way atoms react to a magnetic field.

Just as MRI can help doctors see inside a patient, it can help food scientists see inside food containers. MRI scans have allowed scientists to watch how food reacts to canning, freezing, and drying. MRI can be used to accurately measure heat transfer and food stability during processing.

In the future, MRI may make it possible for food to be inspected without opening and testing random samples. MRI may have the potential to improve the safety and quality of the food supply. It might be used to reduce food losses and lower production costs. MRI will also give food scientists a better understanding of the complex nature of food products.

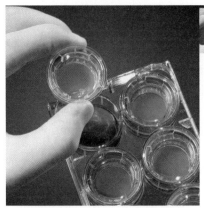

Recent Research
Aseptic Packaging

There are two significant new developments in aseptic packaging. The first is the development of silicon layers to replace the waterproof aluminum foil layer. Since silicon is microwaveable, the package and its contents can be microwaved. Traditional sauces and broths were the first products to use this new technology.

The second development is the ability to successfully process products containing food pieces. In the past, aseptic packaging was limited to liquids and purees that had very small, uniform particle sizes. In 2005 Campbell's released a new soup under the Select Gold label that contains two servings of ready-to-eat soup in a microwaveable container.

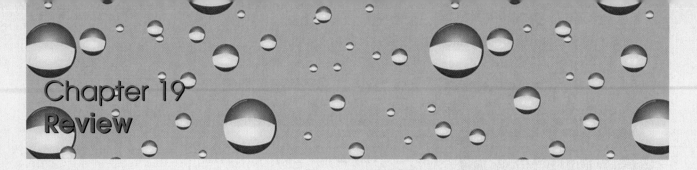

Chapter 19
Review

Summary

Most foods can be preserved through heat or cold processing. These methods involve the transfer of heat energy. Heat processing adds heat energy, which destroys most microorganisms and stops enzymatic activity. Cold processing pulls heat energy from foods, which slows deterioration from enzymes and bacteria.

The food industry uses four levels of heat preservation. Each level stops enzymatic activity and destroys microorganisms to some extent. Heat processing also causes changes to the texture, color, and nutritive value of food. A food processor must consider several factors before choosing a heat-preservation method.

Foods may be heat-processed before or after packaging. In the canning process, food is heat-processed after packaging. Commercial food processors use a retort or hydrostatic cooker and cooler for canning. Heat-sensitive foods are usually processed before packaging. In home canning, two methods of packing and processing may be used. The method of processing depends on the pH of the food.

Refrigeration is the gentlest of all food preservation methods and is ideally begun as soon as possible after harvest or slaughter. Although refrigerated foods have the least change in quality, they have a very short shelf life. Certain variables must be controlled during refrigeration. Manufacturers can extend shelf life by chilling foods according to their unique needs.

Freezing foods extends the shelf life from days to months. Commercial food processors use three basic methods to freeze foods. These are contact with still air, indirect contact with a cooling medium, and immersion into a cooling medium. The faster foods can be completely frozen, the less damage there will be to the food. However, some foods are destroyed by the freezing process.

Check Your Understanding

1. What is the goal of any food preservation method?
2. Describe the four levels of heat preservation used by the food industry.
3. List two of the factors a food producer must look at before choosing a heat-preservation method.
4. What is the cold point?
5. Explain why agitating retorts can process foods faster than still retorts.
6. List three methods of heating foods before packaging.
7. Describe the two packing methods used in home canning and list a food for which each method is recommended.
8. Why is refrigeration the first step in most preservation methods?
9. List the variables that must be controlled during refrigeration.
10. What factors affect the rate at which food freezes?
11. Name two advantages of immersion freezing.
12. Identify four ways freezing can damage foods.

Critical Thinking

1. Why are dented, corroded, and damaged cans of food not a bargain at any price?
2. Can a home canner with a small amount of peas and tomatoes process a few containers of each in the same water-bath?
3. Why should you be skeptical of a refrigerated fruit juice advertised as "all-natural, fresh-squeezed, and free of processing"?
4. Explain why opened canned foods should not be stored in the refrigerator in the original container.

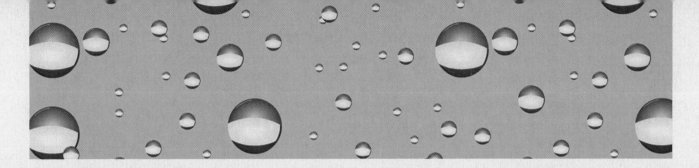

5. Why is it likely that the ears of sweet corn sold at the local supermarket are fresher and of better quality than those sold at a roadside stand?

Explore Further

1. **Technology.** Search the Internet for information about open freezer cases in the supermarket (freezers without doors) and the temperature range at which frozen food products are maintained.

2. **Math.** Compare the cost per serving of canned, frozen, and fresh vegetables. Report the results to the class.

3. **Communication.** Debate the wisdom of using only fresh produce.

4. **Reading.** Learn what impact canned foods had on the military.

5. **Communication.** Contact a manufacturer of home canning equipment to learn what information is provided with the product to promote food safety. Report your findings to the class.

Experiment 19A
Comparing Canned and Frozen Foods

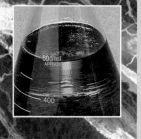

Safety

❖ **Do not taste uncooked food samples.**

❖ **Follow sanitation procedures for food preparation and cleanup.**

Purpose

Heat and cold preservation methods will slow or stop food spoilage. Adding enough heat to a food product will kill bacteria. Cold preservation methods will only slow bacterial growth. Heat will denature enzymes, preventing spoilage due to enzymatic activity. Cold preservation without heat treatment slows enzymes and therefore delays spoilage. Food scientists must consider other factors before selecting heat versus cold processing. In this experiment, you will examine how canning and freezing affect the sensory qualities of food. You will compare and contrast the color, flavor, texture, and cost of foods that are canned, frozen, and chilled.

Equipment

500-mL beaker
wax pencil
white or clear serving dish
serving spoon
1 plate per student
1 fork per student

Supplies

400 mL assigned fruit juice
1 90-mL (3-ounce) paper cup per student
1 package assigned peas or pasta product

Procedure

Part I

1. Clean a 500-mL beaker. Use a wax pencil to label the beaker with your assigned form of juice.

   Variation 1: canned juice

   Variation 2: frozen juice concentrate, reconstituted

   Variation 3: chilled juice

2. If necessary, prepare juice according to package directions. Pour 400 mL of the juice into the labeled beaker and place the beaker in a central location identified by your teacher.

3. Pour approximately 15 mL of one of the juice variations in a 90-mL (3-ounce) paper cup for each student.

4. Sample the juice variation and record your observations of color, mouth feel, and flavor in a data table. Rinse your paper cup.

5. Repeat steps 3 and 4 twice, once with each of the other juice variations.

6. Obtain information on the cost and number of servings per container for each form of juice from your teacher. Record the information in the data table.

Part II

1. Prepare your assigned product according to package directions.

   Variation 1: canned peas

   Variation 2: frozen peas

   Variation 3: canned pasta product

   Variation 4: frozen pasta product

   Variation 5: chilled pasta product

2. Place the prepared food in a white or clear serving dish with a serving spoon. Label the dish and place it in the central location identified by your teacher.

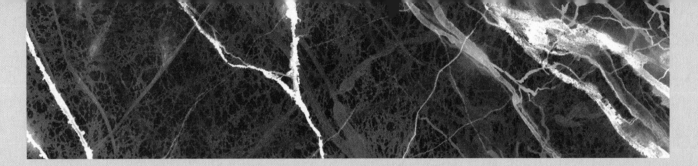

3. Take sample portions of each of the food products. Compare the samples in terms of color, texture, mouth feel, and taste. Enter the information in your data table.

4. Obtain information on the cost and number of servings per container for each food product from your teacher. Record the information in the data table.

Calculations

Calculate the cost per serving for each beverage or food tested and enter results in your data table.

Questions

1. Was there a relationship between cost and taste of the juices?

2. Which sample of peas did you prefer? Explain your choice.

3. Which sample of pasta had the firmest texture? Were any of the pastas too soft?

4. Which form of pasta was the most economical?

5. Which form of pasta was the most convenient?

6. Which pasta did you prefer overall?

7. What other variables were present that could partially account for flavor, texture, and appearance differences among the various forms of each product?

Experiment 19B
Canning Food and pH Levels

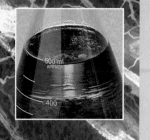

Safety

❖ Do not taste any of the food samples.

❖ Wear safety glasses when heating glass beakers.

❖ Move hot beakers with beaker tongs or hot pads.

Purpose

Foods are canned to kill harmful bacteria and denature enzymes that cause spoilage. Two methods of home canning are water-bath and pressure canning. Water-bath canning is suitable for foods that have a pH of 4.6 or lower. Low-acid foods are at risk for *Clostridium botulinum*. Because *C. botulinum* spores can survive boiling temperatures for hours, low-acid foods must be canned under pressure. Increasing pressure raises the temperature so the spores can be destroyed. In this experiment, you will puree samples of foods. You will test pH levels before and after heating. Based on the data collected, you will recommend the canning method that should be used for each food.

Equipment

electronic balance

blender

2 250-mL beakers

pH meter or pH paper

thermometer

thermometer holder

beaker tongs

Supplies

1 fresh fruit sample per lab group

1 fresh vegetable sample per lab group

200 mL water

Procedure

1. Chop or shred your assigned fruit and vegetable. (Corn and peas do not need to be chopped or shredded.)

   Variation 1: apple, corn

   Variation 2: pear, green beans

   Variation 3: peach, peas

   Variation 4: strawberries, tomatoes

   Variation 5: pineapple, green pepper

2. Mass 100 g of your assigned fruit and 100 g of your assigned vegetable.

3. Puree each sample in the blender with 100 mL of water. Process until the mixture is a slurry.

4. Pour each sample into a 250-mL beaker. Test the pH and record in a data table.

5. Heat the samples to 100°C (212°F).

6. Remove the beakers from the heat with beaker tongs. Allow the slurries to cool to 59°C (138°F) or less.

7. Retest the pH of each slurry and record the results in the data table.

Questions

1. What effect did heat have on the pH of the fruit and vegetable samples?

2. Which samples would you recommend for water-bath canning? Which samples would you recommend for pressure canning?

3. What ingredients, if any, could be added to lower the pH of a food so it could be safely canned in a water bath canner?

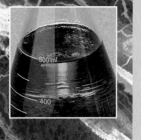

Experiment 19C
Blanching Vegetables

Safety

❖ **Follow sanitation procedures for food preparation and cleanup.**

❖ **Handle hot containers with beaker tongs or hot pads.**

Purpose

You learned in Chapter 12 that enzymes are a major factor in food spoilage. By denaturing enzymes, you can stop enzyme activity and increase the shelf life of a food. In this experiment, you will examine vegetable samples after they have been frozen to determine the benefits of blanching.

Equipment

3 freezer containers or 1-pint resealable plastic freezer bags

1000-mL beaker or 1-quart saucepan

beaker tongs

colander

large mixing bowl

Supplies

masking tape

750 mL (3 cups) assigned fresh vegetable

530 mL (2 cups plus 2 tablespoons) water

1000 mL (4 cups) ice water

plastic wrap

Procedure

1. Write your lab group number and class period on each of three masking tape labels. Afix one label to each of three freezer containers.

2. Wash and cut assigned vegetable into bize-sized pieces.

    Variation 1: green beans

    Variation 2: corn

    Variation 3: carrots

    Variation 4: broccoli

    Variation 5: cauliflower

    Variation 6: snow peas

3. Place 250 mL (1 cup) of the vegetable into a freezer container and label *untreated*.

4. Pour 500 mL (2 cups) of water into a 1000-mL beaker or 1-quart saucepan. Bring the water to a boil.

5. Add 250 mL (1 cup) of the vegetable to the boiling water. Allow the water to return to a boil and cook the vegetable for 3 minutes.

6. Immediately drain the vegetable in a colander.

7. Submerge the blanched vegetable in a large mixing bowl filled with 1000 mL (4 cups) ice water to stop the cooking action.

8. When the vegetable is cool to the touch, drain the vegetable and place it in a second freezer container labeled *blanched*.

9. Place the remaining 250 mL (1 cup) of the vegetable in the 1000-mL beaker with 30 mL (2 tablespoons) of water. Cover the beaker with plastic wrap. Turn back a corner of the plastic wrap to create a vent through which steam can escape. Microwave the vegetable on high power for 4 to 5 minutes, or until tender.

10. Submerge the cooked vegetable in the bowl of ice water to cool quickly.

11. Drain the vegetable and place it in a third freezer container labeled *cooked*.

12. Place all three containers in a freezer for 6 to 8 weeks.

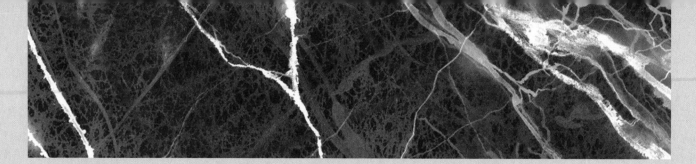

6 to 8 Weeks Later

1. Remove the three containers from the freezer.

2. Record observations of color and appearance of each vegetable sample in a data table.

3. Microwave the untreated and blanched samples until tender. This will take approximately 3 to 5 minutes. Time will vary depending on the wattage of the microwave oven.

4. Allow the cooked sample to defrost as you reheat it in a microwave oven. This will take approximately 2 to 4 minutes.

5. Conduct a sensory evaluation of all three samples. Record your observations of color, texture, and flavor in the data table.

Questions

1. What effect did blanching have on the vegetables?

2. Which method for preparing frozen vegetables resulted in the best color?

3. Which method resulted in the best texture?

4. Which method resulted in the best flavor?

5. Why were the vegetables submerged in ice water?

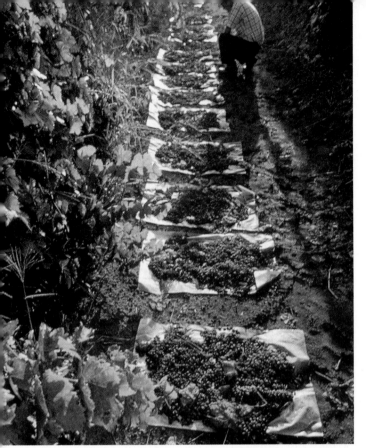

Agricultural Research Service, USDA

Grapes dried by the sun in the field near the grape vines become one of the most popular dehydrated foods—raisins.

Chapter 20

Dehydration and Concentration: Controlling Water Activity

Objectives

After studying this chapter,
you will be able to

explain the relationship between water activity levels and food preservation.

identify factors that affect the quality of dried foods.

list the methods of commercial and home dehydration.

contrast the benefits and problems associated with food concentrates.

describe the role of intermediate-moisture foods in modern food processing.

Key Terms

dehydration

case hardening

sulfiting

sulfuring

dehydrofreezing

concentration

concentrate

intermediate-moisture food

Corn on the cob spoils within days of harvest if it is not canned or frozen. On the other hand popcorn will keep on a pantry shelf for years. The difference in keeping quality between corn on the cob and popcorn is water content.

In Unit V, you discovered the importance of water for the growth of microbes. Water activity (a_w) in a food mixture was identified as an indicator of how perishable a food is. There are three categories of processed foods that are preserved, at least in part, by reduced water activity levels. The categories are dehydrated, concentrated, and intermediate-moisture foods. This chapter will examine the processes used to produce each of these categories. It will also discuss rehydration of dehydrated food products.

Dehydration

Dehydration preserves food by lowering the water content. It is probably the oldest method of food preservation. Researchers have planted dried seed corn sealed in jars thousands of years ago by the Maya and Aztec Indians. After all that time, the seeds still produced a successful corn harvest. Researchers know that people have also been drying beans and fruit for centuries to extend their keeping quality.

In the food industry, dehydration is the artificial drying of a food product under controlled conditions. Protecting food from spoilage is a main function of dehydration. However, it has other benefits for consumers. When water is removed, foods become lighter and take up less space. Lightweight foods are a necessity for space travel and backpacking trips. Their weight and size often make dehydrated foods less costly to package, ship, and store than canned and frozen foods. Another benefit of many dehydrated foods is convenience. For example, instant potatoes are a dehydrated food that provides mashed potato taste and texture in about five minutes. This convenient form of potatoes saves the time-consuming process of peeling, washing, cutting, boiling, draining, and mashing. Dehydrated food products include soup mixes, nonfat dry milk, soy milk powder, raisins, prunes, and instant tea and coffee. See 20-1.

Some dehydrated foods, such as raisins and prunes, are intended to be used in their dry state. Many other dehydrated foods, such as instant mashed potatoes, are designed to be *reconstituted*. This means water is added to the food to return it to its prior state. Food manufacturers want reconstituted foods to have as much of their original flavor and texture as possible. Food processors must understand how dehydration works. They need to know what pretreatments will help foods maintain quality. Processors can then choose the best dehydration method for each food product.

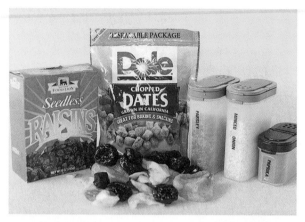

20-1 Raisins, dates, trail mix, herbs, and spices are some of the many foods available as a result of dehydration.

Role of Water Activity (a_w)

Water activity (a_w) is a measure of the free water available to support biological and chemical reactions. In Chapter 7, you studied the role of a_w in foods with a high sugar content. When most of the free water has been removed from a food, molds and bacteria cannot grow. Chemical reactions, including enzymatic activity that leads to spoilage, are slowed or stopped. Dehydration preserves food by lowering the water activity level so food spoilage is prevented.

You can use a_w to compare the free water in a food to pure water. Pure water always has an a_w of 1.00. Microorganisms need an a_w between 0.85 and 1.00 to grow. Most microbes stop growing between 0.70 a_w and 0.85 a_w. In this a_w range, foods' moisture content is at approximately 20%. Most dehydrated foods are below this a_w range with a moisture content of 1% to 15%.

Factors That Affect the Quality of Dried Foods

Dehydration involves transferring heat into a food at the same time water is released. Food processors need to balance processing speed against damage to the food. A number of factors must be studied for successful dehydration. These include the surface area of the food and the circulation of air around the food. The impact of temperature on the food and the control of oxidation and enzymatic activity must also be considered.

Surface Area

Increasing the exposed surface area of the food will speed the travel of heat to the center of the food. The faster the heat reaches the center, the faster the water will move out of the entire food product. Food to be dehydrated is usually cut or sliced into thin, small pieces. In addition, the food pieces need to be uniform in size and thickness. If pieces are not uniform, larger pieces may not complete the dehydration process. If larger pieces are completely dehydrated, smaller pieces will be overcooked and damaged.

If food is thick, there is a greater chance for two problems to develop. The first problem is the outside surface of the food can become damaged. The result can be unpleasant flavor changes and tough, rubbery textures. The second problem is the increased chance of incomplete dehydration in the center of the food. If any portion of the food is not dehydrated enough, there is a risk that bacteria or mold can grow.

Airflow

You may have noticed that your hair dries faster when you use a blow-dryer. The combination of heat and moving air speed the drying process. The same principle is important in food dehydration. Airflow helps move moisture away as it is released from the food. This allows the food to dry more rapidly and evenly.

Commercial and home dehydrators use a heat source, a fan or blower, and a large ventilated drying surface. Food pieces are arranged on the drying surface in such a way that air can circulate. Then a mechanism in the dehydrator draws the moisture from the food out of the system. See 20-2.

Temperature and Case Hardening

Controlling the temperature is critical to successful dehydration. For every 15°C (27°F) rise in temperature, the amount of moisture the air can hold in vapor form doubles. This is because increasing temperature increases heat energy. This, in turn, increases the amount of water that can stay in a gaseous state.

The faster a food is dehydrated, the less change there is likely to be in food quality.

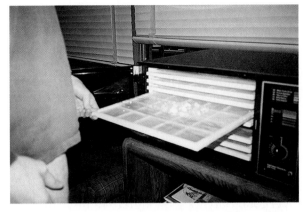

20-2 Trays in a home food dehydrator allow air to pass through to speed the removal of moisture from food.

Raising the temperature will speed dehydration. If a food is heated too quickly, however, a dry skin can form on the outside of the food. This skin will trap moisture in the food. This is known as *case hardening.*

Case hardening is more common in foods that contain dissolved sugars or salts, such as dried fruit and beef jerky. Moisture escapes through tiny pores and cracks in the surface of the food. As the water evaporates, the sugars or salts are left in the pores or cracks. At the same time, the cells on the surface of the food shrink. This causes the sugars or salts to block the openings in the food's surface. Moisture that is still in the food then has trouble escaping. Food scientists must determine the temperature that gives maximum evaporation while preventing case hardening.

Careful monitoring of food temperature during dehydration is also important to avoid damage to the food from high heat. To understand how damage could occur, think about sitting in the shade on a hot summer day. As your skin heats, perspiration comes to the surface. When a breeze begins to blow, the perspiration evaporates and cools the skin. The breeze moves the moist air away from the skin and replaces it with dryer air. The dry air fills with moisture and pulls heat away from the skin in order to cause evaporation. As long as there is moisture to be released, the surface of the skin remains cool. When there is no more moisture, the skin surface will absorb heat from the surrounding air. This will damage the skin, causing it to become dry and flaky.

In a similar way, the surface of food in a dehydrator cools as moving air causes moisture to evaporate. This is due to the latent heat needed for the phase change from liquid to gas. For water to change to steam, heat energy is pulled from the surface of the food and the surrounding air. This can damage the food surface.

Food processors need to move heated air over food only long enough to remove most of the moisture. If exposure to the hot air lasts too long, the food quality will begin to deteriorate. Food processors carefully test each food product. They need to determine how long it takes the temperature of food in the dehydrator to begin rising.

Oxidation

The large surface area and airflow needed for dehydration increase foods' exposure to oxygen. Remember that some enzymes, in the presence of oxygen, will react with a group of phytochemicals called polyphenols. The tannic acid that forms during this reaction is brown. The result is enzymatic browning in foods high in polyphenols, such as apples, grapes, and tea.

The temperatures used for dehydration are not high enough for a long enough time to denature enzymes. Therefore, many foods are pretreated to inactivate the enzymes and prevent browning.

Controlling Enzymatic Activity

Two basic pretreatment methods are used to stop enzyme activity in foods to be dehydrated. These are heating and adding chemicals. The treatment used depends on the type of food product.

Heat Treatment

Pasteurization is a heat treatment used to prepare foods for dehydration. Pasteurization is effective in controlling the growth of microbes in animal-based products like milk and eggs. Pasteurization temperatures are also high enough to stop most enzyme activity.

Blanching is another heat treatment that stops enzyme activity. Food is blanched by being immersed in boiling water or surrounded with steam, 20-3. In commercial settings, foods can also be blanched with microwaves. However, enzyme destruction has been shown to be spotty when microwave blanching is done in home settings.

Blanching is used mainly with vegetables. Fruits are more susceptible than vegetables to flavor and texture changes when heated. Therefore, fruits that are subject to enzymatic browning are most often treated with chemicals instead of blanching.

Sulfiting

Sodium bisulfite is a substance that slows enzymatic browning. This is because oxygen will react with sodium bisulfite before reacting with the polyphenols in foods.

Sodium bisulfite must be dissolved in water to release sulfite ions. The food is then soaked in the solution for 10 to 30 minutes. The soaking time depends on the type and thickness of the food. After soaking, the food is drained and then dehydrated. This process is called *sulfiting.*

Sulfiting has two main disadvantages. The first is the increased drying time. Soaking the food extends the drying time by 15% to 20%. A second disadvantage is that as many as one-third of all consumers are sensitive or allergic to sodium bisulfite. It can cause breathing difficulties in many people. Foods most likely to contain sodium bisulfite are dried fruits, such as figs and apricots.

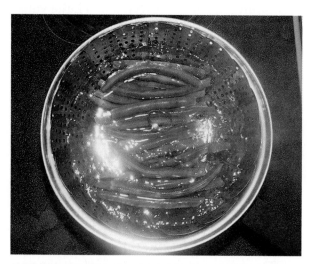

20-3 Plunging fresh vegetables into boiling water for a brief period prevents enzymatic deterioration before the vegetables are dehydrated.

Sulfuring

Most commercial food processors use another antioxidant substance to slow enzymatic browning: sulfur. In a process called *sulfuring,* fruits are exposed to fumes from burning sulfur. As sulfur burns, it combines with oxygen to form sulfur dioxide (SO_2). Food is placed on stacked trays in a covered area where the SO_2 can circulate around the food. The sulfuring process takes one to four hours. After treatment, food must be dried outside to allow the sulfur fumes to escape. Sulfur fumes will damage the lungs if inhaled. An alternative to exposing some foods to sulfur fumes is to dip them in SO_2. A disadvantage of sulfuring is that some people are allergic to SO_2. The advantages of the sulfuring process over sulfiting are listed below.

❖ Sulfuring shortens drying time because there is no soaking needed.

❖ The sulfur's odor repels insects during the drying process.

❖ The sulfur fumes inhibit mold growth. They do this by penetrating the cells and interfering with respiration and enzymatic activity.

Sulfuring and sulfiting have the following two advantages over blanching and pasteurization:

❖ Heat sensitive nutrients like vitamin C are not affected.

❖ Food retains more of its original color and texture because it is not heated and enzymatic browning is stopped.

Sulfur dioxide and sulfites destroy thiamin. Therefore, sulfuring and sulfiting cannot be used on foods that are major sources of this vitamin.

Dehydration Methods

Food processors have several basic drying methods from which to choose. Each method has many variations. To determine which method is best, food scientists consider the type of food and the quality desired. Scientists must also keep in mind how much consumers will be willing to pay for the product. Another factor in selecting the dehydration method is whether the food is whole, divided, pureed, or liquid.

Most dehydrators use heat combined with blowers to circulate the air and remove moisture from the food. A second type of dehydrator adds a vacuum to speed the transfer of moisture from the food. Lowering the atmospheric pressure enables water to escape from the food at low temperatures. It lowers the energy needed for a liquid-to-gas phase change.

Dehydrators can be classified by how the food is held or moved during the drying process. Food may be held on trays, moved by conveyor belts, placed in drums, or sprayed into heated air. When dehydrating some foods, these methods can be combined with freezing or vacuum processing.

Tray Drying

The dehydrators that are easiest and least costly to operate use trays to hold the food. The trays have holes to allow the food to dry evenly on all sides. This type of dehydrator has an enclosed cabinet that holds as many as 50 trays of food on carts or fixed racks. A fan pulls air into the cabinet over heating coils. The air then passes through screens to filter out dirt and small insects. The air is either blown over the food between the trays or rises up through the trays. The moisture-filled air is then vented out of the system. Drying times often range from 10 to 20 hours. Tray drying is usually used in small-scale operations for fruit and vegetable pieces. See 20-4.

Belt Drying

Large dehydration operations often set up drying systems that continuously feed food into a tunnel dehydrator on moving belts. In such systems, food is often placed on trays. The trays may be continually loaded onto the belt at one end of the tunnel and removed at the other. The trays may also be loaded onto carts. The carts are then moved through the drying tunnel on a belt. The drying time in these dehydrators is similar to tray dryers.

Another type of belt drying is the belt trough dryer. In this type of system, food is placed directly on the belt in a thin layer. The belt is made of metal mesh that allows heated air to blow up and around the food. The belt moves the food through controlled areas of heat and airflow. The airflow and the movement of the belt keep the product tumbling for

Tray Dryer

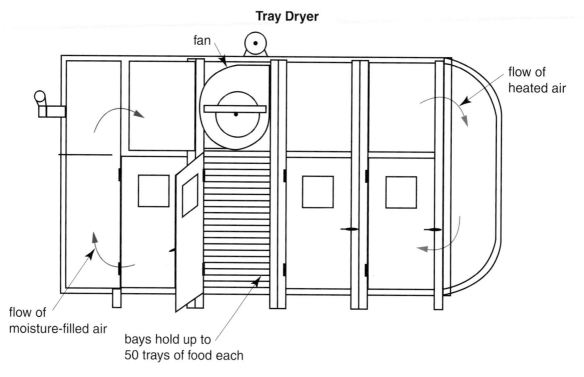

fan

flow of
heated air

flow of
moisture-filled air

bays hold up to
50 trays of food each

20-4 Some tray dryers can be expanded to hold additional tray cabinets to meet the changing dehydration needs of food producers.

even drying. This constant tumbling allows food to reach moisture levels of 5% to 7% in as little as one hour. The movement of the belt is timed so the dried food is ready for packaging as it exits the dehydrator.

Not all foods can be dried in trough dryers. Some sizes and shapes of food will not tumble well enough for even drying. Foods like apple slices are too easily broken. Foods like dates and figs become sticky as they dry. Such foods will tend to clump together, resulting in uneven drying. Grains, peas, and beans work well in this type of dryer.

Drum Drying

Many purees, pastes, and mashed foods are dried on rotating, heated drums. Steam heats the drums from the inside to about 150°C (302°F). The food is picked up by the rotating drum, dried, and scraped off by a blade into a collection system. The size of the drum and the speed of rotation depend on the drying time needed. Most foods can be dried in less than one minute. Drum drying works best with heat-resistant foods that are brittle when dry. Such foods include mashed potatoes, mashed sweet potatoes, and tomato pastes.

Spray Drying

Spray drying is the fastest method of dehydration. However, only liquid and paste foods that can be dispersed in very small drops can be dried by this method. The food is sprayed into the top of a heated tower or chamber. The air of the chamber is heated to as much as 200°C (392°F). The droplets dehydrate and fall to a collection system at the bottom. The height of the chamber is based on how long it will take this process to happen.

In this method, food can be dehydrated in a few seconds. Because of the short exposure to heat, foods are less likely to caramelize or experience nonenzymatic browning of proteins. This method is used for heat-sensitive products, such as milk, eggs, protein powders, and flavorings. Instant coffee is also produced this way.

Vacuum Drying

Vacuum drying produces the highest quality product, but it is costly. Food is placed on heated trays or shelves, which are called *platens*. The platens transfer heat to the food through conduction. The platens are located in a vacuum chamber, which is an area that is sealed so air can be removed. The atmospheric pressure in the chamber is lowered.

Remember that as atmospheric pressure is lowered, the boiling point is lowered. This means the water in food will move to a gaseous state and evaporate at a lower temperature. Fruit juices can be dehydrated in a vacuum system at temperatures as low as 40°C (104°F). This results in a minimum of heat damage. Another advantage of the low atmospheric pressure is that fruit juices do not boil and splatter.

Freeze-Drying

The newest method of vacuum dehydration is freeze-drying. This method is also called *lypholization* or dehydrofreezing. In *dehydrofreezing,* food temperatures and atmospheric pressure are lowered to the point that water will sublimate out of the food. This method is used for foods that may lose volatile flavors or be easily heat damaged.

Food to be freeze-dried is frozen. Then it is placed in a vacuum chamber that is heated slightly. The increase in the temperature speeds the release of water vapor without thawing the food. Microwaves are often used as the heat source for freeze-drying. Freeze-dried foods have many advantages over foods dried by other methods. See 20-5.

With heat-based dehydration, meats must be ground or cut into very thin slices like jerky. Freeze-drying works on steaks with a thickness of up to 2.5 cm (1 inch). Freeze-dried meats have a color and flavor similar to fresh, but they are a little tougher and drier. This drawback can be overcome by tenderizing the meat prior to cooking. Freeze-dried meats can be tenderized by soaking them in a 2% salt solution or a solution with proteolytic enzymes.

Freeze-dried foods are porous because of spaces left by the evaporated ice crystals. If the food is removed from the vacuum into an environment containing oxygen, the pores fill with oxygen. This reduces the shelf life of the food because the oxygen can react with compounds in the food. Therefore, most food processors break the vacuum in the freeze-drying chamber by adding nitrogen. The food is then packaged in lightweight, sealed material in a nitrogen-filled environment. The cost

Advantages of Freeze-Dried Foods

❖ fresher flavors because the food has not been cooked

❖ more original color because oxygen has been removed from the environment

❖ faster rehydration because there is less damage to the surface of the food than with heat-based dehydration

❖ thicker pieces are possible than with other dehydration methods because case hardening is less likely

20-5 Freeze-drying produces high-quality dehydrated foods.

of this process is the main disadvantage of freeze-drying.

Home-Dried Foods

Heat-based methods of dehydration can be done successfully in the home. The methods most often used at home are room or sun drying, oven drying, and drying with a dehydrator.

Room Drying or Sun Drying

The least expensive home dehydration method is room or sun drying. This is also the most unreliable method. Room or sun drying works best in hot, dry climates. However, people living in other climates can use this method during a period of several rain-free days.

For this method of drying, food is arranged in single layers on screens or trays. The trays are left in a warm, dry room or placed outside in the sun until dry. Some foods can be hung from hooks instead of being placed on screens. Fresh herbs are often dried this way. The herbs can be harvested and tied into small bundles. The bundles will dry if hung upside down on a screened porch for several days. See 20-6.

Oven Drying

Oven drying is another dehydration method that can be done at home. Oven drying is more costly than sun drying. It also ties up the oven for several hours and adds heat to the kitchen.

Most ovens can be easily converted into dehydrators. Laying clean stainless steel or

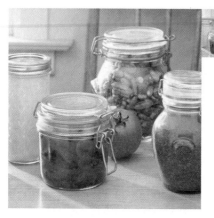

Historical Highlight
Smoking as a Means of Preserving Foods

Many ancient civilizations found they could not dry meat and fish in the sun before spoilage occurred. These peoples discovered that smoking and/or salting these foods during a drying process helped to preserve them. The smoke and salt also added pleasing flavors to the foods.

Smoking and salting work on some of the same principles as dehydration. Historically, the smoking process involved laying moist wood chips on hot coals. Hickory and mesquite were the types of wood that were often used. The smoke would rise up into a closed chamber where the food would be surrounded by the heated smoke. Smoking reduces the moisture content of food by 10% to 40%, resulting in a lowered water activity level. The smoke also contains compounds that act as natural preservatives. Phenols and carbonyls serve as antioxidants and antimicrobial agents. These chemicals, over time, penetrate the food and help prevent spoilage.

When foods are smoked by a traditional process, there is a risk of undesirable compounds getting into the food. Aromatic hydrocarbon compounds may be released in the smoke from some types of woods. The smoking process can break down proteins in foods into cyclic compounds, such as heterocyclic amines (HCAs). Both of these types of compounds have been found to be carcinogenic. Commercial smokehouses carefully control the smoking process to minimize the risk of these compounds entering the food. However, the American Institute for Cancer Research recommends that you limit your use of smoked foods.

Smoked flavor can be added to foods with a natural flavoring called oil of cade. This flavor additive is not a preservative.

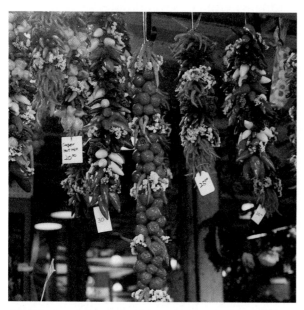

20-6 In some regions, it is common to see chili peppers suspended on strings to dry.

Teflon-coated screening on oven racks can convert them into drying trays. The screen mesh must be small enough to prevent food from falling through as it dries. People who dry large volumes of food or use this method frequently might want to purchase extra oven racks.

Food is pretreated and arranged in single layers on each rack. The racks are placed in the oven, and the oven door is propped open slightly to create airflow. The oven needs to maintain a temperature of 60°C to 66°C (140°F to 150°F) throughout the drying period. Trays must be rotated from bottom to top or food must be rearranged every hour or two.

Microwave ovens can also be used to dehydrate small amounts of some foods. To dry fresh herbs in a microwave oven, arrange single layers of stems with leaves between paper towels. Microwave the herbs on high power in two- to three-minute intervals until dry.

Herbs can be successfully microwaved because they are relatively thin. Other foods require a combination microwave-convection oven. This is because it is difficult to slice other foods thin enough to dry evenly in a microwave oven.

Cooking Tip

One food you might try dehydrating with a combination of microwave and conventional cooking is potatoes. Arrange thinly sliced, salted potatoes in a single layer on a plate or place them upright in a rack. Microwave the potato slices for 3 to 5 minutes per potato. Times may need to be adjusted, depending on the volume of potatoes and wattage of microwave oven you are using. Next, arrange the microwaved potato slices on cooling racks. Bake them in a conventional oven at 150°C (300°F) for 5 to 10 minutes, or until lightly browned and crisp. The microwave oven rapidly denatures the enzymes that cause enzymatic browning and removes most of the water content. The conventional oven allows the potato slices to become golden brown and crisp. The result is fat-free potato chips.

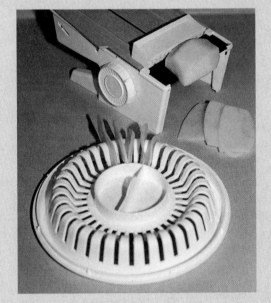

This rack separates thin slices of potato for more even dehydration in a microwave oven.

Using Home Dehydrators

A third method of home dehydration requires an electric dehydrator. The most inexpensive models have an electric heating coil in the base and a lid with air vents. A number of perforated trays stack between the base and the lid. The natural airflow created as heated air rises from the base carries moisture through the vents in the lid. Trays need to be rotated every couple hours to ensure even drying. More expensive dehydrators have a motorized fan, an enclosed chamber with removable trays, and a thermostat. The thermostat needs to be accurate to ±3°C (±5°F). Temperatures used in home dehydrators range from 57°C (135°F) for delicate fruits to 66°C (150°F) for meats.

Maintaining Quality in Home-Dried Foods

The highest quality home-dried foods start out as high-quality fresh foods. Foods to be dehydrated should be clean and free from blemishes. Fruits, vegetables, and herbs should be dried as soon as possible after harvest.

High-quality home-dried foods must be dried to the appropriate texture. The desired texture depends on the type of food. Herbs should be brittle and easily crumbled. Fruits and fruit leathers are pliable and chewy. Properly made jerky has a leathery texture with a spicy flavor. Dried vegetable pieces should be crisp.

Storing dehydrated foods properly can help them maintain their quality. Dried foods can be stored in reclosable plastic bags. After filling a plastic bag with dried food, lay the bag flat on a table or counter. Carefully press out as much air as possible before sealing. Any jar or plastic container with a lid can also be used to store dried foods. To reduce exposure to oxygen, store the dried foods in small containers that can be used quickly after opening. Discard any food that shows signs of mold growth.

Rehydration

Raisins are a dried food that makes a great snack straight from the box. Before most dehydrated foods are eaten, however, they must be *rehydrated*, or have water added back. The

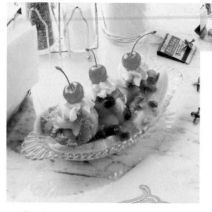

Item of Interest
Making Fruit Leather

Fruit leather is a flexible sheet of dried fruit puree. It makes a tasty, nutritious snack. Because it is compact and lightweight, it is a good choice for backpacking or other activities where space is limited.

Because of their high pectin level, apples add body and pliability to a fruit leather. When

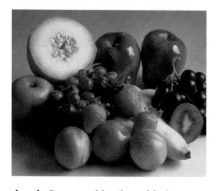

Any fruit or combination of fruits can be used to make fruit leather.

using light colored fruits, such as apples, pears, and bananas, adding lemon juice will help reduce enzymatic browning.

Ingredients:

625 mL (2½ cups) fresh fruit

15 to 30 mL (1 to 2 tablespoons) honey or sugar, if desired

10 mL (2 teaspoons) lemon juice

cinnamon, nutmeg, citrus peel, raisins, coconut, or nuts, if desired

Method:

1. Wash and drain the fruit.
2. Cut fruit in pieces and place in an electric blender or food processor container.
3. Add honey or sugar, lemon juice, and desired flavorings.
4. Puree on high speed for 1 to 2 minutes. Puree should equal 500 mL (2 cups).

5. Prepare a 15 × 10 × 1-inch jelly roll pan by lining with plastic wrap. Tape the plastic wrap in place.
6. Spread the fruit mixture evenly over the entire pan to a thickness of 6 to 7 mm (¼ inch).
7. Dry in a 60°C to 66°C (140°F to 150°F) oven for 4 to 6 hours. Leave the oven door ajar approximately 10 cm (4 inches).
8. Rotate the pan every half hour.
9. Remove the leather from the oven when the surface is no longer sticky. Remove the leather and plastic wrap from the pan. Then peel off the plastic wrap and allow the leather to cool completely. When cool, rewrap and roll.

method of rehydration varies from one food to another. Nonfat dry milk is simply dissolved in cold water before use. Instant potatoes and soup mixes are added to boiling water and cooked until tender. Dried fruits are usually covered with water or fruit juice and allowed to soak until they are plump.

Unwanted rehydration can occur when various dehydrated foods are mixed together, such as in soup mixes. Some foods need a lower moisture level than others to keep from spoiling. When foods are combined in a sealed container, moisture can transfer from one type of food to another. This can cause lumping,

flavor changes, and possible growth of microorganisms. To prevent moisture transfer, moister foods can be coated before being added to a mixture. For instance, raisins are coated with a thin layer of starch before being mixed with bran flakes in breakfast cereal. This keeps the raisins moist and the flakes crisp.

Concentration

Modern processing has created a new category of foods called concentrated foods. Many of these foods are popular convenience foods. Food *concentration* is removing a portion of the water from a food product. In some foods, it is a preliminary step to dehydration. *Concentrates* are foods that are reduced in volume by having part of the water removed. Fruit juice concentrates, condensed milk, maple syrup, and condensed soups are examples.

Concentrates are used in several ways. Fruit juices and soups are reconstituted or have water added before serving. Condensed milk is usually mixed with other ingredients in baked goods. Maple syrup is used in its concentrated form.

Benefits of Concentrates

Concentrates have a number of benefits for food processors and consumers. One benefit of concentrates is they are more economical to ship. Shipping costs are based on two factors: volume and weight. Because most of the mass of a food is in the water, removing water reduces both of these factors. See 20-7.

Most concentrates require additional preservation methods to fully protect them from spoilage. However, removing part of the

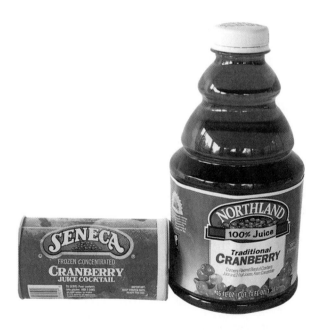

20-7 An advantage of concentrated foods is the savings in shipping and packaging costs. The concentrated juice on the left sells for just over half the price of the ready-to-drink juice on the right.

water often extends a food's shelf life. Jams and jellies will keep much longer than the fruit or fruit juice from which they are made. Jams, jellies, and molasses have a high sugar content as a result of concentration. A high sugar content reduces water activity to 0.7 or lower. At this level, pathogens are destroyed.

Some foods are concentrated before dehydration to simplify handling. For instance, pureed tomatoes are too liquid to drum dry. Concentrated tomato paste has enough viscosity to cling to a drying drum as it rotates.

Problems with Concentrates

Several undesirable reactions can occur in some foods as a result of concentration. One problem is that concentrated foods often have cooked flavors and color changes. As an example, evaporated milk is concentrated milk that is light tan in color and has a slight caramel flavor. This damage is caused by long exposure to heat. Flavor and color changes due to concentration are desirable in some foods. Such foods include caramel candies, maple syrup, and molasses.

Another problem with concentrates is the formation of sugar crystals. Chapter 7 discussed how heated water will hold more sugar than cold water. If too much water is removed from sugary foods, gritty textures can develop as the foods cool. This can be a problem in the production of jams and jellies. Sugar crystals can also form in ice cream if the lactose levels are too high. The lactose crystals make the ice cream have a sandy or gritty texture.

A third problem with concentrates can occur in high-protein foods. The concentration of salts and minerals in these foods can cause the protein to denature. Denatured protein can cause the concentrate to slowly gel over time during storage. This can occur in evaporated and condensed milks. The process is complex and can take weeks or months to develop.

A fourth problem with concentrates is the risk of foodborne illness. The safety concern is due to the low temperatures used for concentration. The temperatures used in some concentration methods will kill microbes but allow bacterial spores to survive. When concentration is done by a vacuum method, the temperatures are even lower. At these low temperatures, many bacteria can multiply in the food. Food safety is not as much of a concern with high-acid foods, such as orange juice concentrate. However, any foods that are susceptible to contamination may require additional preservation treatments. Processing equipment for susceptible foods must also be sterilized often.

Methods of Concentration

Any method used to concentrate foods must perform the basic function of removing water. Commercial systems use three basic types of equipment: kettles, evaporators, and filters.

Open Kettle

The oldest method of concentration is to heat a food product in an open kettle or pan. Heat is applied to the bottom of the kettle, and steam escapes from the open top. This is the method used by pioneers to make apple butter and molasses, 20-8. The high heat and long cooking times result in flavor and color changes. Frequent stirring helps keep food from sticking and burning to the sides and bottom of the large kettles. Some jams, jellies, and condensed soups are made with this method.

Heat Evaporation

Heat evaporators remove water from thin films of food. Food enters and leaves the evaporator in a continuous process. While in the evaporator, the food is exposed to high temperatures for short periods. The concentrated food is then removed from the bottom of the system as water vapor escapes from the top. The time in the evaporator is usually less than one minute. Therefore, heat damage is limited. The result is a product with a fresher flavor than the open kettle method would produce.

Vacuum Evaporation

Adding a vacuum to the evaporator used for concentration can further reduce damage to heat-sensitive foods. Vacuum evaporators are often set up with a series of chambers. Each chamber has a lower atmospheric pressure than the one before. This type of system

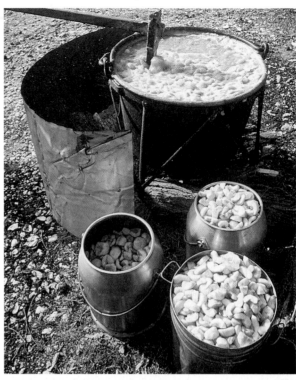

USDA

20-8 The oldest method of concentrating foods is the open kettle method, shown here in the making of molasses at a historic restoration site.

is used for the production of grape and tomato juices and evaporated milk. Grape juice is concentrated from a solution of 15% to 72% solids. This concentration occurs at the rate of 17,034 liters (4,500 gallons) per hour.

Filtration

Another method of food concentration uses filters. Small particles can flow through the filters while larger particles are retained. Some filters allow only water to pass. Filtration allows manufacturers to isolate compounds from their food sources for use in concentrated form. Examples include filtering soy protein from soybeans and flavor extracts from tea and coffee. You will read more about this process in Chapter 23.

Intermediate-Moisture Foods

Dehydrated foods have a moisture level below 15%. Concentrated foods, such as condensed soups, can have a moisture level of as much as 80%. A third category of food products has moisture levels that fall between many dehydrated and concentrated foods. *Intermediate-moisture foods* have moisture levels of 20% to 50% with enough dissolved solutes to prevent the growth of microbes. Because intermediate-moisture foods are concentrated, they can be nutrient and calorie dense. Examples of intermediate-moisture foods include honey, jams, jellies, and fruitcakes. Pepperoni, beef jerky, partially dried figs and dates, and fruit strips are also intermediate-moisture foods.

Some intermediate-moisture foods do not need refrigeration. However, the moisture content of these foods is not low enough to be the only factor that preserves them. Low water activity level works with low moisture content to extend the shelf life of these foods. The low water activity level in intermediate-moisture foods is due to high concentrations of dissolved sugars, salts, or minerals. Lack of free water causes microbes in these foods to dehydrate and die.

Additives may be needed to preserve the quality of some intermediate-moisture foods. For instance, antioxidants may be added to prevent enzymatic activity. Potassium sorbate might be used to prevent mold growth. To be shelf stable, meat-based products, such as sandwich spreads, require additives that will

lower water activity levels. However, the additives must not raise the sugar or salt content of these products to undesirable levels. See 20-9.

Food scientists apply principles used in making food for humans to produce animal feed. An example of this is in the development of intermediate-moisture foods for pets. The low water activity of moist pet food makes it stable at room temperature with minimum packaging. Because this type of food is still moist, rehydration is not necessary.

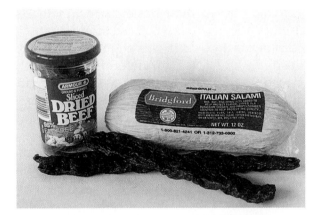

20-9 These meat products are intermediate-moisture foods that contain additives to lower water activity levels and increase shelf life.

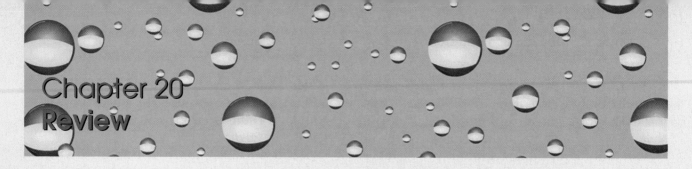

Summary

Dehydrated, concentrated, and intermediate-moisture foods are preserved through lowered water activity levels. Although low water activity levels will stop microbe growth, enzyme activity can still continue. For this reason, many foods must be pretreated with heat or chemicals.

There are several basic drying methods used to dehydrate foods. Food scientists must consider factors such as type of food, quality desired, and cost in determining which method to use. In addition, the speed needed and the heat sensitivity of the food help determine the amount of heat used. Dehydration can also be done in the home. Many dried foods must be rehydrated before being eaten.

Concentration involves removing a portion of water from the food product. Some concentrated foods, such as fruit juices, are reconstituted before serving. Others, such as maple syrup, are eaten in the concentrated form. Intermediate-moisture foods have less moisture than concentrated foods, but more than dehydrated foods. Additives may be needed in these foods to prevent growth of microbes and enzymatic activity.

Check Your Understanding

1. List three advantages of dehydration
2. Describe how dehydration is related to water activity.
3. Name four factors that processors must control during dehydration.
4. Explain how pasteurization and blanching improve the quality of dehydrated foods.
5. What chemicals are used to control enzymatic browning in heat-sensitive foods?
6. List and briefly describe the methods of commercial dehydration.

7. Name two ways foods can be dried at home.
8. Describe how moisture transfer is prevented in mixed dehydrated foods such as raisin-bran flake breakfast cereal.
9. List four undesirable reactions that can occur in foods as a result of concentration.
10. What causes low water activity in intermediate-moisture foods?

Critical Thinking

1. Explain how foods like honey and molasses are naturally protected from most microbial contamination.
2. Name a dehydrated food, a concentrate, and an intermediate-moisture food used to make the following: a dish of pasta with spaghetti sauce and pepperoni.
3. Why does nonfat dry milk have the fat removed as well as the water?
4. Why do food manufacturers face fewer challenges in developing dehydrated foods that are eaten directly rather than those reconstituted before eating?

Explore Further

1. **Communication.** Create a pamphlet to describe proper storage for dehydrated foods before and after opening. Include tips for safe home dehydration of fresh foods.
2. **Science.** Develop a procedure for dehydrating parsley in the microwave oven. Report the results to the class.
3. **Math.** Dehydrate three fresh foods and calculate the water loss. Chart or graph the percentage of water lost for each food.

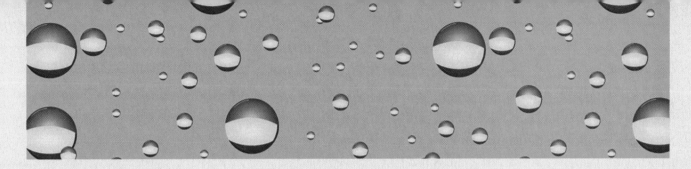

4. **Technology.** Using a nutrition analysis program, compare the nutritive value of one serving of each of the following: grapes versus raisins, plums versus prunes, and mashed potatoes versus instant mashed potatoes. Report the results to the class.

5. **Food and Nutrition.** Plan a day's menu for a backpacker that is lightweight, portable, and fits your MyPyramid plan.

Experiment 20A
Dehydrating Meat

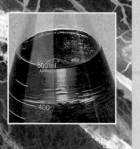

Purpose

One of the oldest food preservation methods is dehydration. When the water activity level is low enough, food will not spoil even at room temperature. Meat, poultry, and fish can all be successfully dehydrated. Flavor can be added by marinating the meat pieces or coating them with a flavoring sauce before dehydration. In this experiment, you will make beef jerky by flavoring thinly sliced pieces of meat and then dehydrating them. It is critical that all pieces be cut to a uniform size and thickness.

Equipment

chef's or utility knife
cutting board
electronic balance
100-mL graduated cylinder
mixing bowl
thermostatically controlled dehydrator

Supplies

round, rump, or sirloin roast or London broil
waxed paper
50 mL (¼ cup) soy sauce
50 mL (¼ cup) Worcestershire sauce
3 mL (¾ teaspoon) hickory smoke flavoring

Procedure

Day 1

1. Cut a section of roast 3 cm thick by 10 cm long. Slice this portion into six 0.5-cm thick slices.

2. Using waxed paper as weighing paper, mass the sliced beef. Record the mass in a data table.

3. Combine 50 mL of soy sauce, 50 mL Worcestershire sauce, and 3 mL hickory smoke flavoring to form a flavoring sauce. Mass the flavoring sauce and record the mass in the data table.

4. Put the flavoring sauce in a mixing bowl. Add the meat strips and toss to coat evenly.

5. Lay the strips on a dehydrator tray so the pieces do not touch each other or the sides of the tray.

6. Dehydrate the meat at 63°C (145°F) for at least 4 to 8 hours. Your teacher will monitor the dehydration process if a timer is not available on the dehydrator. The time needed depends on the dehydrator and the thickness of the slices.

7. Mass any flavoring sauce remaining in the bowl and record the mass in the data table.

Day 2

1. Mass the beef jerky. Record the mass in the data table.

2. Taste a sample of the jerky. Record sensory evaluation regarding texture, appearance, and flavor.

3. Thoroughly clean the dehydrator trays.

Calculations

1. Calculate the mass of flavoring sauce used.

2. Calculate the mass of water lost (original mass of all ingredients minus the mass of the finished jerky).

3. Calculate the percentage of the mass lost in water (mass of water lost divided by the original mass times 100).

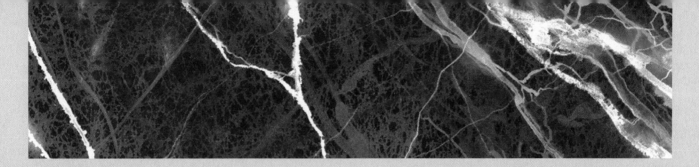

Questions

1. What changes did you observe in the meat after dehydration?

2. What are the advantages of dehydration as a preservation method?

3. What are the disadvantages of this preservation method?

Experiment 20B
Concentrating Soup Stock

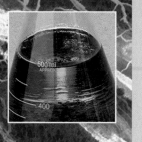

Purpose

During concentration of a food product, water is removed from the product. In this experiment, you will conduct a sensory evaluation of soup stock as it is reduced or concentrated.

Equipment

250-mL beaker

small ladle

small bowl or custard cup

beaker tongs

spoons (1 per lab group member)

Supplies

150 mL (²/₃ cup) canned chicken, beef, or vegetable stock

Procedure

1. Pour assigned stock into a 250-mL beaker.

2. Bring the stock to a boil over high heat.

3. Use a small ladle to remove approximately 1 to 2 mL (¹/₄ to ¹/₂ teaspoon) of stock per lab member from the beaker.

Cool the stock in a small bowl or custard cup. As soon as the broth is cool enough, taste a spoonful. Conduct a sensory evaluation regarding color, flavor, and mouth feel. Record your observations in a data table.

4. Boil the stock left in the beaker until only about 75 mL remain. This will take approximately 15 to 20 minutes. While you are heating the broth, clean the spoons in hot, soapy water and rinse them for the next taste test.

5. Conduct a second taste test as described in step 3.

6. Turn the heat down to medium to reduce the risk of splattering. Heat the stock left in the beaker until only about 35 mL remain. This will take approximately 10 minutes.

7. Conduct a third taste test as described in step 3.

8. Heat the stock left in the beaker until only about 15 mL remain. This will take approximately 5 more minutes.

9. Conduct a fourth taste test as described in step 3.

Questions

1. What changes did you observe in the flavor of the stock as the volume was reduced?

2. What changes did you observe in the color of the stock?

3. What changes did you observe in the mouth feel of the stock?

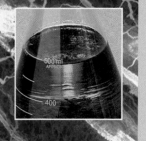

Experiment 20C
Backpacker's Dehydrated Soup

Purpose

Foods contain varying amounts of water. As a result, dehydration times vary from one food to another. Foods must be dehydrated separately before mixing to ensure that all have been dehydrated sufficiently to prevent spoilage. In this experiment, you will prepare a dehydrated vegetable soup that could be stored in resealable plastic bags for a backpacker's use. As a class, decide what size vegetable pieces you desire and what seasonings you will add.

Equipment

chef's or utility knife

cutting board

food dehydrator

mixing bowl

mixing spoon

metric measuring spoons

custard cup

saucepan

Supplies

assigned vegetable or grain product

2 mL (½ teaspoon) herbs (basil, bay leaf, garlic powder, marjoram, oregano, rosemary, thyme)

1 mL (¼ teaspoon) spices (cumin, curry, paprika, pepper)

2 mL (½ teaspoon) salt

5 mL (1 teaspoon) bouillon granules (use low-sodium bouillon or omit salt)

water

Procedure

Day 1

1. Prepare assigned vegetable or grain product. Cut vegetable into pieces of the size determined by the class. If slicing, slice as thinly as possible. Cook grain product according to package directions.

   Variation 1: 1 small potato

   Variation 2: 1 medium tomato or 2 to 3 plum tomatoes

   Variation 3: 1 small onion

   Variation 4: 3 to 4 mushrooms

   Variation 5: 8 to 10 leaves of spinach

   Variation 6: 3 to 4 okra

   Variation 7: 1 small zucchini or yellow crookneck squash

   Variation 8: 56 g uncooked pasta or 75 mL (⅓ cup) uncooked long grain rice

2. Mass assigned vegetable or cooked grain product. Record mass in a data table.

3. Arrange assigned product in a single layer on a dehydrator tray.

4. Dehydrate at 57°C (135°F) for at least 3 to 5 hours. Your teacher will monitor the dehydrator if there is not an automatic timer. Vegetables should be removed as soon as an entire tray is dry.

Day 2

1. Mass your assigned dehydrated food. Record the mass in the data table.

2. In a mixing bowl, combine the dehydrated foods.

3. In a custard cup, combine herbs, spices, salt, and bouillon granules. Add the seasoning mixture to the dehydrated foods.

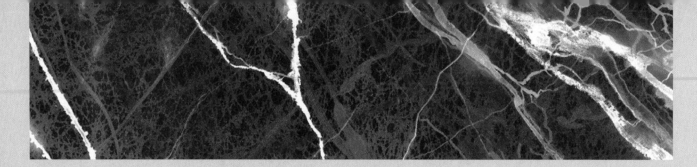

4. In a saucepan, rehydrate the soup in 125 mL (¹/₂ cup) water per 50 mL (¹/₄ cup) of dehydrated product. Simmer about 15 to 20 minutes until the vegetables are tender. Add more water if needed to maintain a soup consistency.

5. Sample the soup and record your observations of the taste, texture, and color of the vegetables and grain product in a data table.

Data

Record your mass data on a class data chart on an overhead projector. Copy the data from the other lab groups into your data table.

Calculations

1. Calculate the mass of water lost from each food product. Record your results in a data table.

2. Calculate the percentage of mass lost from each food product. Record your results.

Questions

1. Which food product had the most water loss? Which had the least?

2. Rank the food products from greatest to least water content.

3. What changes would you recommend for a future soup mix?

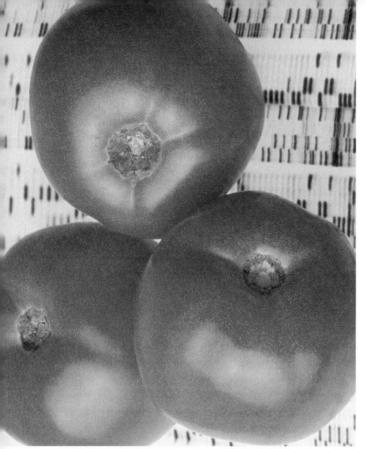

Agricultural Research Service, USDA

These tomatoes have been genetically engineered through a growing field of study called biotechnology.

Chapter 21

Current Trends in Food Preservation: Irradiation, Packaging, and Biotechnology

Objectives

After studying this chapter,
you will be able to

describe the chemical and nutritional changes irradiation creates in food products.

analyze the advantages and disadvantages of food irradiation as a preservation method.

compare reduced oxygen packaging with other food packaging methods.

explain how biotechnology is used in the food industry.

Key Terms

food irradiation

free radical

radiolytic product

rad

gray

kilogray

hermetic

copolymer

ionomer

cellophane

permeable

laminate

reduced oxygen packaging (ROP)

controlled atmosphere packaging (CAP)

modified atmosphere packaging (MAP)

desiccant

biotechnology

Change is one of life's constants. Scientific research and technology are bringing changes to peoples' lives every day. Changes in food production and processing are no exception. Before accepting change, consumers need to ask questions and examine the issues. What are the advantages and disadvantages of the new process? Are there health benefits or concerns people need to investigate? How does

479

the new process work? How should this product be stored to protect the food from spoilage? Only after answering these and other similar questions can consumers make informed decisions.

A number of recent developments in the food industry involve food preservation. One of these is the use of irradiation to preserve foods. Reduced oxygen packaging and biotechnology are also growing trends. Foods produced, preserved, and packaged by these techniques are sold around the world.

Food Irradiation

Food irradiation is a cold food preservation method in which food is exposed to high-energy electromagnetic waves. Food moves from one end of a radiation field to another on a conveyor belt. As the food moves, electromagnetic waves pass through it.

Until lately, irradiation has been used most often for products other than food. For instance, irradiation is used to sterilize hospital equipment, wine bottle corks, and cosmetics, 21-1. More recently, irradiation has been used for spices and on cartons for aseptic food packaging.

The interest in food irradiation increased during the last two decades of the twentieth century. This was due partly to studies about how to provide food for the growing world population. Large volumes of food are currently lost to damage from insects, molds, and

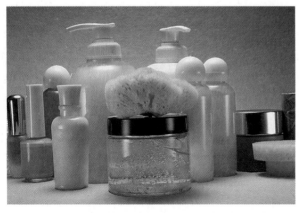

21-1 Cosmetics are among the nonfood products that may be treated with irradiation.

sprouting. (Sprouting causes changes within foods such as potatoes that soften the tissue and result in the production of toxins.) Irradiation can reduce food losses by helping to control these types of damage.

Food irradiation is now approved in over 40 countries for over 60 food products. In the United States, the Food and Drug Administration (FDA) grants approval for irradiating foods. The first foods to receive FDA approval for irradiation were wheat and wheat flour in 1963. Since that time, many other foods have received approval. Wheat is irradiated to reduce losses due to insects and molds. White potatoes were approved to reduce losses caused by rapid sprouting in storage. Spices and herbs are irradiated to lower the risk of contaminants. Treatment of pork was approved to destroy *Trichinella*. Guidelines have been set up for irradiating fruits and vegetables that are susceptible to mold and insect damage. Concerns about salmonellae in poultry and E. coli in red meat have led to the recent approval of these foods.

Effects of Irradiation on Food Products

Foods undergo some chemical and nutritional changes during irradiation. However, irradiation does not cause major changes in flavor, texture, or color of most foods. Dairy products and high-fat foods are the main exceptions. Irradiation can cause these foods to develop some unpleasant flavors.

Chemical Changes

The energy used to irradiate foods is also called *ionizing radiation*. This is because it produces ions in any substance with which it comes in contact.

Food irradiation creates large numbers of short-lived free radicals. *Free radicals* are atoms or compounds that have lost one or more electrons. They are very unstable and quickly react with other substances to form more stable compounds. During their short life spans, free radicals cause chemical changes that result in the death of microbes. The chemical changes started by the free radicals also block some enzymatic reactions. This hinders sprouting in some foods and slows the ripening process in others.

Free radicals are formed during digestion, cooking, freeze-drying, and normal storage. There are more free radicals in a piece of toast than in dry irradiated foods. In other words, irradiation increases the free radicals in food. However, the increase presents no more of a health hazard than other food preservation methods. Because free radicals have very short life spans, most become stable compounds shortly after processing.

During irradiation, electromagnetic waves hit molecules in the food product. The force breaks bonds in the molecules. This causes *radiolytic products* to form. These are chemical compounds that are produced in food as a result of irradiation. A few of the compounds produced include carbon dioxide, formic acid, and glucose. These substances are commonly found in all types of food and food products. The FDA has estimated that total radiolytic products formed during irradiation are less than 3 parts per million.

Radiolytic products are added to irradiated foods. Therefore, the process of irradiation is considered to be a food additive. All food additives are controlled by the FDA. The FDA has over 50 years of data on what happens to food when it is irradiated. Research shows that most of the chemical changes are similar to changes that occur when food is cooked or frozen. Thirty years of testing has failed to find a substance that is unique to irradiated food. See 21-2.

Some foods are damaged by irradiation. High-protein foods are more susceptible to damage. Irradiation can kill salmonellae in poultry without damaging the poultry. If irradiation is used to destroy salmonellae in eggs, however, the protein in egg white will be damaged. The levels of radiation needed to destroy the salmonellae result in a thin, watery egg white. This is partly due to the production of hydrogen peroxide (H_2O_2) from water molecules during irradiation. Damage to high-protein foods can be reduced by irradiating the food while it is frozen. If the food is frozen, the water is unable to react as easily. Much lower levels of H_2O_2 are produced.

Nutritional Changes

Nutrient losses in irradiated foods are similar to those in foods processed by other methods.

The Development of Food Irradiation

1896	Discovery of radioactive material that kills bacteria
1905	U.S. and British patents issued for use of irradiation to kill bacteria in food
1923	First study published about animals fed irradiated foods
1945	First long-term feeding study begins
1950	Food irradiation programs begin in England and some European countries
1958	U.S. Congress requires that FDA evaluates food irradiation as an additive Russia approves use of irradiation for grains and potatoes
1963	U.S. approves canned bacon, wheat, wheat flour, and potatoes for irradiation
1968	U.S. removes canned bacon from list of approved foods due to concerns about *C. botulinum*
1976	FAO/WHO and International Atomic Energy Association recommend that food irradiation be classified as a physical process
1983	U.S. and Canada approve spices for irradiation
1984	FDA sets guidelines for commercial irradiation facilities
1985	U.S. approves pork for irradiation
1986	U.S. approves fruits and vegetables for irradiation
1992	U.S. approves poultry for irradiation
1997	U.S. approves chilled red meat for irradiation

21-2 Every approved use of irradiation is based on years of research and development.

Heating, freezing, and drying can all cause nutrient losses. Food temperature and oxygen levels must be controlled during irradiation. This will help lessen damage to nutrients caused by heat and oxidation.

Proteins, carbohydrates, and fats are stable in the radiation doses used on most foods. Vitamins vary as to how they will react to irradiation. Riboflavin, niacin, and vitamin D are fairly stable. Vitamins A, C, E, K, and B_1 (thiamin) are more likely to be damaged. The damage will vary depending on the temperature and length of the exposure. The packaging material and the type of food will also affect the damage to a given vitamin. Compounds in some foods seem to help protect the vitamins during irradiation.

Energy Used to Irradiate Foods

The process of irradiation uses one of four types of radiant energy. These are gamma rays, electron beams, ultraviolet light, and X rays. These types of electromagnetic waves all differ. Each has a distinct wavelength, frequency, and penetrating power. Each type also has a different effect on living organisms. (Refer to Chapter 5 for an illustration of the electromagnetic spectrum.)

The most common form of energy for food irradiation is gamma rays. Gamma rays are given off by *radioactive* elements. These are elements that release energy as their unstable nuclei break down. The most common material used in food irradiators is cobalt-60. Cobalt is not naturally radioactive. It can be made radioactive when its atoms are blasted by high energy in a nuclear reactor. Cobalt-60 releases high levels of gamma rays. The energy from one container of cobalt-60 can irradiate food for 21 years. Cobalt-60 is the same substance that is used for radiation therapy with cancer patients.

Another source of gamma rays for food irradiators is cesium-137. Cesium-137 is a by-product of the production of plutonium for nuclear reactors. Cesium-137 is not used as much as cobalt-60 because it is more costly.

Gamma ray sources must be stored in specially developed underground storage units. These units lift the energy source up into a processing room when needed. These units can be lowered and sealed off when workers need to enter the processing area for maintenance or repairs. Such units are needed because prolonged exposure to gamma rays can injure or kill humans.

A second form of radiant energy used to irradiate foods is electron beams. Electron beams are made up of high-energy electrons, or beta particles. These beta particles are produced by electronic machinery. An advantage of electron beams is they have no radioactive source material to transport or dump. Radiant energy is present only when the machine is operating. Electron beams are a more costly form of radiant energy than gamma rays. This is due to the expense of running the machines.

Ultraviolet light has limited value in food irradiation. Ultraviolet light cannot penetrate material. Therefore, it is used only for surface treatments. It will kill microbes on the surface of food or in liquid foods that are exposed in thin films. Ultraviolet light is used to treat equipment surfaces, air, and water in some food plants. Many high school science labs have an ultraviolet cabinet to sanitize splash goggles between uses.

X rays penetrate material to varying degrees. The denser a material is, the less deeply the rays will penetrate it. X rays cannot be focused easily. Experiments have been done using X rays to irradiate foods. However, practical uses have not been developed.

Units of Energy

The basic unit used to measure radiant energy is the rad. *Rad* stands for *radiation absorbed dose.* It is the amount of energy absorbed per gram of material. A *gray* equals 100 rads and a *kilogray* (kgray) equals 1,000 grays.

Levels of radiation used in food processing are usually measured in kilograys. Food irradiation damages living tissue so it dies. The more complex an organism is, the lower the dose needed to kill it. This is because it is harder to land a damaging hit on a smaller organism. For example, 500 rads (0.005 kgray) is sufficient to kill humans. However, it takes between 20,000 and 100,000 rads (0.2 and 1.0 kgray) to destroy various insects present in food crops. It takes over 0.01 kgray to slow sprouting in potatoes. Irradiation of spices takes 30 kgrays of energy. See 21-3.

Public Concerns About Irradiation

Many people have concerns about the irradiation of foods. Questions being asked include

❖ Is the food exposed to nuclear radiation?

❖ Does the food contain radioactive material or does the food itself become radioactive?

❖ How much is the food damaged in the process?

❖ Why use this preservation method when so many others exist?

Some people are concerned that eating irradiated foods creates a risk of genetic damage to humans. For over 20 years, millions of research animals have been fed irradiated food. The food was treated at two to five times the radiation levels set by the FDA. None of the animals were found to have transmittable genetic defects due to their diets.

The concern about genetic damage is linked to the issue of radioactivity. Many people have thought that irradiating food would make it radioactive. It is important to know that all substances have traces of radioactivity. An agency that studies the irradiation of food is the International Consultative Group on Food Irradiation (ICGFI). This group studied the effects very high levels of radiation have on foods. They found irradiation did increase the radioactivity of foods. However, this increase was 200,000 times smaller than the radioactivity that was already in the foods. The doses of radiation used for these tests were much higher than the low levels set by the FDA.

A second concern is that irradiation does not decrease the risk of botulism. Irradiation at levels of 10 kgray or less does not destroy *C. botulinum*. However, a number of other microbes that lead to foodborne illness are killed during treatment. These include salmonellae in poultry and *E. coli* in red meat. Also, the risk of botulism for irradiated foods is no greater than for foods preserved by any other method. All foods, including irradiated products, must be handled, packaged, and stored safely.

A third concern involves pesticide residues or additives in foods. Some people worry about the effects irradiation will have on these substances. Tests have shown that pesticides and additives do form radiolytic products. However, these products are formed at levels too low to pose health hazards.

A fourth concern focuses on the radioactive material used to irradiate foods. Consumers want to be sure this material can be shipped and handled safely. In a recent period of over 30 years, more than 870 loads of cobalt-60 were shipped in Canada. There was not a single accident or spill of toxic material in any of these shipments. Food processing plants are equipped with a number of devices to check radiation levels. Many steps are taken to prevent human exposure to radiation. "Meltdowns" or nuclear explosions are just

FDA-Approved Food Irradiation Dosage Levels

Food	Maximum Dose	Approved Use
All foods	1 kGy	Controls insects
Fresh foods	1 kGy	Delays maturation
Poultry	3 kGy	Controls disease-causing microorganisms
Refrigerated meats	4.5 kGy	Controls spoilage and disease-causing microorganisms
Frozen meats	7 kGy	Controls spoilage and disease-causing microorganisms
Dehydrated enzymes	10 kGy	Controls insects and microorganisms
Spices and seasonings	30 kGy	Decontaminates and controls insects and microorganisms

21-3 Approved irradiation dosage levels vary with the type of food being treated.

not possible. This is because the radioactive materials used are of the wrong kind. The amounts of radioactive material are also far too small to pose this kind of threat. Concerns of this type are based on a lack of knowledge about the laws of nuclear physics. See 21-4.

A fifth concern about food irradiation is linked to packaging. Many foods can be irradiated after they are packaged. Packaging material must be chosen with this in mind. Some materials can add unpleasant flavors or toxins to the food.

In spite of many concerns, two factors are helping more consumers to accept irradiation. The first factor is education. Consumers are starting to learn more about the safety of food irradiation. They are also finding out how irradiation can help reduce the risk of foodborne illness. The second factor is support from key organizations. Food irradiation has been backed by the American Medical Association and the American Dietetic Association. The American Council on Science and Health has also shown support for irradiation.

Controlling Irradiation

The FDA has set a number of guidelines to help ensure that irradiating food is a safe process. The FDA requires all irradiated foods to be tested before they are sold. Each food must be tested separately because each food has a unique chemical makeup. The FDA must also approve plans for irradiation plants before they are built. Once these plants are operating, they must be inspected often.

The ICGFI has set guidelines for good irradiation practices that are to be used throughout the world. The ICGFI is made up of experts from three key organizations. These include the FAO and the WHO. Experts from the International Atomic Energy Agency (IAEA) are also part of ICGFI. All food irradiation plants around the world are registered with ICGFI. ICGFI also organizes training for plant workers and managers. Training covers proper processing and packaging methods. It includes record keeping and food inspection, too.

Labeling Irradiated Products

Irradiated foods fall into three groups in terms of labeling requirements. The first group consists of wheat, wheat flour, spices, herbs, teas, and white potatoes. These were the first foods to be approved for irradiation by the FDA in the United States. No labeling requirements exist for these products. The second

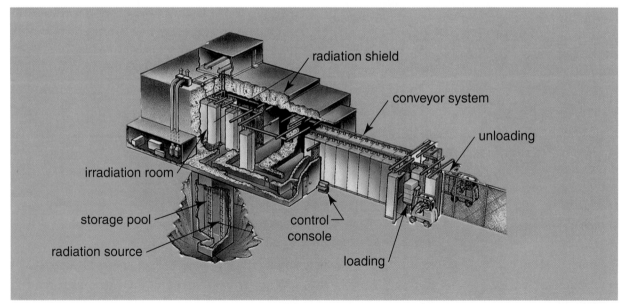

MDS Nordion

21-4 Irradiation facilities have multiple safety features, including an underground water storage tank and thick concrete walls. A conveyor system moves boxes of food into the irradiation room and past a radiation source for treatment.

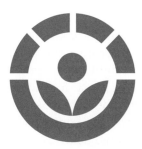

21-5 The radura symbol must appear on irradiated foods.

group of foods is "whole irradiated foods." These are unprocessed foods, such as fresh meats, poultry, fruits, and vegetables. Federal law requires these foods to have the official green and white symbol, called the *radura,* on their labels, 21-5. Whole irradiated foods must also be labeled with the words *treated* *with radiation* or *treated by irradiation.* The third group of foods is processed foods that contain whole irradiated foods as ingredients. Such foods include soups, frozen entrees, and pizza. The labels of these foods do not have to have the radura or any statement about irradiation. If you eat processed food, you have eaten irradiated food.

Packaging

A second area that is the focus of current trends in food preservation is packaging. All methods of food preservation rely on some type of packaging material. Canned, frozen, and dried foods all need to be stored in suitable containers to maintain their quality. Poor or damaged packages can undo the benefits of any food preservation process. See 21-6.

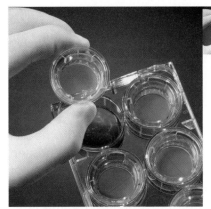

Recent Research
High-Dose Irradiation

High-dose irradiation is defined as radiation at levels of 25 kgray or higher. The International Consultative Group on Food Irradiation (ICGFI) recently studied the use of this technique to preserve foods.

High-dose irradiated foods have been compared to foods preserved by other methods. The high-dose irradiated foods were found to be of higher quality. Foods sterilized with high doses of radiant energy are more stable than foods sterilized with pressurized heat. The high-dose irradiated foods have less change in texture, flavor, color, and nutritive value.

These foods are already used by the NASA space shuttle program. They have an extended shelf life without refrigeration. This makes them especially useful in cases of disaster when there is an extended loss of electric systems. High-dose irradiated foods are also of value to people with rare disorders of the immune system. This is because high-dose irradiation destroys all microbes without the high heat needed for sterilization. Therefore, foods maintain higher quality while being safe for people who cannot consume any microbes.

The ICGFI study found that high-dose irradiation is as safe as approved thermal processing methods for sterilizing foods. The study advised that high-dose irradiation be approved for

❖ spices

❖ dry food ingredients

❖ prepackaged, precooked foods stored for extended periods without chilling

❖ sterilized meals used for disaster victims, campers, and those suffering from chronic immune disorders

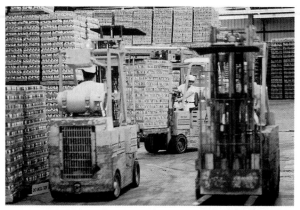

21-6 Packaging material used for individual food containers must withstand the bulk packaging and storage methods used for the product.

Packaging is so complex that it is an industry in itself. Some universities offer degrees in package engineering. When engineers develop new packaging materials, they must assess a number of factors. The material must protect food products. It must be economical to produce. It must not dissolve into the food.

Packaging materials are regulated by the FDA. This is because any packaging that comes in direct contact with a food has the potential to become an additive. Some packaging materials can break down during processing. Others can react with the foods they are holding or covering. This causes leaching of packaging material into the food.

Packaging regulations are based on the type of container. A *primary container* is any packaging that comes in direct contact with a food. A *secondary container* holds the primary container. It does not come in direct contact with the food. An example is the packaging for breakfast cereals. The plastic bag that holds the cereal is a primary container. The box that holds the bag is a secondary container. There are fewer regulations for secondary containers than for primary containers.

Functions of Packaging

Food packaging serves a number of functions. Its main function is to act as a barrier between food and contaminants. Packaging protects food from impact during shipping and storage. Some packaging acts as a dispenser. Such packaging allows consumers to use what they need, close the package, and keep the remaining contents for later use. Packaging may protect foods from moisture, gas, odors, and light. Packaging also identifies the contents. It must follow the guidelines established by the 1993 Nutrition Labeling and Education Act. Some packaging serves multiple functions, such as storage, cooking, and serving. Containers used for frozen, microwavable dinners are an example.

Each food product has unique packaging needs that must be considered. Foods that need a constant environment use a hermetic closure. **Hermetic** refers to a container that is completely sealed. Water, vapor, gases, and odors cannot leave or enter the container. Cans, bottles, and aseptic packaging use hermetic closures.

Some foods need packaging that will allow certain substances in or out of the container. For instance, refrigerated doughs for biscuits and breads release carbon dioxide. If these products had hermetic seals, pressure would build until the tubes holding the products exploded. Instead, small vents in the tubes allow the carbon dioxide to slowly escape.

Types of Packaging Materials

Packaging engineers have hundreds of food packaging options from which to choose. The packaging material selected depends on the functions it must perform. The choice of materials is based partly on the protection needed. The conditions of shipping and storage also affect the type of packaging to be used. Some containers are flexible and others need to be rigid. Lightweight containers work well for some foods, whereas other foods require sturdier packaging. Some packages are disposable and others, like sausage casings, are edible.

Packaging engineers base each choice on the process used to preserve the food. They also consider the chemical contents of the specific food to be packaged. For example, there are at least five categories of steel used to hold canned vegetables. There are also a variety of coatings that might be applied to the insides of the cans. The coating material used depends on the processing machines and how the food interacts with the packaging material. The lining that works well for corn would react with high-acid tomatoes.

Before any material or combination of materials can be used to package food, it must pass thorough testing. Packaging material must pass sanitation and toxicity tests. This checks the packaging material for pathogens or toxins that can contaminate food. The packaging material must also pass a series of "use and abuse" tests. These tests ensure the material will withstand handling at the factory and during shipping. They make sure the packaging will hold up at the point of sale and in the consumer's home, too. See 21-7.

Many of the packaging materials seen in grocery stores today were not used a few decades ago. These include foil-lined pouches and reduced oxygen packaging. Metal, glass, paper, and plastic are all widely used food packaging materials.

Metals

The three most common metals used to hold food are steel, tin, and aluminum. Steel is inexpensive, easily shaped, and can form a hermetic closure. Its main disadvantage is its corrosiveness. This means the material will be eaten away as it reacts with oxygen and acids in food. For this reason, steel cans are coated with a thin layer of enamel or resin.

The name *tin can* comes from the thin layer of tin used to coat the first steel cans. Tin is far less corrodible than steel and is therefore stable for a longer period. Only about 0.25% of the weight of a tin can is actually tin.

Aluminum cans are lightweight, stable against corrosion, and easily shaped. Aluminum's lack of structural strength and rigidity has limited its uses in the canning industry. Because of the high cost of producing aluminum, much of the aluminum used is recycled.

Glass

Glass has long been used as a food packaging material. It is the primary container used for home canning. Glass has the advantage of being chemically inert. It does not react with food and therefore cannot contaminate it.

The major disadvantage of glass is that it is susceptible to breakage. Rapid temperature changes increase the risk of breakage. Therefore, glass is not suitable for rapid heating and cooling preservation methods. Glass will break if the internal pressure from heat processing is too great. If the glass is scratched and weakened, it is more likely to break from impact on assembly lines. Thin glass is more likely to break from internal pressure. However, thicker glass is more likely to break

Testing Packaging Material

A test for	Evaluates
Bursting strength	The amount of pressure it takes before the package bursts open
Compression strength	The number of packages that can be stacked in a shipping container and the number of shipping containers that can be stacked before damage occurs to single packages
Fat permeability	Whether the material will absorb fats and oils
Gas permeability	Whether gases will migrate through the packaging material
Impact strength	The type and amount of damage that occurs when a package is dropped
Print stability	Whether printing on package labels will fade, rub off, or bleed
Seal strength	Whether the material will seal consistently and whether the seal will hold
Tear force	The amount of force needed to pull the package materials apart
Water permeability	Whether water will migrate through the packaging material

21-7 Packaging material is carefully tested to be sure it will meet the requirements of a specific food product.

during temperature changes and from impact with other bottles or machinery.

Thin coatings of wax or silicone on the outside of glass containers reduce damage during the filling process. These coatings protect the glass from scratches. They also result in less breakage and less noise on filling lines.

Another disadvantage of glass is its weight. It is much heavier than paper and plastics. The weight of glass adds to shipping and handling charges. This, in turn, increases the prices consumers must pay for food products.

Paper

Paper has many advantages as a food packaging material. It is lightweight, low cost, and recyclable. Paper must be combined with other substances, such as plastic or aluminum, to achieve a hermetic seal. If the paper comes in direct contact with food, it must meet FDA standards. It must be free of chemical and microbial contaminants.

When paper is used as a primary food container, it is usually coated. Wax, plastics, and aluminum foil are common coatings for paper. The coating material used depends on the needs of the food product. Coatings may be used to increase the strength, grease resistance, sealability, and flexibility of a package.

Plastics

Plastics are made up of long chains of molecules of the same basic compound. Plastics are lightweight, economical, and versatile. They can be manufactured to fit a wide range of needs. See 21-8.

There are three main types of plastics: polymers, copolymers, and ionomers. *Polymers* are constructed of one basic unit of organic molecules formed into long chains. *Copolymers* have two basic units of molecules combined to make one material. *Ionomers* are plastics held together with ionic instead of covalent bonds. Ionomers have stronger bonds that increase the plastic's resistance to dissolving and melting. The development of plastics is a complex field of study. Many chemists specialize in the study of polymers.

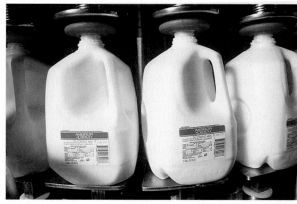

USDA

21-8 Milk cartons are just one of many food containers made from plastic.

Packaging Films

Packaging films cover a broad range of thin, flexible, and often transparent materials. One of the first films to be widely used was cellophane. *Cellophane* is specially processed cellulose. There are over 100 types of cellophane. They vary in terms of thickness, flexibility, and strength.

Films also vary in terms of permeability. A substance that is *permeable* allows liquids and/or gases to pass through or penetrate. Another material used for packaging film is plastic. Plastics can be made to be permeable to a specific gas. For example, plastics have been developed that are permeable to carbon dioxide without being permeable to water vapor.

Edible Films and Coatings

A specialized type of films used with some food products is edible films. An example is an edible rice paper wrapper that has been used for generations to cover Asian seaweed candy. (Some people like the taste of the rice paper package better than the seaweed candy!) It is important that edible films be safe to eat and complement the flavor of the food.

Films generally come as layers or sheets. Edible films may be manufactured from amylose starch and proteins such as casein. Edible films may also be natural materials, such as the animal intestines used as the casings of some sausages.

Food coatings are similar to edible films. Coatings are often liquids, such as wax or oil, in which foods are dipped. Some coatings are sprayed on food products.

Edible films and coatings serve a number of functions, although they may not necessarily be used as packaging materials. The films that cover most hot dogs and formed sausages are used to hold and shape the ground mixture inside, 21-9. Some coatings, such as the wax coating on cucumbers, protect foods from mold and improve keeping quality. Some coatings are used to slow oxidative rancidity. Nuts in mixed foods are often sprayed with a coating of monoglycerides for this purpose.

Another function of coatings is to act as a moisture barrier. Although raisins are dehydrated, they have a higher moisture level than bran flakes. To have raisin bran cereal, the raisins must be sprayed with a thin coating of starch to hold in moisture. Otherwise, the bran flakes would turn stale before a consumer could open the box, and the raisins would be as hard as stones.

Laminates

Better packaging can be achieved by layering a number of flexible materials into one product. Packaging materials made of fused layers of various substances are called *laminates.* A laminate may be made up of the following layers:

❖ an outer covering that is easily printed on, such as cellophane

❖ a moisture barrier, such as plastic

❖ a paper layer to add stiffness

❖ a gas barrier, such as aluminum foil

❖ a plastic that melts to help seal the package

❖ plastics or nontoxic glues between layers to fuse them together

A major use of laminates in food packaging is in retort pouches. These pouches were developed to use in place of metal cans for U.S. military rations. Retort pouches have three layers. The first layer is a strong, printable polyester film. The next layer is aluminum foil, and the third is a polypropylene film that forms the seal. Retort pouches are designed to withstand the high temperatures and pressures of retort pouch canners.

Reduced Oxygen Packaging

One of the newer developments in food packaging involves controlling the air around food. Research has shown this can extend the shelf life of some foods. *Reduced oxygen packaging (ROP)* provides an atmosphere that has little or no oxygen enclosed with the food. ROP is now used for red meat, poultry, seafood, pasta, cheeses, precooked meals, snacks, and dried foods. A category of foods called "fresh chilled" has been developed using ROP technology. These foods, like fresh pasta and sauces, provide consumers with fresh, homemade flavor without all the preparation. See 21-10.

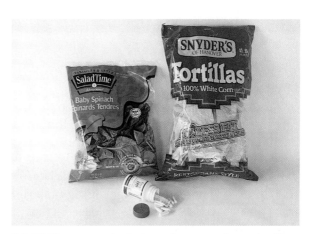

21-10 These products have been packaged with various reduced oxygen packaging methods. The foods inside the packages are surrounded by a gas mixture that differs from the normal composition of air.

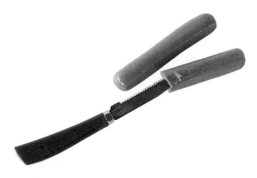

21-9 You can see the knife blade through the thin edible casing on this hot dog.

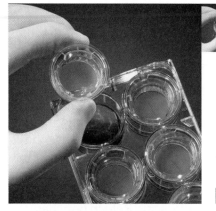

Recent Research
Sensory Evaluation of Package Flavors

Off flavors that result from packaging material are a concern for the food industry. The best way to assess the flavors and aromas added by packaging is through sensory evaluation. (For a review of sensory evaluation, see Chapter 3.) Not long ago, researchers worked to come up with a standardized method for the evaluation process.

The first step was to develop standardized descriptive terms with written definitions. These are the terms evaluators would use to describe flavors and aromas.

Then a 9-point scale, from 0 to 8, was selected for ranking the intensity of flavors and aromas. Higher numbers represent stronger aromas or flavors. Next, chemical references were developed for each term. These references represent the middle intensity of 4 on the scale. For the term *chlorine,* a mixture of 0.05 mL of household bleach in 250 mL purified water was prepared. This mixture was the chemical reference for a rating of 4 on the scale for a chlorine flavor and aroma.

Sensory evaluators must be trained to use the assessment method. They begin by learning the descriptive terms and their definitions. Next, they are exposed to the chemical references for each term. Finally, the evaluators practice testing packages that have been prepared for the training.

Thompson, L.J.; Deniston, D.J.; & Hoyer, C.W. "Method for Evaluating Package-Related Flavors," *Food Technology* January, 1994. pp. 90-94.

The terms used are
acetaldehyde-like
acetone-like
astringent
bitter
cardboard
chemical heat
chlorine
disinfectant-like

fruity
gluelike
metallic
musty
painty
pine/turpentine
plasticlike
pungent
rubberlike

smoky
soapy
solventlike
sour
styrenelike
swampy
vinyl-like
waxy
woody

CAP and MAP

Two main types of ROP are used in the food industry. One type is packaging that uses barriers to control and maintain the desired gases around food. This type of packaging is called **controlled atmosphere packaging (CAP).** Components of the packaging material may absorb oxygen that is released from a food product. Package components may also react to the food itself. This type of CAP is sometimes referred to as *active packaging.*

An example of active packaging is a container lining developed by researchers at Cornell University. This lining will remove bitter flavors from grapefruit juice. The lining contains an enzyme that breaks down the compounds responsible for the bitter taste. The result is a sweet taste without added sugar.

Another type of CAP includes a semipermeable barrier. This barrier "breathes" to control the movement of gases in and out of the package. Precut vegetables, prepared salad greens, and premixed salads are among the most common applications of this type of CAP. Both types of CAP maintain a stable environment as compounds are released from the food.

Fresh fruits and vegetables still respire after harvest. That is, they use oxygen and give off carbon dioxide (CO_2). Sealing these foods in airtight packages would decrease their shelf life. This is because their tissue cells would die once all the oxygen within the package has been used.

CAP will help extend the shelf life of fresh produce. This packaging allows CO_2 inside the package to be slowly replaced with oxygen from the outside. At the same time, water vapor stays in the package to keep the produce from dehydrating. In the case of produce, the CAP must be combined with refrigeration.

CAP can improve the availability and cost of such fragile foods as raspberries, blackberries, and blueberries. These fruits typically have a shelf life of just 4 to 10 days. This shelf life can be extended to three to four weeks through the use of CAP.

Another type of ROP is *modified atmosphere packaging (MAP)*. MAP involves a one-time flushing of a food container with a gas before the container is sealed. The unique needs of the food determine the type of gas used. For example, potato chips are sealed with CO_2 or nitrogen (N_2) gas in the bag. The gas is needed to fill the bag to keep the chips from crushing during shipping and handling. Air cannot be used for this purpose because oxygen causes the fat in chips to turn rancid. By replacing the air in chip bags with CO_2 or N_2, chips stay fresh much longer. See 21-11.

Other ROP Methods

Two other methods of ROP are used in today's market. They are desiccants and enzyme systems. *Desiccants* are compounds that remove substances harmful to food products from the package environment. One type of desiccant is an iron-based compound that is highly reactive in the presence of oxygen. Small packets of this compound may be enclosed with a food that can be damaged by oxygen. The desiccant will react with the oxygen before it can damage the food. The packet is made of material that absorbs the oxygen without releasing the desiccant. Another type of desiccant soaks up extra

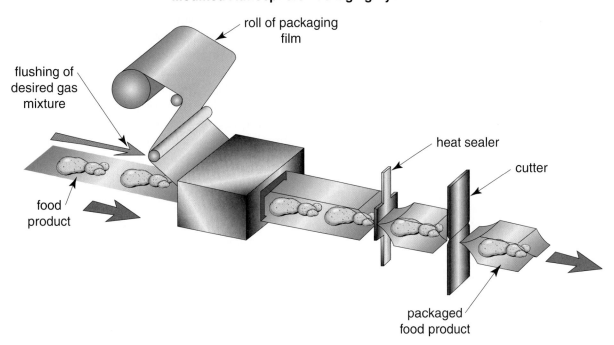

Modified Atmosphere Packaging System

roll of packaging film

flushing of desired gas mixture

heat sealer

cutter

food product

packaged food product

21-11 Modified atmosphere packaging flushes food packaging with a gas mixture to force air out of the package before it is sealed.

water vapor to prevent or slow microbial growth. Desiccant packets are not edible and should never be cooked or served with a food product. These packets are enclosed in many vitamin supplement bottles.

Enzyme systems have very limited uses. Enzymes are added to a food to react with a specific substance before flavors and textures can be altered. An example is the addition of glucose oxidase and catalase to orange-flavored soft drinks. The orange flavor will react with oxygen in the headspace of the drink bottle. If this process is not prevented, the orange drink will develop a "cardboard" flavor. The enzymes react with the oxygen quickly to form gluconic acid. Gluconic acid is harmless and tasteless. In this example, the enzymes alter the atmosphere in the sealed bottle to preserve the flavor.

Functions of ROP

When properly designed, ROP will perform one or more of the following functions:

❖ slow the ripening process

❖ delay maturation and softening

❖ reduce microbial spoilage

❖ slow enzymatic browning

❖ prevent tissue damage from chilling

It is estimated that 25% to 40% of harvested produce spoils before reaching the consumer. ROP can decrease the waste by prolonging the shelf life of many foods.

Biotechnology

Food preservation is just one of many applications being tested in the field of study called biotechnology. *Biotechnology* is the process of using living organisms or any part of these organisms to create new or improved products. The living organisms can be plants, animals, or microbes.

One use of biotechnology is changing the genes in plants to improve certain qualities in the foods the plants produce. For instance, a new tomato that will withstand colder temperatures contains a gene from flounder. This tomato keeps up to two weeks after ripening.

Such uses of biotechnology have sparked a number of questions from consumers. How does changing a gene change the keeping quality? What other changes are being investigated? Are there negative side effects? Can these tomatoes be included in a vegetarian diet? How will all this new technology affect the lives of consumers?

The Old Versus the New

Biotechnology is not new; only the methods being used are new. For thousands of years, people have cultivated plants and bred animals with specific desirable traits. This has led to the development of new reliable plant species and animal breeds. For example, researchers crossbreed plants to strengthen such traits as disease resistance and large size. Most grains, fruits, and vegetables today have been altered by the use of this type of planned cultivation. In the same way, turkey producers have purposely bred turkeys with large volumes of breast meat with other similar turkeys. After generations of breeding, turkeys could be consistently produced to have a high volume of breast meat. These old biotechnology methods require 12 or more years of research before a new seed or breed can be marketed.

New biotechnology methods allow for more precise isolation of desired traits. This isolation can also happen in much less time than old biotechnology methods required. New products can be ready for market in as little as five years.

New biotechnology methods include a technique called *genetic engineering.* This technique allows scientists to identify which gene or groups of genes are responsible for a desired trait. The genes are extracted from the plant or animal that naturally produces them. The extracted genes are then combined with the genes of a host. The host is a plant or microbe that scientists are trying to improve. See 21-12.

The example of the flounder and the tomato can give you an idea of how this process works. Scientists identified the genes in a flounder that allow it to withstand cold water temperatures. They combined these genes

New Species Through Genetic Engineering

Trait-Deficient Host	Natural Source of Desired Trait	Extracted Gene That Controls Desired Trait
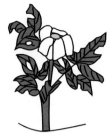	insect-resistant gene 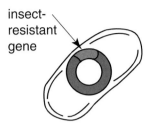	
plant vulnerable to insects	**bacterium**	**insect-resistant gene**
1. Identify the trait desired in a species (insect resistance).	2. Identify a source of the desired trait.	3. Isolate the appropriate gene or group of genes from the natural source.

Altered Host Cell	Genetically Engineered Host
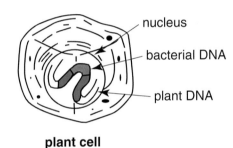 nucleus — bacterial DNA — plant DNA	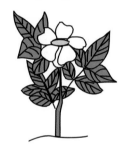
plant cell	**insect-resistant plant**
4. Transfer the extracted gene to the host.	5. Allow the host to develop to see if the desired trait is apparent.

21-12 This simplified illustration shows the basic steps of how new plant and animal species are developed through genetic engineering.

with the genes of a host tomato to develop a frost-resistant tomato. This method of biotechnology can combine genes from any species. This is why a gene from flounder could be used in a tomato.

The tomato about which you have been reading is called the Flavr Savr tomato. It is the first of the new genetically engineered foods to receive FDA approval. Approval was granted in May, 1994. Genetic engineers reversed the gene sequence that is responsible for softening a tomato. This allowed Flavr Savr tomatoes to keep without refrigeration up to 10 days longer that other types of tomatoes. This means the tomato can ripen on the vine before being picked and shipped to market. Although Flavr Savr

tomatoes have not been a marketing success, they have demonstrated the benefits of biotechnology to the food industry and opened the door to other genetically engineered products.

Applications of Biotechnology

Biotechnology is being used to increase the food supply and provide higher-quality foods. Disease- and insect-resistant plants should help increase crop yields and lower costs. They should also allow produce growers to use fewer chemicals.

Another use of biotechnology is to add nutrients to foods that are not normally rich sources. Popular foods such as corn and lettuce could be made more nutritious.

Nutritious foods such as soybeans and spinach could be made tastier.

Some foods already on the market have been altered through biotechnology. There are many examples of the benefits from biotechnology in today's marketplace:

❖ disease-resistant crops (corn, potatoes, papayas)

❖ reduced need for pesticides (corn, soybeans, cotton)

❖ herbicide-resistant crops (corn, canola, cotton, soybeans)

❖ increased nutritional composition of foods (soybeans)

❖ improved flavor and quality of foods (peppers)

Scientists are exploring applications of biotechnology that may benefit the world in additional ways. Growing more food on less land will be necessary as the world population continues to expand. A major concern is finding ways to reduce the risks of foodborne illnesses. Researchers are looking for ways to remove natural toxins from foods such as potatoes and soybeans without altering the food's other properties. There is research underway to develop allergy-safe foods such as peanuts free of the component that triggers allergic reactions.

The goal is to give consumers fruits and vegetables that taste better, last longer, and are more nutritious. Consumers should also be able to buy this improved produce all year long. See 21-13.

Genetically Engineered Foods in the Works

New Product	Trait Adjustment	Benefit
Apples	Increase insect resistance	Reduce use of chemical sprays
Canola	Increase lauric acid content	Provide an alternative source to coconut and palm kernel oils
Coffee bushes	Eliminate caffeine in beans	Decaffeinate without chemicals
Cotton and canola plants	Make oils heat resistant	Allow cooking at higher temperatures without fats breaking down
Potatoes	Reduce fat absorption	Produce lower-fat potato chips with traditional frying methods
Raspberries	Improve keeping quality	Increase shelf life
Soybeans	Reduce palmitic acid content	Produce oil that is nutritionally comparable to canola oil
Sunflowers and canola	Increase oleic acid content	Increase nutritional value
Sweet bell peppers	Eliminate seeds	Increase consumer appeal
Tomatoes	Increase solids	Save the processing industry as much as $100 million per year with each 1% increase

21-13 Researchers are developing a variety of genetically engineered foods that will benefit producers and consumers.

Products currently being developed include tomatoes with more lycopene, garlic with more allicin, rice with higher protein content, and strawberries with increased ellagic acid. Bananas and pineapples that ripen slower, peas that are sweeter, and strawberries with improved flavor and texture may be on grocery store shelves soon.

Regulations Controlling Biotechnology

Some consumer groups have a number of concerns about genetically engineered foods. The FDA has set regulations to control how these foods are developed and sold. The FDA has also held scientific debates and created flowcharts. These resources will help researchers ensure food safety in new varieties of foods.

In 1994, the FDA set up a voluntary process for manufacturers to follow in consulting with the FDA about genetically engineered foods. In 2001, the FDA proposed making this process mandatory. This proposal requires a manufacturer to submit data to the FDA at least 120 days before marketing a genetically engineered food. The manufacturer will also have to prove the product is as safe as its conventional counterpart.

Labeling of genetically engineered foods is required only if altering a food changes the effects of eating it. These effects are of two types. The first is if the new gene is from a food known to cause allergic reactions. For example, a gene from peanuts might be added to corn. People allergic to peanuts would need to know that eating the corn might cause similar allergic reactions. In some foods,

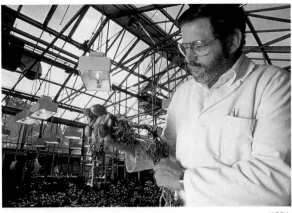

USDA

21-14 This researcher is harvesting genetically engineered potato tubers for field testing.

biotechnologists can transfer a gene without transferring the allergen. If they can prove this is the case, the new food product will not need to be labeled.

The second effect of eating an altered food is when a notable change in the makeup of the food occurs. For instance, an altered fruit may have more or less vitamin A than the unaltered variety. In either case, the altered fruit must be labeled.

Like any new area of study, biotechnology may have some unforeseen drawbacks. Such drawbacks might be due to unexpected interactions when a transferred gene is released to the environment in new ways. Research will be needed to monitor public health. Research will also need to track the impact of new crops on livestock, wildlife, and the environment. See 21-14.

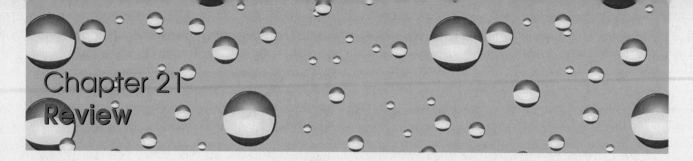

Chapter 21
Review

Summary

Advances in technology are resulting in many changes in the way food is produced, processed, and packaged. To make wise food selections, the consumer needs to be aware of the impact of the new technologies and their applications in the food industry. Three areas of growing concern to today's consumer are food irradiation, packaging, and biotechnology.

Food irradiation uses radiant energy to extend the shelf life of foods. It results in chemical and nutritional changes that are similar to those from thermal food processing methods. Food irradiation is a cold preservation process that kills microbes and consequently reduces the risk of foodborne illness.

Packaging is necessary to maintain freshness and protect food after production. Packaging materials are regulated by the FDA to make sure none leach into the food. Materials used include steel, tin, aluminum, glass, cellophane, plastics, and edible films. Packaging provides a protective barrier for the food. Packaging can have a hermetic seal or a semipermeable one. The type depends on the specific needs of the food, how it will be stored, and the stresses of shipping and handling.

The new methods of genetic engineering in biotechnology have opened up the possibility of a whole new world of food products. By selecting the genetic traits of one organism and transferring them to another, scientists hope to improve foods' keeping quality, nutritional value, and flavor. The Flavr Savr tomato is the first of many genetically engineered foods being developed. Future studies will be needed to monitor the impact of these foods on human health, wildlife populations, and natural habitats.

Check Your Understanding

1. Describe how food irradiation preserves food.
2. Why is food irradiation considered to be a food additive?
3. Name the three types of radiant energy used to preserve food.
4. What irradiated foods must have the radura symbol on the label?
5. List three factors engineers examine when developing new packaging material.
6. Identify four functions of packaging.
7. Name six packaging materials and an advantage of each.
8. Explain the difference between controlled and modified atmosphere packaging.
9. List three functions of ROP.
10. When is labeling required by law on genetically engineered foods?

Critical Thinking

1. Consider the following breakfast and determine the nutrients that would be reduced in each food after irradiation: whole grain cereal with milk and a cup of orange juice.
2. Why do you think the United States, Canada, and many other countries irradiate spices?
3. Identify the primary and secondary containers for smoked sausage in casing.
4. Determine which type of packaging material is used for microwave popcorn.
5. Before the development of the Flavr Savr tomato, describe the appearance of most fresh tomatoes sold at the supermarket.

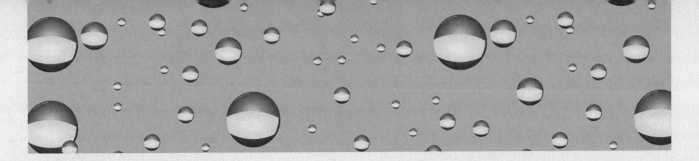

Explore Further

1. **Technology.** Review the current labeling laws for irradiated and bioengineered foods on the Internet. Explain the changes you would recommend in them.

2. **Writing.** Write an editorial for the school newspaper on food irradiation and why it is important for the safety of the food supply.

3. **Science.** Place half a package of fresh berries under an ultraviolet light for 30 minutes. Keep the other half of the package at room temperature for the same amount of time. Place the two halves in separate covered containers. Label and refrigerate. Monitor the berries daily for mold growth and/or signs of spoilage. Report the results to the class.

4. **Communication.** Find out what types of packaging materials are recycled in your community. Report to the class the recycling procedures, pickup locations, and reasons to participate.

5. **Science.** Conduct a sensory evaluation of a carbonated cola stored in glass, aluminum, and plastic. Report the results to the class.

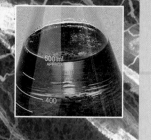

Experiment 21A
Simulating Irradiation

Purpose

Irradiation is the most tested and researched of all the food preservation methods. Electromagnetic radiation is used to destroy bacteria and insect larvae that cause food spoilage. The simplest form of irradiation is ultraviolet (UV) light. In this experiment, you will examine the impact of UV light on bacterial growth.

Equipment

wax pencil
UV light source

Supplies

6 disposable petri dishes with nutrient agar
Serratia marscens or *Bacillus subtilis* bacteria
6 cotton swabs or inoculating loops

Procedure

1. Use a wax pencil to number six disposable petri dishes with nutrient agar as Variations 1 through 6.

2. Remove the lid from one of the petri dishes. Dip a clean cotton swab or inoculating loop into the bacterial culture and then streak the agar in the petri dish in two directions. You may use either of the two methods shown. Immediately replace the lid. Repeat this step with the other five petri dishes.

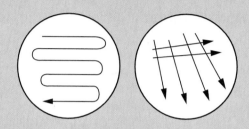

3. Treat the dishes as follows:

   Variation 1: Store overnight in the dark at 22°C (72°F).

   Variation 2: Store overnight in the light at 22°C (72°F).

   For each of the remaining variations, remove the lid during exposure to UV light. The petri dish should be agar side up. Cover the dish at the end of exposure.

   Variation 3: Expose to UV light for 10 seconds. Store overnight in the dark at 22°C (72°F).

   Variation 4: Expose to UV light for 10 seconds. Store overnight in the light at 22°C (72°F).

   Variation 5: Expose to UV light for 40 seconds. Store overnight in the dark at 22°C (72°F).

   Variation 6: Expose to UV light for 40 seconds. Store overnight in the light at 22°C (72°F).

4. The next day, examine each dish. Compare Variations 3 and 5 with Variation 1. Compare Variations 4 and 6 with Variation 2. In a data table, record your observations and draw a sketch of what you see.

Questions

1. Which variation produced the most growth of bacteria?

2. Which variation produced the least growth of bacteria?

3. What difference did the storage in a dark place make?

4. Is exposure to ultraviolet light effective in protecting food from bacteria?

Experiment 21B
Packaging to Prevent Oxidative Rancidity

Purpose

Deterioration of fats in storage can cause *oxidative rancidity*. Oxidative rancidity occurs when oxygen reacts with double bonds in mono- and polyunsaturated fats. The result is an undesirable odor and flavor. Foods at high risk for the development of rancid flavors include potato chips and crackers. In this experiment, you will determine whether exposure to light increases oxidative rancidity.

Supplies

2 1-quart resealable plastic freezer bags
45 potato chips or high-fat crackers
wax pencil
aluminum foil
masking tape

Procedure

1. Conduct a sensory evaluation of the assigned food. Rate the flavor on a scale of 1 to 5, with 1 being strongly dislike and 5 being strongly like. Record your rating.

2. Evenly divide the remaining assigned food into two resealable plastic bags.

3. Seal both bags. Use a wax pencil to label the bags with your lab group number and class period. Mark one bag *unwrapped* and the other *wrapped.*

4. Wrap the bag labeled *wrapped* entirely in aluminum foil. Place a masking tape label with your lab group number and class period on the outside of the foil package.

5. Place both bags on a windowsill or table so they receive as much sunlight each day as possible.

6. Taste test a sample from each bag every other day (Mondays, Wednesdays, and Fridays). Rate the flavor of the samples as described in step 1. Continue testing samples until one of the samples receives a flavor rating of 1 or 2. This will take one to two weeks, depending on the amount of sunshine available. Be sure to carefully rewrap the foil around the bag labeled *wrapped* each time.

Calculations

Create a line graph showing the flavor score on the y-axis and the number of days on the x-axis.

Questions

1. What effect did the aluminum foil wrapping have on the stored food?

2. How are these types of foods packaged by food producers?

3. What other foods could have problems with oxidative rancidity?

Lab Extension

Use a wax pencil to label four 50-mL beakers as follows: *control, Variation 1, Variation 2,* and *Variation 3.* Fill the beakers with the following samples:

Control: 50 mL natural peanut butter

Variation 1: 50 mL natural peanut butter combined with a crushed vitamin A tablet or the contents of a vitamin A capsule

Variation 2: 50 mL natural peanut butter combined with a crushed vitamin C tablet or the contents of a vitamin C capsule

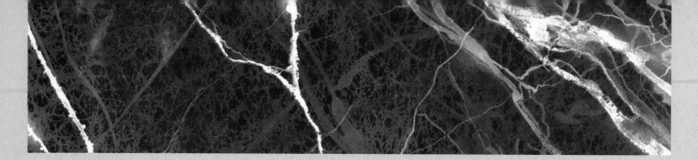

Variation 3: 50 mL natural peanut butter combined with a crushed vitamin E tablet or the contents of a vitamin E capsule

Cover all the beakers with plastic wrap. Secure the plastic wrap with a rubber band. Taste and rate a sample from each beaker every other day for two weeks. Determine which additive best protects peanut butter from oxidation.

Experiment 21C
The Permeability of Plastic

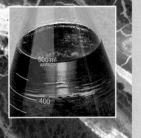

Purpose

Freezing food is a popular preservation method. During freezing, chemical and enzymatic reactions that cause spoilage are slowed almost to a stop. However, poorly wrapped frozen foods will deteriorate through sublimation. Undesired sublimation of frozen foods is called *freezer burn*. Refrigerators and freezers remove moisture from the air during the cooling process. If food is poorly wrapped, moisture will be pulled from the food, which will damage the food's texture, color, and flavor. In this experiment, you will examine how effectively different wrapping materials prevent freezer burn.

Equipment

chef's knife
cutting board
Polaroid or digital camera (optional)
6 saucers
wax pencil
25-mL graduated cylinder

Supplies

fresh fruit or vegetable that is in season and
    freezes well
1 resealable plastic bag
1 resealable plastic freezer bag
1 resealable plastic vegetable bag
aluminum foil
freezer paper
masking tape

Procedure

1. Cut the assigned fruit or vegetable into six equal portions.

2. Record the color, texture, and appearance of the fruit or vegetable. (Optional: Take a picture of the food before freezing.)

3. Place one fruit or vegetable portion on a saucer.

4. Wrap each of the five remaining portions in a different one of the following materials: resealable plastic bag, resealable plastic freezer bag, resealable plastic vegetable bag, aluminum foil, or freezer paper.

5. Place a masking tape label with your lab group number and class period on each sample. Store all six samples in the freezer for 30 days.

30 Days Later

1. Remove the samples from the freezer and unwrap.

2. Use a wax pencil to label five saucers with the five types of wrapping material used. Place the appropriate sample on each labeled saucer. (Optional: Take a picture of the frozen samples.)

3. Record the color, texture, and appearance of each sample in the data table.

4. Cover all six saucers with plastic wrap and place the food in the refrigerator overnight.

Next Day

1. Measure and record the amount of drip (free water found in the saucer) of each sample with a 25-mL graduated cylinder. (Optional: Take pictures of the thawed products.)

2. Record your observations of the color, texture, and appearance of each sample in the data table.

Questions

1. Which packaging material protected the food from freezer burn?

2. Which materials were not acceptable packaging for frozen foods?

3. What changes did freezer burn cause?

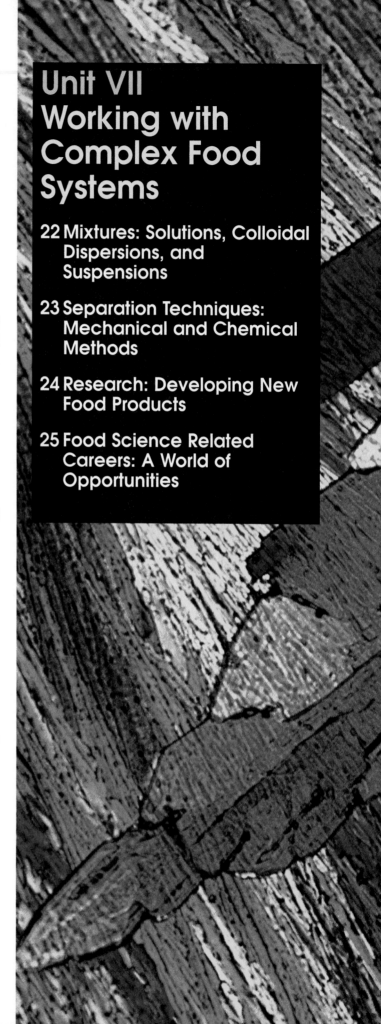

Food scientists must know how the compounds in foods will affect one another. *Complex food systems* are food products that contain most of the types of compounds described in this text. Unit VII explores areas related to the challenges of working with complex food systems.

Some foods exist in nature as complex mixtures. Many other complex mixtures are created by food manufacturers as they develop new food products. Eggs are an example of a complex mixture in nature. Eggs are also an important part of many manufactured mixtures. Chapter 22 examines the different types of mixtures that exist in food products. You will explore how the principles of mixtures are applied to some of your favorite foods.

Many food products result from the separation of complex food systems into parts. For instance, butter is extracted from milk. Vegetable oil is isolated from soybeans, corn, and other seed grains. In Chapter 23, you will examine the physical and chemical methods used to separate food mixtures. You will also study how separation principles apply to your body's metabolism.

Chapter 24 discusses basic research procedures food scientists use to study complex food systems. The steps manufacturers follow in developing new food products are also outlined. After reading this chapter, you may choose to set up a food science research project of your own.

Many people work together to develop and produce all the food products on the market today. In Chapter 25, you will read about the personal qualities, education, and training these people need to do their jobs. You will also explore the employment outlook for careers in food science and other food-related areas.

Do you recognize the popular complex food system in this photomicrograph? It is ice cream, which is an example of a type of mixture called an emulsion.

Unit VII
Working with Complex Food Systems

22 Mixtures: Solutions, Colloidal Dispersions, and Suspensions

23 Separation Techniques: Mechanical and Chemical Methods

24 Research: Developing New Food Products

25 Food Science Related Careers: A World of Opportunities

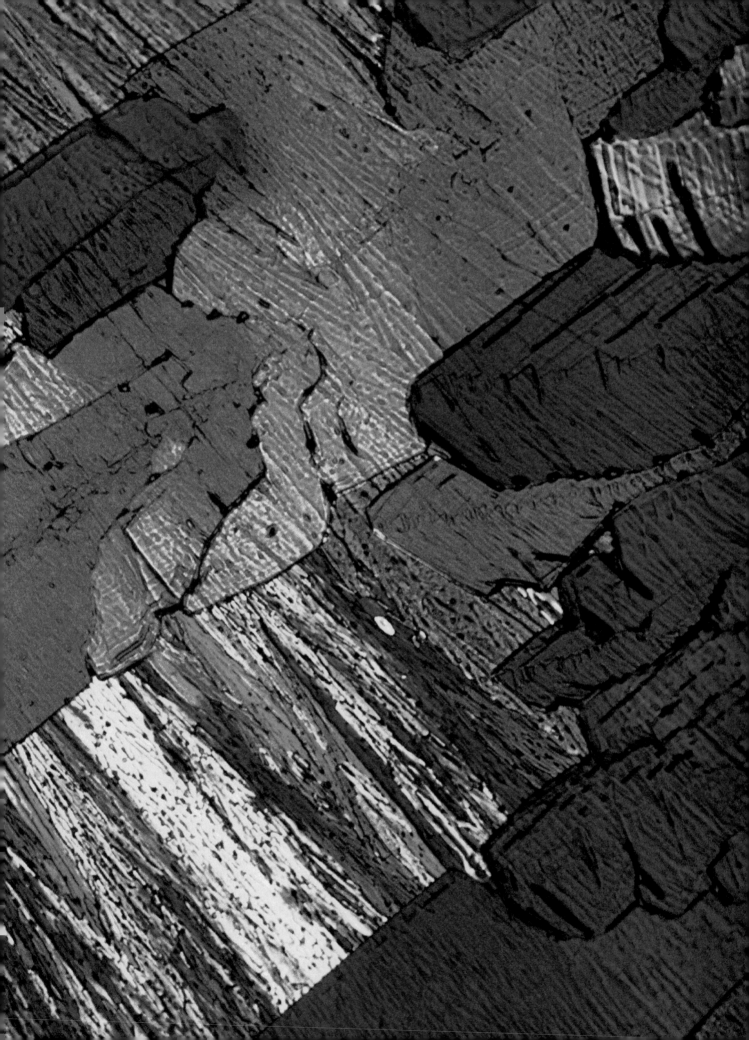

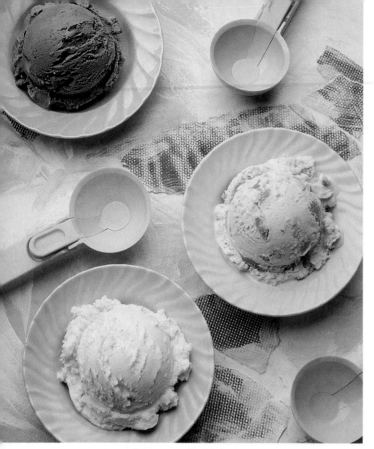

Ice cream is an example of a food mixture called an emulsion.

Chapter 22

Mixtures: Solutions, Colloidal Dispersions, and Suspensions

Objectives

After studying this chapter,
you will be able to

list the factors that affect the solubility of one substance in another.

calculate the mass percent of solute in a solution.

compare colloids and solutes.

differentiate between the two most common types of food emulsions.

describe factors that can affect the stability of a food foam.

explain the properties of suspensions using batters and doughs as examples.

Key Terms

dispersed phase
continuous phase
vapor pressure
mass percent
colloidal dispersion
colloid
Tyndall effect

homogenization
emulsion
temporary emulsion
emulsifier
thermal conductivity
foam
suspension

Foods are not chemically simple elements. Few foods are single elements or compounds. Most foods are complex mixtures of many types of elements and compounds. A glass of milk is a complex mixture of proteins, fats, carbohydrates, enzymes, salts, minerals, vitamins, and water. Understanding how components interact helps food scientists predict how foods will react during processing. See 22-1.

Food mixtures are classified by the size of particles distributed throughout the mixture. The *dispersed phase* refers to the particles that

The Science Behind a Hard-Cooked Egg

Recipe	Rational
Place the eggs in a pan of cold water.	If cold eggs are placed in hot water, the uneven rapid heating can cause the eggshell to crack. This is because the different regions of the shell are of different thicknesses and will expand at varying rates.
Bring to a boil, cover, and remove from heat.	Protein gels become tough and elastic if held at boiling temperatures for an extended period. Covering the eggs holds the heat in the pan, allowing the eggs to cook. The water's temperature quickly drops below the point that would toughen the egg white. The result is a tender but firm white.
Let covered pan sit 15 minutes for large eggs.	There is enough heat left in the water to allow the white and yolk to set up without overcooking.
Rinse the eggs in cold water until they are completely cooled.	Heating causes sulfur and hydrogen to break away from the protein molecules in the egg white. These elements combine to form hydrogen sulfide gas. This gas comes out of the suspension of egg white to the coolest part of the egg. During cooking, this is the yolk. Iron is a solute in the egg yolk. The iron at the surface of the yolk will interact with the hydrogen sulfide. The result is iron sulfide, which is green. If eggs are cooked too long at too hot a temperature, a green ring will develop around the egg yolk. A green ring can also form if eggs are not cooled quickly after cooking. Rinsing the eggs in cold water as soon as the cooking time ends cools the shells. This causes the hydrogen sulfide to move toward the shells.

22-1 Understanding the reactions of complex mixtures such as eggs can help professionals in the food industry develop product preparation procedures.

are scattered throughout a medium. The medium in which particles are distributed is called the *continuous phase*. Mixtures with the smallest particles in the dispersed phase are solutions. Colloidal dispersions have larger particles than those in solutions. The largest particles in the dispersed phase are found in mixtures called suspensions.

Solutions

You read in Chapter 4 that a solution is a homogenous mixture of two or more substances. Solutions consist of two parts: the solute, which is the dispersed phase, and the solvent, which is the continuous phase. The solute cannot be filtered or separated out of the solvent. The particles in true solutions are so small that you cannot see them under a microscope. The particles have high levels of kinetic energy and are therefore in constant motion in the solution. True solutions do not have the ability to form gels.

There are three states of matter, and solutions are possible in any combination of those three states. Most foods that are solutions exist as solids in liquids, liquids in liquids, and gases in liquids. When you prepare a powdered drink mix, you are making a solid-in-liquid solution. You are dissolving sugar and flavoring (solid) in water (liquid). Another common solid-in-liquid solution in food systems is salt in water. Most bottled flavorings, such as vanilla extract, are liquid-in-liquid solutions of alcohol in water plus flavoring compounds. Club soda is an example of a gas-in-liquid solution. It is carbon dioxide (CO_2) gas dissolved in water.

It is possible for solutions to be complex mixtures of more than one solute. An example is carbonated soft drinks. They are solutions of a solid (sugar), a liquid (corn syrup), and a gas (CO_2) in liquid (water).

Factors Affecting Solubility

A solute is soluble when it can be dissolved in a solvent. In Chapter 8, you learned *solubility* describes the amount of solute that will dissolve in a solvent. A number of factors can change how soluble one substance is in another. These factors are temperature, particle size, concentration, agitation, and vapor pressure.

Temperature

The first factor that affects solubility of solids is the temperature of the solvent. As the temperature increases, the amount of a solid solute the solvent will hold increases. For example, 100 g of water at 20°C (68°F) will hold 36 g of sodium chloride (salt). At 100°C (212°F), 100 g of water will hold 40 g of sodium chloride. The type of solute will also affect how much can dissolve in a solution. For example, 100 g of water at 20°C (68°F) will hold 34 g of potassium chloride (salt substitute). At 100°C (212°F), 100 g of water will hold 57.6 g of potassium chloride.

This principle of temperature affecting solubility is used in the candy industry. Sugar syrups, which form the base of many candies, are solutions of sugar in water. As water is heated, it can hold more sugar solute, and the concentration of the sugar syrup increases. The concentration of the sugar syrup affects a candy's sweetness and texture.

The temperature of the solvent also affects the solubility of gases. As the temperature of a solvent increases, the amount of a gaseous solute it will hold decreases. This is why soft drinks lose their carbonation faster at room temperature than when chilled.

The reason solvent temperature affects the solubility of solids and gases is the increased number of molecular collisions. As temperature increases, molecular movement increases. The more the molecules of the solvent collide with the molecules of a solid, the faster the solid will dissolve. The more the gas molecules move, the less energy it takes for the gas to escape into the air.

Particle Size

A second factor that affects solubility is the particle size of the solute. The smaller the particles of solute are, the greater the exposed surface area will be. The greater the surface area is, the faster the solute will dissolve. This is because solute molecules must come in contact with the solvent molecules to dissolve.

You can demonstrate this factor using two glasses of water. You will also need a sugar cube and 2 mL ($\frac{1}{2}$ teaspoon) of granulated sugar. Add the sugar cube to one glass and the granulated sugar to the other glass at the same time. Stir and observe how quickly the granulated sugar disappears as compared to the sugar cube. See 22-2. In the same way, ground coffee beans will flavor a cup of hot water faster than whole coffee beans.

Concentration of a Solution

A third factor affecting solubility is how much solute is in a solution. In Chapter 6, you

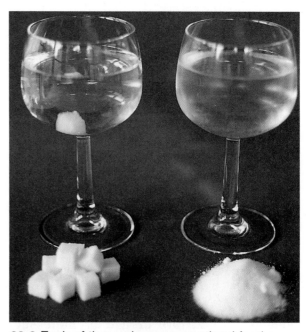

22-2 Each of these glasses was stirred for the same length of time with the same amount of added sugar. The smaller granulated sugar particles on the right dissolved more quickly than the sugar cube on the left.

learned that *concentration* is the measure of parts of one substance (the solute) to the known volume of another (the solvent). A solution holding all the solute that will dissolve in the solvent at a given temperature is *saturated.*

This factor is related to how solutes stay distributed in a solution. Most food solutions are mixtures of polar compounds with water as the solvent. When water molecules come close to other polar molecules, hydrogen bonds will form. This intermolecular bonding keeps the solute distributed in the solvent. Once all the water molecules have bonded to a solute, a solution is at the *saturation point.* No more hydrogen bonds can form. As the saturation point is approached, the solute dissolves at a slower rate. This is because it takes longer for free water molecules to find free solvent molecules.

You can observe this factor by stirring sugar into water. Add sugar, one teaspoon at a time, to a glass of water. Note how long it takes the sugar to disappear after each addition. At what point does sugar remain undissolved in the glass?

You can also use the glass of sugar and water to observe the effects of solvent temperature on solubility. Heat the glass for 30 seconds in a microwave oven. Can you still see any sugar? Adding heat gives the energy needed to break the hydrogen bonds between sugar molecules. The heated solvent can hold more solute. Therefore, a heated solution can have a higher concentration of solute than is possible at a lower temperature.

To form a *supersaturated solution,* a solution must be heated and then cooled. When the solution is heated, it will be able to hold more solute. Then when the solution is cooled, it will have a higher concentration than would normally be possible at that temperature.

The solutes in most supersaturated solutions will form crystals as the solution cools. Removing the crystals from the solution is a separation technique used by some food processors. You will read more about this technique in Chapter 23.

As you read in Chapter 8, candy makers rely on supersaturated sugar solutions.

Supersaturating a sugar solution is possible because sugar will dissolve and liquefy if heated to a high enough temperature. The heat energy breaks hydrogen bonds between sugar molecules. This allows the molecules to flow freely past one another. When handled properly, these solutions can remain stable after cooling. They must be cooled slowly without agitation. This allows the sugar molecules to solidify before they can reform crystals.

The crystallization of saturated sugar solutions is related to the sugar-water ratio, preparation procedure, and additional ingredients. Candies can be divided into crystalline and noncrystalline categories. Rock candy is an example of a mass of large crystals. Fondants and fudges have small, dispersed crystals separated by the action of interfering agents. Noncrystalline candies can be hard, chewy, or gummy. Sourballs are an example of hard candies, which have a glasslike quality. They have a moisture content of 2% or less. Chewy candies like caramels have 8 to 15% moisture. Gumdrops are a gummy candy with 15 to 22% water content.

Agitation

The fourth factor that affects solubility is agitation. Agitation or stirring will speed the dissolving process until the saturation point is reached. Think back to the two glasses of water with the sugar cube and granulated sugar. What happens when the sugars are added but not stirred? Once the water next to the sugar is saturated, dissolving slows or stops. Stirring replaces the saturated water near the sugar with water that is holding less of the solute. Stirring also adds a small amount of energy that raises the temperature slightly.

Vapor Pressure

Another factor that affects the solubility of gases dissolved in liquids is *vapor pressure.* This is the pressure at which gases escape from and dissolve into a liquid at the same rate. Small changes in pressure have little or no effect on the solubility of solids and liquids in solution. However, the concentration of gas in a liquid is directly related to pressure of the gas over the liquid. If you double the pressure over a gas-in-liquid solution, you can double the amount of gas in the solution.

The fizz in carbonated drinks is caused by adding gas to liquid under pressure. The beverages are then sealed in containers. Within the sealed containers, the pressure is in *equilibrium*. This means the pressure of the gas over the liquid equals the pressure of the gas within the liquid. Therefore, the liquid is neither gaining nor losing gas molecules. When the seal on a carbonated beverage is broken, the balance of pressure changes. The pressure above the solution decreases. This allows the gases dissolved in the liquid to bubble, rise to the top, and escape. See 22-3.

Measuring Solute Concentrations

A measure of the concentration of a solution is the mass percent. **Mass percent** is the percentage of the mass in a solution that comes from the solute. The mass of the solute is divided by the total mass of the solution and multiplied by 100. This is the same basic formula used to calculate any percentage.

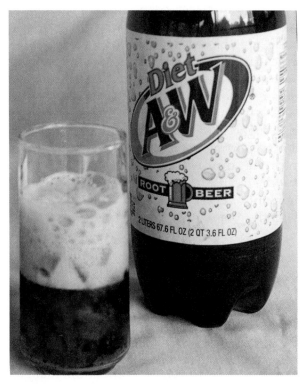

22-3 The foam on root beer results partly from the rapid change in vapor pressure when the bottle is opened.

$$\frac{\text{mass of solute}}{\text{mass of}\ \text{solution}\left(\begin{matrix}\text{mass of} \\ \text{solute}\end{matrix} + \begin{matrix}\text{mass of} \\ \text{solvent}\end{matrix}\right)} \times 100 = \begin{matrix}\text{mass} \\ \text{percent}\end{matrix}$$

What is the mass percent of a solution of 20 g of sugar in 80 g of water? The mass of the solute is 20 g. The total mass of the solution is 100 g (20 g solute plus 80 g solvent).

$$\frac{20\ \text{g}}{100\ \text{g}} \times 100 = 20\%$$

Solutions are usually defined or described in terms of the mass percent of the solute. A 10% salt solution gets 10% of its mass from the dissolved salt.

Solute Concentration Affects Freezing and Boiling Points

Water freezes at 0°C (32°F) and boils at 100°C (212°F). When a solute, such as salt or sugar, is added, the freezing point drops and the boiling point rises. The changes in the freezing and boiling points will be greater as the mass percent of the solute increases. Therefore, a 10% salt solution will have a lower freezing point than a 5% salt solution. The 10% solution will also have a higher boiling point than the 5% solution.

A solution of 1 mole of any solute containing covalent bonds dissolved in 1 kg of water has a freezing point of -1.86°C (28.65°F). Solutes containing ionic bonds will produce solutions with even lower freezing points and higher boiling points. This is because when molecules formed by ionic bonds dissolve, they separate into ions. For instance, sodium and chlorine are ionically bonded to form salt. When a salt molecule dissolves, it separates into one sodium ion and one chlorine ion. Therefore, when 1 mole of salt is added to 1 kg of water, it dissolves into 2 moles of solute. The greater number of particles results in a lower freezing point and a higher boiling point.

You can see the effect of solutes on the freezing points of solutions in the way ice cream freezers work. Solutes such as sugar and milk solids cause an ice cream solution to have a lower freezing point than water. This solution is placed in a metal can, which is surrounded by ice cubes. Salt is added to the ice cubes. The combination of salt and ice is *endothermic*. This means the mixture absorbs heat energy from its surroundings. As a result, the ice melts. The solution of salt, ice, and water that forms has a lower freezing point than pure water. This solution also has a lower freezing point than that of the ice cream solution. The temperature of the saltwater solution is below that of the ice cream mixture. This causes heat energy to be transferred from the ice cream mixture to the saltwater solution through the metal can. As the ice cream mixture loses heat energy, its temperature drops. Heat energy will continue to be transferred until the ice cream freezes.

Solute Concentration Affects Vapor Pressure

The concentration of a solution will affect the vapor pressure of the solution. When the mass percent of a solute increases, the pressure of the solution increases. The solution then tries to equalize the pressure in the solution with the environment around it.

A solution will equalize pressure by either absorbing water from the air or allowing solutes to escape. Molecules will move in the direction that offers least resistance. In the case of a sugar solution, it is easier to absorb water molecules than to release sugar molecules. This is why hard candy that is left uncovered will become sticky. The candy is a concentrated sugar solution. The candy becomes sticky as the solution absorbs water from the air.

A soft drink is a carbon dioxide-in-water solution. In this case, it is easier for the solution to release gas into the atmosphere to equalize pressure. The pressure of the CO_2 in the headspace of a sealed can of soft drink equals the pressure of the carbon dioxide-in-water solution. When the can is opened, the pressure above the solution decreases. The CO_2 collects and forms bubbles as it rises to the top of the solution. The soft drink will fizz until vapor pressure is reached. This is why a glass of soft drink "goes flat" if it sits for a while.

Applications in the Beverage Industry

The solutions that are consumed in the largest amounts are beverages. They include soft drinks, coffee, and tea.

Soft Drinks

Carbonated soft drinks are solutions. Water is the solvent. Sweeteners, flavorings, coloring agents, acids, and CO_2 are the solutes.

Most soft drinks today are sweetened with high-fructose corn syrups and/or sugar. These beverages have a sugar concentration of 8% to 14%. Food scientists cannot simply replace sugar and corn syrup with a nonnutritive substitute to make diet soft drinks. Artificial sweeteners do not give the solution the same body as the sugar and corn syrups. To produce acceptable diet soft drinks, carbohydrate gums or pectins can be added to the solution. These solutes will copy the mouth feel of sweetened carbonated beverages. The most common gums used in soft drinks are alginates, xanthan, and carboxymethylcellulose. Any change in the ingredients in a solution will result in pressure changes. Food scientists must predict the effects of these changes on bottling and storage. See 22-4.

Most carbonated beverages are sold in clear plastic containers that allow exposure to light. They have a pH range of 2.6 to 4.0. The time from production to consumption can be as much as one year. Therefore, flavoring and

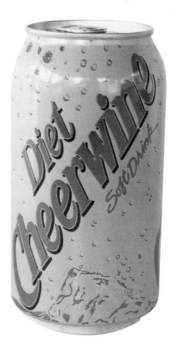

22-4 Added gums or pectins are used to give diet soft drinks the same mouth feel as sugar-sweetened soft drinks.

coloring agents must be tested for stability to light and acids. Artificial and natural flavoring and coloring agents are themselves complex mixtures of chemicals. For example, artificial raspberry flavor contains at least 29 chemicals. Each of these compounds must remain stable in the soft drink solution for the product to meet consumer expectations. If a compound does break down, the resulting products must not make the beverage taste unacceptable.

Carbon dioxide provides fizz to soft drinks. It also adds to the acidity. The acids act as flavor enhancers and preservatives. Citric acid, which is naturally found in many fruits, is the most common acid used in fruit-flavored drinks. Phosphoric acid is used more often in nonfruit flavors, such as colas and root beer. These acids alone are not enough to prevent microbial spoilage during long-term storage. Therefore, sodium benzoate, which converts to benzoic acid in solution, is usually added as a preservative. The mass percent of sodium benzoate in solution is 0.03% to 0.05%. The maximum allowable is 0.10%.

The water used for soft drinks must be examined for quality. Water is a solution. It often contains oxygen, organic matter, and minerals as solutes. These solutes can all affect the finished product. Any variation in pH can alter the microbial stability of the soft drink. Some minerals, like iron, react negatively with many of the coloring and flavoring agents used in soft drinks. Chlorine, which is used by water processing plants, results in unpleasant flavors in drink products if not removed by activated charcoal. Oxygen is also removed from the water by vacuum treatment.

Most beverage manufacturers have a number of bottling plants. These plants cannot each use local water if the product is to be the same from one plant to another. Soft drink bottling plants must treat the water to remove as many solutes as possible. The result is a consistent water quality, whether the drink is bottled in California, New Jersey, or Japan.

This type of quality control is not possible with beverages sold at restaurants and refreshment stands. Most soft drink manufacturers distribute concentrated syrups to these foodservice establishments. These syrups are mixed with water at the point of sale. This is why soft drinks sold in glasses may taste different from the same products sold in cans.

Cooking Tip

In addition to their popularity as beverages, many soft drinks have become cooking ingredients. The phosphoric acid in soft drinks is an excellent meat tenderizer. This makes soft drinks, especially colas, good substitutes for wines, beers, and vinegars in many marinade recipes. The acid content of soft drinks can help protein-based gelatins set. Soft drinks add leavening as well as flavor to many baked goods. Soft drinks can also be used in place of water or milk in many biscuit, muffin, and cake recipes.

Coffee and Tea

Coffee and tea are both nonnutritive beverages. They are consumed for their flavors and stimulating effects. Coffee beans and tea leaves are fermented and/or dried to develop flavors that are extracted or brewed into a water base. These beverages vary with the type of coffee bean or tea leaf and the drying process used. The roasting times, particle sizes, and added flavoring agents affect strength and flavor. When these beverages are brewed, brewing time and temperature will also affect their strengths and flavors. The production of these beverages is a complex industry. Food scientists in this industry must study the effects of many solutes on the finished products. See 22-5.

Colloidal Dispersions

In some mixtures, particles are dispersed in a liquid without being dissolved. *Colloidal dispersions* are mixtures in which microscopic particles of one substance are evenly distributed in another substance. The nature of the particles is what gives colloidal dispersions their unique characteristics. Emulsions, foams, and gels are three types of these mixtures.

Characteristics of Colloidal Dispersions

True colloidal dispersions are made up of a continuous phase and a dispersed phase. The continuous phase is the medium that holds the dispersed particles. The continuous phase is usually made up of small molecules, such as water molecules. The dispersed phase is the particles, or *colloids,* that are distributed all through the mixture. Colloids are macromolecules or clumps of smaller molecules. Starch and protein are examples of colloids that can be distributed in a colloidal dispersion. Jelly, mayonnaise, butter, and gelatin are some foods that are colloidal dispersions.

Comparing Colloids and Solutes

The key factor that distinguishes colloids from solutes is the size of the particles. This factor is why solutions and colloidal dispersions have different properties.

Colloids can be as much as 1,000 times larger than solute particles. Particle size of solutes in solutions is up to 1 nanometer (nm) in diameter. Colloids are usually between 1 nm and 1 micrometer (μm). (There are 1,000 μm to a millimeter and 1,000 nm to a micrometer.)

The small size of solutes allows them to dissolve in other substances. Because colloids are larger, they can be dispersed in another substance, but they will not dissolve. This is why, unlike solutes, colloids do not have a notable impact on the boiling and freezing points of mixtures.

Colloids are large enough to bend or reflect light onto another path. However, solutes are too small to bend light. This fact was discovered by a British physicist named John Tyndall. He was the first to conduct experiments on the scattering of light. He found that when light travels through a solution, no change in the direction of the light rays is noticeable. On the other hand, when light passes through a colloidal dispersion, the light rays scatter and are visible. This phenomenon is called the *Tyndall effect.* See 22-6.

You can do a simple experiment to observe the Tyndall effect. First, shine a flashlight through a beaker of water. Then shine the flashlight through a beaker containing a mixture of water and unflavored gelatin. Notice the difference in what happens to the light as it passes through the beakers.

Factors That Keep Colloids Dispersed

Colloids remain dispersed due to two factors. The first is the motion of the molecules of the continuous phase. The lower mass of the smaller molecules of the continuous phase allows them to move faster than the colloids. The colloids and the molecules of the continuous phase constantly collide with one another. The collisions change the direction of both molecules, depending on their paths before contact. The molecular motion keeps the colloids dispersed.

The second factor that keeps colloids dispersed is their electrical charges. The colloids

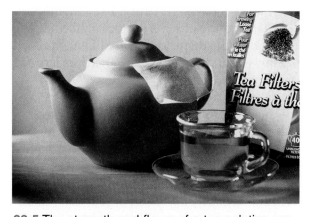

22-5 The strength and flavor of a tea solution are affected by the processing of the tea leaves and the brewing method used.

The Tyndall Effect

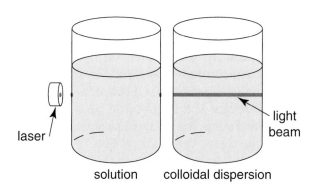

laser

light beam

solution   colloidal dispersion

22-6 Light cannot be seen when it passes through a solution. However, light is scattered when it passes through a colloidal dispersion, causing the light beam to be visible.

are usually molecules of the same substance. Therefore, they all have the same electrical charge. The like charges repel, pushing the colloids away from one another. Because water molecules are polar, they will align themselves around a colloid, forming a water cushion. This cushion helps keep colloids from sticking together and settling out of the mixture.

Effects of Particle Density

In some mixtures, the particles will not remain dispersed. This is due to the density of the particles in the dispersed phase compared to the density of the continuous phase. Examples include flour in water and fat in fresh milk that has not been homogenized.

If the particles are denser than the continuous phase, they will sink as the mixture sits. This is why many sauces must be constantly stirred during the heating process. The starch granules are denser than the water in which they are dispersed. If the mixture is not stirred, it will become lumpy. The starch will sink and burn to the bottom of the pan.

Most colloids in foods are starches or proteins. Chapters 9 and 11 examined how heat can break hydrogen bonds in starch and protein molecules. Once the starch or protein molecules open their molecular structure, intermolecular bonds can form between the molecules. This creates a three-dimensional network. Water becomes trapped between and around the molecules. Once starch molecules have swollen with water, they will stay dispersed, the mixture will thicken, and a colloidal dispersion is formed.

When a thickened colloidal dispersion remains pourable, it is a sol. When pH, temperature, and/or concentrations are altered, the sol can be transformed into a rigid gel. Gelatin is a protein-based colloidal gel. Jams and jellies are pectin-based colloidal gels.

If particles of the dispersed phase are less dense than the continuous phase, they will rise to the top of the mixture. This is why a fat layer forms on the top of gravy. The fat colloids are less dense than the rest of the gravy.

Milk as a Colloidal Dispersion

Milk is an example of a colloidal dispersion. Milk is also a solution. Milk is made up of water, lactose, mineral salts, proteins, and fat. The lactose and mineral salts are solutes. The proteins are colloids. The fats are in suspension. The lactose and mineral salts are dissolved in the water, forming a solution. This solution is the continuous phase in which the proteins are dispersed.

The colloidal dispersion of the proteins in milk is stable. The fat globules in the milk are not a stable dispersion. Like the fat in gravy, the fat particles in fresh whole milk will rise to the top. When they rise to the top, they form a layer of cream. To keep this from happening, milk is homogenized. *Homogenization* is a mechanical process that forces milk through screens or small openings. This ruptures the membranes around the fat globules and breaks the globules into smaller particles. Homogenization alters the chemical nature of the fat particles, keeping them from re-collecting and rising to the top. This is a result of the casein colloids surrounding the fat particles. The charged portions of the casein interact with the continuous phase, keeping the oil droplets apart. This creates a stable colloidal dispersion by causing the fat to remain permanently dispersed throughout the milk. The fat in homogenized milk is an example of a type of dispersion called an emulsion. It is stabilized by colloidal membranes of casein. See 22-7.

Emulsions

An *emulsion* is a mixture of two immiscible liquids, where one is dispersed in droplet form in the other. *Immiscible liquids* are liquids that will separate when combined. Usually one liquid is polar in nature, like water-based vinegar, and the other is nonpolar, like oil. The droplets in the dispersed phase of an emulsion are between 0.1 and 50.0 µm. This is as large as or larger than colloids.

Polar and nonpolar substances repel, or move away from each other. As the molecules in an emulsion move, the molecules of the polar liquid repel the molecules of the nonpolar liquid. At the same time, the molecules of the polar liquid will attract one another and collect. Similarly, the molecules of the nonpolar liquid will gather. This is what causes the liquids to separate. The liquid that is less dense will rise to the top of the mixture.

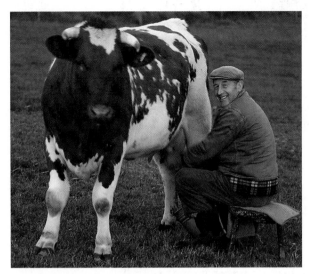

22-7 A layer of milkfat will form on the top of fresh milk that has not been homogenized.

You may have seen this happen in a bottle of vinegar and oil salad dressing. When you shake the bottle, the two liquids combine. As the bottle sets, the liquids separate, and the oil forms a layer on top of the vinegar. This type of salad dressing is a temporary emulsion. *Temporary emulsions* are unstable mixtures of two immiscible liquids. In other words, as the mixture stands, the liquids will separate.

In order for one immiscible liquid to stay dispersed in another, a stabilizing factor must be added. This factor is called an emulsifier. An *emulsifier* is a molecule that has a polar end and a nonpolar end. The polar end is attracted to and forms hydrogen bonds with other polar molecules. In the same way, the nonpolar end is attracted to nonpolar

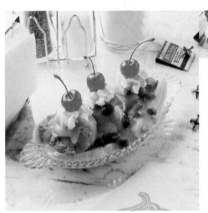

Item of Interest
Emulsifiers

Stabilizers and emulsifiers are a group of additives used to maintain colloidal dispersions in many food products. The emulsifier used depends on the type of emulsion. Many of these additives are gums and alginates from tropical plants. Other emulsifiers are proteins, mono- and diglycerides, and phospholipids. *Phospholipids* are triglycerides that have one of the fatty acids replaced with an acid that contains phosphorus. The fatty acid end is nonpolar. This end attracts fat molecules. The phosphoric acid group is polar. It attracts vinegar and water molecules.

Lecithin is a phospholipid. It is also the emulsifier used in chocolate products. Lecithin and sugar are added to cocoa powder to make a hot cocoa mix.

Cocoa powder does not readily dissolve in water. This is because tiny pockets of air surround the cocoa particles. Lecithin helps water bridge this air gap so the cocoa can dissolve. Lecithin is

also used to keep cocoa powder and sugar evenly suspended in cocoa butter. Emulsifiers such as lecithin have helped make possible the wide variety of chocolate bars and candy.

lecithin

molecules. Most emulsions require agitation, stirring, or beating for the emulsifier to bond to the molecules and stabilize the mixture. For instance, lecithin is an emulsifier that is found in egg yolks. During beating, the lecithin in egg yolks will attach to the molecules of vinegar and oil to form mayonnaise. (See Chapter 11 for an illustration of how an emulsifier works at the molecular level.)

Types of Emulsions

The two most common types of food emulsions are oil-in-water and water-in-oil. The dispersed phase, which is the liquid in droplet form, is listed first. The continuous phase is listed second. Usually, the phase present in the largest amount is the continuous phase. Mayonnaise, salad dressings, ice cream, and cake batters are examples of oil-in-water emulsions, 22-8. Butter and margarine are examples of water-in-oil emulsions.

Butter is a water-in-oil emulsion that is made from whipping cream, which is an oil-in-water emulsion. The fat globules in whipping cream are surrounded by phospholipid membranes containing lecithin. These membranes act as an emulsifier that stabilizes the emulsion and keeps the fat dispersed all through the cream. Churning or agitation breaks the membranes, allowing the fat globules to clump together. As these clumps of butterfat grow in size, they separate from the water phase of the cream. They form an emulsion of oil with small droplets of water trapped in the mixture.

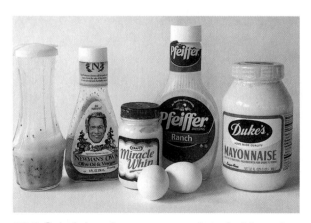

22-8 Salad dressings are examples of oil-in-water emulsions. Those that remain mixed contain an emulsifier, such as lecithin in eggs.

Margarine is made from hydrogenated vegetable oils. Like butter, margarine is 80% fat. Margarine also contains water, emulsifiers, salt, butter flavoring, color, preservatives, and vitamins. All the fat-soluble ingredients are combined with the vegetable oil. The water is mixed with the water-soluble ingredients. These two mixtures are made into an emulsion through vigorous agitation. The emulsion is stabilized by rapid chilling to solidify the mixture.

Butter has a fat content of at least 80%. The remaining 20% of the mass of butter is made up of water and milk solids. Lowfat margarines are made by increasing the percentage of water. You can see this by melting sticks of butter, margarine, and lowfat margarine in separate beakers covered with foil. Let the beakers sit until the fat and water in the melted products have separated. Then compare the water content of the three products. (What do you think will happen if lowfat margarine is substituted for butter in baked goods?)

Factors Affecting the Stability of Emulsions

A number of factors can affect the stability of emulsions. One of these factors is temperature. This is because fats and water have different thermal conductivity levels. *Thermal conductivity* is the ability to transfer heat energy. Water has more thermal conductivity than fat. This means water transfers heat more readily than fat. Therefore, an oil-in-water emulsion will freeze at a higher temperature than a water-in-oil emulsion. An oil-in-water emulsion will also freeze faster than a water-in-oil emulsion. This is because heat begins transferring out of the continuous phase before it begins transferring out of the dispersed phase.

Freezing temperatures can squeeze the water out of an emulsion. This is because the water portion of an emulsion will freeze before the emulsifying agent and the fat. Once the water is in a solid state, the fat droplets can collect and separate from the emulsion. This is why sandwiches and salads with mayonnaise do not freeze well.

High temperatures as well as low temperatures can affect the stability of emulsions. This is especially true when the emulsifier is a protein. High temperatures cause proteins to coagulate. This prevents the proteins from being evenly distributed all through the mixture. The emulsion separates because the protein can no longer act as an emulsifier.

Hollandaise sauce is an example of an emulsion that can easily become unstable and curdle due to high temperatures. Hollandaise sauce is made from a mixture of egg yolk, butter, lemon juice, water, salt, and cayenne pepper. The egg yolk serves as the emulsifier that keeps the butter dispersed in the water and lemon juice solution. Hollandaise sauces are best prepared at 77°C (170°F). Temperatures of 82°C to 88°C (180°F to 190°F) will cause the egg proteins to coagulate. The result is a curdled, separated sauce.

A second factor that can affect the stability of emulsions is electrical charges. Emulsions work because the water-based liquid is electrically attracted to the polar end of the emulsifier. Running electrical currents through an emulsion can disrupt the electrical fields in the emulsion. This can cause the emulsion to destabilize. This principle can be used to separate parts of emulsions.

Ice Cream as an Emulsion

Ice cream is an example of an emulsion that must remain stable during freezing. Ice cream is a water-based sugar solution that forms an emulsion with fat-based cream. The mixing or agitation during freezing adds air to this emulsion. As the water freezes, the concentration of the unfrozen sugar solution increases. Once the solution reaches the saturation point for sugar, lactose and other sugars will begin to settle out as crystals. These crystals can give a gritty, sandy feel to the ice cream.

Emulsifiers give ice cream a smooth, creamy texture. They do this by helping to stabilize the emulsion, which keeps the cream and sugar solution from separating during freezing. Emulsifiers also help keep the sugar, fat, and water particles dispersed so ice and sugar crystals remain small. A sugar molecule cannot bond to another sugar molecule if there is a fat molecule between them.

The emulsifiers used in commercially made ice cream are gums, pectins, and lecithin. They work by thickening the mixture. The more viscous the mixture is, the harder it is for the fat droplets to collect and separate.

Foams

Foams are colloidal dispersions of gas or air bubbles dispersed in a liquid. The froth on top of root beer and other carbonated beverages is an example of an unstable foam. These foams will quickly collapse. Whipped toppings, whipped cream, and meringue are stable food foams that will last for extended periods, 22-9. For a foam to remain stable, four conditions are necessary.

First, the liquid needs to be viscous enough to hold the air. (Whipping cream and egg whites meet this criterion.) The thick texture of the liquid combines with the elastic nature of protein to trap and hold tiny air bubbles.

Second, the dispersion needs to contain a stabilizer that will stretch to form a thin film around air bubbles. Many foams are made by incorporating air into liquid emulsions. The air is trapped by a stable, elastic compound. This is usually a protein, which has polar molecules.

Third, the surface tension of the film should be less than that of water. This will

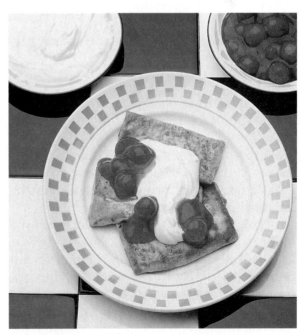

22-9 Whipped cream is a stable foam of air bubbles in liquid cream.

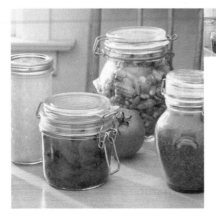

Historical Highlight
Chocolate: A Complex Mixture

Chocolate comes from the seeds or beans inside the yellow, football-shaped pods of the South American cacao tree.

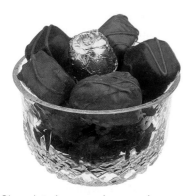

Chocolate is a popular complex mixture and, as such, requires involved preparation processes.

Today's chocolate candy is a complex mixture containing fat, sugar, milk, and over 300 flavor compounds. Developing creamy, high-quality chocolate is an involved process. It entails fermentation, enzymatic activity, and pH adjustment. It also entails altering particle sizes and stabilizing an emulsion. Developing the delicious chocolates of today took over 350 years of experimentation.

The History

❖ In 1519, the Aztecs first offered Hernando Cortez a bitter chocolate drink.

❖ In 1828, a Dutch chemist named van Houten invented the *dutching* process, which gives chocolate a milder flavor.

❖ In 1847, J.S. Fry and Sons produced the first chocolate candy bar.

❖ In 1876, Henri Nestle, a chemist working on condensed milk, and Daniel Peter, a chocolatier, created milk chocolate.

❖ In the late 1800s, conching machines were developed to produce chocolate with a smooth, creamy texture. This process creates a smooth emulsion of cocoa, sugar, and cocoa butter.

❖ Between 1893 and 1903, Milton Hershey used trial and error to develop a process for making milk chocolate. His process was similar to the one used by Nestle and Peter. In

---

keep the air from being squeezed out of the bubbles. Surface tension is the attraction of polar molecules for one another in a liquid. Around a bubble of air, the force of the surface tension pulls inward. If this inward pulling is greater than the pressure of the gas pushing out, the bubble will collapse.

The fourth condition needed for foam stability is a liquid with a low vapor pressure. This will keep the polar films around the air bubbles from readily evaporating into the trapped air. Substances that evaporate easily have high vapor pressures. A liquid with a high vapor pressure would evaporate into the air rather than forming a film around it.

Factors Affecting Foam Stability

A number of factors affect the stability of food foams. One of these factors is temperature. In most cases, the viscosity of a liquid is decreased as the temperature rises. However, egg whites reach the fullest volume when allowed to stand at room temperature for about 30 minutes before beating. Moderate temperatures make it easier for the proteins to denature and form the films necessary to create the air bubbles.

Whipping cream forms the best foam when the cream, mixing bowl, and beaters have been chilled first. This is because the viscosity of the fat is greater when cooled. The

1905, Hershey opened a factory. Through his methods of mass production, he made chocolate affordable for everyone.

The Process

❖ After harvest, the pulp and beans are scraped from the pods of the cacao tree.

❖ Sucrose in the pulp immediately begins to hydrolyze into fructose and glucose.

❖ Yeast is added to ferment the beans. The yeast releases ethyl alcohol into the beans.

$$C_6H_{12}O_6 \longrightarrow 2\ C_2H_5OH + 2CO_2$$

glucose ⠀⠀⠀ ethyl alcohol ⠀⠀ carbon dioxide

❖ The pile of beans and pulp is stirred frequently. The ethyl alcohol oxidizes to acetic acid. This makes up 95% of the many acids that contribute to the flavor of chocolate.

$$C_2H_5OH + O_2 \longrightarrow CH_3OOH + H_2O + heat$$

ethyl alcohol ⠀ oxygen ⠀ acetic acid ⠀ water

❖ Acetic acid plus the heat of fermentation kills the sprouts inside the cacao beans.

❖ Enzymes that break down proteins and sugars are released to further develop the flavor molecules.

❖ Beans are dried and shipped to chocolate manufacturers.

❖ Beans are roasted at 135°C (275°F). The roasting causes browning. Amino acids and sugars form glycosylamines, which in turn become the brown pigments called melanoidins.

❖ Roasting removes most of the volatile acids and loosens the hull.

❖ The hull is removed and the sprout portion is broken into pieces called *nibs*.

❖ Grinding distributes cocoa particles throughout the *cocoa butter*, which is the fat in cacao beans. The friction from grinding melts the mixture. The resulting *chocolate liquor* is cooled to produce unsweetened baking chocolate.

❖ Dutching involves mixing the nibs or chocolate liquor with an alkaline solution of sodium bicarbonate or ammonium hydroxide. The pH is raised from 5.5 to a level between 7.0 and 8.0. Neutralizing the mixture results in a darker, milder flavored chocolate.

❖ Conching machines are shaped like the shell of a sea conch. These machines scrape and stir the chocolate for days. This wears away the rough edges of the cocoa and sugar particles. The result is the smooth, creamy texture of today's chocolate.

❖ The final step is tempering. Tempering is solidifying the chocolate through slow cooling. If chocolate falls below 24°C (75°F) during cooling, unstable fat crystals will form. During storage, these unstable fat crystals change into a more stable form that leaves microscopic cracks in the chocolate. The cracks allow new fat crystals from the inside to move to the surface. The result is a white, greasy film called fat bloom. You have seen the bloom if you have ever cooled a melted chocolate bar in the refrigerator before eating it. The fat bloom does not affect the flavor of the chocolate, only the appearance.

---

foam is formed by the nonfat protein portion of the cream. The fat in whipping cream supports and holds the foam. Heavy whipping cream with a 40% fat content produces the highest foam volume.

The addition of solutes can alter foam stability. Sugar is a common solute in food foams. It helps stabilize the water in the foam. The water molecules hydrogen bond to the sugar molecules. This increases the viscosity of the continuous phase and improves the height and quality of the foam.

Sugar must be added at the right point in foam formation to produce the most stable foam. Protein molecules must bond together to form a film that will trap air bubbles. However, the protein must first be denatured by beating. Adding sugar too early in the beating process will delay the denaturation of protein. Adding sugar too soon will also cause part of the protein to bond to the sugar molecules. This will reduce the ability of the mixture to foam, resulting in a foam that lacks height and stiffness. Adding sugar after a foam is completely formed will cause the air bubbles to be coarse in texture. The best time to add sugar is after a foam begins to form but before it reaches the soft peak stage. This results in a fine-textured egg white foam with maximum height.

The foam needs to be beaten until the sugar dissolves. This is because when granulated sugar is heated, it tends to drop through a foam. This breaks bubbles and causes weeping. Weeping, or syneresis of a meringue, is the result of a foam destabilizing and partially returning to a liquid state. See 22-10.

Acidity is another factor that affects the stability of foams. Whipping cream works best when fresh. This is because as the cream ages, bacteria change the lactose in cream into lactic acid. This causes a decrease in pH, which disrupts the ability of the casein in cream to form an emulsion.

Cream of tartar, or tartaric acid, is used to lower the pH of eggs. The pH range of fresh egg whites is between 7.0 and 8.0. The fresher the egg, the lower the pH. During storage, CO_2 escapes through the porous shell. This causes an increase in pH to over 9.0. The increase in pH causes the protein to begin breaking down, which reduces the egg's ability to foam. The most stable foams from the protein albumin are formed when the pH is between 4.6 and 4.8. The change in pH helps denature the protein. This makes it easier for the protein to coagulate into the film necessary to trap air.

Care must be taken in separating the eggs when making egg white foams. This is because fat reduces the foaming ability of egg whites. The fat in egg yolk will react with the protein and prevent the filming action. The membrane around the egg yolk is less likely to break when the eggs are cold. Therefore, it is easier to separate the eggs while they are cold. Then let the egg whites sit for 30 minutes to reach the best foaming temperature.

Any fat on the bowl or beaters used to beat egg whites will also result in reduced foam volume and stability. Therefore, you should avoid using a plastic bowl for beating egg whites. Plastic bowls are porous. It is difficult to remove all traces of fat from mixtures previously held by plastic bowls.

Suspensions

Clusters or groups of ions and molecules can function as colloids. When the clusters or particles are larger than colloids, the mixture is called a suspension. A *suspension* is a mixture of undissolved particles in a liquid.

Suspensions can be very unstable due to the size of the dispersed particles. The mass of the particles will cause them to sink to the bottom of the mixture. If the particles are lighter than water, they will rise to the top of a mixture. The viscosity of the liquid helps support the particles and keep them from sinking. The larger the particles in a suspension are, the thicker the continuous phase must be to create a stable suspension.

You can easily see the particles in suspensions with an ordinary microscope. In some cases, you can see the particles without the aid of a microscope. Fresh milk contains a suspension of fat globules. When the milk is homogenized, the fat globules decrease in size and a stable colloidal dispersion is created. Hot chocolate is a suspension of cocoa in milk. Stabilized Italian dressings are a suspension of spices and herbs in an emulsion. Pulp in fruit juice, fruit in gelatin, and crushed berries in ice cream are also examples of suspensions.

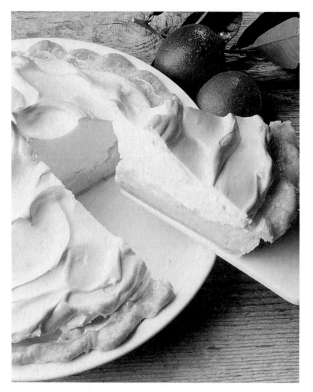

22-10 When making meringues, the sugar needs to be completely dissolved in the egg white to prevent weeping.

Batters and Doughs

Many baked goods are made from batters and doughs that have chocolate chips, chopped nuts, coconut, or raisins suspended throughout. Batters and doughs are the continuous phase of these complex mixtures. See 22-11.

Batters are pourable. The particles most often suspended in batters are air bubbles. These bubbles provide leavening. When they are evenly distributed throughout batters, the result is light, airy baked goods. Too much mixing can cause the air to rise out of a batter suspension. Allowing a batter to sit before baking can also have this effect. When batter loses air, the baked product will be denser and lack height.

Baking coagulates the proteins in batters and creates a stable suspension. Food scientists have to remember that heat will usually reduce the viscosity of a batter before baked goods can solidify. Particles such as chips and nuts must stay suspended in a batter until the product has completed the baking process. The stability of the suspension is one of the many factors evaluated during product

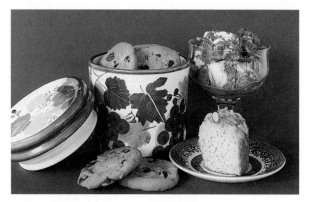

22-11 Chocolate chip cookies and poppy seed cake are examples of coarse suspensions.

development. Stability of a batter can be increased by decreasing the particle size or increasing the viscosity of the batter. Other factors that can be considered are handling procedures and oven temperatures.

The proportion of flour to liquid is higher in doughs than it is in batters. This makes doughs too thick to pour and allows them to be handled and shaped. Doughs are so thick that it is easy to keep large particles evenly suspended.

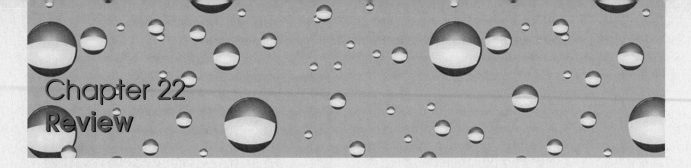

Chapter 22
Review

Summary

Most foods are complex mixtures of many ingredients. These mixtures all consist of at least one dispersed phase of particles scattered through a continuous phase. Knowing the nature of mixtures can help both home cooks and food scientists produce more consistent, high-quality food products.

Solutions are stable food mixtures. A solution is a solute dispersed in a solvent. A number of factors can affect the solubility of a solvent. Solute concentration has an effect on the freezing and boiling points and the vapor pressure of a solution. Knowledge of solutions must be applied in the food industry when producing and preparing soft drinks, coffee, and tea.

A second type of food mixture is a colloidal dispersion. The particles in a colloidal dispersion are called colloids. They are uniformly distributed in the continuous phase, but they are not dissolved. Emulsions are a type of colloidal dispersion. Emulsions contain two immiscible liquids. An emulsifier is often used to stabilize the mixture and prevent the two liquids from separation. Food foams, another type of colloidal dispersion, are composed of gas bubbles distributed in a liquid.

Suspensions are a third type of food mixture. They contain large particles. Batters and doughs form the continuous phase of some food suspensions.

Check Your Understanding

1. Compare the particle sizes of the dispersed phases of three main types of mixtures.
2. Name the three types of solutions and give an example of each.
3. How does increased solvent temperature affect a solvent's ability to hold solid and gas solutes?
4. Explain why it is possible to supersaturate a sugar solution.
5. Why do soft drinks fizz when opened?
6. How many grams of acetic acid are in 100 g of vinegar that is a 5% acetic acid solution?
7. Why do soft drink bottling plants have to treat water from local sources before using it in beverage products?
8. What is the Tyndall effect?
9. What two factors keep colloids dispersed?
10. Why must many sauces be constantly stirred during the heating process?
11. Why is fresh whole milk homogenized?
12. What is the difference between a water-in-oil and an oil-in-water emulsion?
13. What are two factors that can destabilize an emulsion?
14. How do factors affecting the stability of egg white foams differ from factors affecting the stability of whipping cream foams?
15. Identify the suspended particles in three examples of food suspensions.

Critical Thinking

1. Suppose you have two beakers, each containing 10 mL of water at 22°C (72°F). If you stir 5 g of rock salt into one beaker and 5 g of table salt into the other beaker, which will dissolve first? Explain your answer.
2. Which has a lower freezing point, a 1 molar salt solution or a 1 molar sugar solution? Explain your answer.
3. One brand of oil and vinegar dressing needs to be shaken before serving but another brand does not. Explain the difference between these two products.

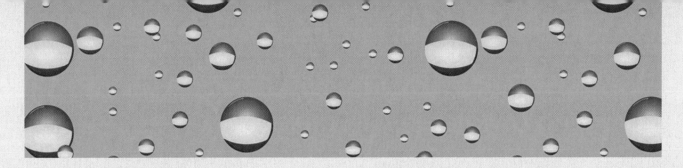

4. Whipped cream and frothed fat free milk served on cappuccino are both food foams made from dairy products. Why does the froth quickly collapse when whipped cream remains stable?

5. Walnut halves used in a trial formulation of a banana bread mix were evenly distributed in the batter. Why did the nuts end up on the bottom of the baked loaf? How could this problem be corrected in a future trial?

Explore Further

1. **Math.** Calculate the mass percent of cocoa and sugar in your favorite homemade cocoa recipe.

2. **Technology.** Create a computer-generated diagram illustrating how emulsifiers work. Then create a table listing common examples of temporary and permanent food emulsions.

3. **Math.** Use the information on food labels to calculate the percentages of fat to water in stick, whipped, tub, and liquid margarine products. Compare these percentages to the fat/water ratio in butter. Which types of margarines, if any, have emulsifiers added?

4. **Science.** Set up and conduct an experiment to answer the following question: When is the best time to add sugar when making whipped cream?

Experiment 22A
Creating a Water-in-Oil Emulsion

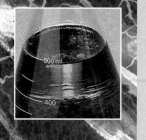

Safety

❖ **Follow sanitation procedures during food preparation and cleanup.**

Purpose

Milk has fat suspended in small droplets or *globules* throughout a water-based solution. It is therefore an oil-in-water emulsion. This emulsion is unstable until the milk has been homogenized. If unhomogenized milk is allowed to sit, the lower-density fat globules will rise and collect on the top. This top milk is cream. Whole milk has about a 3% to 4% fat content. Cream is an oil-in-water emulsion with about a 37% fat content. If cream is beaten vigorously, the fats and proteins in cream will develop a foam. You know this product as whipped cream. If the beating continues, the foam begins to break down. Yellowish granules form. These granules are butter, which is a water-in-oil emulsion with about 80% fat. In this experiment, you will make whipped cream and then butter.

Equipment

mixing bowl with straight sides
electric mixer
clean linen towel
colander
electronic balance
fork

Supplies

500 mL (2 cups) heavy whipping cream
5 to 10 mL (1 to 2 teaspoons) whipped topping per student

waxed paper
NaCl (salt)
commercial butter (1 to 2 teaspoons per student)
bread or crackers (2 pieces per student)

Procedure

1. Empty cold whipping cream into a chilled mixing bowl with straight sides.

2. Beat the cream at high speed until the mixture holds soft peaks.

3. Conduct a sensory evaluation of whipped cream and whipped topping. Record your observations of the flavor, texture, and appearance of each product in a data table.

4. Continue beating the cream until pea-sized granules of fat form.

5. Drain the mixture in a clean linen towel laid in a colander.

6. Rinse the butter granules under cold water. Collect and mass the butter on waxed paper. Record the mass.

7. Add salt to the butter based on the following formula:

mass of butter × 0.0125 = mass of salt to add

8. Work the salt into the butter with a fork, mixing thoroughly until the product is uniform in texture.

9. Wrap the butter in waxed paper and refrigerate it for 15 to 20 minutes. Clean your lab station. Obtain bread or crackers for sensory evaluation.

10. Conduct a sensory evaluation to compare your butter and commercial butter. Record your observations of the flavor, texture, and appearance of each product in a data table.

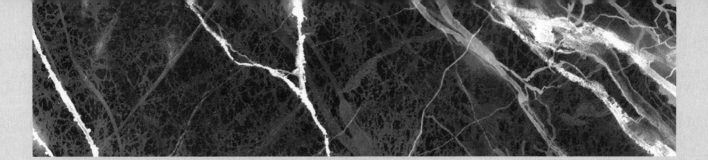

Calculations

Assume you started with 476 g of cream with 37% fat content. What percentage of fat did you recover if the butter is 80% fat? Use the following equations for the calculations:

g cream × 0.37 = g fat in cream
g butter × 0.80 = g fat in butter

$$\frac{\text{g fat in butter}}{\text{g fat in cream}} \times 100 = \% \text{ of fat recovered}$$

Questions

1. How did the texture and flavor of whipping cream compare to commercial whipped topping substitutes?

2. How did the taste and appearance of your butter compare to commercial butter?

3. According to the label, what additional ingredients, if any, are added to commercial butter? Why?

4. Using the cost of butter and whipping cream provided by your teacher, compare the cost of homemade butter to the cost of commercial butter.

5. Why is salt added to butter?

Experiment 22B
Measuring Calories in a Complex Mixture

Safety

❖ Place matches in a nonflammable container after use.

❖ Conduct this experiment on a nonflammable surface.

Purpose

Nuts are a complex mixture of proteins, fats, and carbohydrates. In this experiment, you will be analyzing the fat component of this mixture. You learned in Unit III that proteins and carbohydrates contain 4 Calories per gram. Fat has 9 Calories per gram. In this experiment, you will build a simple calorimeter. A *calorimeter* is a device that measures how much heat energy a food will produce. You will use the calorimeter to evaluate the energy levels created by the mixture of proteins, carbohydrates, and fats in various types of nuts. Fats provide more than twice as many Calories as proteins and carbohydrates. Therefore, the nut that produces the most heat energy per gram has the highest fat content.

Equipment

electronic balance
needle
cork
125-mL Erlenmeyer flask
top plate
plastic gasket
metal cylinder
thermometer
thermometer holder

Supplies

3 assigned nuts
liquid dish detergent
100 mL tap water
matches

Procedure

1. Individually mass your three assigned nuts. Record the mass of each nut in a data table.

   Variation 1: walnuts

   Variation 2: pecans

   Variation 3: Brazil nuts

   Variation 4: cashews

   Variation 5: almonds

   Variation 6: peanuts

2. Create a nut holder assembly by pushing the eye of a needle into the narrow end of a cork. Mass the nut holder assembly and record the mass in the data table.

3. Lightly coat the bottom of a 125-mL Erlenmeyer flask with liquid dish detergent. This will make it easier to clean the soot off the flask after the experiment.

4. Assemble a calorimeter according to your teacher's directions. A typical calorimeter has the top plate positioned on the neck of the Erlenmeyer flask. A plastic gasket attaches to the top of the neck of the flask to hold the plate and flask together. Position the flask so the top plate rests on the top of the metal cylinder.

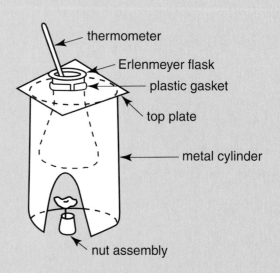

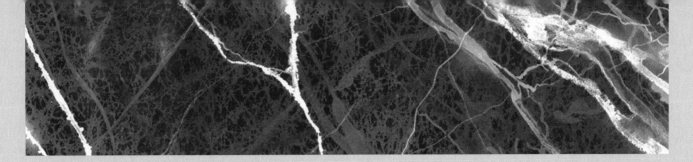

5. Add 100 mL of tap water to the flask. Insert a thermometer into the center of the water and clamp in place with a thermometer holder.

6. In a data table, record the beginning temperature of the water.

7. Mount the first nut on the point of the needle.

8. Position the nut assembly in front of the opening at the bottom of the calorimeter. Ignite the nut with a match and quickly slide the assembly into the cylinder under the flask of water.

9. Allow the nut to burn until it goes out. Stir the water and wait 20 seconds. Record the temperature of the water in the Erlenmeyer flask.

10. Mass the remains of the nut while it is still mounted on the nut holder assembly. Subtract this mass from the mass of the nut holder assembly recorded in step 2. The result is the mass of the nut remains, which you should record the mass in the data table.

11. Repeat this experiment twice, using the other two nuts.

12. Figure the mass lost from each nut and then complete the calculations using the data from your three trials. Record the information on a class data table on the chalkboard or overhead.

Calculations

1. Calculate the average mass lost of the three nuts. Also calculate the average temperature change of the water in the three trials.

2. Calculate the average calories of heat from the burning nuts. Remember that 1 Calorie equals 1 kilocalorie (kcal). One Calorie is the heat needed to raise the temperature of one 1 kg water one degree Celsius (1 kcal = 1°C × 1 L). For 100 mL of water, the formula would be:

$$100 \text{ mL} \times \frac{1 \text{ liter}}{1000 \text{ mL}} \times \frac{1 \text{ kcal}}{\text{degree-liter}} \times \begin{array}{c}\text{average} \\ \text{temperature} \\ \text{change in} \\ \text{degrees}\end{array} = \text{kcal}$$

3. Calculate the kcal per gram by dividing the Calories from calculation 2 by the average mass lost. Record your result in a class data chart on an overhead projector. Copy the data from other lab groups into your data table.

4. Calculate the percent efficiency of the calorimeter using the data from peanuts. The standard or expected caloric value of peanuts is 5.67 kcal/gram.

$$\frac{\text{experimental caloric value}}{\text{standard caloric value}} \times 100 = \% \text{ efficiency}$$

5. Using the percent efficiency from calculation 4, calculate the expected caloric value of each of the other types of nuts tested by the class.

Questions

1. Which compounds are removed through burning? Which compounds remain?

2. Using the class data, rank the nuts in order of highest to lowest fat content.

3. How does a calorimeter show that foods contain energy?

4. Why is the calorimeter not 100% efficient?

5. How do your results in calculation 5 compare to standard Calorie tables?

525

Experiment 22C
Foam Variations

Safety

- ❖ **Keep utensils away from moving beaters.**
- ❖ **Turn off the mixer and unplug it before removing beaters.**
- ❖ **Follow sanitation procedures for food preparation and cleanup.**

Purpose

One popular use of foams in food preparation is in foam cakes, such as angel food cake. The protein in the egg whites used in the cake *denatures* to form a mesh that traps air bubbles. This forms the rigid structure for the cake. A tube cake pan is used to speed the transfer of heat throughout the batter. The pan is ungreased to allow the foam to cling to and climb the sides of the pan. Because of their delicate nature, foam cakes are cooled upside down. Gravity would cause the foam structure to collapse if the cake was cooled in an upright position. Once the cake is cooled, the protein structure is secure, and the cake can be removed from the pan. This experiment will look at factors that affect the height and stability of the egg white foam in an angel food cake.

Equipment

electronic balance

2 mixing bowls

electric mixer

metric measuring spoons

rubber scraper

2-piece tube pan

metric ruler

Supplies

230 g cake flour

340 g powdered sugar

11 large egg whites

6 g cream of tartar (Variations 1 and 3)

1 g salt

227 g granulated sugar

5 mL (1 teaspoon) vanilla

Procedure

Day 1

1. Preheat the oven to 350°F.
2. Combine the cake flour and powdered sugar in a mixing bowl. Set aside.
3. In a large mixing bowl, beat the egg white, cream of tartar, and salt, according to your assigned variation.

   Variation 1: Use cream of tartar and room temperature egg whites.

   Variation 2: Omit cream of tartar and use room temperature egg whites.

   Variation 3: Use cream of tartar and chilled egg whites.

   Variation 4: Omit cream of tartar and use chilled egg whites.

   Beat the ingredients at high speed until soft peaks form. (When the mixer is turned off and lifted straight up, the mixture should form a peak that bends over at the top.)
4. Add the granulated sugar to the egg whites 15 mL (1 tablespoon) at a time. Beat constantly as the sugar is added.
5. Continue beating until stiff peaks form. (Peaks will stand straight up when the mixer is turned off and lifted straight up out of the mixture.)
6. Stir the vanilla into the egg white mixture.

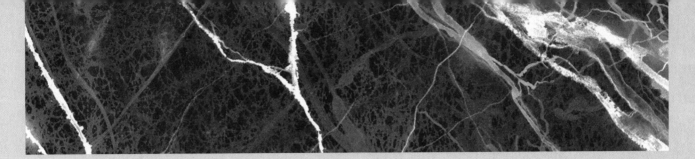

7. Sprinkle one-fourth of the flour mixture over the egg whites. Gently fold the flour mixture into the egg mixture with a rubber scraper 10 times. Turn the bowl one-quarter turn after each fold.

8. Repeat step 7 three times with the remaining flour mixture. After the last addition, gently fold until all the dry flour is blended into the egg mixture.

9. Use the rubber scraper to gently push the batter into the 2-piece tube pan and level.

10. Wash the metric ruler in warm, soapy water. Rinse well and dry. Then use the clean ruler to measure the depth of the batter in centimeters. Record the measurement in a data table.

11. Bake the cake in the preheated oven for 40 minutes or until the cake is delicately browned and the top springs back when lightly touched.

12. Remove the cake from the oven and invert the pan over a long-necked glass bottle. Allow the cake to remain in this position until it is completely cooled.

Day 2

1. Remove the cake from the pan.

2. With a serrated knife, cut the cake in half from top to bottom. Place the metric ruler against the cut surface to measure the height of the cake in centimeters.

3. Conduct a sensory evaluation of each cake variation and record your observations of flavor, texture, and color in the data table.

Calculations

Calculate the percentage increase in the height of the cake during baking.

$$\frac{\begin{array}{l}\text{height} \\ \text{of cake}\end{array} - \begin{array}{l}\text{depth} \\ \text{of batter}\end{array}}{\text{depth of batter}} \times 100 = \% \text{ increase}$$

Questions

1. What difference, if any, did the temperature of the egg whites have on the height and stability of the foams?

2. What effect did the cream of tartar have on the height and stability of the foam?

3. What differences, if any, were there among the colors of the finished cakes?

4. Which variation gave the best overall results?

5. What variables may have affected the data in this experiment?

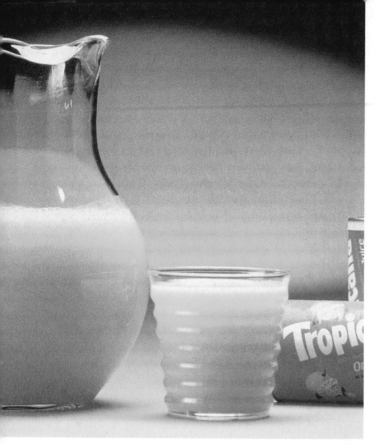

USDA

Fresh orange juice must undergo a separation process to become frozen orange juice concentrate.

Chapter 23

Separation Techniques: Mechanical and Chemical Methods

Objectives

After studying this chapter, you will be able to

classify mechanical methods of sorting or separating foods and food components.

list chemical methods of separating food components.

explain how the principle of osmosis is used to separate food components at the macro-molecular level.

compare osmosis in food products with digestion and metabolism of food components in the human body.

Key Terms

creaming
rendering
sedimentation
centrifugal force
milling
crystallization
precipitation
precipitate
evaporation

distillation
filtration
osmosis
semipermeable
    membrane
osmotic pressure
reverse osmosis
metabolism

Many processes in the food industry involve sorting and separating food. Some types of separation processes are as simple as sorting fruit by size. Others are more involved, such as the process of isolating gluten from wheat flour.

Technology has resulted in many new methods for separating foods. There are two basic types of separation processes: mechanical and chemical. Mechanical methods rely on physical traits of the food. Separation may be based on such qualities as color, size, or density. For example, cranberries are mechanically separated based on their ability to bounce. They are dropped next to a barrier. Berries that meet standards for quality bounce over the barrier. Cranberries that do not meet these standards remain behind the divider. Chemical separations depend on how food components will react on a molecular level.

In this chapter, you will read about the basic methods used to separate foods. You will also study how the separation process of osmosis is related to the way the human body metabolizes food.

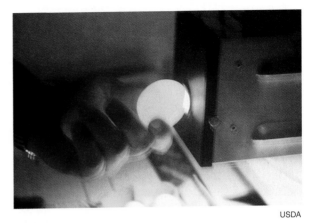

USDA

23-1 One step in the process of sorting eggs is candling to look for impurities inside the egg shell.

Mechanical Separation

Mechanical methods do not rely on chemical changes to separate foods or food components. Some of these methods use machines to physically isolate foods or parts of foods. Other methods rely on nonchemical changes in a food product or the addition of force.

Separation by Physical Properties

A basic separation technique used in many food plants is sorting. *Sorting* separates by physical characteristics, such as size, shape, or color. One example of sorting is separating eggs by sizes such as small, large, and jumbo. See 23-1. Another example is separating ground wheat into bran, germ, and endosperm. This type of sorting is done as food travels on conveyor belts. The food passes over a series of screens. The holes or slits in each screen are smaller than those in the previous screen. Each screen retains items of a different size, from largest to smallest.

Grading is separation based on quality. Meat is inspected and graded based on maturity, muscle firmness, color, and marbling. The meat from older animals usually receives lower grades because it tends to be tougher than meat from younger animals. Meat that has a very dark color indicates the animal was under stress just before slaughter. The chemicals that produce this color result in a lower-quality meat. Marbling, which is fat distributed throughout the muscle tissue, adds flavor and tenderness to meat. Meat that has a lot of marbling often receives a higher grade.

Testing for marbling has typically required cutting into a section of the animal carcass. Researchers are looking at a new way to assess marbling with *ultrasound scanning*. This method uses high-frequency sound waves to produce an image showing the internal structure of the carcass. Studies suggest this technique may be faster and more precise than cutting into the carcass. Ultrasound is also less likely to spread contaminants. This is because a knife can transfer bacteria from the outside of a carcass into a cut made for inspection. A knife can also carry bacteria from one carcass to another.

Some foods are graded and sorted by color. For instance, color indicates ripeness or maturity of many fruits and vegetables. High-speed electronic light sensors can detect the color change that results from mold damage. Food pieces are scanned individually. When the sensors detect a moldy piece, machine-controlled jets of air automatically blow it off the conveyor.

Separation by Density

Another physical property used to separate some foods is density, 23-2. Creaming and sedimentation are two types of mechanical separation based on density. *Creaming* is a separation process in which low-density liquids collect above higher-density liquids. Creaming works best with a cold mixture or a liquid-in-liquid mixture. The cream, or milk-fat, in unhomogenized milk will rise to the top if allowed to sit long enough. Fat is nonpolar

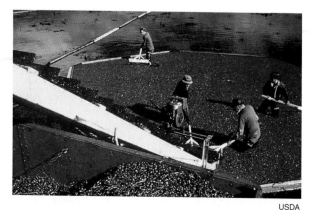

USDA

23-2 Cranberry bogs are flooded so the low-density cranberries can float to the top for collection. Understanding the physical properties of foods can help engineers develop efficient production systems such as this one.

and less dense than water. Therefore, milkfat will separate from the water portion of milk and float to the top. This layer of cream can then be skimmed from the top of the milk.

Rendering is a separation process in which a component is extracted out of a food product by melting. Rendering works on the same principle as creaming. Fat in meat is an example of a substance that might be rendered. Meat can be simmered in liquid until the fat melts and separates from the meat. The cooking liquid can then be chilled, and the fat will rise to the surface and solidify. At this point, the fat can easily be removed from the broth.

Sedimentation uses gravity to pull the denser particles or liquid droplets in a mixture to the bottom. This separation process is used to remove pieces of organic material from many beverages, including beers and wines. The grains and hops used to make beer are allowed to settle after brewing. The liquid, called *wort*, is then drawn off the top without disturbing the sediment. Yeast used to make wine must be removed before the wine is bottled to keep off flavors from developing. The yeast is separated from the wine in a step called *racking*. During this step, the wine sits until the yeast cells and other suspended material settle to the bottom. Then, as with beer, the wine is drawn off without disturbing the sediment.

Separation by the Addition of Force

Allowing fats to rise and sediments to sink can be time-consuming. Many food manufacturers add force to speed such separation processes. Engineers use a knowledge of physics to design force-based equipment to meet the separation needs of each food.

Centrifugal Force

Some foods are separated by the force that acts on objects when they move around a central point. This force is called *centrifugal force*. It tends to propel objects outward from a center of rotation. This force is what makes it necessary to hold on when riding a merry-go-round. An object that is rapidly moving around a central point will move in a straight line when it is released.

A cotton candy machine makes use of this principle. A hot sugar syrup is held in a central tub with very tiny holes in the outside surface. This tub spins inside a large collection tub. As the central tub spins, the hot syrup is forced through the tiny holes and out into the collection tub. The contact with cool air immediately solidifies the syrup into soft, pliable threads, which are wrapped around a paper cone.

The food industry uses centrifugal force in a separation process called *centrifuging*. This process separates particles of different densities. It works on the principle that density affects the speed at which matter moves outward from a center of rotation. Dense objects and fluids will move faster than those that are less dense. Centrifuging is done using a machine called a *centrifuge*. Centrifuges are used to separate cream from milk and oil from water. These fluids are placed in a drum in the centrifuge. The drum spins around a central axis at high speeds. As the drum spins, the denser, water-based particles move out of the drum through small holes on the outside wall. The less-dense cream or oil stays closer to the center and is removed through a pipe.

Pressure

Another use of force to separate foods is in the use of presses. Presses apply extreme pressure to products to squeeze out desired components. Presses work well with foods that have a high moisture or fat content. Molasses is extracted from sorghum and sugar cane with presses.

Pressure can be combined with movement to speed separation. This principle is demonstrated in the way a juicer works. The pressure of pushing a lemon down on a juicer is not enough to remove the maximum amount of juice. By adding a twisting motion against the ridged surface of the juicer, more juice is released. This technique is similar to the commercial process used to extract orange and grapefruit juices. See 23-3.

Pressure is used to prepare some foods for separation. For instance, before the parts of grain kernels can be separated, the grain needs to be ground. The first grain mills ground dried grain kernels between two moving stones. The weight or pressure of the stones crushed the grain into fine particles. Although some small specialty mills still

grind grain between moving stones, most mills use metal rollers. Today, *milling* is moving kernels of grain between a series of rollers. The space between the rollers gets progressively smaller.

The size of the particles produced by milling will vary with the molecular structure of each part of the grain. The bran remains in the largest pieces due to its high cellulose content. Because of its higher fat content, the germ portion remains in larger pieces than the endosperm. The dry protein and starch mixture that makes up the endosperm crumbles into the smallest particles and is called flour.

Once grain is ground, the parts of the kernels are separated for further processing and distribution. For example, ground corn is separated so oil can be extracted from the germ portion. Presses are used to squeeze oil from the germ.

Magnetic Force

Another type of force used to separate some food components is magnetic force. Magnets will attract or pull iron and steel toward them. This force has been used to help separate nutshells from the meats of nuts. The shells are coated with a thin film of an iron solution. The nuts are dried and the shells are broken. The shells are easily separated from the nut meats when the two components are conveyed past magnets. Magnets are also used to remove metal filings that may enter food mixtures during processing.

Combination Separation Processes

The separation of many food components requires a combination of mechanical processes. For instance, olive, corn, canola, and other vegetable oils come from the seed or fruit portion of plants. The oil is suspended in solutions within cell membranes. Presses are used to rupture or break the membranes and separate the oil and juices from the plant solids. Then the liquid is centrifuged to separate the oil from the water-based juices. Chocolate, soy, and sugar cane are among the complex mixtures that must undergo several types of separation processes.

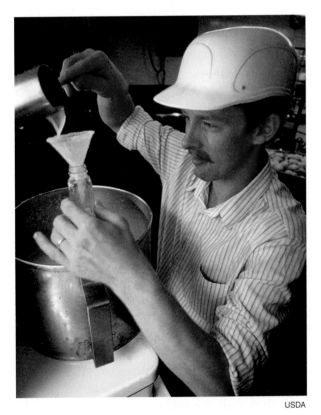

USDA

23-3 Squeezing juice from fruit is one example of separation by pressure. Here, lemon juice is being extracted to conduct a brix test. Brix is the measure of sugar in a solution at a given temperature.

Chemical Separation

Some food components are separated by chemical means. Chemical separation requires a grasp of the physical and chemical properties of foods. Chemical separation methods include the use of solvents, crystallization, precipitation, evaporation, and distillation.

Separating with Solvents

One chemical method of separating foods is treatment with a solvent. Solvents are used to remove a desired component from a food. An example is the use of hexane to maximize the amount of oil removed from plant sources. Hexane is a nonpolar solvent that is percolated through pressed seeds like corn, cottonseeds, and soybeans. The oil dissolves in the hexane and is carried away from the seeds. The hexane is then distilled off the oil and collected to be reused.

Solvents are also used to remove unwanted food components. An example is caffeine in coffee and tea. See 23-4. Caffeine is a mild stimulant that some people wish to avoid. One method for removing caffeine from coffee beans uses water as a solvent. Caffeine dissolves in water but so do many of the flavor compounds found in coffee beans. To remove the caffeine without reducing the flavor of the coffee, green coffee beans are soaked in water. This produces a solution that is saturated with caffeine and flavor compounds. The green, soaked beans are discarded. Then the solution

is passed through carbon filters. The caffeine is attracted to the carbon, but the flavor compounds are not. Therefore, the filtered solution is caffeine free but still saturated with flavor compounds. Next, premium coffee beans are soaked in the filtered solution. Because the solution is saturated with flavor compounds, the flavor from this second batch of beans stays in the beans. However, because the solution has little or no caffeine remaining, it will dissolve the caffeine from the beans. These beans are then dried and roasted. The end product is coffee beans that are 99.9% caffeine free.

Other solvents used to extract caffeine include methylene chloride, ethyl acetate (a compound found in many fruits and vegetables), and carbon dioxide.

Crystallization

Crystallization is a process that separates the solute from the solvent in a supersaturated solution. The atoms of the solute become arranged in a repeating order to form crystals. This happens when water evaporates from salt- and sugar-based solutions. The solute will begin to crystallize. It will settle out of the solution as soon as the saturation point is passed. The solvent does not need to completely evaporate in order to collect the crystals. The crystals can be removed from the solution by centrifuging.

Crystallization is the process used to make rock candy. Crystals form from a supersaturated sugar solution as it cools. The crystals keep forming for a few days at room temperature as water evaporates from the solution.

Precipitation

Precipitation separates two or more compounds from a mixture by causing the compounds to form a precipitate. A *precipitate* is a substance that separates from a solution as an insoluble solid. Food manufacturers add substances to some food mixtures to cause precipitates to form chemically. For instance, acid is added to milk to cause the protein casein to form a precipitate. This precipitate is the curds used to make some types of cheese.

In some cases, no substance needs to be added to cause a precipitate to form.

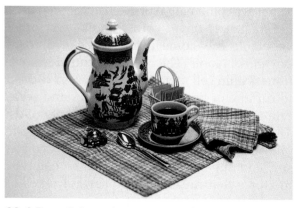

23-4 Decaffeinated teas are made by using solvents to extract the caffeine while leaving behind the majority of the flavor compounds.

Precipitates form in some mixtures because of temperature changes. Precipitation is one step in making decaffeinated instant tea. The first step is brewing tea in water and then evaporating part of the water. If the concentrate is then cooled to 10°C (50°F), the caffeine and tannins will naturally combine to form a precipitate. This precipitate is large enough to be filtered out of the tea concentrate.

Evaporation

When a desired food component is a solute, it may be separated through *evaporation.* This process simply removes all the water from a solution. This separation technique is used to make instant teas and coffees. Tea and coffee are brewed to suspend the flavor compounds in water. The solution is then heated or freeze-dried to evaporate out the water content. What remains are the flavor compounds in a solid state.

Distillation

Sometimes the desired part of a food is so volatile that it quickly evaporates out of a solution. *Distillation* is the collection of vapors and the compounds they carry as they evaporate from a solution. Distillation requires a closed system to carry the steam and/or vapors away from the heated solution. As the collected vapors move away from the heat, they cool and condense. Distillation works because different compounds have different boiling points.

The flavor compounds in tea are volatile. They are often collected as they distill out of the brewed tea that is evaporated to make instant tea. The low boiling point of the flavor compounds enables them to distill out of the tea before water does. These compounds can be collected and mixed back into the tea solids left from the evaporation process. The result will be increased flavor in the instant tea product.

Distilled or purified water has had minerals, salts, and organic matter removed from it. This is done by heating the water. The pure water leaves the solution as steam, and the unwanted solutes and colloids remain behind. The steam is collected, condensed, and bottled for sale. See 23-5.

The making of some alcoholic beverages involves distilling alcohol out of a water-based solution. Alcohol has a higher vapor pressure than water. This causes the alcohol to change from a liquid to a gas state before the water does. The gaseous alcohol is collected in a closed system and condensed back into a liquid.

The oil used to make margarine often contains compounds that can cause unpleasant odors. Steam distillation is often used to remove these compounds from the oils before they are solidified and made into margarine.

In each of these examples, a compound is separated from a food mixture. This separation is possible because different parts of the mixture have different boiling points.

Selective Separation Through Barriers

Some food components are separated by passing the food through barriers. A barrier lets some particles pass through while trapping others. Screens are widely used as barriers in the food industry to sift and sort foods. Filter paper and semipermeable membranes are often used as barriers, too. These barriers are used for the processes of filtration, osmosis, and reverse osmosis.

Water Distiller

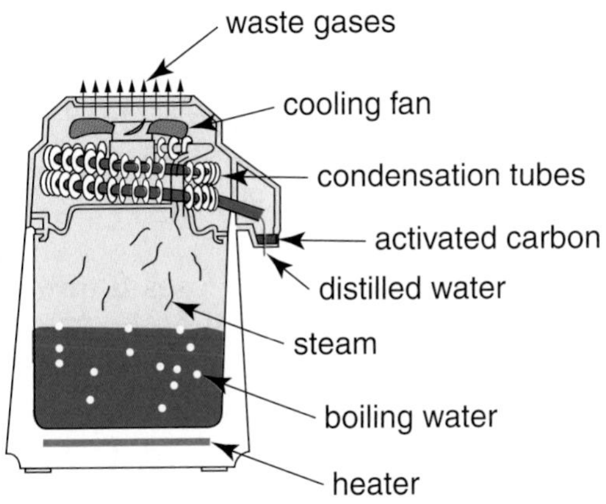

waste gases
cooling fan
condensation tubes
activated carbon
distilled water
steam
boiling water
heater

adapted from Pure-Pro USA Corp.

23-5 This diagram shows how a countertop appliance distills water for home use.

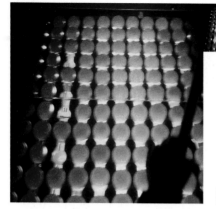

Technology Tidbit
The Chemical Separation of Lactic Acid

Lactic acid is an additive in many foods and beverages. It provides a good example of the procedures that can be involved in separating food components for commercial use. There are seven chemical separation steps involved in producing pure lactic acid from whey.

1. Whey is separated from cheese curds through precipitation.
   - ❖ The whey is placed in sterilized 19,000 to 38,000 L (5,000 to 10,000 gallon) wooden tanks.
   - ❖ The whey is inoculated with Lactobacilli, a specialized strain of bacteria.
   - ❖ Calcium hydroxide is added periodically to keep the mixture from becoming too acidic.
2. Lactic acid is separated from the whey through precipitation and filtration.
   - ❖ Sulfuric acid is added. It reacts with the calcium and lactic acid to form the precipitate calcium lactate. Calcium lactate is a salt that forms crystals.
3. In purer grades, calcium lactate is separated from the whey by concentration and precipitation.
4. The calcium lactate is dissolved in water then recrystallized to purify it.
5. The calcium lactate is dissolved and the solvent, methanol, is pumped through the liquid. Methyl lactate is distilled out of the calcium lactate solution.
6. The methyl lactate is hydrolyzed to produce pure lactic acid and methanol.
7. The methanol is separated from the lactic acid through distillation. The methanol is then recycled. The physical design and careful monitoring of this step are critical as methanol is extremely toxic if consumed in sufficient quantities.

Filtration

Filtration uses porous paper to let liquids and small solutes pass through while trapping *aggregates* (clusters of precipitate). Drip coffeemakers use this type of barrier system. Paper coffee filters let the dissolved flavor compounds and hot water pass through while trapping coffee grounds. Filter papers need to be sanitary and taste-free.

The food industry often uses filtration to remove visible solids from solutions, 23-6. You just read that filtration is used to remove precipitates of caffeine and tannins from tea concentrate. Filtration is also used to remove organic matter from liquids. Fruit juice manufacturers use filtration in this way to make pulp-free fruit juice.

Many colloids and macromolecules can pass through filter paper. Special barriers are often needed to remove these substances from liquids.

New filtration materials do not rely on pore and particle sizes but on the type of polymer and its chemical interactions with the food compounds. For example, scientists could use a polymer that would cause hydrophilic and hydrophobic reactions to block unwanted elements from passing through the filter. This new method is called *nanofiltration*. Though soy contains high quality protein and fat, it also has less desirable compounds. Nanofiltration has allowed researchers to separate the good from the bad. This technology enables engineers to manipulate flavor, color, and other aspects of foods. Scientists hope to use this new technology to isolate phytochemicals from functional foods.

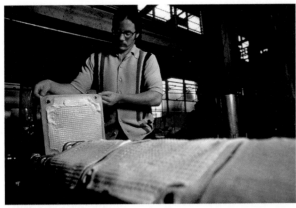

23-6 This worker is removing protein solids that have collected on filter elements. The solution is heated to coagulate the proteins, which can then be filtered out of the solution.

Cooking Tip

In some food preparation procedures, such as making homemade jelly, linen towels are used to separate juices from pulp. To avoid adding unwanted flavors, do not use a linen towel that has had fabric softener added in the laundry.

Osmosis

When separation is needed at the molecular level, osmosis is one process that can be used. *Osmosis* is the movement of a solvent through a semipermeable membrane. The solvent moves from an area of low solute concentration to an area of high solute concentration. A *semipermeable membrane* is a thin layer of material that allows some substances to pass through but not others.

Figure 23-7 shows two sugar solutions separated by a semipermeable membrane. The solution on the left has a mass percent of 10. The solution on the right has a mass percent of 20. The membrane allows water but not sugar to pass back and forth. Because the membrane is semipermeable, the two solutions and the membrane are a connected system.

The different concentrations of the two solutions cause the system to be unstable. A pressure builds up on the side of the membrane with the lower concentration. The pressure caused by two solutions with different

Osmosis

10% sugar solution   20% sugar solution

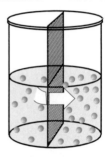

semipermeable membrane

sugar molecules

water

This beaker is divided with a semipermeable membrane. The left side contains a 10% sugar solution. The right side contains an equal amount of a 20% sugar solution.

10% sugar solution   20% sugar solution

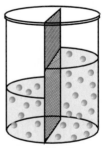

The different concentrations of the two solutions cause osmotic pressure to build up on the left side of the semipermeable membrane. This pressure forces water through the membrane from the solution with the lower concentration toward the solution with the higher concentration.

15% sugar solution   15% sugar solution

When the solute concentrations are the same, water will stop moving through the membrane.

23-7 Osmosis causes water to be drawn across semipermeable membranes to equalize solute concentrations.

concentrations separated by a semipermeable membrane is called *osmotic pressure.* This pressure will force water through the membrane. Water will move from the solution with a low sugar concentration toward the solution with a high sugar concentration. Water will continue to move until osmotic pressure drops and the mass percent of the two solutions is the same.

Osmosis in Food Products

Foods are composed of plant or animal tissue. The cells in this tissue are surrounded by semipermeable walls or membranes. This makes these tissues subject to the effects of osmosis after harvest or slaughter. Therefore, food scientists need to understand how to control osmosis in food mixtures.

To observe the osmotic movement of water through plant cell walls, slice and salt an eggplant. Wait 30 minutes before examining the salted eggplant. Water droplets will have formed on the surface. The salt has pulled water out of the cells of the eggplant to equalize salt concentrations.

Salting eggplant is the first step in making eggplant parmesan. Osmosis reduces the water content in the cells. This makes the eggplant easier to fry and gives it a milder flavor. See 23-8.

Similarly, a first step in making sauerkraut is to put shredded cabbage in brine. The salt in the brine draws water out of the cabbage cells through the semipermeable cell walls. Cell walls are complex systems that use protein molecules to help transport solutes into and out of cells. The cell walls allow sugar to be pulled out of the cabbage cells with the water. This sugar serves as food for the bacteria

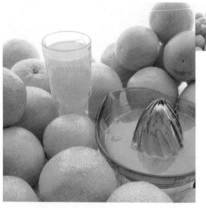

Nutrition News
Athletes Under Pressure

Adequate water is especially important to the athlete. During heavy exercise, the body loses water through perspiration. Perspiration causes a drop in osmotic pressure outside the cells. Water must be consumed. Otherwise, osmosis will move water out of the cells to balance the concentrations on either side of the cell membrane. If these losses are large and the water is not replaced, a chain reaction begins.

❖ Blood volume decreases—blood pressure drops—heart rate increases to compensate.

❖ Transport of nutrients for energy is slowed.

❖ Transport of waste products in slowed.

❖ As water loss increases, perspiration decreases.

❖ Less perspiration results in increased body temperature.

❖ A 2% loss of body weight in fluids decreases performance. (This equals 1.4 kg (3 pounds) for a 67.5 kg (150 pound) athlete.) This much fluid can be lost in 90 minutes of exercise on a cool day.

❖ Heat cramps occur at a 5% loss of body water weight. Heat exhaustion occurs at 5% to 10% water loss. Heat stroke occurs when water loss exceeds 10%.

If you are thirsty, you are dehydrated. However, it is important to remember that thirst is satisfied during exercise before body fluid needs are met. It is a good idea for athletes to weigh themselves before and after an exercise session. For every kilogram (2.2 pounds) lost during exercise, athletes should drink 1 L (4½ cups) of water or sport beverage. During exercise, an athlete should consume 125 mL (½ cup) of water or sport beverage every 20 minutes. Sport beverages provide osmotically balanced water along with sodium, potassium, and glucose. Some athletes find them more appealing than plain water and are therefore more likely to drink them and avoid dehydration.

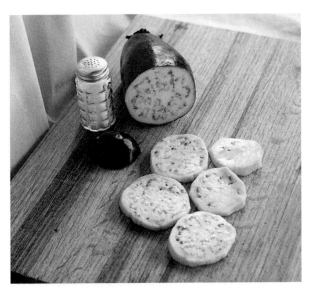

23-8 Sprinkling salt on sliced eggplant pulls water and bitter flavor compounds from the slices.

that ferment the cabbage and turn it into sauerkraut.

Reverse Osmosis

Pressure can be applied to the more highly concentrated of two solutions separated by a semipermeable membrane. This will cause water to flow from an area of high concentration to an area of low concentration. This type of movement is in the opposite direction of osmosis. That is why it is called *reverse osmosis.* Reverse osmosis involves pumping liquids under pressure against a membrane. This process will cause a concentrated solution to become even more concentrated.

Reverse osmosis is used to concentrate fruit juices with limited use of heat. This protects the flavor compounds and vitamin C in the juices, which can be damaged by heat used in evaporation.

Sometimes a series of filters is used to separate several food components. This is how the various components of whey are separated. Whey is the liquid left from the production of cheese. The food industry uses the components of whey for a variety of functions. Whey proteins act as foam stabilizers, gelling agents, and emulsifiers. They are used in meat extenders, processed cheese, pasta products, and snack foods. Lactose from whey is used in icings, toppings, and candies. When combined with sucrose, lactose helps keep foods from being too sweet. It also increases viscosity and reduces crystal size. The result is a smoother mouth feel in candy and confections.

To separate the components of whey, the liquid is first passed through filters that remove the protein molecules. At this point, the liquid is a solution of lactose, lactic acid, and salts. A specially designed reverse osmosis membrane is then used to remove the lactose. See 23-9.

The Role of Semipermeable Membranes

Semipermeable membranes are used to separate many food components. Egg whites, soy proteins, and enzymes are among the substances separated with these membranes.

Semipermeable membranes are designed for the specific solutes that must be trapped

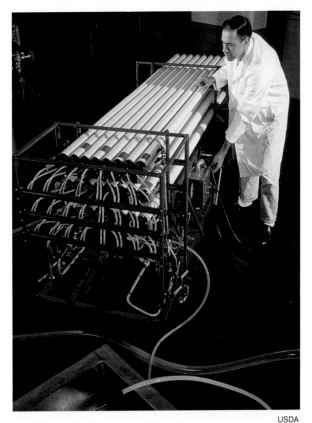

USDA

23-9 This food technologist is examining a reverse osmosis unit. The long white tubes contain the membranes used to concentrate whey. The flexible tube carries the concentrated whey to a collection tank.

and/or allowed to pass through them. These membranes are often designed to allow salts and acids to pass through with the water. This reduces the risk of high salt or acid concentrations damaging the solids in the concentrate. The membranes used to concentrate fruit juices must allow water but not flavor compounds to flow out of the juice. Such factors as the size, polarity, and chemical makeup of solutes determine the type of membrane to be used.

Sometimes a combination of membranes is most effective. Research has shown that deposits of some proteins and polysaccharides can improve the selective nature of semipermeable membranes. For instance, whey protein can be deposited in a gel-like layer on a membrane used for apple juice. This will decrease the flow of flavor compounds

through the membrane with the water. Therefore, the apple juice will be concentrated without loss of flavor.

Digestion and Metabolism

Semipermeable membranes and osmosis play a role in the way your body uses the nutrients from food. Food scientists need to understand how the human body uses food. This knowledge helps them maintain a healthy and nutritious food supply.

Before your body can use the food you eat, the food must be separated into nutrient parts. Digestion is the process of breaking down food into substances that are usable by the body cells. See 23-10. Digestion begins in the mouth where chewing grinds the food into

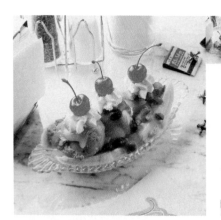

Item of Interest
Cell Walls Versus Cell Membranes

Plants have cell walls and animals have cell membranes. Cell walls and membranes react differently to osmotic pressure.

When the osmotic pressure is higher outside a cell wall, water will move into the cell until it becomes turgid. *Turgid* means swollen and hard. Other pressures from within the cell stop any more water from entering the cell. This is true even if the osmotic pressure is still higher outside the cell. Turgidity is what gives plants a crisp, firm texture that holds the plant upright.

If plant cells are placed in a sugar solution, the osmotic pressure becomes greater inside the

cell. A salt solution would have the same effect. This is because the sugar or salt solution has a high concentration as compared to the fluids in the cells. Water moves through the semipermeable cell wall from the weak solution inside the cells to the strong solution outside. The cell walls become *flaccid*, or limp, because of loss of water. The plant develops a wilted look. If noticed soon enough, wilting can be reversed by increasing the water content in the environment around the plant.

Animal cells have only a thin membrane. If animal cells have a higher osmotic pressure outside

the membrane, the cell will swell with water until it bursts. It is also possible when the reverse pressure exists to dehydrate an animal cell to the point of death. One of the problems with high-sugar and high-salt diets is that fluids surrounding the cells develop a low osmotic pressure. The result is that cells dehydrate and become stressed. Animal cells need the osmotic pressure of fluids around the cells to equal the pressure of fluid in the cells.

small pieces. The ground food and saliva form a solution. One of the components of saliva is the digestive enzyme amylase. Chewing distributes the amylase throughout the food so breakdown of starches into sugars can begin.

From the mouth, food travels to the stomach. The stomach's churning action mixes the food with hydrochloric acid and proteases. The acid denatures the protein molecules. This opens up the molecular structure. The proteases can then begin breaking the peptide bonds and separating the amino acids. (See Chapter 11.)

The stomach and intestinal walls release water into food in the digestive tract. This helps create the liquidity needed for chemical reactions to occur. These reactions will break down protein, carbohydrates, and fat. These macromolecules must be broken into components that are small enough to be absorbed through the intestinal wall for use by the body.

As the partially digested food solution reaches the small intestine, the gallbladder releases bile. Bile is an emulsifier. It suspends the fat molecules in the partially digested food solution. Bile is produced in the liver and stored in the gallbladder until needed. In addition to bile, digestive enzymes from the pancreas are released into the small intestine to break down the macromolecules. The pancreas also releases bicarbonate to neutralize the hydrochloric acid from the stomach. This

Nutrient Breakdown During Digestion

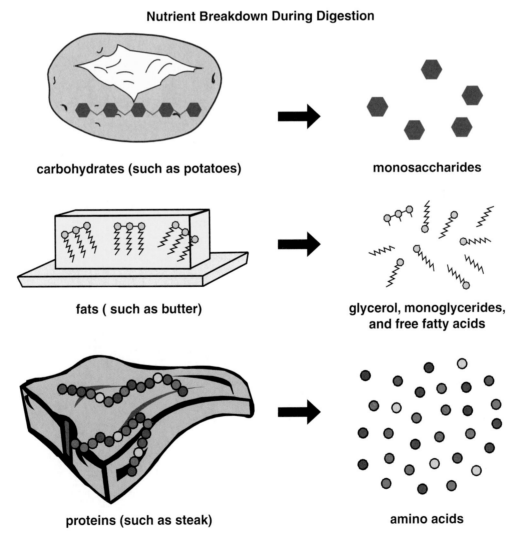

carbohydrates (such as potatoes) → monosaccharides

fats (such as butter) → glycerol, monoglycerides, and free fatty acids

proteins (such as steak) → amino acids

23-10 The body breaks down macronutrients from foods into usable substances through the process of digestion.

raises the pH of the small intestine to about 7.

Food residue moves from the small intestine to the large intestine. Here, water and minerals are removed from digested food. The large intestine also contains colonies of bacteria that produce vitamin K. The remaining wastes from the digestive process are made up mostly of fiber and bacteria.

Metabolism

The small intestines are a semipermeable membrane. This membrane allows nutrient components to be absorbed into the blood and lymph systems. Nutrients are then carried to cells all through the body. Cell membranes are semipermeable. Osmosis controls the flow of nutrients and oxygen into cells. Osmosis also controls the flow of waste products out of cells.

Metabolism is the physical and chemical reactions that constantly occur within cells. Metabolism involves an exchange of energy. There are two basic types of metabolic reactions. The first type is anabolism. *Anabolism* is the bonding of nutrients to make new compounds. This type of reaction absorbs or uses energy. An example is combining amino acids to make enzymes. The second type of metabolism is catabolism. *Catabolism* is the breaking down of compounds into smaller parts. Catabolic reactions release energy. This energy is used for physical activity. The energy is also used to build body tissue and sustain involuntary activities, such as breathing.

Metabolism of Salts

When salt is consumed in the diet, it is catabolized into sodium and chloride. Most sodium in the body is in the fluid that surrounds cells. Large levels of salt in the diet cause sodium levels to rise compared to potassium, which is inside the cells. A key function of sodium and potassium is to control the osmotic flow of substances in and out of body cells.

High intakes of salt in diets around the world have been connected to higher rates of hypertension (high blood pressure). It is believed that as sodium levels in the blood rise, the body pulls water from the cells. This helps maintain a constant sodium concentration in the blood. However, the additional water in the blood increases the total volume of blood. This causes a rise in blood pressure.

Hypertension is a problem for about 10% to 15% of the population. Most people can successfully excrete excess sodium from the diet. Their blood pressure and salt concentrations remain stable. Hypertension appears to be caused by high sodium intakes combined with a faulty ability to remove sodium through the kidneys.

Another problem with a high-salt diet is that it increases the body's need for water. If insufficient water is consumed, water is pulled from the cells to maintain the correct salt concentrations. This puts stress on the cells, reduces water availability for metabolism, and could reduce overall health. See 23-11.

Metabolism and Water

Most metabolic reactions involve the release of or use of water. Water is also the solvent for all metabolic reactions within the cells. When there is insufficient water, reactions slow. Energy is released at a lower rate. Remember that water must be present before carbohydrates, lipids, and proteins can be converted to energy. Water is the solvent that transports nutrients into the cell. It also transports waste products out through the cell membrane. Any separation or movement of compounds through cell membranes requires water.

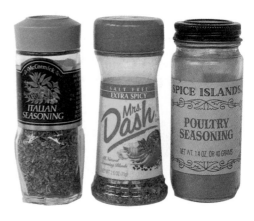

23-11 A variety of salt-free seasoning mixes can be used to flavor foods without adding sodium to the diet.

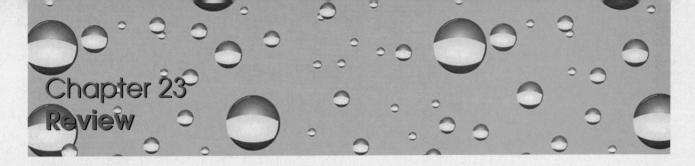

Chapter 23
Review

Summary

Separation processes can be either mechanical or chemical. Mechanical operations are based on physical properties of food. Chemical separations depend on how food components react on a molecular level. Mechanical methods include separation by physical properties, density, and addition of force. Centrifugal force, pressure, and magnetic force can all be used to speed separation processes.

Chemical separation methods include the use of solvents, crystallization, precipitation, evaporation, and distillation. Solvents can be used to remove desired or unwanted food components. Crystallization separates the solute from the solvent in a hypersaturated solution. Creating new chemical compounds in solutions can allow solutes to precipitate out of the solution. Evaporation and distillation involve the removal of water from a solution. In distillation, the vapors are collected.

Some food components are separated by passing through barriers. The barrier processes include filtration, osmosis, and reverse osmosis. Filtration techniques use porous paper to trap solids. When separation is needed at the molecular level, semipermeable membranes are used.

Digestion is the body's complex procedure for separating foods into usable nutrients. Metabolism is the chemical reactions that occur within the cells and involve the exchange energy. As in barrier separation techniques, the body uses semipermeable membranes and osmosis to separate and use nutrients.

Check Your Understanding

1. What is the difference between sorting and grading?
2. Describe three ways foods are separated based on density.
3. How does the food industry speed up the processes of separating foods by density?
4. List two foods that are separated from their sources by pressing or milling.
5. Describe one way solvents are used to chemically separate a food.
6. How are particles chemically removed from a mixture using precipitation?
7. What is the difference between evaporation and distillation?
8. What type of barrier separation method is used to remove visible solids from solutions?
9. Explain what happens during reverse osmosis and give an example of when this process might be used.
10. Why are semipermeable membranes specially designed for each use?
11. List and explain the two basic types of metabolic reactions.
12. What is the solvent for all metabolic reactions within cells?

Critical Thinking

1. Will coffee filters remove caffeine and tannin precipitates from a hot cup of tea?
2. Describe the separation techniques used to convert a cooked batch of home-grown tomatoes into tomato sauce.
3. When a partially opened jar of honey is left in the pantry too long, what causes the honey to become firm?
4. Describe the separation technique at work when oil forms a separate layer in a pourable salad dressing.
5. Salting freshly cut cucumbers as a first step to removing excess water before preparing cucumber salad is an example of what separation technique?

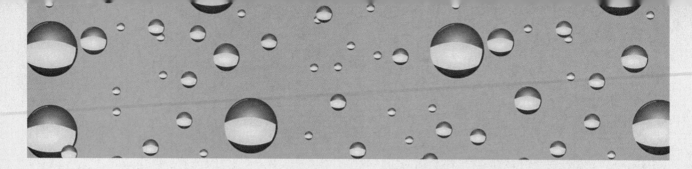

Explore Further

1. **Analytical Skills.** Develop a flowchart that demonstrates the steps to set up for shelling and separating pecans into halves and pieces.

2. **Science.** Research the procedure for making rock candy. Test the procedure and the product that results.

3. **Communication.** Write an article for the school newspaper explaining the importance of athletes drinking enough liquids during and after sports events.

4. **Science.** Distill the alcohol from vanilla flavoring. Describe the results.

5. **Analytical Skills.** Select one complex food system (corn, milk, soy, or wheat) and identify the separation technique used to develop each of five different products produced from the complex food.

Experiment 23A
Filtration

Purpose

One method of separating complex food mixtures uses a variety of filters. Many homes use filtration devices every day. One common device is a pitcher or faucet attachment that filters water with activated charcoal. Another common type of household filter is the filter papers used for brewing coffee. In this experiment, you will determine what types of ingredients can be separated by each of these common filters.

Equipment

permanent marker
drip coffeemaker or strainer and mixing bowl
metric measuring spoons
small bowl
100-mL graduated cylinder
filtration pitcher with filter

Supplies

3-ounce plastic cups (3 per lab group member)
3 coffee filters
2 mL (½ teaspoon) vanilla extract
550 mL (2¼ cups) water
50 mL (¼ cup) soft drink
50 mL (¼ cup) Italian-seasoned chicken broth

Procedure

1. Use a permanent marker to label three plastic cups with the name of each lab group member.
2. Place a coffee filter in the basket of the coffeemaker or in a strainer over a mixing bowl.
3. Combine 2 mL of vanilla extract and 50 mL of water in a small bowl.
4. Pour 2 to 3 mL of the flavored water into a plastic cup for each lab group member. Sample the liquid and record your observations of the flavor and appearance in a data table. Rinse and dry your plastic cup.
5. Pour half the remaining vanilla-flavored water through the coffee filter positioned over the coffeepot or mixing bowl.
6. Pour the second half of the vanilla-flavored water into a filtration pitcher.
7. After the water has passed through the filtration devices, pour 2 to 3 mL of one of the variations into each lab group member's plastic cup. Sample the liquid and record your observations of the flavor and appearance.
8. Rinse and dry your plastic cup and sample the second variation. Record your observations.
9. Wash the filter basket and coffeepot or mixing bowl and strainer. Pour 250 mL of water into the filtration pitcher to flush residues from the filter, then wash the pitcher.
10. Repeat steps 2 through 9 once with the soft drink and once with the Italian-seasoned chicken broth. Use a clean coffee filter and a new set of plastic sampling cups each time.

Questions

1. Which method was the most effective in removing flavors?
2. Which method was the most effective for removing particles?
3. Which method was the most effective in removing coloring agents?
4. How can you apply this information to other food preparation procedures?

Extracting Gelatin and Fat

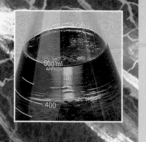

❖ Wear safety glasses when heating glass beakers.

❖ Use beaker tongs to move hot beakers.

❖ Sanitize all surfaces that come in contact with raw meat products.

Purpose

The greatest solvent is water. Because of water's polar nature, many compounds can be dissolved in it. Some compounds can be pulled out of or extracted from their source by soaking and/or simmering the source in water. This is known as rendering. In this experiment, you will simmer chicken wings in a variety of solutions to determine which solution is most effective for extracting gelatin.

Equipment

electronic balance

1000-mL beaker

100-mL graduated cylinder

metric measuring spoons

beaker tongs

wax pencil

tongs

hot pad

knife

glass pie plate

viscosity ring

Supplies

5 chicken wings

assigned solution

paper towels

waxed paper

line-spread sheet

Procedure

Day 1

1. Mass five chicken wings. Record the mass in a data table.

2. Arrange the wings in a 1000-mL beaker.

3. Add your assigned solution.

   Control: 300 mL distilled water

   Variation 1: 300 mL distilled water and 15 mL vinegar

   Variation 2: 300 mL distilled water and 5 mL salt

4. Place the beaker over medium-high heat and bring the mixture to a boil. As soon as the mixture boils, turn the heat down to simmer.

5. Simmer the mixture for 50 minutes to 1 hour (or until 10 to 15 minutes before the end of the class period).

6. Remove the beaker from the heat with beaker tongs. Use a wax pencil to label the beaker with your lab group number, class period, and variation.

7. Remove the chicken wings from the liquid with tongs. Carefully blot the hot wings dry with paper towels and mass. Record the mass in your data table.

8. Record the approximate volume of liquid in the beaker. Record the approximate volume of the yellowish fat layer on top of the liquid.

9. Place the beaker on a hot pad in the refrigerator.

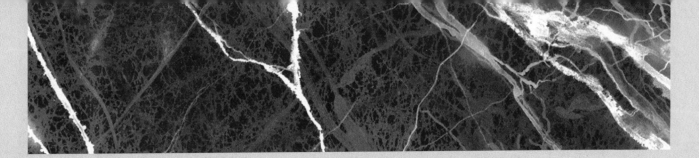

Day 2

1. Carefully remove any fat from the top of the liquid in the beaker. The fat should form a solid layer. Loosen the edges with a knife and lift the fat layer from the beaker.

2. Place the fat layer on waxed paper that has been tared. Mass the fat. Record the mass in your data table.

3. Place a glass pie plate over a line-spread sheet and use a viscosity ring to conduct a viscosity test on the chilled liquid. Record the average of four viscosity readings. (See Experiment 9A.) The more viscous the liquid is, the more gelatin it contains.

Calculations

1. Calculate the total mass lost from the chicken wings during cooking.

2. Calculate the total percentage of mass lost from the chicken.

3. Calculate the percentage of mass lost from the chicken in the form of fat.

4. Calculate the mass lost from the chicken in the form of substances other than fat.

5. Calculate the percentage of mass lost from the chicken in the form of substances other than fat.

Data

Record the results of your calculations on a class data chart on an overhead projector. Copy the data from the other lab groups into your data table.

Questions

1. Which solution was the most effective for extracting gelatin? How did you determine this?

2. Were other compounds extracted during the simmering process? How do you know?

3. What principles made it possible to extract fat during simmering?

4. How does the percentage of mass lost in the form of substances other than fat compare among the three variations?

5. How can this information be applied to food preparation?

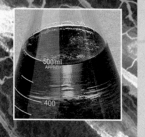

Experiment 23C
Osmosis and Egg Membranes

Purpose

Eggs have a membrane that separates the shell from the egg white. This membrane is similar in structure to cell walls. In this experiment, you will observe the movement of solutions through the membrane of the egg. To achieve this, the shell must first be removed. The shell is composed largely of calcium carbonate, which will slowly dissolve in vinegar.

Equipment

1000-mL beaker
1 250-mL beaker per student
100-mL graduated cylinder
wax pencil

Supplies

1 egg per student
1 to 2 L white vinegar
100 mL corn syrup
100 mL cider or red wine vinegar
100 mL 1 M NaCl solution
100 mL distilled water with food coloring
plastic wrap

Procedure

Day 1

1. Place one egg per lab group member in a 1000-mL beaker.
2. Cover the eggs with white vinegar.
3. Wait 5 minutes and record your observations.

Days 2 and 3

1. Turn any eggs that have risen above the surface of the vinegar. If necessary, add more vinegar to keep the eggs covered. Record your observations.

Day 4

1. Under cool running tap water, gently rub your egg in a circular pattern. The eggshell will slowly dissolve in the water and be lifted off the egg. Be very patient with this step. It takes as much as 10 minutes to remove all the shell. If your hands are callused, cover them with plastic gloves. The egg membrane will rupture easily.
2. Place your egg in a 250-mL beaker. Record your observations regarding the egg's size in comparison to the beaker.
3. Cover your egg with 100 mL of the assigned liquid.

   Student 1: corn syrup

   Student 2: cider or red wine vinegar

   Student 3: 1 M NaCl solution

   Student 4: distilled water with food coloring added
4. Use a wax pencil to label the beaker with your name and assigned liquid. Cover the beaker with plastic wrap.

Day 5

1. Record your observations regarding changes in the egg's size in a data table. Also note any other changes in the egg.
2. Copy the data from the other lab group members into your data table.

Questions

1. Which liquids caused the eggs to shrink?
2. Which liquids caused the eggs to swell?
3. Did any substances move into the egg? How do you know?
4. How can you apply this information to food preparation?
5. How can you apply this information to your diet?

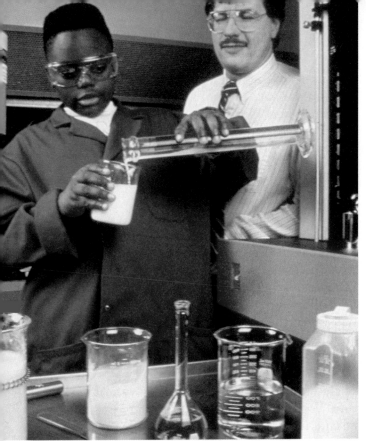

USDA

Under the supervision of a research technician, this student is conducting tests on a newly developed milk product.

Chapter 24

Research: Developing New Food Products

Objectives

After studying this chapter, you will be able to

contrast descriptive research and analytical research.

list the steps in developing food science experiments.

develop an experiment to examine one of the characteristics of a complex food system.

describe the steps involved in developing a new food product.

create a new food product or new variation of a food product.

Key Terms

research
descriptive research

analytical research
ethics

A popular story for children promotes a breakfast of green eggs and ham. Food scientists who study consumer trends would predict that most people would eat the ham but skip the eggs. Although grocery stores may not stock green eggs, they do carry frozen, cholesterol-free, and powdered eggs. Food scientists conducted research to develop each of these alternatives to fresh eggs.

Developing new products is an ongoing venture in the food industry. In 1906, the first cold breakfast cereal was introduced. Today, there are over 125 varieties of cold cereal in most stores. These cereal products are flaked, puffed, popped, shredded, and extruded in fancy shapes.

The example of cereal is typical of nearly all food products found in modern grocery stores. One hundred years ago, grocery stores stocked an average of 500 different food products. Today, most grocery stores stock over 12,000 different products. Each new product that is introduced represents millions of dollars and thousands of hours used for research and market analysis. See 24-1.

Research in the Food Industry

Research in the food industry follows the same basic standards of any scientific research. *Research* is an organized method of examining a question, issue, or theory to improve understanding. The goal of research is to apply new knowledge in ways that can help society.

Research is based on the scientific method, which was discussed in Chapter 2. It is important to understand that steps of the method are not always followed in sequence. Scientists may start at any point and work forward or backward. They may go back and forth between the steps or work on two steps at the same time. This is because research is a continuing process. Experiments designed to test a hypothesis or solve a problem often reveal new hypotheses to be tested. Sometimes experimental results do not match

expectations. In these cases, scientists often go back and seek more base information or develop a new hypothesis.

Research requires patience and attention to details. Researchers must remain objective and avoid being influenced by biases and emotions. Good researchers must conduct their studies carefully. They begin by gathering any information that relates to their problem so they can learn as much as possible. Researchers also need to study how others have investigated the problem. They must keep detailed and accurate records.

Following guidelines for good research will make the research *replicable*. This means another scientist should be able to follow the written record to repeat the procedure and achieve similar results. Most experiments conducted in high school science labs were at one time someone's original research. This research has been verified by many scientists who replicated the procedure. Science teachers have students repeat the procedure so the students can see scientific principles at work.

Results of research are reported so others can use and apply the knowledge gained. An exception to this is research by a company to develop a secret recipe. This type of research would not be shared in order to maintain an advantage over a competitor.

Research is divided into two main types: descriptive and analytical. Both types of research are used to develop new food products.

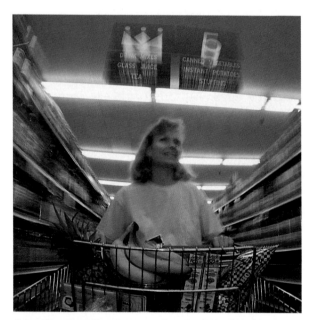

24-1 Each of the thousands of products on grocery store shelves is the result of extensive research and development.

> ### Cooking Tip
> You need to keep notes whenever you try new recipes or experiment with small changes in recipes. This will allow you to repeat changes that are successful and avoid repeating changes that are unsuccessful. Your cookbooks can become ongoing research journals if you record successes, failures, and specifics about changes made.

Descriptive Research

Descriptive research involves collecting data that describes the natural course of events or opinions of people at a given time. Descriptive research uses observations, surveys, and interviews to collect data. The data is then used to make decisions or keep track of changes over time. See 24-2.

Food scientists use descriptive research to assess people's opinions. This type of research is taking place when food scientists conduct taste tests. The scientists are collecting information on consumer opinions about food products. Doing research on opinions is critical to see whether consumers will purchase a product. The panel must be made up of people for whom the product is designed. For example, if a new cereal is being designed to appeal to children, taste panels will need to include children.

A taste test must allow testers to respond in a way that can be measured scientifically. For instance, simply observing the facial expressions of children tasting cereal may not provide accurate data. Their expressions and moods may be caused by many factors other than the cereal's taste.

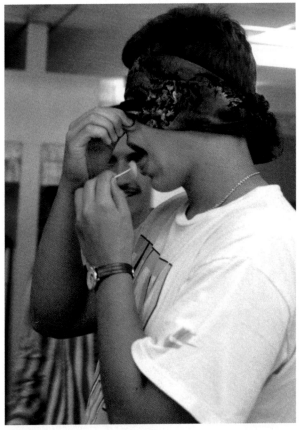

24-2 Descriptive research might involve gathering people's opinions about the taste of new food products.

Written surveys can be designed to allow for responses that can be measured scientifically. However, a written survey would not work with a panel of preschoolers who cannot read or write. For preschoolers, a better survey might be made up of pictures illustrating a range of responses, from pleasure to dislike. Each child could circle or point to the picture that represented his or her opinion.

Another option when working with a test panel made up of children would be to interview the children. This would allow the children to provide oral feedback on what characteristics of the cereal may need to be changed. In such a case, interviewers would need training on how to ask questions. They would need to avoid showing bias through their tone of voice or body language.

Questions need to be designed carefully to gather information that will be truly useful. Just asking a child if the new cereal is good does not give enough information. Manufacturers need to know if the child will choose the cereal over other favorites. Manufacturers also need to know if the child's parents will buy the product.

Food scientists can use descriptive research to study trends in food consumption. Scientists can also collect data from consumers about the types of new products that interest them. Researchers then use this information to help their companies decide what products to develop. For instance, research showed an increased awareness of the importance of a healthful diet as a trend among U.S. consumers. Through surveys and interviews, researchers learned that consumers were interested in more options for healthful snack foods. This information led food scientists to develop many new food products that are low in fat and/or sugar. Baked potato chips, lowfat cheeses, and sugar-free cookies are just a few of the foods introduced in the 1990s. See 24-3.

Another example of the use of descriptive research is in the study of functional foods. In Chapter 14, you read that functional foods are modified foods or food ingredients. These foods and ingredients may provide health benefits beyond the traditional nutrients they contain. Research has been conducted on the growing area of functional foods. Functional

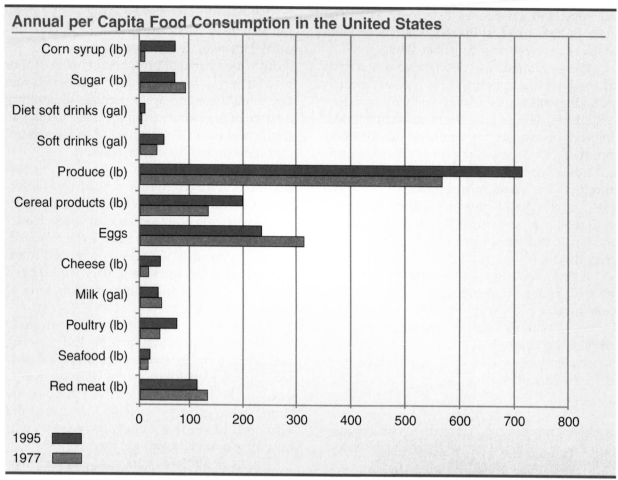

Annual per Capita Food Consumption in the United States

Corn syrup (lb)	
Sugar (lb)	
Diet soft drinks (gal)	
Soft drinks (gal)	
Produce (lb)	
Cereal products (lb)	
Eggs	
Cheese (lb)	
Milk (gal)	
Poultry (lb)	
Seafood (lb)	
Red meat (lb)	

0   100   200   300   400   500   600   700   800

1995
1977

24-3 Food scientists use information about consumer eating patterns to help companies decide what types of products to develop. This chart indicates increased consumer interest in healthful food options.

foods were introduced in the early 1990s. They have grown to a $10 billion a year industry since that time. This growth is expected to continue for the next 10 to 15 years. Such information from descriptive research is valuable to food science research teams. It helps researchers meet the consumer's demands for new foods and the company's demands for a profitable product.

Analytical Research

Analytical research determines cause and effect through observation and testing. This type of research involves exact measurements of mass, volume, time, length, and/or chemical makeup, 24-4. However, this type of research goes beyond just collecting information. Research leads to the development of theories. These theories can then be used to solve problems.

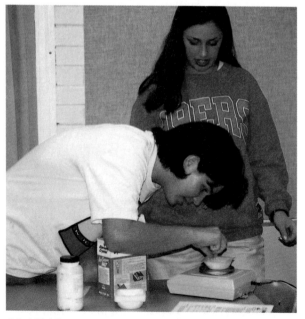

24-4 Taking accurate measurements is an important part of analytical research.

Analytical research is used to test hypotheses. It is also used to find out why reactions occur as they do. For instance, in the past, soybeans had limited use in the United States. Consumers did not like the "beany" flavor. Analytical research was used to find out what caused the unpopular flavor. Researchers learned the flavor is caused by the enzyme lipoxidase. By conducting experiments, food scientists developed a process for neutralizing the enzyme. This process allowed scientists to maintain the nutritional value of the soybean while keeping the unpleasant flavors from forming.

Analytical research is key to the development of a new food product. Once descriptive research has revealed trends, researchers look for ideas. New food product ideas can come from anywhere. Ideas may come from food scientists, marketing analysts, management, or consumer feedback. Once a decision to develop a new product is made, the research team comes up with recipe variations to test. Hundreds of mixtures are carefully prepared and tested. Careful records of each trial are needed to determine which will be the final product. Once analytical research has narrowed the choices, taste tests are held to check for consumer approval.

Usually, descriptive research is used to reveal trends. The results of the descriptive research are used to set up analytical research. The analytical research is used to develop a new product. Before the new product is mass-produced, descriptive research is used again. This time, the research helps assess consumer opinion about the product.

Developing Food Science Experiments

A food science experiment is designed to solve a problem or answer a question about food. Experiments are a key part of any analytical research. In recent years, much research has centered on the problem of finding new uses for the microwave oven. Food scientists have conducted experiments to answer such questions as "How can popcorn be cooked in the microwave oven?" Through experiments, food scientists have solved this problem and developed hundreds of microwaveable food products. See 24-5.

Stating the Problem

The first step in developing an experiment is to state the problem. This step may seem very elementary. However, many people repeatedly do tasks the same way. They never stop to consider how or why to do the tasks differently. If the problem is not recognized or stated, it cannot be solved.

What questions have occurred to you as you conducted experiments throughout this class? Was there a problem related to food you would like to have answered? As you study this chapter, you may have the chance to conduct research to answer a question about food.

Forming a Hypothesis or Research Question

The second step in developing an experiment is to form a hypothesis or research question. A hypothesis is an educated guess about how or why something happens. You can form a hypothesis about a phenomenon you have observed. Food scientists observed that soybeans had an unpleasant flavor. The scientists hypothesized that some compound in the beans caused the unpleasant flavors to develop. This hypothesis could be stated as a research question: *What compound in soybeans causes the unpleasant flavor?*

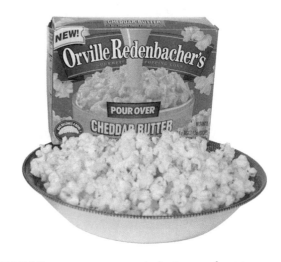

24-5 Microwave popcorn is just one of many products food scientists developed through experiments to find new uses for microwave ovens.

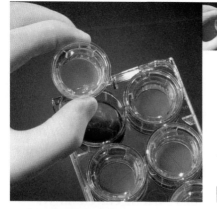

Recent Research
The Connection Between Fruit and Flowers

The following three seemingly unrelated events puzzled researchers:

❖ A chrysanthemum grower turned on a gas heater to protect his flowers from cold weather. The next day, the greenhouse was warm, but the plants had lost their

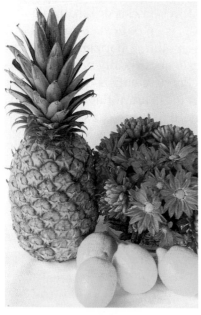

By observing the effects of ethylene on chrysanthemums, pineapple, and lemons, scientists have developed an understanding of the role of ethylene in ripening. This understanding has allowed scientists to help control fruit crop losses.

leaves. The grower lost his entire crop of flowers.

❖ Pineapple growers sometimes use smudge pots in their fields to protect the young plants from frost. In years when growers have used smudge pots, the plants have budded earlier and flowered together. Harvesting has been easier because all the fruit has ripened at the same time.

❖ During winter, a grocer placed a box of green lemons near a kerosene stove to keep them warm. He hoped the heat would ripen the lemons faster. The next day, the lemons were already turning yellow. The grocer continued to place green citrus fruits near the stove for a faster color change.

It took researchers several years to discover the heater in the greenhouse was not working properly. Incomplete combustion in the heater resulted in the release of ethylene into the air. More research revealed that many plants produce ethylene during the final stages of maturing. Because the chrysanthemums were close to full maturity, the ethylene sped up the aging process. The ethylene caused the flowers to grow old overnight.

Ethylene also accounted for the changes in the pineapples and lemons. The ethylene from the burning smudge pots sped up and evened out the flowering process of the young pineapple plants. Ethylene from the kerosene stove caused the chlorophyll in the lemon peels to disappear, leaving a bright yellow color.

Today, ethylene is used to ripen bananas and kiwifruit after they reach their destination. Refrigeration slows the ripening process in these fruits during shipping. Once they have reached the United States, the fruits are exposed to ethylene to speed ripening. They become ready to eat in just a couple days. If ethylene exposure is left unchecked, fruit will go from ripe to overripe to rotten.

The shelf life of fresh apples is extended by suppressing their natural ethylene production. When apples are chilled and stored in air with high levels of carbon dioxide, the apples will keep for months. However, this storage process has caused a new problem. Chemicals responsible for flavor in the apples are lost during storage. Although the apples look and feel fresh, they do not taste like fresh-picked apples. This shows how solving a problem through research often leads to new problems that need to be solved.

Sometimes the question will come before the hypothesis. Then a hypothesis is formed as a possible answer to the question. For instance, you may have noticed the pizza in your school cafeteria has grease on top. The problem is, the grease looks unappetizing and can drip on your clothes, 24-6. Your research question might be *What causes grease to collect on top of pizza in the school cafeteria?*

Brainstorming sessions are often used in this step of experiment development. Exchanging ideas in this way can help researchers narrow their hypothesis. This gives them more focus for designing an experiment. In the case of the soybeans, researchers might have listed compounds that could cause the unpleasant flavors. To do that, the researchers needed to know what components make up soybeans. After listing various options, the researchers might have hypothesized that lipoxidase caused unpleasant flavors in soybeans. This new hypothesis could be stated as a research question: *Does lipoxidase in soybeans cause unpleasant flavors?*

In the pizza example, you could brainstorm a number of hypotheses to answer your question. You might hypothesize that the type of cheese used causes grease to collect. Perhaps you think the pizza in the school

cafeteria is made differently from pizza served elsewhere. You may suppose the cooking method is causing the fat to separate from its food source. You could use any of these hypotheses as the basis for setting up an experiment.

Gathering Information

The next step is to gather information that is already available about the question or problem. Food scientists must learn as much as they can about the components of the proposed food product. They must study the chemical and physical nature of the components. Food scientists must also look at the availability and cost of ingredients. Researchers need to study how ingredients interact in food systems similar to the new product, too. If a new flavor is being developed, scientists must compare natural and artificial flavors. The scientists also need to study how the flavorings react to other food components.

Such research is usually done by a team of specialists. Each member of the team uses his or her expertise to ensure the success of the product. Many research teams will have a food scientist who specializes in microbiology and another whose strength is chemistry. Another member of the team might be a family and consumer sciences professional. This specialist would be familiar with the cooking process and the quality of food to be attained. An engineer who understands the mechanics of mass production and equipment design might also be part of the team. A marketing and advertising specialist will examine how to promote the new product. Someone who knows about packaging will assess options that can be used with the new product. Chapter 25 will discuss these and other career options. See 24-7.

In gathering information on pizza, you discover your school uses the same type of cheese as the local pizza parlor. You also learn the cafeteria and the pizza parlor use the same oven temperature when baking the pizza. However, you discover the cafeteria holds pizza in warmers longer than the pizza parlor does. You have learned in foods and nutrition classes that fat in cheese will separate. This

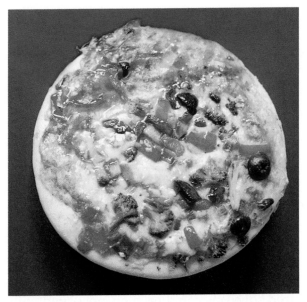

24-6 The problem of grease on pizza might be the focus of a food science hypothesis or research question.

Food Product Research Team Members

Position	Responsibilities
Researcher	Identifies food components, finds formulas (recipes) for similar food products, predicts reactions of ingredients, and recommends proportions. (In a company setting, this would be a subteam of food scientists. The subteam would include specialists in biology, chemistry, and physics as appropriate to the project.)
Librarian	Conducts literature searches for previously conducted research and information. Issues and retains research books.
Technician	Identifies the variables to control, develops recipe variations, and records product trial data. May be focused on the laboratory and/or pilot plant.
Evaluator	Conducts consumer taste tests, evaluates data, and recommends the final formulation.
Registered dietitian	Analyzes food components, develops an ingredient list, and monitors nutritional value of the food. Also creates the nutrition label according to the Nutrition Labeling and Education Act.
Packaging specialist	Evaluates preservation methods, develops packaging, and finalizes the food label.
Engineer	Arranges for equipment and supplies and plans, sets up, and oversees production.
Quality control director	Tests and monitors for safety and practicality. Uses HAACP principles to examine each point at which contamination could occur. Recommends procedures to avoid contamination at each critical risk point in the food production process.
Advertising executive	Develops graphics for the label, creates the product name, and develops an advertising campaign proposal.
Accountant	Keeps the financial records, prepares production cost analysis, monitors budget, and oversees supplies.
Manager	Runs the business meetings and brainstorming sessions and assigns tasks. Also monitors progress of the entire team and oversees presentation of the product proposal to the management team.

24-7 Each member of a food product research team plays an important role in the development of a new food product. Test kitchen home economists or family and consumer sciences professionals often fill the roles of researcher, technician, and evaluator.

happens when cheese is cooked at too high a temperature for too long a time. This information helps you choose which hypothesis will be the focus of your experiment. Your research question becomes *Does holding pizza in a warmer for an extended time cause grease to collect on top?*

Designing the Experiment Procedure

After studying as much information as possible, the researcher designs an experiment to test the hypothesis. What procedure could you set up to test the hypothesis about grease on pizza? Think about the case of the soybeans. The microbiologist may propose the flavor change is caused by some microbe feeding on the soybeans. The microbiologist would use his or her knowledge of microbes. He or she might design a way to isolate and identify all the microbes found on a soybean. Next, the microbiologist would grow cultures of each microbe in petri dishes. Sets of sanitized soybeans could each be inoculated with a different microbe and allowed to sit. Then the beans would be cooked and tasted to check for flavors. In this case, the taste test panel would be composed of the researchers in the lab or trained testers.

An important part of designing the experiment is controlling for variables. Which variable would be altered in each variation and how? Which variable must remain constant for accurate testing? With the soybeans, the variable being altered is the type of microbe. The amount of time the beans are allowed to sit must be the same for each variation. The cooking time and temperature must be the same, too. Otherwise, researchers would not know if flavor changes were caused by changing the microbes, the sitting time, or the cooking method.

Before a researcher can conduct an experiment, he or she must write the procedure in detail. The written procedure should be clear enough that someone else could conduct the experiment without the researcher's assistance. The written format will be similar to that used in experiment procedures you have followed in this class.

Collecting Data

Before starting the procedure, the researcher must write the questions he or she expects the experiment to answer. This will help the researcher think through what type of data he or she needs to collect. He or she must be certain the procedure will provide the data needed to answer the research question.

The researcher must next determine how to record the data. The researcher must also think about how the data will be analyzed. This will allow him or her to gather the data in a suitable format. For instance, lengthy verbal descriptions will not be useful if variations are to be ranked numerically. Preparing data tables ahead of time makes it easier to conduct the procedure accurately. This is especially true when the steps must be timed.

In food science experiments, collecting data often means measuring length, mass, temperature, time, and volume. Observations about texture, color, flavor, and aroma may also be recorded. To obtain accurate data, a researcher must follow the steps of the procedure exactly as they are written. The researcher must be sure to record the data neatly. Carefully gathered data should make sense a week or year after it is gathered. See 24-8.

Analyzing and Interpreting Data

After conducting the experiment and recording the data, the researcher must be able to interpret the results. The questions the researcher wrote before starting the procedure will help guide his or her analysis. How do the results relate to present information? Do the results give a new or greater understanding? In the case of the soybeans, which microbe gives the beans an unpleasant flavor? If none of the variations answers the research question, the researcher may need to change the hypothesis. He or she may need to rewrite the experiment procedure to test a different variable.

Sharing Results

Food scientists share results with other researchers. Scientists may present findings on the Internet or at professional meetings. Food scientists may also share results through research journals, such as *Food Technology* and *Journal of Food Science*. By reading journals and attending meetings, food scientists learn what other researchers have discovered. These are the same resources researchers use to gather information about their research topics.

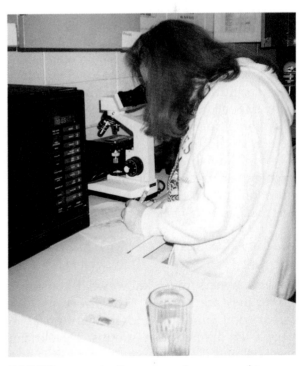

24-8 When conducting research, you need to carefully record your data and observations.

Developing a New Food Product

Consumers constantly demand more choices and new taste experiences. Consumers also want improved convenience and more healthful foods. This demand prompts manufacturers to develop 12,000 to 16,000 food products each year. All this product development increases the need for trained food scientists.

Some items food scientists work on developing are new products. Other items are variations of established products. Olean is an example of a new food product. It was developed to give consumers the taste and feel of fat without the calories. White cheddar microwave popcorn is an example of a variation of an established product. It was developed to give consumers a new flavor option of a popular convenience food.

The best way to understand a process is to work through it. This section examines the process a food product development team could take to develop a new product, 24-9. The team may develop ideas for a new product. It is also possible that management could give the team an assignment. Whatever the case, the team's first step is to identify the problem or need.

Identify the Problem or Need

Imagine a frozen food company is losing sales. The marketing department believes the loss is due to a new line of lowfat frozen desserts introduced by a competitor. The company's food product development team must now come up with a product that will compete with the frozen desserts. The team discusses a number of options before stating the problem as a research question. The research question is *What desserts in our current product line could be made in lowfat versions?*

Identify the Consumer Group Being Targeted

Researchers must know what consumer group they are targeting. This is because different food products and flavors appeal to people in different age groups. Developing multicolored ice pops would waste time and money if the target group is older adults. Ice

Research and Development Tasks

❖ identify the type of food mixture—solution, emulsion, colloidal dispersion, coarse suspension, or a combination

❖ identify types of carbohydrates and their functions

❖ identify types of fats and their functions

❖ identify protein and amino acid components

❖ list additives and their functions

❖ identify factors that affect pH

❖ develop formulations for trial and large-scale productions

❖ identify equipment and develop process for trial and large-scale production

❖ keep records of formulation variations attempted with sensory evaluations

❖ prepare charts on taste evaluations, growth of contaminants, and production costs

❖ evaluate preservation options

❖ determine shelf life

❖ determine a serving size

❖ calculate calories per serving

❖ list ingredients by weight

❖ list vitamins and minerals that exceed 1% of RDA

❖ design a mock-up of label and packaging

❖ prepare a storyboard of advertising campaign

24-9 Food product development team members would be responsible for completing all these tasks as they prepare to introduce a new food product.

pops would appeal to children. However, older adults are likely to prefer a lowfat New York-style cheesecake. See 24-10.

To identify the target group, food scientists work with marketing analysts. They study descriptive research to look for trends about who buys most lowfat desserts.

Conduct Research

Once food scientists have selected the type of food product, they must research formulations. Food scientists need to study the chemical and physical properties of the ingredients.

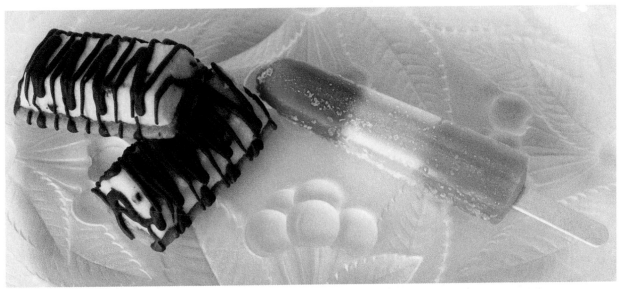

24-10 Each of these products would appeal to a different group of consumers. Food scientists need to keep their target market in mind when developing new products.

Researchers must also gather information on the best way to preserve the product. In the case of cheesecake, researchers must gather all the information they can find on mixing and baking cheesecakes. Which ingredients are high in fat? What lowfat ingredients might they be able to use as substitutes? What are the chemical and physical properties of the substitutes? How do these properties differ from the properties of the original ingredients? What changes might the substitutes cause in production and packaging?

Develop the Product

Once the information is gathered and examined, the experimental procedure can be designed. During this stage of the process, trial batches are prepared. These batches are small to save money and reduce waste. Each batch and formulation is numbered. Team members taste and examine the trial batches. Then they discuss what changes are needed to improve the product in the next set of trials. Accurate records of every trial are a necessity.

The team working on a lowfat cheesecake may start this step by looking at the original cheesecake formulation. They identify cream cheese as a main source of fat in the original formulation. In the first set of trials, the researchers decide to simply replace part of the cream cheese in the filling. They decide to

try replacing one-fourth, one-half, and three-fourths of the cream cheese. The researchers have found three possible substitutes: lowfat cottage cheese, Neufchâtel, and tofu. It would take nine trials to test all three ratios on all three substitutes. It is common for food development teams to test hundreds of variations of each new food product.

A critical part of the development process is record keeping. With hundreds of variations to monitor and remember, accurate records are essential. Researchers use a variety of methods to record data, from handwritten logs to electronic files.

Pilot Manufacture the Product

Once team members have agreed on the final formulation, they must pilot manufacture it. This means they produce and evaluate a larger batch. Pilot manufacturing includes choosing and testing packaging for the product. This is the first step in sealing up the formula and process for the product.

The pilot manufacturing step helps production managers estimate manufacturing costs. This step helps engineers figure out what kinds of machines are needed for mass production. See 24-11. This step allows food scientists to see if mass production alters the quality of the product. Pilot manufacturing also allows food scientists to see how they

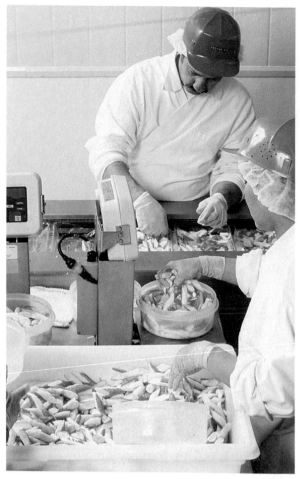

24-11 Making a large test batch of a food product helps food scientists analyze what adjustments they will need to make for full-scale production.

may need to change production methods. For instance, the recipe for a trial batch of jelly cannot simply be increased to make a larger batch. The larger volume requires a longer heating time. A longer heating time will alter the ability of the mixture to gel.

Consumer panels taste samples from the pilot manufacturing. Panel members complete surveys about the product. Responses from the consumers help researchers decide if the product will sell.

Receive Management Approval

Before a food product is mass-produced, a complete report is presented to a management team. This report would include

❖ a sample product with a complete description

❖ the formulation or recipe
❖ a cost analysis broken down by ingredient and individual market unit
❖ an analysis of the pilot manufacturing and taste test results, including any new or redesigned equipment needed
❖ a recommendation for packaging materials and storage requirements
❖ a description of market competition with similar products
❖ an advertising proposal
❖ an explanation of why the company should develop this product

It is the management team's task to study the information. The team must decide if the company will invest millions of dollars to mass-produce the food. The team must also approve the advertising campaign needed to promote the product to the public.

Mass-Produce the Product

Once the management team grants approval, a test market is chosen. This is a region of the country in which the product will be introduced. Equipment is set up for a small production run. The product is then advertised and marketed in the test region for several months. Descriptive research is conducted on sales. Then the company makes a decision about whether to develop the assembly lines needed for nationwide distribution.

Market and Advertise the Product

An advertising campaign is usually being put together at the same time a company is preparing to manufacture a product. The campaign needs to be ready to go when the food is ready to place in stores. Advertising experts must know what is unique about the product. They need to know the target consumer group to whom the advertising should appeal. They need to be aware of how the product will be packaged. It is also helpful for them to know the preparation requirements and storage needs of the new product. All this requires the marketing and advertising team to work closely with the food product development team.

Apply Professional Ethics

In the food science profession, negligence and intentional actions can put the health and well-being of people at risk. The public trusts foods to be safe to consume. The scientific community trusts that reported research is carefully and accurately documented and analyzed. Therefore, food science professionals, like all workers, have a responsibility to follow a code of ethics in the workplace. *Ethics* are the principles of conduct and character that distinguish right from wrong. Ethical issues in research relate to experimental and human error. Honest mistakes can be accepted if they are handled promptly and properly. See 24-12.

Fraud and deliberate misrepresentation are against the law. Unethical behavior includes

❖ concealing relevant data that contradicts a hypothesis

❖ revising data

❖ creating false data

❖ failing to inform human subjects of potential risks of products they are testing

❖ keeping sloppy records

Failing to apply professional ethics can cause a worker to be fired, fined, and/or sentenced to jail. However, a lack of ethics is not just a matter of law. It is a matter of safety for all future customers.

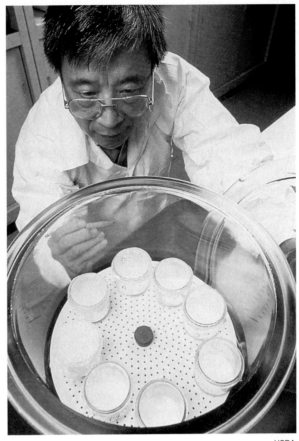

USDA

24-12 Food scientists have a responsibility to conduct their research in an ethical manner.

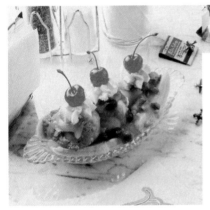

Item of Interest
Flavor Trends Guide Food Research

One factor that helps direct the development of a new food product is market analysis of current and future flavor trends. Trends that researchers have observed in the 21st century include:

❖ preference for darker, less-sweet chocolates

❖ interest in caramel-, orange-, cream-, and cherry-flavored dairy

❖ regional and ethnic trends like Greek olives and Chinese parsley

❖ demand for low-carbohydrate foods

❖ combinations of familiar flavors with exotic ones such as vanilla-cranberry and papaya-poppyseed

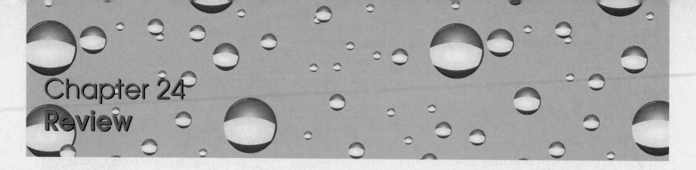

Summary

Research is central to the development of every new food product. Two types of research are used in the food industry—descriptive and analytical. Experiments are a part of analytical research. Certain steps are followed in conducting scientific experiments. These steps help food scientists make sure the results of experiments are valid.

Developing a new food product or variation of a food product is a time-consuming process. It involves many experts working as a team to brainstorm ideas, research information, and develop procedures. After a product is developed, other steps are taken to make the product a success. Professional ethics must be applied in all aspects of research and development.

Check Your Understanding

1. Explain the difference between descriptive and analytical research.
2. Describe one way food scientists can use descriptive research.
3. Describe how descriptive research and analytical research are used together in the creation of a new product.
4. What is the purpose of a food science experiment?
5. List the steps in developing a food science experiment.
6. How must variables be controlled when designing an experiment? Why must they be controlled in this way?
7. Why must a researcher determine how to record data before the data is collected?
8. List two ways food scientists share results of experiments with other researchers.
9. List the steps a food manufacturer may go through to develop a new product.

10. Why is it important for researchers to identify the consumer group being targeted?
11. List two reasons a research team pilot manufactures a product.
12. Give three examples of unethical behavior.

Critical Thinking

1. Keeping notes at home about the successes and failures resulting from experimenting with recipes is an example of what type of research?
2. Developing preparation directions for the package of a food product sold nationally is the result of what type of research?
3. If all available packaging materials were unsuitable for a new product, what questions might the product developers ask?
4. Suppose everyone in the class makes the same package of basic muffin mix at home tonight. It calls for combining an egg, milk, and oil together and mixing that with the package ingredients just until blended. Even if directions are followed exactly, what variables may possibly result in product differences?

Explore Further

1. **Technology.** Search the Internet for information about the number of new food products introduced to the market each year and the percentage that succeed.
2. **Application Skills.** Design a survey to assess your classmates' taste preferences in ice cream products and similar frozen desserts. Based on the results of your survey, what new dessert product might be worth developing?

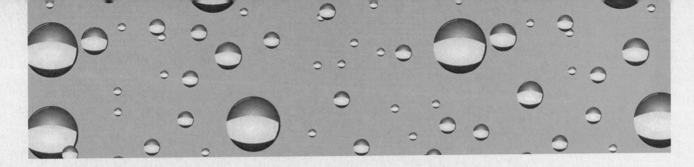

3. **Math.** Survey your classmates to determine the following statistically: What new food products were tried this year? Of those, how many were a repeat purchase (purchased more than once)?

4. **Application Skills.** Develop an experimental procedure to determine the proportion of melted chocolate to whipping cream needed to make a chocolate sauce for ice cream sundaes, called ganache. Design a data table for the ganache research that records amounts, heating time, heating temperature, cooling temperature, and viscosity.

5. **Communication.** Create a packaging design and an advertising campaign for a new low-calorie, lowfat breakfast bar. What would your new TV commercial show? How would your advertisements look and in which publications would they appear?

Activity 24A
Developing a Food Science Experiment

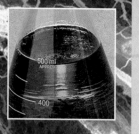

Purpose

Developing a new experiment can begin in several ways. One way is to first review experiments you have conducted in this class. Have any of the experiments raised questions that were not answered? For example, in Experiment 10C, you tested the effect of different fats on dropped cookies. You may have wondered what difference fat makes in bar cookies or cakes. A second approach to developing a new experiment is to identify a topic of special interest to you or your lab group. Which chapter or unit in this text most grabbed your attention? After you have identified an area of interest, focus your thoughts on what you want to learn more about in that area. Other people can also be a source of ideas for developing a new experiment. Ask what problems others have found with food preparation. Select a problem that interests you. After you have chosen a topic for your experiment, state the problem you want to solve as a result of your experiment.

Procedure

1. Use the scientific method to develop your experiment. (See Chapter 2.)
2. Determine which variable you will be testing.
3. Determine what your control will be.
4. Outline the steps in the procedure needed to test your hypothesis.
5. Estimate the time needed to conduct each step of your experiment.
6. List all the equipment needed for your experiment.
7. List all the supplies needed for your experiment.
8. List what data you will be collecting.
9. List what types of observations you should record.
10. Determine what calculations, if any, will be needed to interpret your data.
11. Construct a data table to fit your procedure.
12. Submit your written experiment to your teacher for approval.

Later

1. Conduct your experiment as planned.
2. Record all the data you collect.
3. Make any necessary calculations.
4. Analyze your data.
5. Form a conclusion that explains your results.
6. Write your report.
7. Present your results to the class.

Activity 24B
Analyzing a Complex Food System

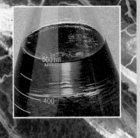

Purpose

An important aspect of any research project is the review of literature. This part of research provides you with information about discoveries others have made related to your problem or project. In this activity, you are to learn all you can about a complex food system that interests you. You will then develop a nutritious snack for teens that uses the complex food system as a major ingredient.

Equipment

computer with Internet connection

Procedure

1. As a class, determine which complex food system you want to study. The following are complex food systems commonly used in foods: corn, eggs, milk, soybeans, chocolate, and wheat.

2. Visit the Web sites of growers' associations, trade organizations, and/or major producers for information. Focus your research on one of the following aspects of your complex food system (each lab group should choose a different aspect):

   ❖ Identify the types of organic compounds (proteins, carbohydrates, and fats) in the basic food product. Also,

identify other components in the food system that affect the nutritional value, flavor, and/or production of products containing the complex food system as a major ingredient.

   ❖ Prepare a detailed nutritional analysis of your complex food system. Identify nutrients for which the system is considered a good source and nutrients for which it is considered a poor source. Also, identify any potential health benefits and/or concerns associated with consuming foods made with the food system.

   ❖ List solutions, foams, emulsions, and gels typically made from your complex food system. Describe the properties of your food system than support these mixtures.

   ❖ Analyze which food preservation methods are most effective with the food products resulting from your complex food system.

   ❖ Identify the major by-products that are based on your complex food system. Also, identify any separation techniques used to produce the by-products.

   ❖ Compile a list of items of interest related to your complex food system. The list may include recommended preparation procedures, recipes, production procedures, current research, and biotechnology applications.

3. Give an oral presentation to the class. Prepare a computer-generated visual and a handout or worksheet that covers information gathered through your research in step 2.

4. Develop a formulation for a nutritious snack that uses your complex food system or a by-product of the complex food system as a major ingredient. Keep in mind what you learned through your

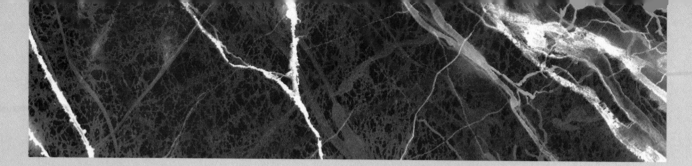

research and the oral presentations given by the other lab groups as you develop your formulation. Each lab group should develop a different formulation for the same type of snack food. (You might want to use the FCCLA Star Events NutriSnack event as a guideline.) Refer to Activity 24A for an experimental procedure to use in developing your formulation.

5. After receiving approval from your teacher, prepare your formulation.

6. Conduct a sensory evaluation with classmates so all students can sample all formulations. Write a concluding recommendation regarding your snack product. Determine which formulation you would choose for the class snack product.

7. Distribute copies of your formulation to your classmates and explain why it was or was not chosen as the final snack product.

Activity 24C
Developing a New Food Product

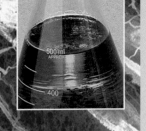

Purpose
This activity will provide the opportunity for your class to simulate the experiences of a food science product development team.

Problem
You are employed by the Frozen Gourmet Food Company. At the last departmental meeting, your boss reported company sales as compared to your main competitor, Frozen Delights, Inc. Frozen Gourmet ranked a poor second. Your product development team is to present a proposal for a new frozen entrée. This entrée will be the first in a new line of products designed to appeal to health-conscious consumers. The new entrée must

❖ be cost competitive (Consider developing a vegetarian entrée or using a protein analog for up to 50% of the meat content.)

❖ be nutrient dense to attract the largest possible number of health-conscious consumers

❖ meet FDA standards for nutrition labeling and label claims

❖ be able to be sold as a functional food

Procedure
1. Hold a brainstorming meeting to develop product ideas.

2. Determine who will fill each committee position. Complete a chart listing all the tasks that need to be accomplished by your committee. List the name of the committee member who is responsible for completing each task. Also, identify the deadline by which each task must be completed in order to finish the class project on time. (See Charts 24-7 and 24-9 in the text.)

3. Have the manager keep meeting minutes and explanations of all decisions.

4. Have the research committee conduct research as outlined in Activity 24B. Look for information on government regulations related to your food product. Investigate what nutrients are popular in functional foods. Find recipes for similar homemade products to use as guidelines.

5. Have the technicians prepare small trial formulations of the product and keep logs of raw data from trials and experiments. (See Activity 24A.)

6. Have the accountants keep financial reports.

7. Have the evaluation committee conduct sensory evaluations among committee members.

8. Have the advertising committee name the product. This committee will also prepare a package design for the front of the package and an advertising campaign for TV commercials.

9. Have the dietetics committee assemble a nutrition and ingredient label that meets FDA labeling standards.

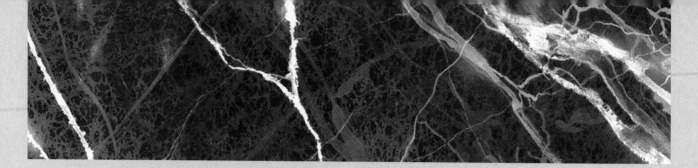

10. All class members should provide input for a report of project results to the company board of directors. The report is to include the following:

❖ demonstration of how this product fills a void in the market without just copying competitor selections

❖ formulations with supply lists and production procedures

❖ sensory evaluation results of the pilot production

❖ cost projections

❖ samples for tasting

❖ sample packaging

❖ advertising campaign proposal

❖ proposals for expansion of the product line if this entrée is successful

Proposed Timeline

Day 1: hold organizational and brainstorming meetings

Day 2: finalize product idea and begin research

Day 3: research and develop formulation ideas, submit supplies list

Day 4: conduct trials on formulations

Day 5: conduct trials and sensory evaluations

Day 6: continue trials as needed, develop packaging and advertising

Day 7: complete trials, packaging, and advertising campaign

Day 8: assemble reports

Day 9: complete reports and determine presentation format

Day 10: give presentation to board of directors

Questions

1. What do you feel you learned from this activity?

2. How could you apply this experience to food preparation at home?

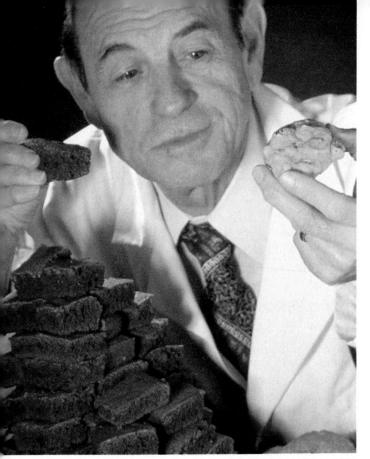

Agricultural Research Service, USDA

This chemist specializes in developing food ingredients. He is preparing to sample baked goods made from a reduced-fat ingredient he invented.

Chapter 25

Food Science Related Careers: A World of Opportunities

Objectives

After studying this chapter, you will be able to

describe personal qualities and training needed for success in food-related occupations.

compare the working conditions and employment outlook of food-related careers with other career areas.

list career opportunities related to food science, foodservice, and dietetics.

evaluate career opportunities related to foods in business, education, and government.

Key Terms

finished food

dietitian

registered dietitian

entrepreneurship

You may have a career goal in mind that defines what you want to be and do someday. If you are like most teens and young adults, however, you have not yet chosen a career. You may not even have given the subject more than a passing thought.

As you look toward the future, you might want to consider the broad range of career opportunities related to food. The food industry is the largest industry in the United States. It encompasses job opportunities from the farm to the table. People who work in development, production, inspection, marketing, distribution, and education are all tied to food in some way. This chapter will help you examine whether a food-related career can provide the opportunities you want.

Careers, Food, and You

The first step in exploring career opportunities is to examine who you are. What are your likes and dislikes? What kinds of skills and talents do you have? What do you enjoy doing? How much education and training are you willing to undertake? What kind of work environment suits you best? Examining all these aspects about yourself can help you find the career pathway that is right for you. See 25-1.

Personal Qualities

Some qualities are needed for success in most jobs. If you are dependable, good-natured, and cooperative, you are likely to do well in any job you choose.

The food industry offers a broad range of careers. There is a position to suit every personality type. Whether you are curious,

precise, artistic, or mechanical, the food industry has a place for you.

Are you analytical and detail oriented? These traits are vital for many positions in the food industry. Food scientists in research must study every aspect of the development of a new food product. They must keep detailed records of each step of the research process. Food technologists and inspectors must carefully run tests at various steps in the production process.

Education and Training

You can develop many of the skills you will need in the work world while you are in high school. These include skills in problem solving, teamwork, and communication. You should also acquire basic computer keyboarding skills and a knowledge of applications software. Many jobs will require you to have abilities in these areas.

Before choosing a career, an important factor to consider is the type of training you will need beyond high school. How much and what kind of education do you prefer? How long can you afford to stay in school? How much time are you willing to spend on formal training?

The food industry has positions for every level of training, from high school to graduate school. Many positions simply require a willingness to learn and on-the-job training. In 1996, 70% of all jobs required only on-the-job training or postsecondary vocational training. However, experts project that most jobs in the next decade will require at least an associate's degree.

Many school systems offer opportunities for internships, apprenticeships, and job shadowing. These opportunities give high school students a chance to experience career options firsthand. This is an excellent way to explore a career before you spend time and money on formal training.

Professional organizations provide many opportunities for members to develop leadership skills. Members can serve on committees, executive boards, or hold office. They can help advance their profession by conducting workshops and lectures on their areas of expertise. Attending meetings and participating in training

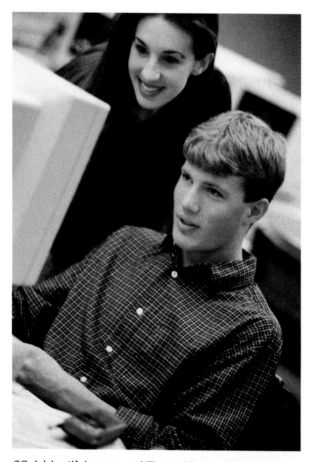

25-1 Identifying your skills and interests while you are in high school can help you choose the right career for your future.

sessions helps members establish important professional networks. Students can begin this process by joining and participating in the student organizations available at their campus. Family, Career, and Community Leaders of America (FCCLA), SkillsUSA, and Future Business Leaders of America-Phi Beta Lambda (FBLA-PBL) are some of the student organizations that provide opportunities to acquire leadership skills, develop professional skills through competition, increase service skill through community service, and expand career related scholarship and internship opportunities.

College and university programs in food science are comprised of a challenging set of courses. The core food science courses include a study of food chemistry, food analysis, and food microbiology, 25-2. Courses in food processing and food engineering are also at the heart of a food science program. Students in the program will be required to take courses

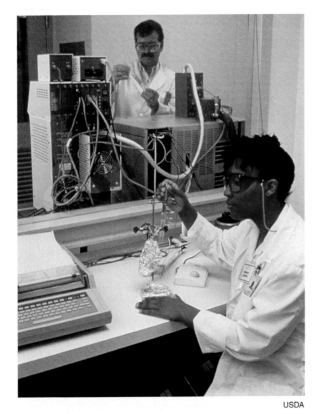

USDA

25-2 Education in food science involves working with ongoing research projects. Here, a chemist is preparing samples of peanut butter for aroma evaluation by a student.

in calculus, physics, biology, nutrition, communications, and statistics. They will be expected to use computers and develop thinking skills. General courses, such as history, ethics, economics, literature, foreign language, and fine arts, are required, too. In addition, students may be urged to take special interest courses. Students might study such areas as food law, sensory evaluation, biotechnology, or waste management.

Working Conditions

Working conditions include many factors that can affect your comfort in the environment in which you are employed. Working conditions include such issues as location, schedule, transportation, parking, and the number of employees. The work environment also involves smells, noise levels, lighting, and temperature. Working part-time during high school can help you determine the type of environment in which you will feel most comfortable.

You may be able to change some working conditions that you find uncomfortable. You will have to simply accept other conditions if you are going to hold a certain job. For instance, you might be able to bring a portable heater into an office that is cold. However, you would not be able to install a window in an office that does not have one. You will have to decide which working conditions you can and cannot accept.

One working condition over which you will not have much control is whether the work is done inside or outside. Professionals who work indoors in the food industry range from accountants to food scientists. Those who hold outdoor positions span from farmers to agricultural scientists.

Another working condition that you may not be able to change is your schedule. The workweek may be Monday through Friday, or it may change from one week to the next. Hours can be flexible or set. Many food production plants have shifts that work set hours. Other companies rotate days off each week. Many jobs in the foodservice industry require employees to work evenings and weekends. Workers who have to travel, such as distributors and salespeople, are often away from home for days at a time. It is important to think about how your schedule might affect your personal life. When conflicts arise, you will have to decide what events will be scheduling priorities.

Employment Outlook

Employment outlook refers to the number of jobs expected to be available in an occupation. You can find information about employment outlook in *The Occupational Outlook Handbook.* This book is published by the U.S. Department of Labor. A copy should be in your local library.

Many jobs in the food industry have an employment outlook rating of very good to excellent. This means job forecasters are predicting there will be more job openings than qualified candidates. Some jobs have positive outlooks due to high turnover. This means people do not stay in the positions very long. Low wages, unpleasant working conditions, and few chances for advancement are circumstances that often lead to high turnover. If you take a job in a field with high turnover, you must be prepared to accept challenging working conditions.

The employment outlook for some jobs indicates there will be keen competition. This means the number of people applying for jobs will be greater than the number of job openings. If you are interested in such a field, you will need to be prepared for stiff competition. Being willing to move or taking classes may help you get a job in a competitive area. You may also qualify for your "dream job" after spending several years learning lesser positions and moving up through a career.

Food Science Careers in the Food Industry

The total food-producing system generates 20% of the U.S. gross national product. This system employs one-fourth of the U.S. workforce. It includes a broad range of careers. People working in this industry grow, process, manufacture, and distribute all the foods you eat. Food industry workers also produce additives and packaging used for all types of food products. All these workers

could benefit from some knowledge of food science. See 25-3.

Production

Food production refers to the growth of basic foodstuffs, such as grains, vegetables, fruits, nuts, and livestock. Careers in this area include farmers and farm managers. These workers oversee the management of farms, orchards, and/or herds and flocks.

Most people in food production put in long hours and have few days off work. Their work is often seasonal. People working in this field often view living in a rural area, being self-employed, and working outdoors as advantages.

Many jobs in food production do not require special education and training. However, some farmers choose to get at least an associate's degree. Studying business and economics can help farmers with such skills as managing money and predicting crop futures. Courses in agriculture can help farmers learn about the physical and chemical nature of their product. Farmers also need to know about the chemistry of crop fertilizers and pesticides. Farm workers need mechanical skills to repair and maintain farm equipment. See 25-4.

The employment outlook in food production is declining. Before the industrial

Employment in Food-Related Occupations	
Occupation	**Employees Nationwide**
Foodservice	5 million
Raw food materials production	3 million
Food distribution	2 million
Retail sales	2 million
Food manufacturing	1.7 million
Wholesale sales	700,000
Dietetics and nutrition	58,000
Research, development, and quality control	25,000

25-3 The food industry employs millions of people in a broad range of careers.

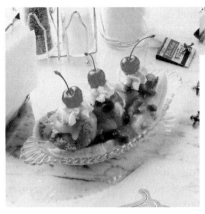

Item of Interest
Defining the Food Industry

The food industry is divided into three main categories based on product type.

❖ Raw food products are uncooked items in their natural state. Raw products include meat, fish, poultry, milk, grains, vegetables, fruits, nuts, spices, and herbs.

❖ Manufactured foods are raw materials converted into finished products. These foods include canned fruit, frozen vegetables, and baked bread.

❖ Highly processed foods have had significant changes to the raw material or one or more ingredients in the food

product. Highly processed foods include high-fructose corn syrup, nondairy whipped topping, fat-free cheese, and microwavable entrees.

---

revolution, about 90% of the U.S. workforce was farmers. Today, about 2% of the workforce runs farms. This large drop is due to advances in science and technology. These advances have made it possible for each farmer to produce enough food for thousands of people.

One type of farming that is expected to increase in the future is aquaculture. Aquaculture farms raise fish and shellfish. Commercial fishing has placed a strain on

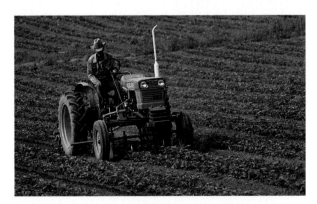

25-4 Many farmers take classes to study the chemistry and biology behind the crops they raise. They also study business management and acquire skills in equipment maintenance and repairs.

some natural fish resources. A growing awareness of the role fish can play in a healthful diet has increased consumer demand for fish. These combined factors have led to this relatively new area of farming. Aquaculture farmers need to know what water conditions will support the type of fish they are producing. They must run tests on the temperature, pH, and oxygen levels of the water.

A number of fields are related to food production. Botanists and biologists are among the professionals who work with farm crops and animals. These workers study ways to improve the quality and quantity of basic foods. They use the principles of science to solve problems in their research. Most food scientists and farmers work mainly with one type of crop or livestock. Other workers who support food production are employed by manufacturers of pesticides, animal feed, and farm equipment and tools.

Biotechnologists are also professionals who work with crops. Their research involves developing new forms of crops. New hybrid crops are developed by removing genes from one variety of a species and splicing them onto another variety or species. Many varieties of grain crops grown in the United States have been developed through biotechnology.

Manufacturing

Although many foods are sold and consumed immediately after harvest, most undergo changes. Raw foods are processed, preserved, and packaged. See 25-5. Manufacturers refine, combine, and alter foods to make thousands of different products. Some employees at each step in the manufacturing process must know about the physical and chemical nature of foods. They must also know how the foods will react in mixtures.

It takes the expertise of many people to manufacture food products. Frequently, teams of professionals work together to try to anticipate the needs and desires of consumers. They strive to develop new food products that will sell well. Food engineers and microbiologists are often part of such a team. The knowledge of packaging specialists and marketing experts is also needed. Food scientists, family and consumer sciences professionals, and technicians work together to help prepare formulations of new products. These professionals conduct tests on batches of processed

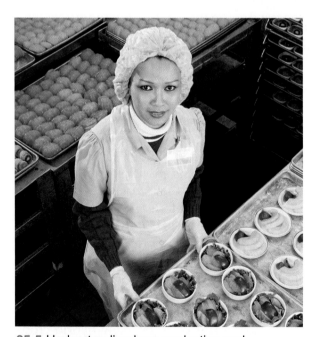

25-5 Understanding how production and packaging processes affect foods can help people in the manufacturing area of the food industry produce quality products.

foods. Family and consumer science professionals also work in test kitchens to assess products as they are developed. They write package directions and develop prototype formulations, too.

Another career in the area of manufacturing is food science. Food scientists study the basic properties of foods and help develop new products. They check factors that affect food safety. They hold sensory evaluations. Food scientists also monitor the quality of the mass-produced foods.

The terms *food scientist* and *food technologist* are often used interchangeably by the food industry. In some companies, however, *food scientists* focus on researching the nature of foods and principles of processing. *Food technologists* may be more involved in applying what others have learned through research to the development of new food products. People from a variety of backgrounds may hold either of these positions in industry. Food scientists and food technologists may have degrees in chemistry, agriculture, or family and consumer sciences.

A food scientist must have an inquiring mind. He or she must be good with details, technical work, and written and oral communication. A food scientist in research must enjoy conducting experiments, solving problems, and exploring the unknown. He or she needs an interest in how and why reactions occur the way they do. Some food science problems take years to solve. Therefore, a food scientist needs patience. He or she also needs creativity to develop experiments and new food product ideas.

Working in lab teams may have made you aware of how important teamwork skills are to the food scientist. For any group of people to work together for an extended period, each member of the group must respect others. Being tactful and having good communication skills are critical. Good team members will stay on task. They will perform their share of responsibilities while looking for ways to help other team members. Treating others as you would want others to treat you is always a good rule to follow.

Working conditions in the field of manufacturing vary with each food product. Processing plants are often noisy in areas where machinery is used. Workers must maintain a clean environment. Most food handlers are required to wear uniforms, which may include hair restraints, lab coats, shoe covers, aprons, and gloves.

Education and training for manufacturing positions depend on the job. Many positions require on-the-job training for a specific skill, such as cutting meat or running a grinder. Technicians often have an associate's degree in food science or technology. A food scientist must have at least a bachelor's degree in food science, food technology, or food engineering. See 25-6. Half of all food scientists have a master's degree or a doctorate. An advanced degree is required for most jobs in research.

Professional Profile: Food Science Laboratory Manager

Mike is the head chemist and manager of the food science lab for Midstate Mills. The food science lab conducts tests on all the flour products the mill produces to ensure consistent quality. The tests analyze the physical and chemical properties of each batch of flour ground and mixed at the mill.

Mike started his career by working as summer help on the construction of a bakery plant at age 17. After the construction was completed, Mike was offered summer work at the bakery as a baker's assistant. Mike had other career plans. "I wanted to become a veterinarian like my father," says Mike. However, he accepted the job with the goal to raise money for his college expenses. Mike spent the summers of his college years at the bakery.

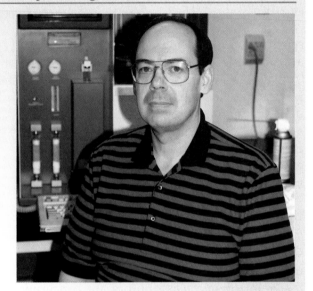

When Mike's plans for veterinary medicine did not work out, he returned to the bakery. He was offered a job as laboratory assistant, provided he learned how every product of the plant was made. At the completion of training, Mike was offered the job of setting up and developing the bakery's testing laboratory. After eight and a half years, Mike transferred to a mill. At his new job in the mill, Mike learned about the milling and mixing industry. After several years, he transferred to Midstate Mills to assume his current position as laboratory manager. Mike's recommendation to today's teen is: "Learn all you can from any job you have. You never know for sure what you will need in the future."

Mike's background is well suited for his position. He has the necessary college degree in chemistry combined with on-the-job training in bakery products and business skills. He understands all the testing procedures from a chemical standpoint. He also knows about the quality standards of products from a baker's perspective.

Skills needed in Mike's position include knowledge of chemical composition of milled products and their ingredients. Mike needs decision-making skills. The manager decides what analytical chemical tests are needed. He or she chooses the procedures for each test and follows any needed safety precautions. The manager needs business and administration skills, too. These include abilities in accounting, budgeting, and supervising others. A manager needs to be able to effectively communicate with and relate to people. The manager must be aware of all the federal regulations regarding the food industry. These include codes about additives, labels, and potential food hazards. The manager also needs taste and odor identification skills.

Maintaining the skills needed to be a food science laboratory manager requires a lifelong commitment to learning. Mike must be willing to study and attend seminars on new legislation, alternate testing procedures, and other relevant scientific developments.

25-6 A food science laboratory manager needs an educational background in business topics as well as a knowledge of the chemistry of foods.

Many management positions are filled by people with a master's degree in business administration in addition to a foods backgrounds.

Over 20,000 food processing plants in the United States have more than 20 employees each. Job opportunities exist in the food industry in every region of the United States. There is more job stability in the food industry than in the manufacturing of most nonfood products. The demand for trained employees to help manufacture food products is fairly steady.

The employment outlook for trained food scientists is increasing. Consumers are more aware of the importance of a healthful diet. Consumers are also selecting more convenience foods. In response, the food industry is developing more tasty, healthful products that are ready to eat in under 30 minutes. The development of these products has created a growing need for people with food science knowledge.

Distribution

Food distribution involves hauling and storing foods. Distributors move food products from the farm to the processing plant to the point of sale. Distributors are concerned with the weight and form of food products. They are also concerned about how stable the products are. Distributors must work closely with manufacturers and retailers to keep foods safe. Everyone working in this area of the food industry must be aware of how to maintain food quality and safety.

Many of today's foods must be held and moved in controlled atmospheres. Care must be taken to keep temperatures and air quality at proper levels. Engineers work with food scientists to design packaging that will protect food from damage during shipping. For example, they might figure how many bags of pretzels can be packed in a box without damaging the pretzels. They would also need to determine how many boxes could be stacked without crushing the bottom box.

The number of job openings is expected to grow slightly in many areas of distribution. Training and education needed vary from on-the-job training to a master's degree in business management.

Quality Control

Inspectors and testers are needed at each step in the food production process to maintain quality control. These workers ensure that every food product is safe and meets federal regulations. They also make sure products meet a standard of quality. Quality control workers are the people who make sure potato chips are crunchy and bread is soft and moist.

Some workers in the field of quality control work for federal, state, and county agencies. Many of these workers are inspectors who are required by law to check food processing plants. The inspectors look at processing methods and sanitation procedures. They must also check production and testing records. Inspectors need a thorough understanding of the food product and processing methods they are examining. See 25-7.

Many people who work in the area of quality control work directly for food manufacturers. These workers are often food scientists and technicians. They run tests on samples of each batch of food that is processed and keep records of test results. Food scientists and technicians may have to conduct and keep track of several tests at the same time. These workers need speed and accuracy when test results are required before the next step in processing can be started. Testers must approve the quality of each batch of food before it is packaged for distribution.

The types of quality control tests run on food products will vary depending on the product. For example, self-rising flour is

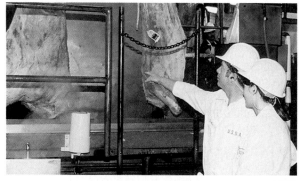

USDA

25-7 Inspectors receive training for the specific foods they inspect. Part of this training involves learning how to keep careful records for HACCP.

tested for physical contaminants, such as metal filings and small pieces of stone. It is then tested for pH, toxic residues, and nutrient content. Samples of each batch of flour are used in typical recipes for foods like pancakes and biscuits. These foods are then examined for density, height of rise, color, and overall appearance. Country ham, on the other hand, must have careful monitoring of curing room temperatures and humidity. Curing salts and sugars are mixed and tested before being applied to the meat. Tests are also run to monitor potentially hazardous mold growth.

Educational requirements for quality control workers depend on how technical the work is. Workers who conduct simple pass-fail tests may need only a high school diploma. These workers will receive on-the-job training about how to use test equipment and record results. Food scientists who manage labs often have business and management training. Technicians in the lab may have associate's or bachelor's degrees in food science or a related field.

Working conditions in the area of quality control vary with the type of food processing plant. Inspectors and testers often work in laboratories. They may have to wear lab coats and safety apparel.

Implementation of HACCP and improved technology are leading to more automated inspection of food products. (HACCP is a food safety system that examines the food production process at every point where contamination can occur.) Manufacturers are also shifting some inspection tasks to production workers. As a result, the number of job openings in the field of quality control is projected to decline. However, trained testers will continue to be used to assess the taste, smell, appearance, and performance of products.

Other Food-Related Career Areas

Other food-related career areas include jobs that involve providing a service. *Service* is labor that does not produce a product. Consumers of services are paying for workers' knowledge, skills, and time.

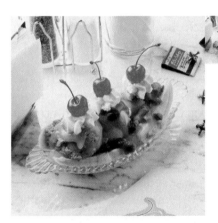

Item of Interest
The Importance of Quality Control

Profit margins in the food industry can be as low as a fraction of a cent per food container. This is possible because of the high volume of food sold. However, errors in safety or quality can result in losses large enough to put a company out of business. Two recent incidents illustrate this point.

A milling company in North Carolina orders a peppery spice blend from a processing plant in

Mexico. The spices are used in a coating mix for meat. The spice blend is formulated based on degrees of heat desired.

On one occasion, the processing plant prepared a batch of the spice blend that had too much heat. This error was not caught until the milling company had mixed over $100,000 worth of the coating mix. Because the processing plant was at fault, it had to cover the cost of the

ruined coating mix. This was a staggering loss for the small processing plant.

In a separate event, an E. coli outbreak was traced to ground beef. The beef had been improperly handled at a meat processing company. An investigation of the company resulted in a recall of 2.5 million pounds of hamburger. The losses caused the company to go out of business.

Two food-related career areas focus on services instead of or in addition to products. One area is foodservice. Foodservice involves preparing meals and serving them to customers. See 25-8. The second area is dietetics. Dietetics involves planning meals to meet nutritional needs. A basic knowledge of food science can be of value to anyone working in either of these areas.

Foodservice

A foodservice worker turns raw and manufactured food products into finished food. *Finished food* is a food item or meal that is ready to eat.

The foodservice industry provides entry-level job opportunities for teens in almost every community in the United States. Foodservice workers held over 3.4 million jobs in 1996. These jobs included hosts, servers, chefs, cooks, and buspersons. Twenty percent of food preparation workers are ages

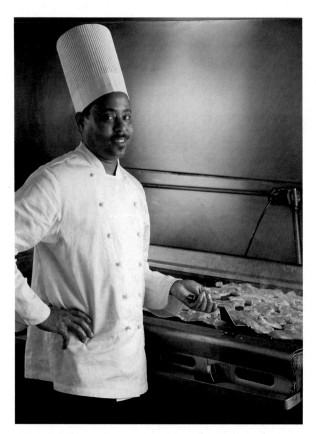

25-8 Restaurants, cruise ships, and other businesses that serve foods hire chefs to prepare delicious, attractive foods for customers.

16 to 19. As many as half of the foodservice workers work part-time hours.

Chefs are responsible for preparing meals that are pleasing in taste and appearance. To advance in this field, a chef needs to be creative and artistic. The reputation and success of a restaurant will depend on the abilities of the chefs and cooks.

Skills needed for many positions, such as short-order cooks and kitchen workers, are acquired through on-the-job training. Chefs are the most highly trained foodservice workers. Most chefs complete a two- to four-year degree in culinary arts. Most culinary arts programs involve some training in food science. It is also possible to advance to a chef's position after thorough on-the-job training through apprenticeship programs. Advancement does not depend only on culinary skills. An executive or head chef must also be able to manage workers, supplies, and time schedules.

The foodservice industry does not always provide the most comfortable working conditions. Kitchens are often warmer than other work environments. Many foodservice workers spend much time on their feet. Some jobs require workers to lift and move heavy containers of food. Chefs often work under time pressure.

Jobs in foodservice are projected to offer higher than average pay. The number of job openings is expected to be much higher than in other areas. Foodservice includes 11 out of the 25 careers identified as having fast growth and low unemployment for the next decade. The growth is expected as a result of more people eating more meals away from home. This trend is due to the larger number of two-career and single-parent households. The strength of the U.S. economy also has a positive effect on the foodservice industry. Greater household income and more leisure time are factors that increase how often people eat away from home.

Dietetics

One more career area linked to food is dietetics. Many of the people who work in this field are dietitians. *Dietitians* are professionals who assess diets and plan nutrition programs. They may also supervise the preparing and

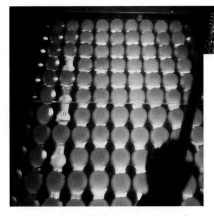

Technology Tidbit
The Cook/Chill Foodservice System

Many hospitals prepare and serve over a thousand meals a day. Preparing this much food is a challenge. However, the real problem is to plate and deliver

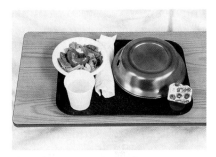

Cook/chill technology allows hospitals to deliver hundreds of hot meals to patients all over the building.

the food to patients throughout the hospital without loss of heat.

The solution is cook/chill technology developed by 3M for the Apollo lunar spacecraft. With this technology, plates are designed to cook the food they hold. A special coating on the bottom of the plates converts electrical energy to heat on contact. The plates have built-in sensors that separately monitor and control the temperature of each food item. The plates are double-walled and insulated so they stay cool to the touch on the outside.

The hot portions of meals are cooked a day or more in advance. The food is then chilled in bulk containers. On the day a

meal is served, the cold food is placed on the plates. The plates are placed in special carts and stored in a refrigeration unit until shortly before serving. The carts can be plugged into a power source in the kitchen to heat the food. In 24 minutes, the food has been heated to the desired temperature. Milk, puddings, and other cold foods on the same cart remain cold.

Another application of this technology is airline foodservice. Food served on airplanes must be prepared in advance and safely held during transport and loading. The food must then be easily heated and quickly delivered by flight attendants.

serving of meals. Many dietitians work for hospitals and nursing homes, 25-9. These professionals plan menu options to meet the special dietary needs of the patients. Some dietitians work in doctors' offices. Others work for public schools, colleges, and fitness centers. A number of dietitians are also in private practice.

Consumer interest in nutrition has led to more jobs for dietitians in the food industry. These dietitians may work as part of a product development team. They assess the nutritional value of food products. They may also prepare nutrition facts and tips for consumers.

Most dietitians are not directly involved in food preparation. However, they need to be aware of how preparation methods affect the

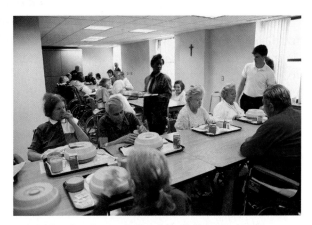

25-9 Nursing homes employ dietitians to plan meals that will meet the nutrient needs and address the health concerns of older adults.

nutritional value of food. They must know what nutrients are found in different foods. Dietitians must also know how food affects health.

Dietitians need skills that will help them communicate and interact with people. These skills help dietitians who work closely with chefs and cooks. These skills also help dietitians who counsel with patients one-on-one.

Dietitians have at least a bachelor's degree in dietetics or foods and nutrition. Many jobs require a master's degree. Forty states have laws that regulate dietitians. In 27 states, dietitians must be licensed. Dietitians usually have to pass a national exam before a state will issue a license. This certification exam is given by the American Dietetic Association (ADA). Dietitians who have passed the exam are called *registered dietitians.* To remain certified, registered and licensed dietitians must stay up-to-date in their field. They do this by taking classes and going to professional meetings.

Dietitians usually work out of an office. Their jobs may involve research, counseling, and teaching. For instance, a dietitian at a large hospital might have to study the links between nutrients and health conditions. He or she would meet with individual patients to discuss their nutritional needs. When a number of patients have the same needs, the dietitian might hold classes. Many hospital dietitians conduct classes on diets for people with diabetes or heart disease.

Salaries for dietitians are close to salaries for food scientists. The job outlook is favorable. The number of job openings is expected to grow at an average rate for the next few years. One factor hindering job growth is the limits on insurance coverage for nutrition counseling.

Advertisement

Food-related career opportunities exist in advertising. Ad agencies, publishers, and product boards need people with training in journalism and food science. Food photographers are in demand to take pictures of food for use in advertising. Food stylists are also needed to attractively arrange food before it is photographed.

Entrepreneurship

Entrepreneurship is owning and running a business. Many food-related businesses offer opportunities for people who want to be entrepreneurs. Food scientists and dietitians can open private consulting firms or do freelance work. People who like to prepare food might start a catering, cake decorating, or home baking business, 25-10. Many specialty food companies began as home-baking ventures.

It can take time before this type of work becomes profitable. Entrepreneurs often work long hours. However, many people like the flexibility of being self-employed.

Types of Employers

When choosing a career, you need to think about the type of organization for which you would prefer to work. Employers can be grouped in different areas, or *sectors*, of the economy based on their main goals. The central goal of the business sector is to produce goods and services for profit. The chief goal of the education sector is to teach students. The broad goal of the government sector is to protect the well-being of the citizens in a specific region. All these sectors have positions for food scientists. Job security, salaries, and benefits tend to vary with the type of employer.

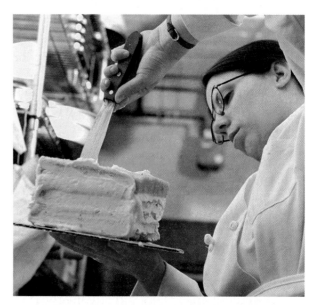

25-10 Someone who enjoys baking and decorating cakes might use those interests to start a business.

Business Sector

The business sector is made up of all privately owned food companies. This sector also includes companies that make food-related products. Food manufacturers in the business sector hire about 75% of all food scientists. These professionals may have such job titles as sensory scientist, development scientist, director of research, and fermentation manager.

Many food scientists who work in the business sector deal with only one type of food. Some scientists form a specialization while they are in school. Others become focused on the types of products they work with in their first professional jobs. However, food scientists in some positions work with all kinds of foods.

The business sector has a greater wage range than the education and government sectors. Salaries vary with the type of food product and the region of the country. The expertise a job requires and a worker's educational level will also affect his or her income.

Education Sector

The education sector employs people who teach food science in public and private schools. Food science developed as a field of study at the university level in the mid 1900s. There are now about 40 colleges and universities in the United States that offer food science programs. Food scientists who are interested in research and teaching are best suited to work in these institutions. Many high schools also offer introductory courses in food science. These courses are often taught by trained family and consumer sciences (FCS) instructors. Educators need to enjoy learning, studying research, and working with young people. See 25-11.

As long as there is a need for food scientists, there will be a need for people to train them. Therefore, job security is highly stable in the education sector for both private and public schools. High school and college teaching positions are expected to be two of the fastest growing jobs for the next decade. Job forecasters estimate that two million more teachers will be needed just to fill the demands of public schools. One of the subjects

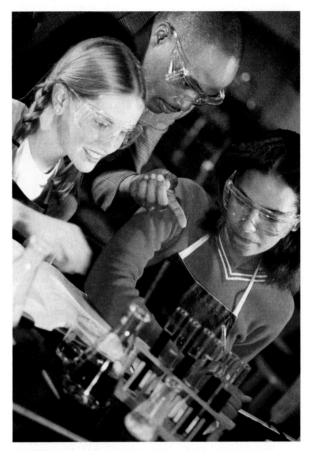

25-11 A teacher in a food science class helps students understand how scientific principles relate to the production, processing, preservation, and packaging of foods.

already experiencing a severe shortage of teachers is FCS. Many states are only graduating one trained FCS teacher for every 10 to 15 job openings.

Education does not offer as many chances for advancement as the business sector. Salaries also tend to be lower in education. However, pay scales in public schools and colleges have improved over the last decade. They are expected to continue to rise as the demand for teachers increases. Education offers some of the best insurance and retirement benefits. In the education sector, work hours are somewhat flexible outside of class. Time off is greater than in any other full-time occupation.

Government Sector

About 20% of all food scientists work for federal, state, or local governments. Most of these workers are researchers or inspectors. At the federal level, food scientists might work for the United States Department of Agriculture (USDA). The Food and Drug Administration (FDA) and the Commerce Department also employ food scientists. At the state and local levels, departments of health often hire food scientists. Job openings at the international level are found with such agencies as the World Health Organization (WHO).

Many systems used by the food industry are a result of research sponsored by the government space program. Lightweight, flexible foil pouches and aseptic packaging were initially developed for NASA. The HACCP system was developed to ensure the safety of food prepared for space travel. HACCP is now used throughout the food industry for quality control. Candy makers use controlled atmosphere warehouses to store peppermint candies. These warehouses keep the red and white stripes from bleeding together. The warehouses are based on climate control technology developed for the space program.

Food scientists employed by the space program are currently working on such projects as growing food in outer space. This project evolved out of the space station program. Long-term space travel will not be possible until food scientists can successfully grow fruits and vegetables in zero gravity.

An area of government work that is easily missed is the Department of Defense. The Defense Department works with industry to develop food products for the armed forces. During combat, troops need foods that are easy to transport and require little or no preparation. See 25-12.

Government jobs are fairly secure. They include good benefit packages, and wages compete well with the business sector.

Professional Associations

People who love science and communication or have strong administrative skills can find job opportunities within the professional associations and watchdog groups. These organizations can be found in the business, education, and government sectors. Examples include the Institute of Food Technologists (IFT) within the business sector and the Food and Drug Administration (FDA) within the government sector. The American Association of Family and Consumer Sciences (AAFCS) is a professional association that connects business and education sectors. FCCLA is a student organization that functions like a professional association at the secondary education level.

Professional associations rely heavily on dues from members and volunteer labor. These organizations provide networking and professional training opportunities for their members. The regional, state, national, and international meetings they organize provide opportunities to share research and new developments in the field. Most professional organizations also publish research journals and/or magazines on a monthly or quarterly basis. These magazines keep members and students informed of the newest research, trends, and statistics. Organizations hire staff to oversee the administration of the association, edit the publications, and organize meetings and workshops. Professional publications often have a section listing job opportunities in the field.

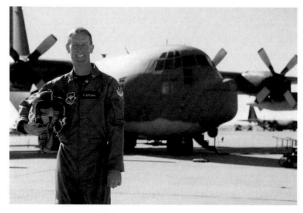

25-12 The government employs food specialists to meet the food needs of military personnel.

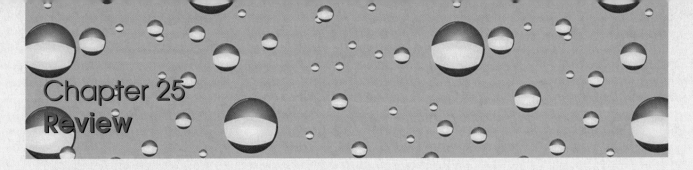

Summary

The food industry is the largest industry in the United States. One in four jobs will be connected in some way to the production, distribution, or sale of food. The first step in selecting a food-related career is to examine your personal traits and preferences. Other factors you should consider include required education and training, working conditions, and employment outlook for the occupation.

An understanding of basic food science principles is beneficial to anyone who works in the food industry. Food science careers can be found in the areas of production, manufacturing, distribution, and quality control. Other food-related career areas include foodservice, dietetics, and advertising. Many entrepreneurship opportunities are also available.

Food science positions can be found in each of the sectors of the economy. The business sector produces goods and services for a profit. The education sector teaches students. The government sector protects the well-being of citizens. Each sector has advantages and disadvantages in terms of job security, salaries, and benefits.

Check Your Understanding

1. List three basic skills you can develop in high school.
2. Where can you find information about employment outlook?
3. What type of farming is expected to increase in the future?
4. List five qualities necessary to food scientists.
5. What two factors are causing a decrease in the projected number of job openings in the field of quality control?
6. What is a finished food?
7. What education and certification are required of registered dietitians?
8. Name three food-related business opportunities for entrepreneurs.
9. Which sector of the economy is made up of all privately owned food companies?
10. List three advantages of jobs in the education sector.

Critical Thinking

1. What are your personal qualities and how will they most likely affect the type of career you will pursue?
2. How would a job that required you to work every Friday and Saturday night affect your personal life?
3. What are three specific questions about food safety for which a fresh meat distributor would need answers?
4. When you pay a restaurant bill, you are paying for more than just the food you eat. Give three specific examples of knowledge, skills, and time for which you are paying restaurant workers.
5. The government sponsors research and works with industry to develop foods for use during space travel and combat. Why would the government not leave this development solely up to the business sector?

Explore Further

1. **Writing.** Check with your school guidance counselors to find out if they offer personality tests. If available, take one of these tests and review the results with your counselor or teacher. Write a paper describing your personal qualities and the types of jobs for which you are best suited.

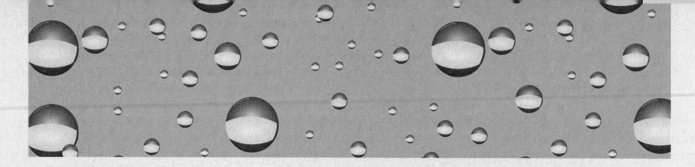

2. **Reading.** Use the want ads from a local newspaper to identify career opportunities in food production and processing facilities in your geographic area.

3. **Technology.** Collect employment outlook statistics on food science and food-related careers. Compile the information using a computer and a spreadsheet program. Use the computer to generate at least two types of graphs to illustrate or explain the statistics. Report your results to the class.

4. **Communication.** Work in a team to create a brochure that promotes food science related careers in the business, education, or government sector. The brochure should cover the types of opportunities available and education needed. The brochure should also identify salary ranges, job security, benefit packages, and advantages and disadvantages as compared with the other sectors. Publish the brochure and distribute it to class members.

Activity 25A
Developing a Resume

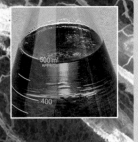

Purpose

An important tool to have when applying for jobs is a personal resume. A resume is a concise description of your experiences, education, awards, and skills. It is wise to keep an updated resume on file. The information on your resume can be useful when you are filling out application forms for jobs, scholarships, and colleges and universities. The average worker in the United States changes jobs five to seven times during the course of his or her lifetime. This figure does not include the part-time employment experiences that many people have as teenagers. Each job change will require an updated resume. A resume that is stored on a computer disk can be quickly updated by adding new information and deleting unrelated or outdated data.

Equipment

computer with word-processing software
printer

Supplies

sample resumes
high-quality paper

Procedure

1. Assemble information regarding your community service experiences, positions of employment, education, and awards.

2. Examine sample resumes for content organization and formatting styles.

3. Explore template and auto formatting options that are available with your word-processing software. (Templates and auto formatting will automatically space and format the information you enter. However, you have to organize the data to be entered by categories.)

4. Select an organizational style that fits your needs.

5. Organize your information by category and date. Information on resumes is usually listed with the most recent data first. Categories are

   ❖ Work Experience – employer's name and address, job title, responsibilities, dates of employment (List volunteer experience under this category, too.)

   ❖ Education – school name and address; degree earned or expected graduation date; subjects in which you excel, if any; grade-point average, if high

   ❖ Activities – names of organizations, school clubs, sports teams, and music groups; leadership positions held, responsibilities, dates of membership

   ❖ Skills – job-relevant skills you have acquired through means other than employment or volunteer work

   ❖ Honors and Achievements – types of awards, dates

   ❖ Hobbies and Interests

6. Enter relevant data into the computer. Save your work.

7. Check the resume for grammatical, typing, and spelling errors. Double-check all addresses and dates for accuracy. A resume should be error free.

8. Print a copy on regular paper. Turn it in to your teacher for inspection.

9. Make any corrections needed to the file. Save corrections.

10. Print at least one copy on high-quality paper. Save the file to a disk.

11. Store the printouts and the disk where you keep important papers and records.

12. Take a copy of your resume with you to any job interview. Mail a copy with job application forms and cover letters.

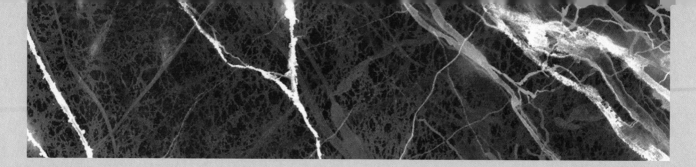

Questions

1. What areas, if any, are blank on your resume?

2. How can you gain experience in these areas that will benefit your career search in the future?

3. What skills do you need to acquire to achieve your career goals?

4. What types of part-time and summer employment will have the most benefit for your career goals at this point?

5. In what organizations can you become involved that will provide opportunities to develop skills related to your career goals?

Activity 25B
Preparing for a Job Interview

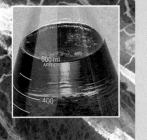

Purpose

Resumes often help employers determine who they will interview for a position. For most positions, employers decide who to hire based on an interview. A face-to-face meeting can tell an employer a lot about how your skills might meet the needs of his or her company. You can increase your chances of receiving a job offer by doing some homework before an interview occurs. Practicing with someone who is willing to give honest and constructive criticism can help you avoid first impression mistakes. Knowing the kinds of questions you are likely to be asked can help you prepare for a successful interview.

Equipment

computer with word-processing software
printer

Procedure

1. Arrange to interview someone who is responsible for hiring employees for his or her company. If possible, the person should be from a business related to your future career goals.

2. When you schedule the interview, explain your assignment briefly and thank the person for being willing to assist you. Good manners are always an important part of the interview process. Begin to practice now.

3. Use a word-processing program to type a list of questions you want to ask. Leave space after each question so you can note the person's answers. List one to three questions unique to the type of position being discussed. Other possible questions might include

   ❖ What do you consider appropriate attire for an interview?

   ❖ What do you look for in the first 30 seconds of an interview?

   ❖ What body language presents a positive image to you?

   ❖ What body language presents a negative image to you?

   ❖ What questions do you typically ask at an interview?

   ❖ When you have several qualified candidates, what factors help you make a final decision about whom to hire?

   ❖ What types of questions do you expect a candidate to ask you?

   ❖ What kind of follow-up or contact do you appreciate from a candidate after an interview is over?

4. Print your list of questions. Save your work.

5. Dress neatly for the interview.

6. Shake the person's hand at the beginning of the interview. Thank the person again for his or her time.

7. Stay focused on your questions at the interview. Avoid taking up too much of the person's valuable time.

8. After the interview, open the word-processing file containing your list of questions. Type the answers provided by the person you interviewed.

9. Type answers you might give to the questions listed by the person you interviewed.

10. Print your work and submit your finished project to your teacher.

Questions

1. What wardrobe changes do you need to make for future interviews?

2. Is there a uniform or style of wardrobe expected for the type of career you are presently pursuing?

3. Are there personal grooming habits you need to work on improving?

4. What should you practice to improve the first impression you make in an interview?

5. What should you avoid doing during an interview?

Activity 25C
Developing Career Goals

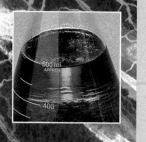

Purpose

According to an old saying, "You can't hit what you don't aim for." This saying can apply to your future career. It means you will not be able to do the type of work that interests you unless you set some career goals. Many of your career goals may change during the next few years. However, setting goals now will help you acquire skills needed to succeed in any career path. Perhaps you have already determined a career goal. For instance, you may already know you want to be a research scientist for a biotechnology firm. Reaching a career goal involves many steps. Knowing those steps and focusing on what is needed to accomplish each one can help you succeed.

Procedure

1. Determine a career goal you believe you want to achieve.

2. Research information on the Internet and in occupational handbooks at your school library. List the skills, education, and on-the-job training needed to reach your goal.

3. Research technical schools, training programs, community colleges, and colleges that offer programs in your chosen field of study.

4. Select three programs you are interested in applying to attend.

5. List each program, the cost to attend, the location, and special circumstances that are relevant.

6. List the advantages and disadvantages of each option.

7. Use the *Occupational Outlook Handbook* to help you list the types of positions that would best assist you in gaining the skills you need. Also list intermediate positions you would need to hold between now and reaching your goal.

8. Find entry-level job opportunities in your area through your local Chamber of Commerce.

9. Develop a timeline showing education needed, part-time employment possibilities, and goals for each step from entry-level position to the position you hope to achieve.

Questions

1. What skills are needed for any career that you can work at developing now?

2. What opportunities are available for you to develop career-specific skills while you are still in school?

3. List the steps you need to complete to reach your final goal. Identify a preliminary goal you would need to achieve each year for the next 10 years to reach your final career goal.

Measurement Conversion Charts

Common U.S. to Metric Measures (Approximate)

Length

Abbreviation	When You Know	Multiply by	To Find	Abbreviation
in	inches	2.5	centimeters	cm
ft	feet	30	centimeters	cm
yd	yards	0.9	meters	m
mi	miles	1.6	kilometers	km

Area

Abbreviation	When You Know	Multiply by	To Find	Abbreviation
in^2	square inches	6.5	square centimeters	cm^2
ft^2	square feet	0.09	square meters	m^2
yd^2	square yards	0.8	square meters	m^2
mi^2	square miles	2.6	square kilometers	km^2
	acres	0.4	hectares	ha

Mass

Abbreviation	When You Know	Multiply by	To Find	Abbreviation
oz	ounces	28	grams	g
lb	pounds	0.45	kilograms	kg
	short tons (2000 lb)	0.9	metric ton	t

Volume

Abbreviation	When You Know	Multiply by	To Find	Abbreviation
tsp	teaspoons	5	milliliters	mL
Tbsp	tablespoons	15	milliliters	mL
in^3	cubic inches	16	milliliters	mL
fl oz	fluid ounces	30	milliliters	mL
c	cups	0.24	liters	L
pt	pints	0.47	liters	L
qt	quarts	0.95	liters	L
gal	gallons	3.8	liters	L
ft^3	cubic feet	0.03	cubic meters	m^3
yd^3	cubic yards	0.76	cubic meters	m^3

Temperature (exact)

Abbreviation	When You Know	Multiply by	To Find	Abbreviation
°F	degrees Fahrenheit	subtract 32, multiply by $5/9$	degrees Celsius	°C

Metric to Common U.S. Measures (Approximate)

Length

Abbreviation	When You Know	Multiply by	To Find	Abbreviation
mm	millimeters	0.04	inches	in
cm	centimeters	0.4	inches	in
m	meters	3.3	feet	ft
m	meters	1.1	yards	yd
km	kilometers	0.6	miles	mi

Area

Abbreviation	When You Know	Multiply by	To Find	Abbreviation
cm^2	square centimeters	0.16	square inches	in^2
m^2	square meters	1.2	square yards	yd^2
km^2	square kilometers	0.4	square miles	mi^2
ha	hectares (10,000 m^2)	2.5	acres	

Mass

Abbreviation	When You Know	Multiply by	To Find	Abbreviation
g	grams	0.035	ounces	oz
kg	kilograms	2.2	pounds	lb
t	metric ton (1,000 kg)	1.1	short tons	

Volume

Abbreviation	When You Know	Multiply by	To Find	Abbreviation
mL	milliliters	0.03	fluid ounces	fl oz
mL	milliliters	0.06	cubic inches	in^3
L	liters	2.1	pints	pt
L	liters	1.06	quarts	qt
L	liters	0.26	gallons	gal
m^3	cubic meters	35	cubic feet	ft^3
m^3	cubic meters	1.3	cubic yards	yd^3

Temperature (exact)

Abbreviation	When You Know	Multiply by	To Find	Abbreviation
°C	degrees Celsius	multiply by $^9/_5$, add 32	degrees Fahrenheit	°F

Glossary

A

acesulfame K. An organic salt used as an artificial sweetener. (15)

acid. A substance that creates a surplus of hydrogen or hydronium ions. (6)

activation energy. The energy needed to start a reaction. (12)

active site. The location where an enzyme attaches to a substrate. (12)

adulteration. Lowering the quality and safety of a product by adding inferior or toxic ingredients. (1)

aerobic. Describes something that must have oxygen to function. (17)

agitation. The beating and stirring of a candy solution. (8)

albumin. A protein found in egg whites and milk. (11)

alcohol. An organic compound that contains at least one -OH group. (8)

aldehyde. An alcohol that has been dehydrogenated. (11)

allyl sulfides. A group of compounds that contain sulfur and increase enzyme reactions. (14)

amine group. A nitrogen and two hydrogens bonded to a carbon, which is represented by the chemical formula $-NH_2$. (11)

amino acid. An organic acid in proteins that has three basic parts to its structure: a side chain of carbon and hydrogens, a carboxyl group, and an amine group. (11)

amylopectin. Starches that have a branched structure. (9)

amylose. Starches that have the glucose units linked in a line. (9)

anaerobic. Describes something that functions best in an oxygen-free environment. (17)

analytical research. A type of research that determines cause and effect through observation and testing. (24)

anhydrous. Free of water. (7)

animal fat. A lipid that is found in meats and poultry. (10)

anticaking agent. A food additive that absorbs moisture so powdered food ingredients remain free flowing. (16)

antimicrobial agent. A preservative that prevents growth of microbes in food. (16)

antioxidant. A compound that will quickly react with oxygen to form new substances. (10)

appearance. The shape, size, color, and condition of a product. (3)

applied science. The process of putting scientific knowledge to practical use. (2)

aroma. Odor. (3)

aseptic. Describes something that is free of pathogens. (19)

aspartame. A dipeptide made from the amino acids aspartic acid and phenylalanine with a sweetness 200 times that of sucrose. (15)

astringency. The ability of a substance to draw up the muscles of the mouth. (3)

atherosclerosis. A hardening of the arteries caused by a buildup of plaque deposits. (10)

atmospheric pressure. The force of the weight of gases in the air pressing down on a surface. (7)

atom. The smallest unit of any elemental substance that maintains the characteristics of that substance. (4)

atomic mass. Approximately the sum of the masses of all protons and neutrons in an atom. (4)

atomic mass unit. A measure approximately equal to the mass of one proton or neutron. (4)

atomic number. The number of protons in the nucleus of each atom of an element. (4)

auto-oxidation. A complex chain reaction that starts when lipids are exposed to oxygen. (10)

Avogadro's number. 6.02×10^{23}. (6)

Note: Numbers in parentheses refer to the chapter in which each term is defined.

B

bacilli. Rod-shaped bacteria. (17)

bacteria. Extremely small single-celled organisms that multiply through cell division. (17)

base. A substance that produces a surplus of hydroxide ions. (6)

beaker. A deep, wide-mouthed container with a pouring lip used to hold substances during experiments and take inexact volume measurements. (2)

beta-carotene (β-carotene). The precursor for retinol. (13)

bioactive component. A compound in food that has physiological benefits. (14)

bioavailability. The body's ability to absorb and use a nutrient in the form consumed. (13)

biodegradable. Describes a substance that biological systems will eventually break down into chemical parts that nature can safely recycle. (18)

biotechnology. The process of using living organisms or any part of these organisms to create new or improved products. (21)

blanching. Briefly plunging food in boiling water to stop enzymatic activity. (12)

blast freezer. A freezer that uses airflow to speed freezing. (19)

botulism. The deadliest type of foodborne illness, which is caused by a toxin produced by the bacteria *Clostridium botulinum.* (6)

bound water. Water that is tied to the structure of large molecules like protein and starches. (7)

brine. A mixture of salt and water. (17)

brittleness. A texture quality based on how easily a food shatters or breaks apart. (3)

Bronsted-Lowry theory. A scientific explanation of the nature of acids and bases that identifies acids as proton donors and bases as proton acceptors. (6)

buerre manie. A ball of equal amounts of solid fat and starch mixed together often used by professional chefs to thicken soups and sauces. (9)

buffer. A compound that helps stabilize pH by absorbing excess acids or bases in a solution. (6)

bulking agent. A substance added to foods to enhance texture or thicken the consistency. (15)

burette. A graduated glass tube with a control valve at the bottom used to pour an accurate amount of liquid. (2)

by-product. A substance that is produced in addition to the main product of a reaction. (17)

C

calibrate. The process of adjusting a measuring instrument to a standard. (2)

calorie. The heat required to raise the temperature of one gram of water one degree Celsius. (5)

capsid. The protein coating that surrounds a virus particle. (18)

caramelization. The changing of sugar into a brown liquid when it is subjected to high or prolonged heat. (8)

carbohydrate. A group of organic compounds that contain the elements carbon, hydrogen, and oxygen in the basic structure $C_x(H_2O)_y$. (8)

carbohydrate gum. Water-soluble polysaccharides that are extracted from plants. (9)

carboxyl group. A carbon atom, two oxygen atoms, and a hydrogen atom. (10)

carcinogen. A substance that is known to cause cancer. (14)

carotenoids. A family of compounds that can function as antioxidants. (14)

case hardening. The formation of a dry skin on the outside of a food, which traps moisture inside the food and occurs when the food is heated too quickly. (20)

casein. A hydrophobic globular protein found in milk. (11)

catalyst. A substance that starts a reaction between substances without being affected by the reaction. (12)

cellophane. A film made from specially processed cellulose. (21)

cellulose. A carbohydrate made from large amounts of β-D-glucose, which is indigestible. (9)

Celsius degree. A unit of temperature equal to 0.01 of the difference between the boiling (100°C) and freezing points (0°C) of water. (2)

centrifugal force. The force that tends to propel objects outward from a center of rotation. (23)

chemical bond. The force that holds two atoms together. (4)

chemical change. A transformation that occurs whenever new substances with different chemical and physical properties are formed. (4)

chemical energy. Energy generated by the forming and breaking of chemical bonds during a chemical change. (5)

chemical formula. A combination of symbols that represents the elements that make up a compound. (4)

chemical leavening agent. An ingredient that is added to baked goods to lighten or aerate the finished product. (6)

chemistry. The study of the makeup, structure, and properties of substances and the changes that occur to them. (4)

chewiness. A texture quality based on the ease with which one part of a food slides past another without breaking. (3)

coagulation. A permanent denaturation that results when a liquid or semiliquid protein forms solid or semisoft clots. (11)

cocci. Spherical bacteria. (17)

coenzyme. A substance that must be present for an enzymatic reaction to occur. (12)

cold pack method. A method of packing canning jars in which food is prepared and then packed in sterilized containers without preheating the food. (19)

cold point. The point in a can or mass of food that is the last to reach the desired temperature. (19)

cold water paste. A paste formed by quickly stirring a small amount of cold water into starch until the mixture is smooth. (9)

collagen. A protein in connective tissue. (11)

colloid. A particle that is suspended in the continuous phase of a colloidal dispersion. (22)

colloidal dispersion. A mixture in which microscopic particles of one substance are uniformly distributed in another substance. (22)

colorimeter. A device that measures the color of foods in terms of value, hue, and chroma. (3)

complete protein. A food that contains all eight essential amino acids. (11)

compound. A substance in which two or more elements have chemically combined. (4)

concentrate. A food that is reduced in volume by having part of the water removed. (20)

concentration. The measure of parts of one substance to the known volume of another. (6) Removing a portion of the water from a food product. (20)

conclusion. An analysis and application of data in an experiment that answers the question how, what, where, when, or why and describes what data and observations mean. (2)

condensation. The phase change when a substance changes from a gas to a liquid. (5)

conduction. A transfer of heat energy through matter from particle-to-particle collisions. (5)

consistency. The thinness or thickness of a food product, which can be measured in terms of pourability. (3)

consumer taste panel. A group of untrained consumers who evaluate products after they have been developed to determine what the average consumer will prefer. (3)

contaminant. Anything that makes a substance impure or unsuitable. (7)

contamination. Making food unfit or impure for use by introducing unwholesome or undesirable elements. (18)

continuous phase. A medium in which particles are distributed. (22)

control. The standard against which all changes in an experiment are measured. (2)

controlled atmosphere packaging (CAP). Packaging that uses barriers to control and maintain the desired gases around food. (21)

controlled-use substance. A food additive that does not appear on the GRAS list and must be used within set guidelines. (16)

convection. A transfer of heat energy by the motion of fluids, such as water or air. (5)

copolymer. A type of plastic that has two basic units of molecules combined to make one material. (21)

covalent bond. A chemical bond formed when one or more pairs of electrons are shared between two atoms. (4)

creaming. A separation process in which low-density liquids collect above higher-density liquids. (23)

cross-contamination. The tainting of a food that occurs when a contaminated substance comes in contact with another food. (18)

cross-linked starch. A type of modified starch that is changed chemically so cross-bonding or cross-linking takes place between starch molecules. (9)

cruciferous vegetable. A member of a group of plants, including broccoli, cabbage, kale, and cauliflower, that has cross-shaped flower petals. (14)

cryogenic liquid. A substance that is in liquid form at extremely low temperatures. (1) A liquefied gas that has a very low boiling point. (19)

crystallization. The phase change when a substance changes from a liquid to a solid; also known as freezing. (5) A separation process in which the atoms of the solute in a supersaturated solution become arranged in a repeating order to form crystals, which can be removed from the solvent. (23)

curd. A clump of coagulated protein. (17)

cytoplasm. A gelatinous liquid that fills the rigid cell walls of bacteria. (17)

D

data. Measurable facts that are collected during an experiment. (2)

dehydration. A method of preserving food by lowering the water content. (20)

dehydrofreezing. A method of vacuum dehydration in which food temperatures and atmospheric pressure are lowered to the point that water will sublimate out of the food. (20)

Delaney Clause. Legislation that prohibits the approval of any food additive found to cause cancer in humans or animals. (16)

denaturation. Any change in the shape of a protein molecule that does not break peptide bonds. (11)

deposition. Changing a substance directly from a gas phase to a solid phase. (5)

descriptive research. A type of research involving the collection of data that describes the natural course of events or opinions of people at a given time. (24)

desiccant. A compound that removes substances harmful to food products from the package environment. (21)

dextrose. The name for glucose used by the confectionery trade. (8)

diabetes mellitus. The body's inability to move glucose from the bloodstream to the cells. (8)

dietitian. A professional who assesses diets, plans nutrition programs, and supervises the preparing and serving of meals. (25)

diglyceride. A glycerol with two fatty acids attached at the site of a hydroxyl group. (10)

disaccharide. Two monosaccharides joined together. (8)

dispersed phase. The particles scattered throughout a medium. (22)

distillation. A separation process that involves collecting, cooling, and condensing vapors and the compounds they carry as the vapors evaporate from a solution. (23)

disulfide cross-link. A covalent bond that forms between two protein molecules at side chains that contain sulfur. (11)

double bond. A chemical bond formed when two atoms share two pairs of electrons. (4)

E

electrical energy. Energy produced by the movement of electrons. (5)

electrolyte. A positively or negatively charged ion in solution. (12)

electron. A subatomic particle that has a negative charge that is equal to, but opposite of, the positive charge of a proton. (4)

element. A substance that contains only one kind of atom. (4)

emulsifier. A stabilizing substance that has a polar end and a nonpolar end. (22)

emulsion. A mixture of two immiscible liquids where one is dispersed in droplet form in the other. (22)

endothermic reaction. A reaction whose products have less total heat than the reactants. (5)

endpoint. The point at which there is an equal number of acid and base molecules. (6)

energy. The ability to do work. (5)

enrichment. The process of restoring to refined grain products some of the nutrients removed during processing. (13)

entrepreneurship. Owning and running a business. (25)

enzymatic browning. A color change that occurs when the enzyme polyphenol oxidase (phenolase) reacts with oxygen. (12)

enzyme. A protein that starts a chemical reaction without being changed by the chemical reaction. (12)

enzyme inhibitor. Any substance that will prevent an enzyme-substrate complex from forming. (12)

equivalence point. The point at which there is an equal number of acid and base molecules. (6)

Erlenmeyer flask. A flat-bottomed, cone-shaped container used to mix and hold liquids and take inexact volume measurements. (2)

essential amino acid. An amino acid that must be supplied by foods in the diet. (11)

essential fatty acid. A fatty acid that cannot be produced by the human body. (10)

ester. An organic compound produced by combining an organic acid and an alcohol. (16)

ethics. The principles of conduct and character that distinguish right from wrong. (24)

evaporation. The phase change when a substance changes from a liquid to a gas. (5) A separation process that removes all the water from a solution. (23)

exothermic reaction. A reaction during which energy is released. (5)

experiment. A controlled situation that allows a scientist or researcher to determine what causes a change to occur. (2)

external energy. Energy applied to an object by another source. (5)

F

facultative. Describes something that can function in an environment with or without oxygen. (17)

fat. A lipid that is solid at room temperature. (10)

fat-soluble vitamin. A vitamin that has a nonpolar molecular structure and dissolves in fats and oils. (13)

fatty acid. An organic molecule that consists of a carbon chain with a carboxyl group at one end. (10)

fermentation. An enzymatically controlled change in a food product brought on by the action of microorganisms. (17)

filtration. A separation process that uses porous paper to let liquids and small solutes pass through while trapping aggregates. (23)

finished food. A food item or meal that is ready to eat. (25)

firmness. A texture quality based on a food's resistance to pressure. (3)

flash point. The temperature at which lipids will flame. (10)

flavonoids. A group of compounds responsible for many of the flavor characteristics of foods. (14)

flavor. The combined effect of taste and aroma. (3)

fluid. A substance that has characteristics of a liquid and a gas. (4)

foam. A colloidal dispersion of gas or air bubbles dispersed in a liquid. (22)

food additive. A substance that is added to a food to cause a desired change in the characteristics of the food product. (16)

food analog. A natural or manufactured substance that is used in place of a traditional food or food component. (1)

foodborne illness. A sickness caused by eating contaminated food. (18)

food infection. A foodborne illness caused by a microbe releasing digestive enzymes that begin to damage body tissue. (18)

food intoxication. An illness caused by a toxin released in food by microbes. (18)

food irradiation. A cold food preservation method in which food is exposed to high-energy electromagnetic waves. (21)

food science. The study of the nature of food and the principles of its production, processing, preservation, and packaging. (1)

food spoilage. A change in a food that causes it to be unfit or undesirable for consumption. (18)

food vehicle. A specific food to which a fortificant is added. (13)

formulation. The term for a recipe used in the food industry. (2)

fortificant. A nutrient that is being added to a food. (13)

fortification. The process of adding nutrients, such as vitamins, to food whether or not it is normally contained in the food for the purpose of correcting a nutritional deficiency in a population. (13)

free radical. An atom or compound that has lost one or more electrons, causing it to become very unstable and likely to quickly react with other substances to form more stable compounds. (21)

free water. Water that is easily separated from food tissues. (7)

fructose. A monosaccharide that is found widely in fruits and honey. (8)

functional food. A modified food or food ingredient that may provide a health benefit beyond the traditional nutrients it contains. (14)

Fungi. A kingdom of organisms in which yeasts and molds are classified. (17)

fungus. A plant that lacks chlorophyll, has a filament structure, and reproduces through spores. (17)

fusion. The phase change when a substance changes from a solid to a liquid; also known as melting. (5)

G

galactose. A monosaccharide that can only be found in animals and humans and is one of the basic sugars found in milk. (8)

gel. A rigid starch mixture composed of molecules bound together in a three dimensional network that keeps the molecules from shifting in comparison to one another. (9)

gelatinization. Thickening a liquid with starch while heating. (9)

gelatinization point. The temperature at which maximum swelling of starch granules occurs; the point at which starch will hold the most water and have the greatest thickening power. (9)

genus. A group of living organisms that have similar characteristics. (17)

glucose. A monosaccharide that is the most abundant of the sugars, which is the basic energy source of humans. (8)

gluten. The network of elastic protein strands that give bread dough its structure. (11)

glyceride. A molecule that has a glycerol base. (10)

glycogen. Multibranched chains of glucose. (8)

graduated cylinder. A tall container used to accurately measure the volume of liquids to the nearest milliliter. (2)

graininess. A texture quality based on the size of the particles in a food product.

gram (g). The mass of 1 cubic centimeter (cm^3) of water at 4°C (39°F). (2)

Gram's stain. A staining process used to identify bacteria. (17)

granules. Packets of starch produced by plants. (9)

GRAS list. A list of all food additives that are generally recognized as safe. (16)

gray. A unit used to measure radiant energy that equals 100 rads. (21)

H

HACCP (Hazard Analysis Critical Control Point). A food safety system that examines the food production process at every point where contamination is possible. (18)

halophilic. Describes microbes that require high salt concentrations to function. (17)

headspace. The space left after adding food to a container to allow for the expansion of the food during heating. (19)

heat. An energy transfer from one body to another caused by a temperature difference between the two bodies. (5)

heat capacity. The ability of a substance to absorb heat. (5)

hepatitis. A viral infection that attacks the liver cells. (18)

hermetic. Refers to a container that is completely sealed to prevent water, vapor, gases, and odors from leaving or entering the container. (21)

heterogeneous mixture. A blend of substances that have a nonuniform distribution of particles throughout a sample. (4)

high-density lipoproteins (HDL). Clusters of lipid and protein molecules that transport unneeded cholesterol in the body to the liver. (10)

homogeneous mixture. A blend of substances that have a uniform distribution of particles throughout a sample. (4)

homogenization. A mechanical process that forces milk through screens to rupture the membranes around the fat globules and break the globules into smaller particles. (22)

host. An animal or plant from which a parasite receives nutrients. (18)

hot pack method. A method of packing canning jars in which foods are heated in syrup, juice, or water prior to packing in containers. (19)

humectant. A food additive that is used to help products retain moisture. (16)

humidity. The measure of water vapor in the air compared to how much water vapor the air can hold at a given temperature. (19)

hydrate. Any chemical compound that is loosely bound with water. (7)

hydrated. Full of water. (7)

hydrogenation. The process of adding hydrogen atoms to an unsaturated lipid to increase its saturation level. (10)

hydrogen bond. An attraction of the positively charged hydrogen atom of one molecule toward the negative end of another molecule. (7)

hydrogen ion. A positively charged hydrogen atom. (6)

hydrolysis. A process that occurs when a molecule, such as a disaccharide or larger molecule, is split into its composite parts by adding water. (8)

hydronium ion. A hydrogen ion bonded to a water molecule to form H_3O^+. (6)

hydrophobic. A water-repelling interaction between nonpolar side chains of proteins. (11)

hydroponic crops. Plant foods grown with their roots suspended in liquid nutrient solutions. (1)

hydrostatic cooker and cooler. A modified U-shaped tube filled with water and steam that has a conveyor belt to transport filled cans from one end to the other. (19)

hydroxide ion. A negatively charged ion composed of one atom of oxygen and one atom of hydrogen (OH^-). (6)

hydroxyl group. An oxygen and hydrogen atom bonded together, which is represented by the chemical formula –OH. (8)

hyphae. Filaments or tubes that form the basic structure of most fungi. (17)

hypothesis. A possible solution to a problem based on available evidence. (2)

I

impurity. Substance other than water. (7)

incidental food additive. A substance that unintentionally enters a food product during production, processing, storage, or packaging. (16)

incomplete protein. A protein that is missing one or more of the essential amino acids for human growth. (11)

indicator. An organic dye that demonstrates through color change the degree of acidity of a solution. (6)

indoles. A family of compounds found in large amounts in cruciferous vegetables. (14)

ingredient. A substance that is generally recognized as safe and is a component part of a food. (16)

inorganic compound. A substance that does not contain carbon or has only a single carbon atom. (4)

insulin. A hormone produced by the pancreas that allows glucose to move into the cells where it can be used for energy. (8)

intentional food additive. A substance purposely added to a food product to give the product a specific characteristic or help it resist spoilage. (16)

interfering agent. A substance that can prevent or slow crystal growth. (8)

intermediate-moisture food. A food that has moisture levels of 20 to 50 percent with enough dissolved solvents to prevent the growth of microbes. (20)

intermolecular. Between molecules. (7)

internal energy. Energy within an object. (5)

International System of Units (SI). The internationally accepted version of the metric system used by scientists all over the world. (2)

invert sugar. A mixture of glucose and fructose that results from the hydrolysis of sucrose. (8)

ion. An atom or group of atoms that has a positive or negative electrical charge. (4)

ionic bond. A chemical bond in which electrons are transferred from one atom to another. (4)

ionization. The process of forming ions. (6)

ionomer. A type of plastic held together with ionic instead of covalent bonds. (21)

isoflavones. A subgroup of flavonoids found mainly in soy products. (14)

isomer. One of two molecules with the same chemical formula but slightly different structures. (14)

isothiocyanates. A subgroup of indoles found in cruciferous vegetables that protect against cancer by affecting enzyme reactions. (14)

J

junction. A connection formed when two molecules of hydrogen bond together. (9)

K

ketone bodies. A by-product of ketosis. (9)

ketosis. The process the body uses to turn fat into energy when carbohydrates are not present. (9)

kilogram (kg). The mass of 1 liter of water at 4°C (39°F). (2)

kilogray. A unit used to measure radiant energy that equals 1,000 grays. (21)

kinetic energy. The energy of motion. (5)

L

lactose. A disaccharide composed of one glucose and one galactose molecule that is the sugar found in milk. (8)

laminate. Packaging material made of layers of a variety of materials fused together. (21)

latent heat. The energy needed to complete the rearranging of molecules that occurs at the point of a phase change of a substance. (5)

latent heat of fusion. The energy needed to melt or freeze a substance. (5)

latent heat of vaporization. The energy needed to evaporate or condense a substance. (5)

lauric acid. The main component of a group of lipids found in palms such as coconut. (10)

law of conservation of matter. A scientific principle stating that matter can be changed but not created or destroyed. (4)

length. The distance between two points. (2)

Lewis structure. A shorthand method of diagramming electrons that are likely to be shared between atoms. (4)

linolenic acid. A lipid that is found in large amounts in soybeans and wheat germ. (10)

lipid. An organic compound that is insoluble in water and has a greasy feel. (10)

lipolytic. Describes microbes that produce enzymes to digest fats. (17)

lipoprotein. A cluster of lipid and protein molecules. (10)

liquefaction. The phase change when a substance changes from a gas to a liquid. (5)

liter (L). A unit of fluid volume in the metric system, which equals the space in an area 1 decimeter high by 1 decimeter wide by 1 decimeter deep (1 cubic decimeter). (2)

low-density lipoproteins (LDL). Clusters of lipid and protein molecules that transport cholesterol from the liver throughout the body. (10)

M

macromolecule. A very large molecule that contains hundreds or thousands of atoms. (9)

magnetron. An electron tube in a microwave oven that converts electrical energy to microwaves. (5)

Maillard reaction. The reaction between proteins and carbohydrates that causes food to brown when cooked. (11)

major mineral. A mineral that is needed by humans in amounts of 100 mg or more each day. (13)

maltose. A disaccharide made of two glucose molecules that is commonly found in grains such as malt. (8)

mannose. A monosaccharide that is a component of long chains of sugars found in some plants. (8)

marbling. The specks or streaks of fat in muscle tissue of animals used for meat. (10)

margin of safety. The zone between the concentration in which a food additive is normally used and the level at which a hazard exists. (16)

marinate. To soak food in a flavorful liquid. (12)

marine oil. Fish oil. (10)

mass. A measure of the quantity of matter. (2)

mass percent. The percentage of the mass in a solution that comes from the solute. (22)

matter. Anything that occupies space and has mass. (4)

maturing and bleaching agent. Chemical that speeds the aging process and whitening of flour. (16)

mechanical energy. The total kinetic and potential energy of a system. (5)

melting point. The temperature at which a lipid is completely liquid. (10)

meniscus. The curve at the surface of a liquid in a container. (2)

meta-analysis. When the results of several individual studies are pooled to yield overall conclusions. (2)

metabolism. The physical and chemical reactions that occur continuously within cells. (23)

meter (m). The standard unit of length in the metric system. (2)

microbe. A living organism that is only visible through a microscope. (17)

microbiology. The study of living organisms too small to be seen by the unaided human eye. (17)

micrometer. One-thousandth (0.001) of a millimeter. (17)

microorganism. A living organism that is only visible through a microscope. (17)

microwave. A low-frequency electromagnetic wave of radiant energy. (5)

milkfat. A lipid that comes from the milk of cows, goats, and other mammals. (10)

milling. The process of moving kernels of grain between a series of rollers to grind the grain into fine particles. (23)

mixture. Substances that are put together but not chemically combined. (4)

modified atmosphere packaging (MAP). A type of food packaging that involves a one-time flushing of a container followed by sealing. (21)

modified starch. A starch that has been changed structurally by chemical or mechanical means. (9)

molarity. A measure of solute concentration expressed as moles per liter. (6)

molasses. The crude, boiled liquid pressed from sugar cane. (8)

mold. A fungus that forms a mycelium structure with a fuzzy appearance. (17)

mole. Avogadro's number of particles of any substance. (6)

molecule. The basic unit of any compound. (4)

Monera. A kingdom of organisms in which most biologists classify bacteria. (17)

monoglyceride. A glycerol with one fatty acid attached at the site of a hydroxyl group. (10)

monosaccharide. A simple sugar molecule that cannot be broken down into a smaller molecule without changing its basic nature. (8)

monounsaturated. Describes a fatty acid that has one double bond in the carbon chain. (10)

mycelium. A branched network of hyphae. (17)

myoglobin. The iron-containing protein pigment in muscle tissue that provides color. (11)

N

neutral. A term describing a substance that has an equal number of positive and negative charges. (6)

neutralization. The point at which all ions in a solution have combined chemically; also the process of reacting an acid and a base to form a salt and water. (6)

neutron. A subatomic particle located in the nucleus of an atom that has about the same mass as a proton and is electrically neutral. (4)

nomenclature. Naming system. (12)

non-Newtonian fluid. A substance that has characteristics of a solid and a liquid. (4)

nonpolar. Neutral in nature. (10)

nonpolar covalent bond. A bond within a molecule in which there is an equal sharing of electrons. (7)

nuclear energy. The result of splitting or combining atoms of certain elements, which then give off radiation. (5)

nucleus. The central core of an atom. (4)

nutrient. A food component necessary to sustain life. (7)

nutrition. The study of components of food and how they are used by the body to sustain life and health. (1)

O

oil. A lipid that is liquid at room temperature. (10)

oleic-linoleic acids. Lipids that make up the largest group of triglycerides. (10)

olestra. A sucrose polyester designed to act, feel, and hold onto flavor compounds like fat without providing any calories. (15)

olfactory bulb. A bundle of nerve fibers located at the base of the brain behind the bridge of the nose. (3)

omega-3 fatty acid. A polyunsaturated fatty acid that has a double bond between the third and fourth carbon from the end with the methyl group (CH_3). (10)

opacity. The degree to which an object blocks light. (9)

orbital. The space occupied by a pair of electrons in an atom. (4)

organic compound. A substance that contains chains or rings of carbon. (4)

organic dye. A naturally occuring color pigment that changes color when exposed to acids or bases. (6)

osmosis. The movement of a solvent through a semipermeable membrane from an area of low solute concentration to an area of high solute concentration. (23)

osmotic pressure. The pressure caused by two solutions with different concentrations separated by a semipermeable membrane. (23)

oxidase. An enzyme that reacts only in the presence of oxygen. (12)

oxidation. The reversible chemical reaction that adds oxygen to a compound. (11)

P

parasite. An organism that lives in and feeds on a host. (18)

paste. A thickened mixture of starch and liquid that has very little flow. (9)

pasteurization. A process in which a liquid is heated until spoilage bacteria have been destroyed. (17)

pathogen. A microorganism that can cause illness in humans. (18)

pectin. A complex carbohydrate that is found in plant cells and made of chemical derivatives of a monosaccharide called sugar acids. (9)

peptide bond. The bond that is formed between two amino acids. (11)

permeable. Refers to a substance that allows liquids and/or gases to pass through or penetrate. (21)

phase change. A physical change in the visible structure of matter without changing the molecular structure. (4)

pH control agent. A food additive that alters or stabilizes the pH of a mixture. (16)

phenolic acids. Weak acids that have a hydroxyl group attached to an aromatic ring. (14)

phenols. Weak acids that have a hydroxyl group attached to an aromatic ring. (14)

phenomenon. A fact, occurrence, circumstance, or process that can be observed. (2)

phospholipid. A glycerol base with two fatty acids and a phosphorus-containing acid attached. (10)

photosynthesis. A process through which plants convert the energy from the sun into glucose. (8)

pH scale. A range used to express the degree of concentration of hydrogen or hydronium ions present in a solution. (6)

physical change. A transformation of a substance involving a shift in shape, physical state, size, or temperature without a shift in chemical identity. (4)

phytochemical. A compound produced by plants. (14)

phytoestrogens. Plant hormones that are weaker versions of the human hormone estrogen. (14)

plaque. Deposits of lipids and cholesterol on artery walls. (10)

polar covalent bond. A bond within a molecule in which there is an unequal sharing of electrons. (7)

pollutant. Anything that makes a substance impure or unsuitable. (7)

polymer. A large molecule that consists of large numbers of small molecular units, which are linked. (9)

polyols. A group of low-calorie sweeteners found naturally in apples, berries, and plums. (15)

polypeptide. A molecule with many peptide bonds. (11)

polyphenols. Phenol compounds with more than one carbon ring. (14)

polysaccharide. A molecule that consists of many sugar units. (9)

polyunsaturated. Describes a fatty acid that has two or more double bonds in the carbon chain. (10)

potential energy. Energy that is stored; the energy of position; the measure of work done. (5)

precipitate. A substance that separates from a solution as an insoluble solid. (23)

precipitation. A separation process in which two or more compounds can be removed from a mixture after they have combined to form a precipitate. (23)

precursor. A chemical compound that the body changes into the active form of a vitamin. (13)

preservative. A substance added to food to prevent or slow spoilage. (16)

pressure processing. A canning method recommended for low-acid foods that involves heating containers of food under pressure. (19)

product. A substance that is formed as a result of a chemical reaction and is written on the right side of a chemical equation. (4)

protein gel. A mixture of mostly fluids locked in a tangled three dimensional mesh made of denatured and coagulated proteins. (11)

proteolytic. Describes microbes that produce enzymes to digest protein. (17)

proton. A subatomic particle located in the nucleus of an atom that has a positive electrical charge. (4)

proton acceptor. A compound that easily accepts protons. (6)

proton donor. A compound that easily gives up protons. (6)

pure culture. A large volume of one type of microbe that has purposely been grown in a nutrient medium. (17)

pure substance. An element or compound in which all the basic units in the substance are the same. (4)

R

rad. The basic unit used to measure radiant energy. (21)

radiant energy. Energy transmitted in the form of waves through space or some medium. (5)

radiation. A transfer of heat energy by electromagnetic waves. (5)

radiolytic product. A chemical compound that is produced in food as a result of irradiation. (21)

rancidity. A form of food spoilage that occurs when the addition of oxygen causes the formation of new compounds, which have an unpleasant flavor. (10)

reactant. A substance found at the start of a chemical reaction and written on the left side of a chemical equation. (4)

reduced oxygen packaging (ROP). A type of food packaging that provides an environment in which little or no oxygen is enclosed with the food. (21)

reduction. The reversible chemical reaction that removes oxygen from a compound. (11)

refrigerant. A fluid that can be used to remove heat energy from its environment. (19)

registered dietitian. A dietitian who has passed the national certification exam given by the American Dietetic Association (ADA). (25)

rendering. A separation process in which a component is extracted out of a food product by melting. (23)

replicable. Term used to describe an experiment that meets the scientific standard of being repeatable. (2)

research. An organized method of examining a question, issue, or theory to improve understanding. (24)

respiration. The process in which animal and plant tissues absorb and give off gas. (19)

retinol. The active form of vitamin A found in animals and humans. (13)

retort. A huge pressure canner that is used by commercial food processors. (19)

retrogradation. The firming of a gel during cooling and standing. (9)

reverse osmosis. The movement of water through a semipermeable membrane from an area of high concentration to an area of low concentration due to the application of pressure on the more highly concentrated solution. (23)

ribonucleic acid (RNA). The material that carries the genetic code in the cells and is used for the production of DNA. (8)

ribose. A sugar that contains only five carbons. (8)

ripening. Allowing candy to sit for a period of time. (8)

roux. A gravy that has had the starch heated in fat until it turns a rich red-brown. (9)

S

saccharide. The name given in organic chemistry to all carbohydrates that are classified as sugars. (8)

saccharin. An artificial sweetener that is stable in a wide variety of foods under extreme processing conditions, such as high heat. (15)

salmonellosis. A foodborne illness caused by salmonellae bacteria. (18)

salt. A combination of acids and bases that form a compound with ionic bonds. (6)

saponins. Molecules formed from a sugar reacting with an alcohol. (14)

saturated. Describes a fatty acid that has the maximum number of hydrogen atoms. (10)

science. The systematic knowledge of natural and physical phenomena. (2)

scientific method. A system of steps used to solve problems. (2)

sedimentation. A separation process that uses gravity to pull the denser particles or liquid droplets to the bottom of a mixture. (23)

semipermeable membrane. A thin layer of material that allows some substances to pass through but not others. (23)

sensory evaluation. The human analysis of the taste, smell, sound, feel, and appearance of food. (3)

sharp freezing. A method of freezing food in which food is brought in contact with still cold air. (19)

shelf life. The time a food can be stored and still be safe to eat. (19)

shell. An area of space surrounding the nucleus of an atom that has one or more orbitals. (4)

Simplesse. The trade name of a fat substitute made from protein. (15)

slurry. An uncooked mixture of water and starch. (9)

smoke point. The temperature at which fatty acids begin to break apart and produce smoke. (10)

sol. A thickened liquid that is pourable. (9)

solidification point. The temperature at which all lipids in a mixture are in a solid state. (10)

solubility. The ability of a solute to dissolve in a solvent. (8)

solute. A material that is dissolved in another material. (4)

solution. A homogeneous mixture of one material dissolved in another. (4)

solvent. A material in which another material is dissolved. (4)

species. The basic category of a classification of living organisms. (17)

specific heat. The ability of a substance to absorb or transfer heat as compared to water's ability to absorb or transfer heat. (5)

spirilla. Spiral-shaped bacteria. (17)

spore. A seed of a fungus. (17)

stability. The ability of a thickened mixture to remain constant over time and temperature changes. (9)

starch. Molecules that are composed of sugar units or saccharides linked in branched or straight chains. (9)

starter. A substance containing microorganisms that is added to food to bring about desired flavor, texture, and/or color changes. (17)

sterol. A complicated molecule derived or made from lipids. (10)

subatomic particle. A small part of an atom. (4)

sublimation. Changing a substance directly from a solid phase to a gas phase. (5)

substrate. A substance on which an enzyme acts. (12)

sucralose. A sugar substitute made by adding chlorine atoms to sugar. (15)

sucrose. Table sugar; a disaccharide that contains one glucose and one fructose molecule. (8)

sulfite. A salt containing sulfur that is used by the food industry to help prevent browning of cut fruits and vegetables. (16)

sulfiting. Soaking food in a solution of sodium bisulfite before dehydration to prevent enzymatic browning. (20)

sulfuring. Exposing fruit to fumes from burning sulfur to prevent enzymatic browning. (20)

supersaturated. Describes any solution that has been heated to dissolve more solute than the water would normally hold. (8)

surface tension. The force between molecules at the outside edge of a substance. (7)

suspension. A mixture of undissolved particles in a liquid. (22)

syneresis. Water leaking out of a gel in storage. (9)

T

tannins. A group of polyphenols that contribute to the astringency of foods and are involved in the enzymatic browning process. (14)

taste bias. A tendency to like or dislike a food based on positive or negative experiences, respectively. (3)

taste test panel. A group of people who evaluate the flavor, texture, appearance, and aroma of food products. (3)

temperature. The measure of the average kinetic energy of a group of individual molecules; an indirect measure of molecular motion. (5)

temporary emulsion. An unstable mixture of two immiscible liquids. (22)

terpenes. A group of compounds responsible for the flavors of citrus fruits and many seasonings and herbs. (14)

texture. The way a product feels to the fingers, tongue, teeth, and palate. (3)

thermal conductivity. The ability to transfer heat energy. (22)

thermal death curve. The line plotted on a graph that shows how long it takes to destroy a microorganism at a given temperature. (19)

titration. Process of adding a base with a known pH to an acid or adding an acid with a known pH to a base. (6)

toxin. A substance that is released by a microbe and is harmful to humans. (18)

trace mineral. A mineral that is needed by humans in amounts less than 100 mg per day. (13)

translucency. A measure of how much light an object will let through. (9)

trichinosis. An infection caused by *T. spiralis.* (18)

triglyceride. A glycerol with a fatty acid joined at each of the three hydroxyl sites. (10)

Tyndall effect. The bending or scattering of light rays as they pass through a colloidal dispersion. (22)

U

unsaturated. Describes a fatty acid that does not contain all the hydrogen it could contain. (10)

V

valence electron. An electron in a partially full shell that is likely to be shared or transferred between atoms. (4)

vaporization. The phase change when a substance changes from a liquid to a gas. (5)

vapor pressure. The pressure at which gases escape from a liquid at the same rate as gases dissolve or condense into the liquid. (22)

variable. A factor that is being changed in an experiment. (2)

variation. Each change that is made in an experiment. (2)

vegetable butter. A lipid that comes from the seeds of tropical plants. (10)

virus. A microscopic disease-causing agent made up of genetic material surrounded by a protein coating. (18)

viscosity. The resistance of a mixture to flow. (9)

vitamin. An organic compound that is needed in small amounts in the diet. (13)

volatile. The property of evaporating quickly. (3)

volume. The amount of space occupied by an object. (2)

W

water activity. The measure of the partial water pressure over a food as compared to the vapor pressure (gaseous water) over pure water at a given temperature. (7)

water-bath processing. A canning method recommended for only high-acid foods that involves submerging containers of food in boiling water. (19)

water-soluble vitamin. A vitamin that has a polar molecular structure and dissolves in water and water-based liquids. (13)

weight. The measure of the force of gravity between two objects. (2)

whey. A by-product of cheese production that looks like watery milk and is mainly composed of a group of water-soluble proteins, lactose, and minerals. (11)

Y

yeast. A single-celled fungus that reproduces by budding. (17)

Index

A

Acesulfame K, 340
Acetic acid fermentation, 396, 397
Acids
    antimicrobial agents, 361
    concentration, 129
    definition, 121
    enzyme denaturation, 272
    identifying, 123-125
    in water, 160
    measuring, 125-130
    molarity, 129, 130
    pH control agents, 368
    pH, 127, 128
    theories, 122, 123
Activation energy, 266
Active site, 268
Additives, 355-371
    antimicrobial agents, 360, 361
    antioxidants, 361-363
    benefits and risks, 370, 371
    coloring agents, 363, 364
    consistency control, 365-369
    definition, 356
    Delaney Clause, 358, 360
    flavor enhancers, 364, 365
    flavoring agents, 364
    functions, 360-370
    GRAS list, 357, 358
    guidelines, 357
    incidental, 356
    intentional, 356
    international regulation, 360
    nutritive value, 369, 370
    preservatives, 360
    regulations, 356-360
    sensory characteristic enhancement,
        363-365
    sweeteners, 365
Adulteration, 21
Advertising
    careers, 578
    product development, 558
Aeration, 228
Aerobic, 382
Agitation, 182

Albumin, 252
Alcoholic beverages, yeast fermentation,
    391, 392
Alcohols, 174, 175
Aldehydes, 256
Amine group, 242
Amino acids, 241-244. *See also* Proteins
    classification by side chain, 243, 244
    definition, 242
    essential, 242, 243
Amylopectin, 197
Amylose, 197
Anaerobic, 382
Analogs, 336-347
    fat substitutes, 342-346
    functions, 337-339
    pros and cons, 338, 339
    salt substitutes, 346, 347
    sugar substitutes, 339-342
Analytical research, 550, 551
Anhydrous, 156
Animals, transmission of pathogens, 419, 420
Anticaking agents, 365
Antimicrobial agents, 360, 361
Antioxidants, 226, 362, 363
    controlled-use, 362
    GRAS list, 361, 362
    sulfites, 362, 363
Appearance, 61
Applied science, 36
Aroma, 62, 63
Aseptic, 441
Astringency, 62
Atherosclerosis, 232
Atmospheric pressure, 147
Atom, 79
Atomic mass, 80
Atomic mass unit, 81
Atomic number, 80
Auto-oxidation, 226
Avogadro's number 129

B

Bacilli, 381
Bacteria, 381, 382
    characteristics, 384, 385
    scientific names, 386

Baking, 132-135
    batters and doughs, 134, 135
    chemical leavening agents, 133, 134
    pH, 132-135
Baking powder, 133, 134
Baking soda, 133
Barriers, separation through, 533-538
Bases
    concentration, 129
    definition, 122
    enzyme denaturation, 272
    identifying, 123-125
    measuring, 125-130
    molarity, 129, 130
    pH, 127, 128
    pH control agents, 368
    theories, 122, 123
Batters, pH, 134, 135
B-complex vitamins, 291
Beaker, 41
Belt drying, 463, 464
Beta-carotene, 289
Beverage industry, 509, 510
    contaminants, 160
Bioactive components, 326
Bioavailability, 300
Biodegradable, 408
Biological pollutants, 159, 160
Biotechnology, 26, 492-495
    applications, 493, 494
    old versus new, 492, 493
    regulations controlling, 495
Blanching, 271, 435
Blast freezers, 447, 448
Bonds, 145, 146
    hydrogen, 146
    nonpolar covalent, 145
    polar covalent, 146
Botulism, 132
Bound water, 154
Bran, 206, 207
Bread, yeast fermentation, 390
Brine, 392
Brittleness, 64
Bronsted-Lowry theory, 122, 123
Buerre manie, 204
Buffers, 130-132
    pH control agents, 368
Bulk, 206, 207
Bulking agents, 342
Buret, 41

Business sector, 579
By-product, 389

C
Calcium, 293
Calibrate, 39
Calorie, 107
Candy making, 180-182
CAP, 490
Capsid, 417
Carbohydrases, 275
Carbohydrates
    alcohols, 174, 175
    complex, 196-208. See also Complex
        carbohydrates
    definition, 171
    disaccharides, 173, 174
    monosaccharides, 172, 173
Carbohydrate gums, 198
Carboxyl group, 217
Carcinogens, 314
Careers, 567-580
    advertisement, 578
    business sector, 579
    dietetics, 576-578
    distribution, 574
    education and training, 568, 569
    education sector, 579
    employment outlook, 570
    entrepreneurship, 578
    foodservice, 576
    government sector, 579, 580
    manufacturing, 572-574
    personal qualities, 568
    production, 570-572
    professional associations, 580
    quality control, 574, 575
    working conditions, 569, 570
Carmelization, 182-184
Carotenes, 315, 316
Carotenoids, 315, 316
Case hardening, 461, 462
Casein, 246
Catalyst, 266
Cellophane, 488
Cellulose, 197
Celsius degree, 42
Centrifugal force, 530, 531
Cheeses, fermentation, 395, 396
Chemical bonds, 83-86
    covalent bonds, 85, 86
    ionic bonds, 84, 85

Chemical changes, 88-91
    chemical equations, 90, 91
    identifying, 89, 90
    permanent and reversible, 90
Chemical contaminants, 408, 409
    in water, 160
Chemical energy, 102, 103
Chemical equations, 90, 91
Chemical formula, 81
Chemical leavening agents, 133, 134, 366
Chemical separation, 532, 533
Chemical structure, lipids, 217, 218
Chemistry, 78-91
    chemical bonding, 83-86
    chemical changes, 88-91
    definition, 79
    identifying changes, 89, 90
    matter, 79-83, 86-88
    phase changes, 88, 89
    physical changes, 88
Chewiness, 64
Chloride, 293-295
Cholesterol, 232, 233
Choline, 292, 293
Clostridium botulinum, 412, 413
Clostridium perfringens, 410, 411
Coagulation, 247
Cocci, 381
Coenzymes, 269
Coffee, 154
Cold pack method, 442
Cold point, 437
Cold processing, 442-450
    freezing, 446-450
    refrigeration, 443-446
Cold water paste, 204
Collagen, 255
Colloidal dispersions, 510-518
    characteristics, 511
    definition, 510
    foams, 515-518
Colloids, 511
Colorimeter, 61
Coloring agents, 363, 364
Color of foods, maintaining, 321, 322
Commercial heat processing, 438-441
Commercial sterilization, 435
Complete proteins, 242, 243
Complex carbohydrates, 196-208
    functions in food preparation, 198-200
    nutritional impact, 206-208
    physical properties of starch and liquid

mixtures, 200-204
    thickening sauces with starch, 204-206
    types, 197, 198
Complex food systems, 502-580
    careers, 567-580
    mixtures, 504-529
    research, 547-559
    separation techniques, 528-540
Compounds, 81
Concentrates, 469
Concentration
    benefits of concentrates, 469
    effects of freezing, 449, 450
    enzyme activity, 271
    filtration, 470
    heat evaporation, 470
    methods, 470
    open kettle, 470
    problems with concentrates, 469, 470
    solute, 508, 509
    vacuum evaporation, 470
Conclusion, 47
Condensation, 111
Conduction, 108, 109
Consistency, 64, 65
Consistency-controlling additives, 365-369
    anticaking agents, 365
    emulsifiers, 365, 366
    humectants, 366
    leavening agents, 366
    maturing and bleaching agents, 366-368
    pH control agents, 368
    stabilizers and thickeners, 368, 369
Consumer groups, target, 556
Consumer taste panels, 66
Contaminants, 159, 160
Contamination, 406-423
    chemical contaminants, 408, 409
    definition, 407
    food industry sanitation procedures,
        421-423
    foodborne illness, 410-418
    microbial contaminants, 409, 410
    physical contaminants, 407, 408
    transmission of pathogens, 419-421
    types, 407-410
Continuous phase, 505
Control, 45
Controlled atmosphere packaging, 490
Controlled-use antioxidants, 362
Controlled-use substances, 358
Convection, 109, 110

Copolymers, 488
Corn syrup, 178
Covalent bond, 85, 86
Creaming, 529
Cross-contamination, 420
Cross-linked starch, 204
Cruciferous vegetables, 318, 319
Cryogenic liquids, 27, 449
Crystallization, 111, 532
Crystallizing agents, 180-182
Cultural influences on food likes and
     dislikes, 60
Cultured dairy products, 394, 395
Curds, 395
Cytoplasm, 381

D
Dairy products, cultured, 394, 395
Data, 46, 47
     collecting and interpreting, 555
Dehydration, 459-468
     airflow, 461
     belt drying, 463, 464
     case hardening, 461, 462
     definition, 460
     drum drying, 464
     enzymatic activity, 462, 463
     factors that affect quality of dried foods,
          461, 462
     freeze-drying, 465
     home-dried foods, 465-467
     methods, 463-467
     oxidation, 462
     rehydration, 467, 468
     spray drying, 464
     sulfuring, 463
     surface area, 461
     temperature, 461
     tray drying, 463
     vacuum drying, 464, 465
     water activity, 460
Dehydrofreezing, 465
Delaney Clause, 358, 360
Denaturation, 247-249, 271, 272
Dental caries, 184, 185
Deposition, 111
Descriptive research, 548-550
Desiccants, 491
Dextrose, 178
Diabetes mellitus, 186, 187
Dietary recommendations, lipids, 233
Dietetics, 576-578

Dietitians, 576
Digestion, 538-540
Diglyceride, 217
Disaccharides, 173, 174
Dispersed phase, 504
Distillation, 533
Distribution, careers in, 574
Disulfide cross-links, 246
Double bond, 86
Doughs, pH, 134, 135
Drum drying, 464

E
Edible films and coatings, packaging
     materials, 488, 489
Education, 568, 569
Education sector, 579
Eggs, principles of cooking and storing, 253
Electrical energy, 130
Electrolytes, 272
Electron, 79
Elements, 79, 80
Employment outlook, 570
Emulsifier, 365, 366, 513
Emulsions, 512-515
     lipids, 229
     proteins, 251
Endothermic reaction, 102
Endpoint, 128
Energy, 99-112
     chemical, 102, 103
     definition, 100
     electrical, 103
     flow in phase changes, 111, 112
     forms, 101-106
     heat, 106, 107
     kinetic, 100, 101
     measuring, 106-108
     mechanical, 101, 102
     nuclear, 105, 106
     potential, 100, 101
     radiant, 103-105
     reaction rates in food preparation, 112
     temperature, 107, 108
Enrichment, 298-300
Entrepreneurship, 578
Environmental influences on food likes and
     dislikes, 61
Enzymatic activity, dehydration, 462, 463
Enzymatic browning, 277-279
Enzyme inhibitors, 272, 273
Enzymes, 265-279

activity in reactions, 266, 267
carbohydrases, 275
changes produced, 273-275
coenzymes, 269
concentration, 271
definition, 265
denaturation, 271, 272
electrolytes, 272
factors affecting activity, 270-273
food supply, 273-279
lipases, 275
naming, 269, 270
proteases, 275-277
water availability, 270
working models, 267-269
Equivalence point, 128
Erlenmeyer flask, 41
Escherichia coli, 413, 414
Essential amino acids, 242, 243
Essential fatty acids, 231
Ester, 364
Ethics, 559
Evaluation forms, 68, 69
Evaporation, 111, 533
Exothermic reaction, 102, 103
Experiment, 36, 44-46, 551-555
    analyzing and interpreting data, 555
    collecting data, 555
    conducting, 45, 46
    definition, 36
    designing the procedure, 44, 45, 554, 555
    developing, 551-555
    gathering information, 553, 554
    hypothesis, 551, 553
    results, 555
    stating the problem, 551
External energy, 100

F
Facultative, 382
Fats, 220
Fat-soluble vitamins, 289-291
    vitamin A, 289, 290
    vitamin D, 290
    vitamin E, 290
    vitamin K, 290, 291
Fat substitutes, 342-346
    manufactured fats, 345, 346
    protein-based fat replacers, 345
    starch-based fat replacers, 344, 345

Fatty acids, 217
FDA, 356
    monitoring food safety, 422, 423
Fermentation, 380-398
    acetic acid, 396, 397
    bacteria, 381, 382
    bacterial fermentation, 392-396
    benefits, 397, 398
    characteristics of microbes, 384, 385
    definition, 389
    lactic acid, 392-396
    microbe growth, 386-389
    microbial enzymes, 385, 386
    mold fermentation, 396
    nutritional changes, 398
    single-celled organisms, 381-386
    two-step, 396, 397
    yeast, 384, 389-392
Fermenting agents, 184
Fiber, 206, 207
Filtration, 534
Finished food, 576
Firmness, 64
Flash point, 227
Flavonoids, 316-318
Flavor, 62
    maintaining, 322, 323
Flavor enhancers, 364, 365
Flavoring agents, 364
Fluoride, 297
Foams, 251, 252, 515-518
Food additives, 355-371. *See also* Additives
    definition, 356
Food analogs, 336-347. *See also* Analogs
    definition, 27
Food and Drug Administration, 356
Food industry
    research, 548-551
    sanitation procedures, 421-423
Food infection, 414-416
    Listeria monocytogenes, 414
    salmonellosis, 414-416
Food intoxication, 410-414
    Clostridium botulinum, 412, 413
    Clostridium perfringens, 410, 411
    Escherichia coli, 413, 414
    Staphylococcus aureus, 411, 412
Food irradiation, 479-485. *See also* Irradiation
    definition, 480
Food likes and dislikes, 59-61
Food preservation and packaging, 432-495.
    See also Preservation and packaging

Food processing, phytochemicals, 321-324
Food product development, 556-559. *See also*
     Product development
Food safety, 406-423. *See also* Safety
Food science
     definition, 19
     expanded food supply, 26
     history, 20, 21
     new processing techniques, 27, 28
     new products, 26, 27
     reasons to study, 29
     recent contributions, 26-29
Food spoilage, 409
Food vehicle, 299
Foodborne illness, 410-418
     definition, 410
     food infection, 414-416
     food intoxication, 410-414
     parasitic infections, 416, 417
     viral infections, 417, 418
Foodservice careers, 576
Formulations, 36
Fortificant, 299
Fortification, 299, 300
Free radicals, 480
Free water, 154
Freeze-drying, 465
Freezer burn, 450
Freezing, 446-450
     changes during, 449, 450
     factors affecting rate of, 446, 447
     immersion, 449
     indirect contact, 448
     methods, 447-449
     shelf life of frozen foods, 447
     still air contact, 447, 448
Fructose, 172
Fruit maturity, pH, 135, 136
Functional foods, 326
Fungi, 381-384
     characteristics, 384, 385
     definition, 381
     molds, 384
Fungus, definition, 382
Fusion, 111

G
Galactose, 173
Gas-in-water solutions, 151, 152
Gelatinization, 199
Gelatinization point, 199
Gels, 201
Genus, 386

Glass, packaging materials, 487, 488
Glucose, 172
Gluten, 248, 252, 253
Glycerides, 217, 218
Glycogen, 184
Government regulation of food industry,
     21-26
     early regulation, 21, 22
     food labeling, 25, 26
     food safety, 422, 423
     regulation today, 22, 24, 25
     timeline chart, 23, 24
     watchdog groups, 25
Government sector, 579, 580
Graduated cylinder, 41
Graininess, 64
Gram (g), 39
Gram's stain, 381
Granules, 197
GRAS list, 357, 358
GRAS list antioxidants, 361, 362
Gray, 482
Gums, carbohydrate, 198

H
HACCP, 421-423
     meat industry, 422
Halophilic, 385
Handling procedures, 420, 421
Hazard Analysis and Critical Control Point,
     421-423
HDL, 232
Headspace, 439
Health benefits of phytochemicals, 324-327
Health concerns related to sugar, 184-187
Heat, 106-112
     conduction, 108, 109
     convection, 109, 110
     energy flow in phase changes, 111, 112
     enzyme denaturation, 271, 272
     radiation, 111
     transfer, 108-112
     water as a medium, 150
Heat capacity, 107
Heat processing, 435-442
     after packaging, 438-440
     before packaging, 439-441
     blanching, 435
     commercial methods, 438-441
     commercial sterilization, 435
     degrees of preservation, 435, 436
     food components, 437, 438
     heat transfer, 436, 437

home canning, 441, 442
  pasteurization, 435
  pH, 438
  retorts, 438, 439
  sterilization, 435, 436
  time versus temperature, 437
  variables affecting method, 436-438
Hepatitis, 418
Hermetic, 486
Heterogeneous mixture, 87
History of food science, 20, 21
Home canning, 441, 442
  packing food, 442
  processing, 442
Home-dried foods, 465-467
  home dehydrators, 467
  maintaining quality, 467
  oven drying, 465-467
  room or sun drying, 465
Homogeneous mixture, 87
Homogenization, 512
Honey, 178, 179
Hosts, 416
Hot pack method, 442
Humectants, 366
Humidity, 445
Hydrate, 156
Hydrated, 159
Hydrogenation, 223
Hydrogen bond, 146
Hydrogen ion, 121
Hydrolysis, 174
Hydronium ion, 121
Hydrophobic, 246
Hydroponic crops, 26
Hydrostatic cooker and cooler, 439
Hydroxide ion, 121
Hydroxyl group, 172
Hyphae, 383
Hypothesis, 44
  in experiments, 551, 553

I
Ice crystal damage, 450
Impurities, 149
Incidental food additives, 356
Incomplete proteins, 243
Indicators, 127
Indoles, 318, 319
Induction cooktops, 105
Industrial revolution, 20, 21

Influences on food likes and dislikes, 59-61
  cultural, 60
  environmental, 61
  physical, 59, 60
  psychological, 60
Ingredients, 355
Inorganic compounds, 86, 87
Insulin, 186
Intentional food additives, 356
Interfering agents, 181, 182
Intermediate-moisture foods, 470, 471
Intermolecular, 146
Internal energy, 101
International regulations, 29
  additives, 360
International System of Units, 37
Invert sugar, 174
Iodine, 297
Ionic bond, 84, 85
Ionization, 121
Ionomers, 488
Ions, 120-136
  defining acids and bases, 123-125
  definition, 84
  measuring acids and bases, 125-130
  pH applications, 130-136
Iron, 296
Irradiation, 479-485
  chemical changes, 480, 481
  controlling, 484, 485
  definition, 480
  effects, 480-482
  energy used, 482, 483
  labeling products, 484, 485
  nutritional changes, 481, 482
  public concerns, 483, 484
Isoflavones, 317, 318
Isomalt, 179
Isomer, 322
Isothiocyanates, 319

J
Junction, 201

K
Ketone bodies, 206
Ketosis, 206
Kilogram (kg), 39
Kilogray, 482
Kinetic energy, 100, 101

L

Labeling, 25
Lab safety, 48
Lactic acid fermentation, 392-396
  cultured dairy products, 394, 395
  meats, 394
  olives, 393, 394
  pickles, 393
Lactose, 173
Laminates, 489
Latent heat, 111
Latent heat of fusion, 111
Latent heat of vaporization, 111
Law of conservation of matter, 91
LDL, 232
Lead, 408, 409
Leavening agents, 133, 134, 366
Length, 40
Lewis structure, 85
Lipases, 275
Lipids, 216-233
  categories, 218-224
  chemical structure, 217, 218
  cholesterol, 232, 233
  definition, 217
  dietary recommendations, 233
  dietary sources, 223, 224
  essential fatty acids, 231
  functions in food preparation, 226-229
  functions in the body, 230, 231
  glycerides, 217, 218
  hydrogenated vegetable oils, 223
  molecular structure, 218-220
  omega-3 fatty acids, 231, 232
  phospholipids, 218
  physical characteristics, 224-226
  physical state, 220-223
  sterols, 218
  unsaturated oils, 233
Lipolytic, 385
Lipoproteins, 232
Liquefaction, 111
Liquid-in-water solutions, 152, 153
Listeria monocytogenes, 414
Liter (L), 41

M

Macromolecules, 197
Macronutrients, 168-285
  complex carbohydrates, 196-208
  enzymes, 265-285

lipids, 216-233
proteins, 241-259
sugar, 170-195
Magnesium, 295, 296
Magnetron, 103
Maillard reaction, 256
Major minerals, 293-296
Malted, 391
Maltose, 173
Mannose, 172
Manufactured fats, 345, 346
Manufacturing, careers, 572-574
MAP, 491
Maple syrup, 178
Marbling, 224
Margins of safety, 357
Marinated, 276
Marketing, product development, 558
Mass, 37-40
  equipment for measuring, 39
Mass percent, 508
Matter, 79-83, 86-88
  classification, 86-88
  definition, 79
  elements, 79, 80
  periodic table, 80-82
  subatomic particles, 79
Maturing and bleaching agents, 366-368
Measurements, 37-43
  length, 40
  mass, 37-40
  temperature, 42, 43
  time, 42
  volume, 40-42
Meat
  principles of cooking, 255, 256
  fermentation, 394
Mechanical energy, 101, 102
Mechanical separation, 529-532
  addition of force, 530-532
  density, 529, 530
  physical properties, 529
Melting point, 221
Meniscus, 42
Meta-analysis, 49
Metabolism, 540
Metal ions, 160
Metals, 81
  packaging materials, 487
Meter (m), 40
Microbes, 381-389

bacteria, 381, 382
    common characteristics, 384, 385
    definition, 381
    factors affecting growth, 386-389
    food supply, 386
    fungi, 382-384
    growth, 386-389
    pH, 387, 388
    scientific names, 386
    water, 386, 387
Microbial contaminants, 409, 410
Microbial enzymes, 385, 386
Microbiology, 378-423
    contamination and food safety, 406-423
    definition, 381
    fermentation, 380-398
Micrometer, 381
Microorganisms, 381
Microwaves, 103-105
Milk
    colloidal dispersion, 512
    principles of cooking, 253, 254
Milling, 531
Minerals, 293-297
    as additives, 302, 303
    calcium, 293
    chloride, 293-295
    effects of processing and preservation,
        297-301
    enrichment and fortification, 298-300
    fluoride, 297
    iodine, 297
    iron, 296
    magnesium, 295, 296
    major, 293-296
    nutrient stability, 300, 302
    phosphorus, 293
    potassium, 293-295
    preserving at home, 303, 304
    sodium, 293-295
    sulfur, 295, 296
    trace minerals, 296-298
    zinc, 297
Mixtures, 87, 504-519
    colloidal dispersions, 510-518
    solutions, 505-510
    suspensions, 518, 519
Modified atmosphere packaging, 491
Modified starches, 204
Molarity (M), 129, 130

Molasses, 177
Mold fermentation, 396
Molds, 384
Mole, 129
Molecule, 81
Monera, 381
Monoglyceride, 217
Monosaccharides, 172, 173
Monounsaturated, 220
Mycelium, 383
Myoglobin, 246

N
Neotame, 341
Neutral, 122
Neutralization, 128
Neutron, 79
Nitrites, 361
Nomenclature, 269, 270
Nonmetals, 81
Nonnutritive sweeteners, 339-341
Nonpolar, 218
Nonpolar covalent bond, 145
Nonpolar molecules, lipids, 225, 226
Norwalk virus, 418
Nuclear energy, 105, 106
Nucleus, 79
Nutrient stability, 300, 302
Nutrients, definition, 145
Nutrition
    complex carbohydrates, 206-208
    definition, 19
    fermentation, 398
    irradiation, 481, 482
    proteins, 256-259
    starches, 207
    sugar, 184-187

O
Oils, 221
Olestra, 345, 346
Olfactory bulb, 63
Olives, fermentation, 393
Omega-3 fatty acids, 231, 232
Opacity, 203
Orbital, 79
Organic compounds, 86, 87
    shorthand chart, 314
Organic dyes, 125
Osmosis, 535-537

Osmotic pressure, 535
Oven drying, 465-467
Oxidases, 277
Oxidation, 246, 290
    dehydration, 462

P
Packaging, 485-492
    edible films and coatings, 488
    functions, 486
    reduced oxygen packaging, 489-492
    types of materials, 486
Paper, packaging materials, 488
Parasites, 416
Pastes, 201
Pasteurization, 388, 435
Pathogens, 410
    transmission, 419-421
Pectins, 198
Peptide bond, 242
Periodic table, 80-82
Permeable, 488
Personal qualities, 568
pH
    applications, 130-136
    baking, 132-135
    buffers, 130-132
    digestion, 130
    eggs, 135
    food preservation, 132
    fruit maturity, 135, 136
    heat processing, 438
    measuring, 127, 128
    microbes, 387, 388
pH control agent, 368
pH scale, 125, 126
Phase changes, 88, 89
Phenolic acids, 319, 320
Phenomenon, 35
Phospholipids, 218
Phosphorus, 293
Photosynthesis, 171
Physical changes, 88-91
    identifying, 89, 90
    permanent and reversible, 90
    phase changes, 89, 90
Physical contaminants, 160, 407, 408
Physical influences on food likes and dislikes,
        59, 60
Phytochemicals, 312-327
    allyl sulfides, 314, 315

carotenoids, 315, 316
    definition, 313
    families, 313
    flavonoids, 316-318
    food processing, 321-324
    health benefits, 324-327
    increasing in diet, 324-326
    indoles, 318, 319
    phenolic acids, 319, 320
    preserving, 323, 324
    saponins, 320, 321
    terpenes, 321
Phytoestrogens, 318
Pickles, fermentation, 393
Pilot manufacturing, 557, 558
Plaque, 232
Polar covalent bond, 146
Pollutants, 159, 160
Polymer, 197
Polyols, 341, 342
Polypeptides, 242
Polyphenols, 320
Polysaccharides, 197
Polyunsaturated, 220
Potassium, 293-295
Potassium chloride, salt substitutes, 346, 347
Potential energy, 100, 101
Precipitate, 532
Precipitation, 532, 533
Precursors, 289
Preservation and packaging, 432-495
    biotechnology, 492-495
    concentration, 468-470
    dehydration, 459-468
    intermediate-moisture foods, 470, 471
    irradiation, 479-485
    packaging, 485-492
    pH, 132
    thermal, 434-451
Preservatives, 360
    sugar, 179
Pressure processing, 442
Procedures, experiments, 554, 555
Processing
    preservation, effects, 298-302
    techniques, new, 27, 28
Product development, 556-559
    conducting research, 556, 557
    ethics, 559
    identifying products or needs, 556
    management approval, 558

marketing and advertising, 558
mass production, 558
pilot manufacturing, 557, 558
target consumer groups, 556
Production, careers, 570-572
Products, 91
new, 26, 27
Pofessional associations, 580
Proteases, 275-277
Protein-based fat replacers, 345
Protein gel, 249
Proteins, 241-259
amino acids, 241-244
cooking high-protein foods, 253-256
denaturation, 247-249
emulsions, 251
foams, 251, 252
functions in food, 249-253
health concerns, 259
molecular interactions, 245-247
nutrition, 256-259
primary structure, 244
protein pigments, 246, 247
secondary structure, 244, 245
tertiary structure, 245
Proteolytic, 385
Proton, 79
Proton acceptors, 122
Proton donors, 122
Psychological influences on food likes and
dislikes, 60
Pure culture, 384
Pure substance, 86

Q

Quality control, careers, 574, 575

R

Rad, 482
Radiant energy, 103-105
Radiation, 111
Radiolytic products, 481
Rancidity, 226
Reactants, 91
temperature, 112
Reaction rates in food preparation, 112
Reduced oxygen packaging, 489-492
CAP, 490
functions, 492
MAP, 491
Reduction, 246
Refrigerant, 448

Refrigeration, 443-446
food changes during, 445, 446
role in food processing, 446
storage temperature chart, 444
variables to control, 443-445
Registered dietitians, 578
Regulations
biotechnology, 495
food additives, 356-360
government, 21-26
international, 29
Rehydration, 467, 468
Rendering, 530
Replicable, 37
Research, 547-559
analytical, 550, 551
definition, 548
descriptive, 548-550
developing experiments, 551-555
food industry, 548-551
product development, 556-559
scientific method, 44
Respiration, 445
Results
evaluating, 47
reporting, 47, 49, 50
Retinol, 289
Retorts, 438, 439
Retrogradation, 201, 202
Reverse osmosis, 537
Ribonucleic acid, 173
Riboses, 173
Ripening, 182
RNA, 173
ROP, 489-492
Rotavirus, 418
Roux, 205

S

Saccharide, 172
Saccharin, 339, 340
Safety, 406-423
food industry sanitation procedures,
421-423
foodborne illness, 410-418
handling procedures, 420, 421
lab, 48
transmission of pathogens, 419-421
types of contamination, 407-410
Salmonellosis, 414-416
Salt, 122
Salt solutions, 153, 154

Salt substitutes, 346, 347
Sanitation procedures, 421-423
Saponins, 320, 321
Saturated, 220
Science, definition, 35
Scientific evaluation, 35-50
    measurements, 37-43
    science in the food industry, 36, 37
    scientific studies, evaluating, 49, 50
Scientific method, 43-50
    ask questions, 43
    conduct experiment, 45, 46
    conduct research, 44
    define problem, 43, 44
    design experiment, 44, 45
    evaluate results, 47
    report results, 47, 49, 50
    state hypothesis, 44
Scientific names, microbes, 386
Scientific studies, evaluating, 49, 50
Sedimentation, 530
Semipermeable membrane, 535
Sensory evaluation, 58-70
    acids and bases, 123-125
    characteristics of food products, 61-66
    definition, 59
    influences on food likes and dislikes, 59-61
    taste test panels, 66-69
Separation techniques, 528-540
    chemical separation, 532, 533
    digestion and metabolism, 538-540
    mechanical separation, 529-532
    selective separation through barriers,
        533-538
Sharp freezing, 447
Shelf life, 435
Shell, 83
SI, 37
Simplesse, 345
Single-celled organisms, 381-386
    bacteria, 381, 382
    fungi, 381-384
Slurries, 201
Smoke point, 227
Sodium, 293-295
Soft drinks, 509, 510
Solidification point, 224
Solid-in-water solutions, 153, 154
Sols, 201
Solubility, 180
Solute, 88
Solutions, 151-154, 505-510

beverage industry, 509, 510
    definition, 88
    factors affecting solubility, 506-508
    gas-in-water, 151, 152
    liquid-in-water, 152, 153
    salt, 153, 154
    solid-in-water, 153, 154
    solute concentrations, 508, 509
    sugar, 153, 154
Solvents, 88
    separating with, 532
    water, 151-154
Sorghum, 178
Soy sauce, 396
Species, 386
Specific heat, 107
Spirilla, 381
Spoilage, 409
Spores, 383
Spray drying, 464
Stability, 203
Stabilizers, 368, 369
Staphylococcus aureus, 411, 412
Starch-based fat replacers, 344, 345
Starches, 200-207
    cold water paste, 204
    definition, 197
    modified starches, 203, 204
    nutritional functions, 207
    opacity and translucency, 203
    physical properties of mixtures, 200-204
    retrogradation, 201, 202
    stability, 203
    starch and fat, 204, 205
    starch and sugar, 206
    texture, 203
    thickened sauces, 204-206
    types of mixtures, 201
    viscosity, 202, 203
Starter, 385
Steam, cooking with, 150
Sterilization, 435, 436
Sterols, 218
Stevioside, 340, 341
Subatomic particles, 79
Sublimation, 111
Substrate, 268
Sucralose, 341
Sucrose, 173
Sugar, 170-187
    alcohols, 174, 175
    caramelizing agents, 182-184

carbohydrate production, 171, 172
corn syrup, 178
crystallizing agents, 180-182
dental caries, 184, 185
diabetes mellitus, 186, 187
disaccharides, 173, 174
fermenting agents, 184
functions in food preparation, 179-184
health concerns, 184-187
honey, 178, 179
isomalt, 179
maple syrup, 178
monosaccharides, 172, 173
nutritional value, 184-187
preservatives, 179
sorghum, 178
sources, 176-179
structure, 172
sugar beets, 178
sugar cane, 177
sweeteners, 179
tenderizers, 179, 180
weight gain, 187
Sugar solutions, 153, 154
Sugar substitutes, 339-342
acesulfame potassium, 340
aspartame, 340
bulking agents, 342
neotame, 341
new developments, 342
nonnutritive sweeteners, 339-341
nutritive sweeteners, 341, 342
saccharin, 339, 340
stevioside, 340, 341
sucralose, 341
Sulfites, 362, 363
Sulfiting, 462
Sulfur, 295, 296
Sulfuring, 463
Supersaturated, 180
Surface area, reaction rates, 112
Surface tension, 146, 147
Suspensions, 518, 519
Sweeteners, 365
bulking agents, 342
new developments, 342
nonnutritive, 339-341
nutritive, 341, 342
sugar, 179
Syneresis, 201
effect of freezing, 450
Systems, complex. *See* Complex food systems

T
Tannins, 323
Taring, 39
Taste bias, 60
Taste test panels, 66-69
environmental factors, 67
evaluation forms, 68, 69
influences from other testers, 67
psychological biases, 68
setting up, 66
Tea, 154
Tempeh, 396
Temperature, 42, 43, 107, 108
heat processing, 437
in reaction rates, 112
microbes, 388, 389
Temporary emulsions, 513
Terpenes, 321
Texture, 63-66
measuring objectively, 66
Thermal conductivity, 514
Thermal death curve, 437
Thermal preservation, 434-451
cold processing, 442-450
heat processing, 435-442
Thickeners, 368, 369
Thickness of food, reaction rates, 112
Thirst, 158, 159
Time, measuring, 42
Titration, 127
Toxic substances, 408
Toxins, 410
Trace minerals, 296-298
Training, jobs, 568, 569
Translucency, 203
Transmission of pathogens, 419-421
Tray drying, 463
Trichinosis, 416
Triglyceride, 217
Two-step fermentation, 396, 397
Tyndall effect, 511

U
Unsaturated, 220
Unsaturated oils, 233
USDA, monitoring food safety, 422, 423

V
Vacuum drying, 464, 465
Valence electrons, 85
Vaporization, 111
Vapor pressure, 507

Variable, 45
Variation, 45
Viruses, 417, 418
Viscosity, 202, 230
Vitamins, 289-292
    as additives, 302, 303
    definition, 289
    effects of processing and preservation,
        297-301
    enrichment and fortification, 298-300
    fat-soluble, 289-291
    nutrient stability, 300, 302
    preserving at home, 303, 304
    water-soluble, 291, 292
Volatile, 63
Volume, 40-42

W
Water, 144-160
    acids, 160
    contaminants and beverage industry, 160
    content in foods, 154-157
    covalent bonds, 145, 146
    dehydration, 459-468
    functions in food, 150-154
    functions in the body, 157-159
    heat medium, 150
    hydrogen bonds, 146
    impurities, 149
    ionization of, 121, 122
    metal ions, 160

    microbes, 386, 387
    pollutants and contaminants, 159, 160
    pressure, temperature, and phase changes,
        147-149
    solvents, 151-154
    structure, 145-149
    surface tension, 146, 147
    thirst, 158, 159
Water activity, 157
    role in dehydration, 460
Water availability, enzyme activity, 270
Water-bath processing, 442
Water-soluble vitamins, 291, 292
    definition, 289
Weight, 39
Weight gain, sugars, 187
Whey, 246
Wine, yeast fermentation, 390, 391
Working conditions, 569, 570

X
Xanthophylls, 316

Y
Yeast, 384
Yeast fermentation, 389-392
    alcoholic beverages, 391, 392
    bread, 390
    wine, 390, 391